Community health care
and
the nursing process

Community health care
and
the nursing process

MARGOT JOAN FROMER

R.N., M.A., M.Ed.

SECOND EDITION

with **63** illustrations

The C. V. Mosby Company

ST. LOUIS • TORONTO • LONDON   1983

MOSBY

A TRADITION OF PUBLISHING EXCELLENCE

Editor: Michael R. Riley
Assistant editor: Susan R. Epstein
Manuscript editor: Mary Dolan
Book design: Staff
Cover design: Suzanne Oberholtzer
Production: Mary Stueck, Jeanne A. Gulledge

SECOND EDITION

Copyright © 1983 by The C.V. Mosby Company

Printed in the United States of America

The C.V. Mosby Company
11830 Westline Industrial Drive, St. Louis, Missouri 63141

Library of Congress Cataloging in Publication Data

Main entry under title:

Community health care and the nursing process.

   Includes bibliographies and index.
   1.   Community health nursing.   I.   Fromer,
Margot Joan.   [DNLM: 1.   Community
health nursing.   WY 106 F931c]
RT98.C654   1983   610.73′43   82-2130
ISBN 0-8016-1725-1   AACR2

GW/VH/VH   9 8 7 6 5 4 3 2 1   02/C/243

CONTRIBUTORS

MARJORIE J. KELLER, R.N., M.S., C.A.G.S.

Associate Professor,
Department of Community Health Nursing,
Virginia Commonwealth University
Medical College of Virginia, Richmond, Virginia;
Robert Wood Johnson Fellow, Indiana School
of Nursing, Indianapolis, Indiana

GEORGIA P. MacDONOUGH, R.N., M.A.

Arizona Department of Health Services,
Children's Hospital Bureau of Maternal and Child
Health, Tempe, Arizona

DOLORES T. MAZURKEWICZ, M.A., Ph.D.

Assistant Professor, Department of Psychology,
Camden College, Rutgers University,
Camden, New Jersey

ANITA GOLDEN PEPPER, M.S.W., M.P.H., M.Phil., Ph.D.

Associate Professor of Epidemiology for Nursing,
St. Louis University School of Nursing and Allied
Health Professions, St. Louis, Missouri

LAURA J. REILLY, R.N., M.S., J.D.

Attorney, Office of General Counsel,
University of Texas System, Austin, Texas;
formerly Assistant Professor of Community Health
Nursing, University of Oklahoma College of
Nursing, Norman, Oklahoma

WILLIAM HARRIS TUCKER, M.A., Ph.D.

Assistant Professor of Psychology,
University College, Rutgers University,
Camden, New Jersey

GRACE WYSHAK, M.S.Hyg., Ph.D.

Department of Preventive and Social Medicine,
Harvard Medical School,
Boston, Massachusetts

To the memory of
Beatrice Neuman Fromer

PREFACE

Health care and the systems involved in its delivery are changing rapidly. In years past community health nurses were generalists who happened to work in a community agency rather than in a hospital. As increasing technology has forced hospital nurses to become specialists, so has increasing knowledge in the social and behavioral sciences forced community nurses to become specialists in family therapy, epidemiologic research, primary health care, community planning, consultation, ambulatory care, mental health, and other aspects of community nursing. Nursing education in general is shifting from a disease-oriented curriculum that seemed to be based primarily on hospital geography to curricula that stress primary health care, health maintenance, prevention of illness, and the theoretical concepts of health, illness, and wellness. *Community Health Care and the Nursing Process* is an introduction to community nursing, a field that is occupying an increasingly large place in the curriculum.

This text is not meant to be a "cookbook" for community nursing. There are no specific recipes on how to make a home visit or manage a well-baby clinic. Rather it is an overview of what is happening today in community health in general and in community nursing in particular. Each author who has contributed a chapter is an expert in his or her field, and although not every chapter is necessarily concerned with nursing per se, each one is included because the subject matter is essential reading for community nurses.

Curricula in schools of nursing have begun to reflect the holistic approach to human development. *Community Health Care and the Nursing Process* mirrors this approach and stresses three basic concepts: (1) the health-illness continuum, (2) human beings as persons who think about and do things that directly and indirectly affect their health and the way they relate to their environment, and (3) the effects of various situations, health problems, and stressors on the health and development of the individual, the family, and the community.

As curricula change, so do students. More and more collegiate programs require students to take a large proportion of liberal arts courses. This fact, coupled with the increasing political and social awareness of students today, is leading more graduates into community nursing, where they plan to function as change agents. Their education has provided them with the intellectual skills needed to assess the health problems of families and communities and to deal with them realistically.

Health care is not only big business in the United States today, it is also an area of political concern and action. The number and the complexity of organizations providing this care have escalated enormously in recent years, and the provision of care has become increasingly mechanized and dehumanized. The problem of providing health care to the masses while keeping the delivery of that care personal is one that is taxing the minds and ingenuity of all health professionals. This book will focus on family and community development and dynamics and the effort to maintain healthy functioning. The purpose and function of nursing intervention in a variety of situations will be stressed. The addition of chapters on aging and on cross-cultural nursing in the community in this new edition of *Community Health Care and the Nursing Process* reflects the reality of community health. The proportion of elderly people in the United States is increasing rapidly, and the nurse must be prepared to care for them as well as to deal with the wide variety of cultural diversity that exists in this country.

It is believed that all human beings have personal dignity and worth and that health care is as much a right as all other social, civil, and political rights that a free society must guarantee its citizens. The health care system as it exists in this country today does not meet all the needs of the people it seeks to serve, and with changing political climates it may do so to an even lesser degree in the future. This text is designed to help prepare the practitioner of professional nursing to become a change agent in the system so that the client—the individual, the family, and the community—ultimately will benefit from professional nursing intervention. *Community Health Care and the Nursing Process* will also help students to seek new relationships among various fields of study and will demonstrate that nursing theory, research findings, and professional concepts can be practically applied to real-life situations. Since the community nurse is very much an organizer and coordinator of health care activities, principles of management are included.

A note here about the book's semantics. It has generally been accepted that the term *community nurse* has replaced the term *public health nurse,* although the meaning remains the same; this practice will be continued here. The terms *nurse, community nurse,* and *professional nurse* are synonymous (it is hoped that all nurses practicing in the community will be functioning as professionals); each of these terms is used in this book, sometimes for clarity and sometimes for variety.

Although men are still a tiny minority in nursing, their presence is being increasingly felt. Many people think it is no longer acceptable to refer to the nurse only as "she." Neither is it acceptable, to me and to the vast majority of nurses, to refer to the nurse only as "he." The use of the term "she/he" or "her/him" is awkward, and the reader soon becomes irritated. In the interest of readability, the nurse will be referred to as "she," and I hope that the male readers will not be offended.

The traditional term *patient* has been eliminated; *client* is used instead. It is believed that the designation of a person as a patient connotes passivity to the will of others, in this instance to health professionals. The term client denotes active participation in whatever decisions will be made. Clients seek advice and counsel and then make their own decisions.

The inclusion of case situations is designed to develop students' ability to think and to stimulate the process of making creative judgments. I hope that teachers will use the situations as a stimulus for class discussions, research assignments, and other learning experiences. The case studies can enhance learning by providing practice in group work, planning and studying, using various interviewing techniques, understanding mental health concepts and communication, and independent study. The situations have been developed to mirror reality as much as possible. The families described are in all stages of development and in all socioeconomic strata. They each have complex needs and require mature nursing judgments. The situations should also focus students' attention on the dynamics of family interaction.

Acknowledgment is gratefully made to all contributors of chapters. Their effort and cooperation greatly exceeded their monetary rewards, and this text would not be what it is without them. My thanks go to Susan Petrillo for some ideas and examples in Chapter 13 on the nursing process as it applied to community nursing.

I am also deeply indebted to Nancy Evans. Her confidence in me and her continued encouragement during the creation of this book were more valuable than I can possibly acknowledge.

Margot Joan Fromer

The following verse comes from the files of the National Defense Education Act Institute on Counseling and Guidance of Purdue University. As professional health workers we must recognize that not everyone wants to sit at a square brown desk.

ABOUT SCHOOL

Author unknown

He always wanted to say things. But no one understood.
He always wanted to explain things. But no one cared.
So he drew.

Sometimes he would just draw and it wasn't anything. He wanted to carve it in stone or write it in the sky.
He would lie out in the grass and look up in the sky, and it would be only him and the sky and the things inside him that needed saying.

And it was after that, that he drew the picture. It was a beautiful picture.
He kept it under the pillow and would let no one see it. And he would
look at it every night and think about it. And when it was dark, and his eyes were closed, he could still see it.
And it was all of him. And he loved it.

When he started school he brought it with him. Not to show anyone, but just to have it with him like a friend.

It was funny about school.
He sat in a square brown desk like all the other square brown desks, and he thought his should be red.

And his room was a square brown room. Like all the other rooms. And it was tight and close. And stiff.

He hated to hold the pencil and the chalk with his arm stiff and his feet flat on the floor, stiff, with the teacher watching and watching.

And then he had to write numbers. And they weren't anything. They were worse than the letters that could be something if you put them together.
And the numbers were tight and square, and he hated the whole thing.

The teacher came and spoke to him. She told him to wear a tie like all the other boys. He said he didn't like them, and she said it didn't matter.

After that they drew. And he drew all yellow, and it was the way he felt about morning. And it was beautiful.

The teacher came and smiled at him. "What's this?" she said. "Why don't you draw something like Ken's drawing? Isn't that beautiful?
It was all questions.

After that his mother bought him a tie, and he always drew airplanes and rocketships like everyone else. And he threw the old picture away.

And when he lay out alone looking at the sky, it was big and blue and all of everything, but he wasn't anymore.

He was square inside and brown, and his hands were stiff, and he was like everyone else. And the thing inside him that needed saying didn't need saying anymore.

It had stopped pushing. It was crushed.
Stiff.
Like everything else.

CONTENTS

Community health care
and
the nursing process

1

HEALTH CARE DELIVERY SYSTEMS

Health care has become a multi-billion dollar industry in the United States, one of the two or three largest and probably the one that affects the greatest number of people. Indeed, it is almost impossible to find a person in the United States today who has not at some time been a consumer of health care. Succeeding chapters will discuss specific aspects of the system and how nurses and nursing agencies function within it, but in this chapter we shall look at health care delivery systems as a whole: how they are presently working (or not working), what some of their strengths and weaknesses are, why they exist, and what could be done to improve them.

To look at health care as an industry as we look at steel or automobile manufacturing as industries may seem a bit jarring to our sense of social and professional propriety. But when there are enormous amounts of money and numbers of people involved in the provision of a service, there is no other way to look at it (Table 1-1). As an industry it is unique and can be compared with other institutions of comparable size *only* in terms of money and personnel. In terms of function and organization there is no way to compare the health care industry with any existing industry of comparable size. The automobile industry, for example, has the goal of manufacturing and selling a product and making a profit. In the United States this goal is achieved by four large companies that are designed to compete with each other to the theoretical ulti-

mate benefit of the consumer. Each of the four companies is organized in a similar fashion, and each has the same goal: to sell more cars and make more money. The health care industry is just the opposite. Its goal is to provide a service, and, except in a few instances, there is no profit motive involved. The system is loosely arranged into thousands of organizations, each trying to provide a

Table 1-1. Similarities and differences in two large American industries

AUTOMOBILE INDUSTRY	HEALTH CARE INDUSTRY
Goals	
Manufacturing product	Maintaining and improving
Selling product	health
Making profit	Providing services to that end
Organization to achieve goals	
Four domestic companies	Thousands of organizations
Each company organized in approximately same way	Different organizational structure to achieve different subgoals
All companies in private sector	Organizations in both public and private sector
Consumer	
Actively solicited	Solicited only in minority of instances
Quickly ignored after sale is made	Kept in system once initial contact is made

service; sometimes the services are the same, and sometimes they differ. This can lead to an overlap in the provision of service, needless competition between organizations, fragmentation of service, and frustration for the consumer. The ultimate goal of all health organizations is the same: provision of service for improvement and maintenance of health.

Some health professionals believe that a secondary goal of all organizations is the preservation and survival of the organization itself. Hence, the consumer's needs are subordinated to those of the organization. In some communities similar organizations provide the same service: for example, a voluntary nursing agency (Visiting Nurses Association) and a proprietary one (Homemakers UpJohn) could find themselves competing for clients. This happens more and more frequently.

The consumer of the auto industry is wooed, won, then mostly forgotten. In the health industry it is again the opposite. Consumers in most cases are not actively solicited, but once they are in the system, they are often encouraged to stay. Physicians, nurses, and some other health care practitioners are forbidden by their code of ethics to advertise. Other health care practitioners, such as optometrists, chiropractors, and pharmacists, do advertise, so there is conflict in *how* the consumer enters the health care system. Other consumers are actively solicited, for instance, black people for sickle cell screening and mothers of infants for well-baby clinics. The philosophy of how to treat the consumer in each industry has similarities and differences, but the end result is largely the same: the consumer is often ignored, with needs unmet and dissatisfaction not heeded. When a new car turns out to be a "lemon," it often takes months of frustrated letter writing and angry telephone calls to achieve any kind of satisfaction. Hospitalized clients can experience the same frustration when they realize that the system is designed to serve and meet the needs of its employees rather than its customers. For example, community nurses do not make home visits in the evening when it is more likely that all family members will be available and

the nurse can observe the functioning of the family unit. Some families who need it receive no community nursing service at all because the adults of the family are at work all day.

A client in both industries may have the basics— a new car and a hospital bed or a physician's office appointment—but the finer points of automobile service and health maintenance may be neglected.

The web of the health care industry and its delivery systems is so large that more than 90% of the total population is served by it in some capacity. It is impossible to estimate what portion of people's health needs is being met by current methods of delivering health care and what portion is not. Years of observation of and participation in the delivery of health care in a variety of settings have indicated that the vast majority of the health needs of people in this country are not being met. The main reason is the very nature of the system itself. The system is fragmented in such a way that coordination of services is often difficult, if not impossible. This may be best illustrated by an example.

Jonathan Daniels had an accident at work and broke his leg so severely that he was in the hospital for six weeks. He was finally discharged in a smaller cast but was confined to a wheelchair and could not leave his third floor walk-up apartment for another two months and then only slowly and with great pain. The hospital had no discharge planning service, but he remembered one of the nurses making a vague reference to visiting nurses. Even if he had known how to contact the local Visting Nurses Association, he would not have done so because he did not see himself as sick, only greatly inconvenienced and very annoyed.

When his cast was removed (he had to be taken to and from the hospital by private ambulance for this), he was referred to a private physical therapist who came to Jonathan's apartment for a few weeks until the latter's leg was strong enough to bear weight. He lived mostly on sandwiches and beer because cooking was too much effort and because he asked his friends to go grocery shopping for him as seldom as possible.

There was no central person who coordinated all

his needs, and although he had private health insurance, he eventually received bills from the following: the hospital, the orthopedist, the Emergency Department associates, the anesthesiologist, the ambulance company, the physical therapist, and the surgical supply company.

In this chapter the two methods of delivery of health care currently in use will be discussed, followed by some suggestions for improving and modifying the system. The two existing systems are the familiar fee for service and the relatively new concept of health maintenance organizations (HMO), or prepaid health care.

FEE-FOR-SERVICE SYSTEM
Private practitioners

The structure and philosophy of the fee-for-service system is quite simple: one receives health care service, and one pays for the service received. This is the way most health care is given in the United States today, and it takes several forms:

1. The private practitioner (e.g., physician, dentist, physical therapist, or hospital) provides health care (all the way from a simple office visit to open heart surgery) and bills the client directly. The fee is paid directly by the client to the private practitioner for services rendered.

2. Third-party payers, which are basically private insurance companies, reimburse the client for services rendered by the private practitioner. Most often the client is billed by the practitioner. The client must fill out and submit the forms to the insurance company and then wait for reimbursement. This assumes that the client can understand and fill out the forms. Many cannot and therefore do not receive the insurance benefits to which they are entitled. Another way in which third-party payments work is that the insurance company is billed by the practitioner who then receives the part of the fee that the insurance company chooses to pay, then bills the client for the remainder. The client pays for the care received in two ways: by purchasing (or working for a company that purchases for him) health insurance with a variety of types of coverage and by paying for the remainder of

care himself. Even though part of the fee is paid directly by someone other than the consumer, it is still the consumer's own money that paid for the health care; the consumer must purchase the insurance in the first place. Charity and industry may also be third-party payers. People who cannot afford care may be eligible for the benefits of an organization (the American Cancer Society will pay for an artificial leg if the amputation was the result of carcinoma but not if it was the result of trauma), or they may be employed by companies large enough to provide some health care benefits. There is still a fee for the service rendered; it is simply the charity or the company who is billed and not the individual client.

3. Various kinds of government assistance programs such as Medicare and Medicaid provide a way for indigent people to receive health care. The private practitioner or hospital still bills for services rendered, but they bill a government agency (e.g., Medicare, Medicaid, or local welfare administrations) instead of the recipient of the health services. These funds are provided by taxation and Social Security deductions. But the fee-for-service system remains the same: a service is provided and a bill is rendered.

Public and private sectors

The health care delivery system can also be divided into public and private sectors. The private sector is based on the private physician in a one-to-one relationship with the client. This base has expanded in recent years to include group practice. Third-party payments cover various kinds of extended health care services, paramedical and nonprofessional personnel, suppliers of equipment and prostheses, laboratory and diagnostic services, and other agencies involved in restoring and maintaining health. But the private sector is still primarily disease and cure oriented and has its major emphasis on medical therapy.

Although the American Medical Association (AMA) and other organizations have encouraged people to have annual physical examinations for the purpose of health maintenance and disease prevention, there is little practical incentive to do this. Most private insurance plans do not cover routine checkups, so the cost of a physical examination must be paid by the client, and this can become extremely expensive. Following is the cost of the most fundamental kind of health maintenance in an eastern metropolitan area:

Annual physical examination, including CBC and urinalysis	$120
Electrocardiogram	40
SMA-12 and other chemistry tests	50
Semiannual dental prophylaxis and annual x-ray film	60
Annual (semiannual for women over 30) gynecological examination and Pap test	40
Biannual eye examination	25
Biannual chest x-ray film	20
TOTAL	$375

Not many people will easily part with $375 if they are feeling well. It is not much fun to hand a physician $160 to hear what you already knew: that you are in good health. There has recently been in the public press and in professional journals a good deal of speculation about the advisability and worth of a physical examination. Most diseases cannot be detected merely by the thumping and prodding that goes on in a physician's office, and it is a well-known fact that an ECG is not a predictor of heart disease; it shows only damage that has already taken place. People are notoriously reticent about going to the dentist until they are in excruciating pain, and the ophthalmologist is usually not seen until vision begins to dim. Women, for a variety of reasons, avoid gynecological examinations. Blood and urine tests, which are the best initial indicators of a health problem, are not done unless ordered by a physician. The private sector is disease oriented, and the fee-for-service system tends to discourage health maintenance. This is one of its many disadvantages.

The public sector of the health care delivery system is only slightly better. It is still fee for service, but it encompasses various official and voluntary health agencies, which, to some extent, encourage health promotion and public education about health maintenance and disease prevention. There are various kinds of public screening programs, some funded by the government and some by private foundations, to detect certain diseases. Examples of this are multiphasic screening done by health departments, well-elderly clinics held by the Commission on Aging, classes in breast self-examination sponsored by the American Cancer Society, television commercials about tooth decay paid for by the American Dental Association, mass Pap test clinics sponsored by local health departments, mobile chest x-ray units owned and operated by the Lung Association, and venereal disease clinics operated by health departments. These services are supported by taxes or by voluntary dollars contributed through various organizations. They *do* affect the public health as a whole.

Characteristics

Although the fee-for-service system is philosophically appropriate for a capitalist society and there is no reason why professional health workers, including nurses, should not profit from their professional efforts, the system has often been accused of being class oriented and run as much for the benefit of the providers of health care as for its consumers.

The present health care system is closed, controlled by medical physicians, and does not distribute services equitably. There is little interchange among doctors, other health care professionals, and health institutions or agencies, on one hand and the person, family, or community on the other. Health workers other than doctors of medicine cannot function in an independent, open manner, and thus have to work around the system to provide the kinds of services the public deserves and expects. Presently, medical doctors control entry into and the pathway through the health care system.*

The system "grew like Topsy" from a series of only distantly related programs, legislative acts,

*From Murray, Ruth, and Zentner, Judith: Nursing concepts for health promotion, Englewood Cliffs, N.J., 1975, Prentice-Hall, Inc., p. 20.

technological advances, services, and facilities. The people providing health care and those receiving it often seem in conflict with each other, and each health professional who charges a fee is a private entrepreneur, which tends to create further fragmentation.

The use of the term *patient*, which has been traditional, implies a passive subservience to authority. The word *client*, while still denoting dependence, implies a more active participation in the system. Health care workers are often separated by a caste system of professional versus nonprofessional and of various occupational levels. Lines of communication have been vertical: orders are handed down; obedience is returned. The goals of the professionals may not always be those of the client; hence the needs of the client may not be met in the most effective manner.

The fee-for-service system is in a trap of ever-accelerating costs for ever-diminishing services. Inflation slowly eats away at the value of the dollar, and the cholecystectomy that cost $361 in 1950 cost $839 in 1965 and $2208 in 1975.[1] Hospital care today in major metropolitan areas costs the system a total of about $1000 a day.*

The rising costs of labor, services, and manufactured products threaten to exceed the consumer's ability to pay. Medical malpractice insurance premiums alone (which can exceed $50,000 per year for some specialties like neurology and anesthesiology) have caused the cost of surgery to skyrocket. Physicians seem to feel they have no choice but to pass these costs along to the consumer. "Along with the overall rise has come a substantial shift in the distribution of expenditures among different types of services reflecting, primarily, the changing technology of health care."[2,p.42] Physicians' services used to be the largest share of health care costs. Today hospitals have this majority share, and the proportion of their share is increasing every year. Nursing homes increased their share of the cost, but to a very small extent, as did medical research. Price increases and inflation are the greatest single cause of the increase in health care costs, but improvements in the quality of care, population increase, and greater use of existing facilities and services also contribute to the increase.[2] Private health insurance, public programs, and other forms of third-party payment were devised to take some of the burden off the consumer in the fee-for-service system. The goal of transferring the pocket from which the money is taken has been achieved, but while relieving the consumer, third-party payments have added to the cost of delivering health care. Insurance companies make a profit from each premium dollar paid. As the insurance companies' costs increase, they must increase the price of the premiums: more money out of the consumers' pockets that is not destined to pay for actual health care.

Medicare and Medicaid

The government thought it had at least a partial answer to the problems of the fee-for-service system: Medicare and Medicaid. Medicare is health insurance for people ages 65 and over and is provided by Title 18 of the Social Security Act of 1965. It went into effect on July 1, 1966, after bitter opposition by the AMA, which feared it as the beginning of socialized medicine. It is now a generally accepted and mostly popular part of the health care system that, despite problems, has given medical coverage to many elderly people who would receive little or no health care without Medicare.

Medicare has provided far better benefits to this age group than do private insurance companies; it has drastically reduced the cost of health care to the individual aged person who frequently lives on a fixed income and can least afford it. It has contributed to the overall improvement in the kinds of care available to the elderly. According to an article in *Time* on June 13, 1977, the cost of health care for the elderly is about 250% of what it is for the general population; it was the inability of the private sector to pay these costs that led to the development of Medicare. The quality of care in hos-

*Public Relations Office, University of Maryland Hospital, Baltimore.

pitals and nursing homes has improved, particularly in those which had never been inspected by the Joint Commission on the Accreditation of Hospitals (JCAH).[3] The providers of care, notably physicians, hospitals, and nursing homes, have benefited by Medicare because they are now guaranteed payment for the care of clients who previously could not afford to pay. The costs of Medicare, which is financed partly through Social Security contributions and partly through general tax revenues, have risen drastically and far faster than the planners had anticipated. These costs have been passed on to the elderly consumer and to people still on the work force through increases in Social Security deductions. The reader is referred to Chapter 17 on Aging for a full discussion of the administration and benefits of Medicare.

Medicaid is almost the opposite of Medicare. It is a public assistance medical care program provided under Title 19 of the Social Security Act of 1965 and a federal insurance program paid for by prospective beneficiaries and their employers through general taxes and administered by state welfare boards. There are some federal eligibility standards, but there are wide state and regional variations with entitlement based on a state-administered means test, very much like eligibility tests for public assistance. The amount of available funds fluctuates greatly with frequent changes in political and economic policy. Only about one third of the medically indigent have benefited from Medicaid since its inception. This is a result mainly of greatly underestimated costs of providing care, poorly managed administration of funds and services, and the ever-present inflation. Because Medicaid is so unpopular and the financing so shaky, it has become a political football. Funds are frozen and unfrozen in many states with depressing regularity, and people often do not know from week to week whether they will be able to receive medical care. Hospitals, particularly those in metropolitan areas with large numbers of poor clients, depend on Medicaid funds for operating expenses and are thrown into frequent fiscal turmoil. The

Department of Health, Education, and Welfare (DHEW) Secretary's Task Force on Medicaid and Related Programs made the following recommendations for the reorganization and improvement of Medicaid[4]:

1. It should be converted to a program of a uniform minimum level of health benefits financed 100% by federal funds. There should also be federal matching funds for certain supplementary benefits and for individuals not covered under the minimum plan.

2. Both the basic federal benefit and the supplementation should provide incentive for improved organization and delivery of service. Beneficiaries should be given the option to select a group practice prepayment plan (HMO).

3. The commitment to provide medical care to all the indigent should be reaffirmed, and priorities should be established to extend coverage to additional groups by abolishing the income level limit as a requirement for participation in Medicaid.

4. States should be required to simplify methods for determining eligibility, and there should be some stipulation for provisional certification in an emergency before final eligibility is established.

For all of Medicaid's administrative and financial problems, it has done some good. It has brought medical care to millions for the first time; it has helped to relieve many providers of health care from the burden of caring for the indigent by themselves with no outside financial help. There are reports that it has slowed the exodus of physicians from poverty areas, both urban and rural.[2] It is, however, large, unwieldy, and much too complex to continue in an effective manner in its present form.

It serves little purpose simply to say that it should be abolished in favor of national health insurance. The need for Medicaid could be greatly reduced through such a program, or even through the improvement of Medicare and private health insurance—the most urgent next steps. It is most unlikely, however, that any insurance scheme that could be passed in the foreseeable future would be comprehensive enough to permit total abolition of Medicaid, at least for a number of years. Thus, ways must be found to strengthen the residual programs.*

Faults

There are many inequities inherent in the fee-for-service system. The most obvious one is that health care is available only to those who can afford to pay the fees, either directly to the providers of care or indirectly through third parties. If we as health professionals believe that health care is the right of all people instead of the privilege of a few, then we are obligated to do what we can to improve and change the system. The fee-for-service system exacerbates the three major problems of health care delivery: the high cost of care, uneven accessibility of health resources, and shortage and poor distribution of health care workers.

Little can be done by health professionals about inflation itself, but much can be done about the health industry's contribution to its own skyrocketing costs. Because private (nongovernmental and fee-for-service) institutions are run independently of each other, there is enormous duplication of services. There is no reason for four or five hospitals in a metropolitan area to each have radioactive cobalt therapy equipment, which is used infrequently and at tremendous cost. Annie Oakley would be proud of this "anything-you-can-do-I-can-do-better" philosophy, but it has no place in hospital administration when it is the consumer who pays for the poorly utilized equipment.

Uneven accessibility of health services is another inequity in the system, and consumers are becoming angry. The great technological advances of the past decades are available almost exclusively to people who live near them, have the sophistication to know about them, and can pay for them. There is little likelihood that a coal miner's wife living in Appalachia will ever benefit from mammogra-

phy when she first notices the lump in her breast. There is even the possibility that she has had so little exposure to health education that she will not know that the lump is anything out of the ordinary. Even in large cities where people are a bus ride or two away from x-ray equipment, their health problems are undiagnosed because they do not have access to the information that such help exists. Despite increasing public awareness, through the use of mass media, of the advances in health technology, the utilization of resources remains uneven. The fault lies with health professionals who do not make enough effort to reach out to the potential consumers of health care. An image comes to mind of Paul Revere galloping frantically from house to house warning people about the coming of the British. The colonists needed this information for their self-protection and their very survival. So do people need information about health, illness, and disease for their self-protection and very survival. Our methods of communication are much more effective and sophisticated than a midnight horseback ride. Why are we not using them? Literally everyone listens to the radio; almost everyone watches television; a smaller number read the newspapers; everyone converses. There is no reason why intensive multimedia and even door-to-door campaigns cannot be initiated about various kinds of health problems. Through a variety of outreach programs, *every person* in this country could have access to health education and health care *if* health professionals choose to make it possible.

The shortage and uneven distribution of health care personnel is a reason why care is not available to all and is a function of the fee-for-service system. The shortage of physicians is due partly to the incredibly high cost of medical education and partly to the fact that the medical community has traditionally kept itself small and elite. It is only recently that the fraternity of physicians has begun to accept members of minority groups—blacks, women, and people from lower socioeconomic classes—into its ranks.

*Reprinted with permission from Health care in transition: directions for the future (p. 68), by Anne R. Somers, copyright 1971 by the Hospital Research and Educational Trust, 840 North Lake Shore Dr., Chicago, Ill. 60611.

Physicians distribute themselves in uneven clumps for two main reasons: cities are where the great medical centers and technological resources are, and the affluent suburbs are where the money is. Rural areas, city ghettos, and other sectors of the country do not offer sophisticated medical facilities and consequently suffer from a lack of physicians (Fig. 1-1). It is in the nature of our health care system that other health workers follow the physicians, so where there are no doctors, there are few nurses, laboratory technicians, physical therapists, or any of the other ''support'' people in the system. There *are* isolated exceptions to this statement. In city ghettos and in rural areas there are nurse practitioners (e.g., the famous Frontier Nursing Service in Kentucky) who function more

or less independently and do what they can to bring health care to the people. But their efforts are the exception rather than the rule and are miniscule in comparison with what needs to be done. If we continue to insist that the primary care provider is always a physician, then other health personnel will never have the opportunity to meet health needs of the client that do not require a physician. The *majority* of the general population's needs can be met by various other members of the health team. Although the total number of physicians has increased, the trend is toward specialization, and the number of primary care physicians (family care practitioners, pediatricians, and internists) per total population has decreased.

Another related reason for the uneven distribu-

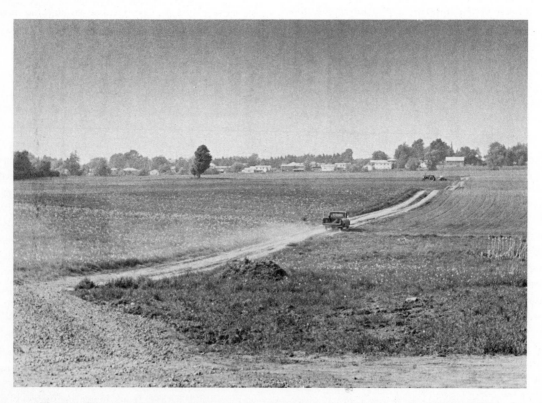

Fig. 1-1. The poor distribution of professional health workers frequently leaves people in rural areas without access to health care. (Photograph by Susan McKinney; courtesy Editorial Photocolor Archives, Inc., New York.)

tion of health care is that illness is more "glamorous" and exciting than wellness and therefore attracts more physicians. Medical journal articles are mostly concerned with disease and cure, not with maintaining wellness.

In 1971 DHEW issued a *White Paper* on the delivery of health care called "Towards a Comprehensive Health Policy for the 1970s." Following are summarized some of the proposals for improved health strategy[4]:

1. Prevention of disease, including welfare reforms, nutrition and family planning, occupational health and safety, research into automobile accidents, and alcoholism; pollution control; prevention of communicable disease; product safety; personal responsibility for health; and financial incentives for preventive health care
2. Innovation and reform of health care delivery and the development of health maintenance organizations
3. Improvement of health manpower by the distribution and use of manpower resources, the provision of student assistance, improving the financial stability of health professional schools, and increasing the supply of health manpower
4. Improving the financing of health services by providing some form of health insurance for everyone, most likely national health insurance

Ten years after publication of the *White Paper* little progress can be noted in the implementation of many of the proposals. True, there has been some research and improvement in a few of the areas, but by and large the health care delivery system is in the same sorry state it was when the proposals were written.

The fee-for-service system evolved and continues to be useful to some for largely political reasons. Power has a great deal to do with the delivery of health care. The "medical elite" have power over the "helpless sick." If one is forced to pay for health care, then one is put into the position of supplicant, and the philosophy of caveat emptor prevails. Those who can pay for health care and those who control the purse strings of the system have power over everyone else. Those who administer and perpetuate the system have power over those who seek to change it: the establishment over the upstarts.

There is also a beneficial use of power in the system. Knowledge about how the system works imparts the power to manipulate it for the benefit of clients. But it seems that most of the power flows in a downward rather than an upward or lateral direction, and health professionals should not have to waste valuable time and energy figuring out ways to manipulate the system so the client is helped. A system where the power automatically flows from the providers of care *to* the client would be preferable.

Special interest groups also perpetuate the fee-for-service system. The best known, and the most successful, is the AMA. The system obviously benefits the individual physician, and the AMA strongly opposes any program or proposed legislation that will take financial control out of the hands of the physician and give it to the consumer or the government.

Representatives of pharmaceutical manufacturers and suppliers of hospital equipment have powerful lobbies in Washington who also oppose any move to change fee for service. The advent of some form of national health insurance will surely curtail these manufacturers' profits.

Cater and Lee [editors: *Politics of health*, New York, 1972, MEDCOM, Inc.] define an interest group they call the "subgovernment of health." It is composed of certain political executives, that is, persons appointed to high level positions by elected officials; career bureaucrats, such as civil servants and Commissioned Corps Officers who serve in the HEW; key congressional committee persons . . . who have carved out empires as health advocates; interest group professionals who, like those from the AMA, seek governmental influence; and the public interest elites . . . who do research and prepare information for use by the other groups.*

*From Archer, Sarah, and Fleshman, Ruth: Community health nursing, N. Scituate, Mass., 1975, Duxbury Press, p. 166.

The adroit use of politics would help us to understand the motives of these special interest groups so they can be encouraged or opposed on an intelligent and practical basis.

Economics

Economics is probably the most potent force behind the fee-for-service system. The vested interest of individual physicians has already been discussed, as has the profit motive of private insurance companies. There is a finite amount of money available for the provision of health care (Fig. 1-2), and the allocation of all resources for one system precludes the formation of another—and we are right back to power politics (Tables 1-2 and 1-3). There is a reason why health care costs so much,

and inflation is not the entire answer. Advanced technology involves millions of dollars' worth of "hardware," chemicals, and other supplies. Someone is manufacturing these things, and in accordance with the American economic tradition of free enterprise, profits are being made. Pharmaceutical manufacturers, drug wholesalers, and retail pharmacists together account for the approximately 300% markup of most prescription drugs. That is, a tablet that costs 10¢ to manufacture will cost the consumer 40¢ to purchase. This is not to say that manufacturers and suppliers should not make a profit—they should. But one wonders if it is absolutely necessary to have thirty or forty brands of aspirin, ten or twelve manufacturers of essentially the same fetal monitor, twelve or so differently colored cap-

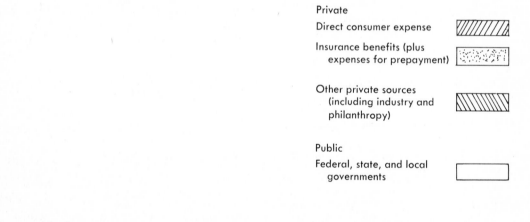

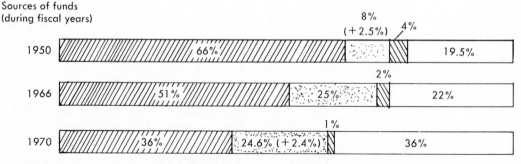

Fig. 1-2. Financing of health services in United States: sources of funds for personal health expenditures. (Reprinted with permission of Macmillan Publishing Co., Inc., from The care of health in communities, by Nancy Milio. Copyright © 1975 by Nancy Milio.)

Table 1-2. Financing of health services in United States: changes in total national expenditures, including personal health services, 1950 to 1972*

	FISCAL YEARS			
	1950	**1965**	**1971**	**1972**
Total health expenditures†	$12.1	$38.9	$75.0	$83.4
Percent of GNP	4.6	5.9	7.5	7.6
Personal health expenditures‡				
Percent of total	89.4	89.3	89.9	91.2
Per capita	$79.0	$198.0	$358.0	$394.0

*Reprinted with permission of Macmillan Publishing Co., Inc., from The care of health in communities, by Nancy Milio. Copyright © 1975 by Nancy Milio.
†In billions; does not include expenditures for health care training and education or air and water pollution control and treatment.
‡Does not include government public health expenditures, medical research, or medical facilities construction; includes administrative overhead.

sules of the same tetracycline, and dozens of brands of fever thermometers that all perform the same function. There is no easy solution to this situation, short of disturbing the entire economic system, but it is the consumer who pays for the advertising, marketing, promotion, and transportation of yet another brand of aspirin.

Another economic consideration in keeping the fee-for-service system intact is people's attitudes about money and its power. There is a common belief that something is worthwhile only if it costs money, and the more it costs, the more worthwhile it must be. This belief is, of course, upheld by health workers in private practice, but it is erroneous in theory. Unfortunately, the constant reinforcement of it in practice makes it appear to be true. Private "paid-for" health care is generally of superior quality than "charity" care, but there is no reason why this should continue to be so. If the fee-for-service system did not exist, there would be no *financially based* inequities in the delivery of health care. Perhaps it is the Protestant work

ethic so prevalent in our way of life that makes us think that people we perceive to be slothful do not deserve a reasonable standard of health care. Perhaps it is the constant emphasis on spending money with which we are bombarded at every turn that makes us need to spend money on health care. We are so used to the high cost of living that we have grown to distrust anything that is either free or reasonably priced.

We are a nation of immigrants, most of us springing from ancestors who faced poverty and struggled to exist and survive in the New World. We are the recipients of the tradition that we must give our children what we did not have ourselves, which almost always involves the spending of money: on things, on education, on cultural improvements like singing and piano lessons, and on expensive medical care. If Grandpa was delivered by a lay midwife at home, then the expected baby will be born in a gleaming hospital with an expensive obstetrician in attendance. If Papa received his "baby shots" at a public health clinic for free, then this child will receive his immunizations in a Park Avenue pediatrician's office.

It has become painfully evident that the fee-for-service system of delivering health care is not working. It is expensive (prohibitively so), inequitable, and it is not meeting the needs of the people it seeks to serve. There are several possible ways in which the situation might be remedied or at least the process of rectification begun. There is

the challenge to create a system that will give us the best of both worlds—the world of advanced science, technology, heavy capital investments, sophisticated management, specialized personnel, and systems engineering, and also the world of individual freedom, individual responsibility, respect for privacy and human dignity, understanding of the holistic or psychosomatic nature of health and disease, and appreciation of the need of human beings for other human beings.*

*Reprinted with permission from Health care in transition: directions for the future (p. 88), by Anne R. Somers, copyright 1971 by the Hospital Research and Educational Trust, 840 North Lake Shore Dr., Chicago, Ill. 60611.

Table 1-3. Financing of health care in United States: allocation of total national expenditures (in billions) by payers and purpose, 1972*

SOURCES OF PAYMENTS

			Administrative expense
For personal health services	$71.9	(86.2%)	
Direct	$25.1	(30.1%)	
Indirect	$46.8	(56.1%)	
Private	20.0	(24.0%)	
Insurance companies	19.0‡	(23.0%)	
Philanthropy and industry	1.0	(1.0%)	
Public§	26.8	(32.1%)	
Federal government	17.7	(21.2%)	
State and local government	9.1	(10.9%)	
			$3.3 (4.0%)
For public health services	**$2.1**	**(2.5%)**	
Public sources	$2.1	(2.5%)	
Other payments	**$6.1**	**(7.3%)**	
Private	$3.0	(3.6%)	
Research	0.3	(0.4%)	
Construction	2.7	(3.2%)	
Public	$3.1	(3.7%)	
Research	1.8	(2.1%)	
Construction	1.3	(1.6%)	

Total national health expenditures† $83.4 (100%)

Additional amounts for

Education of health workers

Environmental protection

Shares of national health expenditures

Direct, consumer	30.1%
Other private	27.6%
Public sources	38.3%
Administrative	4.0%
	100.0%

BENEFICIARIES OF PERSONAL CARE EXPENDITURES

Providers of services	$71.9	(100%)
Hospitals	32.5	(45%)
Physicians	16.2	(23%)
Dentists	5.0	(7%)
Other profiles	1.7	(2%)
Drugs	7.9	(11%)
Eyeglasses, etc.	2.0	(3%)
Nursing homes	3.5	(5%)
Other (including volunteer agencies)	3.1	(4%)

Consumers of services

Under 19 years		
Private	73%	} 100%
Public	27%	
19 to 65		
Private	77%	} 100%
Public	23%	
65 years and over		
Private	32%	} 100%
Public	68%	

*Reprinted with permission of Macmillan Publishing Co., Inc., from The care of health in communities, by Nancy Milio. Copyright © 1975 by Nancy Milio.
†Does not include expenses for air and water pollution control and treatment or private and public costs of education and training in health occupations.
‡Includes about $1 billion for prepaid group practice plans.
§Includes Medicare ($8.4 billion), Medicaid ($7.3 billion), and $11.1 billion for other programs such as workmen's compensation medical benefits, military and veterans medical and hospital care, temporary disability insurance, and school health.

Suggestions for change

There are some practical ways to meet this challenge. The supply of health personnel must be increased. The physician/population ratio is too low, and we depend too heavily on foreign-trained doctors. Medical education must be reformed in content and philosophy so that more physicians can be trained quickly. The cost of medical education is prohibitive except to a very few who are wealthy or lucky enough to receive scholarships, so the pool of potential medical students is very small.

Nurses are not in as short supply as physicians for three main reasons. Nursing education has never been as elitist as medical education and is becoming even less so; the cost of the preparation to practice nursing is far less than medical school, and it takes only about a third as long. The major nurse/population problem is distribution. Nurses tend to want to work near major health care centers and, because they are mostly women, are, or feel they are, less mobile. Married nurses are restricted by husbands and children from moving to a challenging new job in a different area, and single women usually want to be in or near big cities where the "action" is.

There is nothing to be done about the reluctance of nurses to move, but there are things that could be done to attract nurses to work in certain areas. Hospitals could provide protection when walking to cars or they could provide transportation to and from work; community health nurses could institute media campaigns about what they carry with them, so the fear of assault for drugs would be lessened. There should be cooperation between community health agencies and police departments and neighborhood protective associations. Community health agencies do not do much about public relations: informing neighborhood people (other than direct clients) exactly what their purposes and goals are and what they are *not*. People see nurses as authority figures, part of the establishment, and they need to be informed that we do not have most of the power attributed to us: to cut off welfare checks, to report to some authority that unmarried people are living together, or to garnish wages.

The health care system needs to make use of paraprofessionals such as physicians' assistants, various technicians, and home health aides. The Department of Health and Human Services (DHHS) lists over 200 health-related occupations, many of which could be a direct help to professionals. There seems to be a mounting feeling of fear and jealousy among professional health workers when they contemplate the growing number of paraprofessionals. Physicians grudgingly delegate some of the routine tasks to physicians' assistants, but they become very nervous when nurses begin to use the word "diagnosis." The American Nurses Association and the American Medical Association have a committee working on these "territorial" problems, so perhaps some of the conflict will be resolved. Nurses resent physicians' assistants taking away what they see as *their* jobs (often for larger salaries), but then they don't know what to do with all that extra time. Nurses have been saying that they want time to do "real nursing," but now, with the coming of paraprofessionals, they seem "at loose ends." This situation is slowly being remedied by more precise definitions of nursing, but there is still a great deal of conflict between nursing and other health professions.

And what kind of paraprofessionals are needed? Should there be technologists with bachelor's degrees, or is three months of on-the-job training sufficient? The answer depends, of course, on what function is to be served. In some health jobs human warmth counts most. The personality and humanity of a hospital aide, who is always under the direction of professionals, is as important as a high school diploma. A home health aide, on the other hand, who needs to function on a much more independent basis (she will be under the direction of professionals but not under their constant physical surveillance) should have a stronger educational background and a longer training. There is in Philadelphia an organization called Wheels, Inc. It relies solely on volunteers to drive people to and from health care appointments at hospitals, clinics, and physicians' offices. The only requirements for the volunteers are the willingness to help (very often the transport is done on the way to and from the volunteer's job) and a few hours of learning how to help people into and out of wheelchairs. These people might be considered paraprofessional health workers; they certainly fill a desperate need, and they receive a tremendous amount of satisfaction from doing it.

In Colorado there is a new kind of pediatric practitioner. She could be defined as a kind of "maxinurse," although she is not a registered nurse. Her training lasts for five years after high school: two years of liberal arts, two years of special pediatrics training in a medical school, and one year of internship. She is licensed by the state and will have considerably more authority than the pediatric nurse practitioner. This could be the start of a whole new classification of health workers, filling the gap between physicians and nurses. If we as nurses feel it is our function to fill this gap between medicine and traditional task-oriented nursing practice, then we had best do something to assert ourselves before our functions become more downgraded.

Something else that must be done for the revitalization of the health care delivery system is to change and improve the relationship between the health professional and the client. Dehumanization and impersonal treatment are becoming so widespread and so accepted that people are loath to enter the system. They are not equipped to understand what is happening to them, and there is no one to interpret the technological data. The AMA, in recognition of the problem, instituted the specialty of family practice, which has helped somewhat. But the physician is only a small part of the entire system, and there is still the situation in which one individual is referred to three or four different clinics—which may be held on three or four different days—for a single health problem. This does not include the number of offices that must be visited and the number of lines waited in to receive financial assistance or social work help of some kind. Every interviewer asks basically the same questions, so the client may spend three entire days just having low back pain diagnosed. This is an intolerable way to provide health care. It is inhumane, inefficient, and costly. There is no reason why care could not be coordinated in hospitals, group practices, and community health agencies by experts in management and business administration.

Evaluation procedures for the health care system as a whole are rarely undertaken. Each profession and occupation, in theory at least, engages in ongoing evaluation, but there is no coordination and comparison of the effectiveness of the total delivery of care. A community health agency, which is a microcosm of the entire health care system, is administered by a director who is ultimately responsible for the quality of the care provided by the agency. Administration implies not only responsibility for the care provided by individual practitioners but also for overall staffing and the effective distribution of staff. Achieving a balance between professional capability and utilization of that capability is the primary function of an agency administrator.

If public health agencies can be administered, then the entire health system can also be. True, it is an enormous job and could not be done by one person, but without some method of quality control, there will not be much quality. Quality is difficult to measure in an area where there is no definable product, but there must be certain standards of care for the system in general and methods of recourse for the consumer who is receiving care that is below the standard. Lay participation, which will be discussed in detail later in the chapter, is absolutely essential if the quality of health care is to be raised and maintained.

One suggestion for the improvement of health care delivery is the "forced" redistribution of health personnel. If health workers will not voluntarily move to where they are needed, and if society demands excellent health care for everyone, then there is no reason not to redistribute what is readily available. As citizens we are used to being forced to pay for our services (although we don't like it and complain constantly). There are few people who would volunteer a portion of their salaries to pay for highway construction, garbage removal, national defense, prison upkeep, the administration of justice, and the thousands of other services without which we could not function. If we will not voluntarily give up our money, it must be taken from us in the form of taxes, and laws have been devised to do just this.

Involuntary taxation is a socially workable, albeit unpopular, means of paying for the societal goods and benefits that people have come to expect. If a society decides that it wishes to provide health care to those who are in need, then perhaps a similar system can be devised, that is, providing nonvoluntary health workers for those consumers who would otherwise not be served. There are two major and practical ways in which this can be done. One way involves professional workers; the other involves nonprofessionals.

Professional education is becoming more and more expensive, and it is not just medical students who are in financial crisis. As education takes longer and becomes more complex, the cost rises. The number of students who do not need any kind of financial assistance are in a minority, and for those who do, government loans should be provided for *all* who need them. There should, however, be a stipulation: interest on the loans should be high, but *if* the student promises to devote a period of time (two or three years) after graduation to serve where needed, the entire loan will be forgiven. High interest rates on government loans should discourage students from not taking the offer; underserved areas will be guaranteed a constant flow of professional health workers, and students will have a free professional education. The inexperience of the new graduates can be offset by professional health workers who are paid premium salaries for working and living in places that some might consider undesirable: ''combat pay'' for health service.

One solution might be that nonprofessional health needs can be met by a ''draft,'' although admittedly this would not be a popular idea, particularly in view of the current furor over reinstatement of the military draft. However, when socially important choices must be made in a democracy, certain portions of the population will be dissatisfied. Health care is certainly no less important than military defense, and if this country supported a military draft for over thirty years, it can support a health draft. The recruitment, organization, and administration could be similar. Everyone would be required, on graduation from high school or on reaching age 18, to spend two or three years serving the people of a given community, meeting their health needs in a variety of ways. On-the-job training would be done, and individual preferences for work could be honored. The pay scale would be minimal, but, as in the military draft, the basic needs of the health workers would be met by government subsidy. They would be under the direction of professionals, and after their term of service was completed, they could stay on if they wished as ''nondraft'' workers with salaries and benefits competitive with those in the private sector.

There is a reasonable argument to be made that people who are forced or coerced into doing a particular job do not do it well, and the hostility engendered might result in a poor quality of care or even outright harm to clients. This is definitely a factor to be considered, and safeguards would have to be built into the system. Effective supervision, massive public education about the merits of the draft, competent peer counselors, and a workable grievance procedure could be used to try to ensure a high standard of work.

Another incentive would be government-sponsored training for those who wanted to stay after their term of service and begin to climb the occupational/professional ladder. Perhaps the time served as a draftee could be used to partly offset the time required to have a professional educational loan forgiven. There are all kinds of creative ways in which the system could be managed, and there are variations on all the ''enforcement'' themes discussed, but it seems essential that there is some way to ensure that people who need health care receive it. And if people are ''inconvenienced'' for a few years of their lives, it is the price we must pay for living in a democracy and espousing certain universal rights.

This coercion, subtle or not-so-subtle, to provide health care to people who would not ordinarily receive it, creates a dilemma. A democracy does not ordinarily force citizens to work in occupations or in locations unless a grave national emergency, such as war, were to exist. A society that did so would be less than democratic. On the other hand, war is not the only imaginable national emergency. The lack of an adequate health care system could reasonably be considered a justification for a draft of professional health workers.

HEALTH MAINTENANCE ORGANIZATIONS

Probably the greatest innovation in the health care system in the past thirty or forty years, and a practical alternative to fee for service, is the health maintenance organization (HMO). An HMO is a prepaid (by a monthly or quarterly membership fee) organized system of health care providing basic and supplemental services to its members. The concept is aimed at preventing illness and maintaining health by close observation, routine health examinations, early detection of disease, and health teaching (Fig. 1-3).

The essential ingredients of all HMOs include the following:

1. Prepayment
2. Group practice by primary physicians and specialists (some smaller HMOs do not employ specialists; clients are referred to them, they bill the HMO, and the client has no extra charge)
3. A unified medical center that includes offices, laboratories, x-ray facilities, inpatient hospital beds, and satellite clinics (again, the number of these facilities is determined by the size of the population to be served)
4. Voluntary enrollment
5. Payment of physicians', nurses', and hospital fees on the basis of capitation or a fixed fee per time period for each member, regardless of the amount of care provided; that is, brain surgery or the removal of a wart are each covered by the same membership fee
6. Coverage includes a full spectrum of comprehensive health care from prevention to diagnosis, treatment, and rehabilitation

There is strong emphasis on the prevention of disease because it is a medically sound philosophy and a fiscally sound one as well. It is much less expensive to keep persons healthy than it is to cure them once they become ill. A diagnostic office visit and routine health examination are much cheaper than a stay in the hospital.

Primary health care, which is one of the major functions of an HMO, is the provision of accessible and equitable health services; it updates the family doctor concept with modern support services such as x-ray and laboratory procedures and physical therapy. This should be continually available to a specific group of people and should drastically reduce the fragmentation, gaps, and duplication of service present in the fee-for-service system.

Each client, once he becomes a member of the HMO, is entitled to all the services provided. He must choose his primary physician from those on the HMO's staff, but there is usually a sufficient variety to satisfy almost everyone. The physicians may work only for the HMO, or they may also be in private practice. But while they are employed by the HMO, they receive a salary that remains the same whether they see five clients a week or 500. And the member's fee remains the same, whether he sees the physician once a year or once a week. All basic health services are provided at a central location, and some very large HMOs have their own hospital. Most, however, have contractual arrangements with a hospital to provide such services as inpatient care, some sophisticated diagnostic services like brain scans or thermography, and certain outpatient therapeutic services like radiation or cobalt therapy or the use of very expensive physical therapy equipment. HMOs have 24-hour emergency telephone service. Emergency calls are screened by a physician who either recommends that the client come to the health center the following day or go immediately to the hospital emergency room. Clients are on the board of directors and have direct representation in the policy

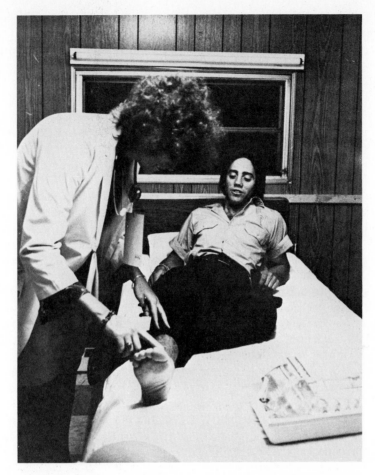

Fig. 1-3. The major advantage of an HMO is emphasis on primary care and health maintenance. (Photograph by Ann Chwatsky; courtesy Editorial Photocolor Archives, Inc., New York.)

and decision-making process of the HMO, and there is usually an active, well-run grievance procedure. The rate structure of most HMOs is controlled by the state insurance department, which also enforces the health insurance rules and regulations that apply to HMOs.

A variation on this health care concept is the individual practice association HMO (IPA). This is a partnership, association, corporation, or other legal entity that has entered into a service agreement with private health practitioners. The client joins an HMO group, but services are provided by physicians in their own offices instead of at a cen-

tral health center. There is still an annual membership fee, but the client does not have the convenience of "one-stop shopping." Any additional services that are required are provided on a contractual basis by the IPA.

There are problems inherent in operating an HMO and in the system concept itself. When more HMOs are organized, there could be competition for members, and costs could rise. This could lead to a reduction in the services offered and a consequent lowering of the level of care. Even now, before competition is a real problem, costs are escalating, and cutting of essential corners is a problem that must be avoided. Most HMOs are administered by nonhealth professionals and are run as the businesses they essentially are. HMOs can be a threat to physicians, both those working for the HMO and those in private practice. The provider of primary care in an HMO may not always be a physician. Very often it is a nurse, and this can create ego problems for the physician and interpersonal conflicts in the nurse/physician relationship that can affect the quality of care. Some HMOs, however, have personnel policies and interdisciplinary team conferences to try to avoid this kind of conflict. Physicians in private practice could feel that the HMO may take away their business, or at least a part of it, and well it may. If HMOs meet the needs of the people, they may very well be the health care system of the future and could absorb up to 90% of the private practice clients. Being an HMO physician, however, is not an unattractive life. Salaries are excellent, and fringe benefits such as retirement plans and personal health benefits are paid by the HMO, as are malpractice insurance premiums, one of the biggest items in a physician's overhead. Emergency call is taken on a rotating basis, and there is a liberal paid vacation every year. More and more physicians are forming group practices, and from there it is only a small step to the adoption of the HMO concept.

Nurses are an integral part of the functioning of an HMO. They are primary health practitioners who define problems, assess needs, implement and coordinate care, educate clients and other health workers, and evaluate results. The nurse functions *with* the physician, not *for* him. Although there are legal restrictions on what nurses may and may not do, most HMO physicians (probably because they themselves are committed to the concept of primary care) view nurses as colleagues, not as subordinates. Following are some examples of the kinds of things that nurses do in an HMO: coordination of the care of a person with a stable chronic illness such as diabetes or hypertension; history taking and physical assessment of well adults and children; initial screening of clients with acute illness; family

planning (contraception) counseling; all kinds of health teaching; and various interdependent functions with other members of the HMO and outside agencies, such as making referrals, planning home visits, coordinating inpatient services, hospital visits, and dietary planning with nutritionists. Nurses in HMOs, however, are still not paid what they are worth. They work equally as hard and as long as physicians, and perform functions that are different from but as important as those of a physician. Their salaries are usually about 25% of that of the physician. In this respect nurses have not made any more progress in an HMO than they have in any other area of practice.

Murray and Zentner,[6] in their discussion of the delivery of health care, list several concepts and proposals for change in the present health care system. It appears that they can all be incorporated into the HMO system and that the nurse can play a large role in their implementation. Following are some of the concepts that have not been previously mentioned:

1. Separation of the well from the sick, using a screening plan to meet specific needs of clients.

2. Consideration of the cultural, social, psychological, and physiological aspects of the person.

3. Avoidance of care that is hospital based and physician controlled by delivering care in the community with focus on the individual, wellness behavior, and on ways to maintain or restore a healthy state.

4. More deliberate use of health screening, health education, counseling, and referral.

5. Encouraging health personnel to assume personal responsibility for their own decisions and actions.

6. Encouraging social and natural scientists, humanists, health professionals, and consumers to become active participants in planning and evaluating care and distributing authority and control.

7. Emphasis on group approaches and demographic planning to maximize individual potential and health care services.

8. Avoidance of hasty planning and quick, easy answers that lead to the abandonment of problems

too soon when immediate results are not forthcoming. Epidemiological data and scientific problem solving will help prevent the tendency to rely on fast, unrealistic answers.

A discussion of three kinds of HMO models follows. Two are large and well known; the small regional one probably typifies HMO development going on all over the country.

Cronkhite-OEO model

In April, 1970, the Cronkhite-OEO model was launched in Boston. Its name derives from its director, Dr. Leonard Cronkhite of the Children's Hospital Medical Center in Boston, and from the basic OEO (Office of Economic Opportunity) neighborhood health center concept. The OEO neighborhood health centers are discussed in detail in Chapter 7. The system would serve approximately 300,000 people and include neighborhood health centers, hospitals, nursing homes, and a home care plan, all under a single management. The cornerstone of the system is a primary care center that accepts total responsibility for providing comprehensive, personal health services. The system would function as any other HMO but would be managed by a nonprofit corporation. More than sixty of these centers have now been funded across the country (some with DHHS money), and they are a significant factor in the evolution of a new health care delivery system. Following are some of the most important features of the Cronkhite-OEO model:

1. It is directed at a disadvantaged population living in a strictly defined geographical area.

2. The programatic focus is on primary care, and the organizational focus is a primary care unit: the neighborhood or family health center.

3. Funding so far has been almost entirely through the government (DHHS, government grants, and a small amount from Medicare and Medicaid), and all care is free to clients.

4. Heavy emphasis is placed on the development and use of nonprofessional indigenous personnel and on involvement of the community in program planning and operation.

5. The hospital is not viewed as part of the system: its use in emergencies or in acute care is generally on a "backup basis," and there are no close organizational or financial ties between the hospital and the HMO.

6. Physicians are salaried, and institutions are paid on the basis of cost.

7. No one is forced to come to a center, but the care *is* free for the target population. For the time being there is no choice of physician within the system. Individual clients and families are simply assigned to a health care team.

There are several advantages to the Cronkhite-OEO model. Poor people, who formerly had to rely on clinics for the indigent or a kindly physician who would take them on as a charity client, now have access to quality health care on an ongoing basis, and they have a sense of participation and involvement in their own care. The system touches only peripherally on the "mainstream" providers of health care who could feel threatened by the provision of free care on such a large scale. In racially segregated urban ghettos this is not a minor consideration, and it has proven easier to establish an entirely new neighborhood health system than to reorganize ambulatory care services that already exist in large hospitals.

There are also drawbacks. One of the major ones is the break that occurs in the provision of care when the client must be hospitalized. This underscores the already existing fragmentation of service and is particularly disastrous in the disadvantaged population who have less knowledge of and confidence in the system. A traumatic hospital stay, with no ties to the neighborhood health center, could frighten the client right back out of the system. The maintenance of two complete systems, one for primary care and one for hospital care, leads to higher costs and lower quality for both. Another disadvantage is that the separation from the mainstream of health care will discourage excellent physicians, nurses, and other health personnel from working there. Thus the quality of care could diminish. Long-term financing of these neighborhood health centers will be a problem. If the centers keep expanding across the country, as many as 25% of all Americans could receive absolutely free medical care, and it seems likely that the 75% who are still paying would resent this. ''Either the free care would have to be discontinued, or it would have to be made available to the entire population. In other words, we would then be committed to an eventual national health service supported by general taxes rather than a national health insurance scheme based primarily on contributory financing.''[2,p.113] Yet another disadvantage of the Cronkhite-OEO model is that the client does not have a choice of primary caregiver. This further fragments health care and gives impetus to the charge that the poor receive care that is inferior to that received by the nonpoor.

Kaiser model

The second major model is the Kaiser system on the west coast. It is a private program with over 2 million members, and its success has led it to be a model for the development of HMOs all over the country. It incorporates most of the HMO characteristics already discussed, and there are some important contrasts with the Cronkhite-OEO model:

1. It is used by a cross section of the population living in a certain geographical area but with less rigid geographical or income limits.

2. Almost the whole spectrum of comprehensive care is provided (except for dental care and extended mental health benefits). There is no special emphasis on primary care, but neither is it discouraged as it is in fee for service.

3. Funding is almost entirely private. The hospitals are financed out of the operating surplus of the health centers. This is highly unusual.

4. Paramedical and nonprofessional personnel are used more than in conventional practice but less than in an OEO center. Community involvement was almost nil in the beginning but is now increasing. Community representatives are on the governing board.

5. The hospital is viewed as the center of the delivery system, and physicians' offices are either there or at a satellite clinic. The hospitals and the medical group depend on the insurance plan for capital expansion.

6. Physicians are organized into a separate legal entity, a group, and contract with the HMO to provide services for a fixed fee per member per year, regardless of the amount of service provided. The amount of money available to pay physicians depends on the amount required to pay hospitals. Consequently, the incentive to hold down hospital admissions is high.

7. Within the plan, members are free to choose their own physicians, who then refer them to specialists as needed.

With its broad community-wide orientation, a substantial degree of consumer free choice, effective integration of most major hospital and ambulatory services, effective managerial controls combined with considerable provider freedom, and the well-documented lesser use of expensive hospital care and lesser costs, there are many today who believe the Kaiser model is the ideal for the United States as a whole.*

The Kaiser model, however, is not a panacea for the health care ills that beset us. Only 4% of the population now belong to a Kaiser type of HMO, and, although the number is steadily increasing, the rate is very slow. It is still a seller's market for physicians' services, and, no matter how inefficient the practice, private practitioners still enjoy very high earnings, and they are not likely to give up easily. Starting a Kaiser type of system takes a tremendous amount of capital, and finding major investors is difficult. Consumers are reluctant to lock themselves into a system about whose quality they are not certain.

Small regional HMO

The Cumberland Regional Health Plan (CRHP) in Vineland, New Jersey, is an excellent example of a small regional HMO that is serving the health

*Reprinted with permission from Health care in transition: directions for the future (p. 114), by Anne R. Somers, copyright 1971 by the Hospital Research and Educational Trust, 840 North Lake Shore Dr., Chicago, Ill. 60611.

needs of the city in which it is located plus nearby towns and the surrounding rural countryside. Vineland is a city of about 50,000 people in south central New Jersey about midway between Philadelphia and Atlantic City. It is surrounded by several smaller towns and very rich farmland. It is a fairly middle class community with a large population of Spanish-speaking people (Cubans and Puerto Ricans). The CRHP began enrolling members in April, 1975, and in August, 1980, there were 9,590 members. The projected goal is 10,000. It is a nonprofit corporation with a fourteen-member board of directors from area communities. The health center is in the middle of Vineland in a modern building that is fully equipped with examining rooms, office space, laboratories, an x-ray department, children's play room, conference rooms, and a medical records library. The center employs several physicians (family practitioners, internists, pediatricians, a gynecologist, and a urologist), a pediatric and an adult nurse practitioner, a nursing supervisor, an x-ray technician, a laboratory technician, a medical records librarian, and a variety of clerks and secretaries. Specialists are available if necessary. The center is open six days a week, two evenings, and there is a 24-hour emergency call service.

Newcomb Hospital in Vineland is small (150 beds) but modern and well run and is used for the majority of acute illnesses and surgery. Atlantic City Medical Center is an hour's drive, and a bit further in the other direction is Philadelphia with its outstanding medical facilities. There is a capitation arrangement with Newcomb Hospital, and all hospital charges are covered by the HMO membership. All CRHP physicians are salaried, and the medical director is a pediatrician with an evident commitment to health maintenance.

There are four classifications of membership (Table 1-4): group I, employees of companies who pay for membership on a group basis; group II, individual members and families; group III, low-income members whose fees are on a sliding scale; and group IV, the largest, Medigroup. This is a new program developed by Blue Cross and Blue Shield of New Jersey as an option to the traditional Blue Cross/Blue Shield membership plan. Group IV members receive the same services as other members, but their fees are paid by Blue Cross/Blue Shield, and they must enroll as part of an employee group. There are no individual Medigroup members. The purpose seems to be to give a choice to employees who formerly accepted Blue Cross/Blue Shield health insurance or nothing.

The health benefits covered by the CRHP are broad indeed. At the medical center they include physicians' office visits, physical examinations, regular pediatric care and immunizations, prenatal and postnatal care, specialists' care when referred by the CRHP physician, nursing care, diagnostic x-ray and laboratory services, vision and hearing screening, family planning services, health education, minor surgery and anesthesia, mental health care, medical social services, and ambulance service. In the hospital or other approved institution there are 365 days a year of semiprivate bed and board, services of all hospital employees, surgery, anesthesia, therapeutic solutions, oxygen, dressings and casts, drugs, physical therapy, consultation, diagnostic x-rays, laboratory and pathology services, radioactive isotope studies, surgically implanted cardiac pacemakers and batteries and replacements, and oral surgery. Maternity benefits are seven days for a normal delivery and nine days when there is a cutting procedure (cesarean section or other complication) plus additional benefits for postpartum complications. Mental health care includes thirty days a year of hospitalization and twenty outpatient visits a year for short-term therapy or crisis intervention. There are sixty home care visits a year by a home health aide or nurse, and physicians will make house calls when medically necessary for a nominal fee. Extended care in nursing homes is available for thirty days a year. Emergency care outside the service area and not in Newcomb Hospital is covered if the member notifies CRHP within 48 hours of the receipt of care.

Services not covered are those which are not authorized by a CRHP physician; prescription

Table 1-4. Cumberland Regional Health Plan: rates, options, and services

	MONTHLY RATES*	NUMBER OF SUBSCRIBERS	SERVICES COVERED
Group I (companies)	$22.90 per person 50.81 employee and one dependent 74.55, family of three or more	1,000	All services listed in text
Group II (individual)	30.02 per person 50.98 person and one dependent 77.05, family of three or more	650	
Group III (low-income)	Sliding scale of $4 to $15/month No charge if there is dire need	2,950	Same as groups I and II
Group IV (Medigroup)	Same as group I	4,600	Same as groups I and II except: 1. Service to people age 65 and over 2. Prosthetic devices 3. Service provided under any other insurance contract 4. Hospital services primarily for rehabilitation

*As of August, 1980.

drugs; general dental care; cosmetic surgery; long-term psychiatric care; use of durable medical equipment and artificial aids (e.g., hospital beds, crutches, and walkers); military service-connected or war-related illnesses or injuries; services covered by any governmental agency; blood or plasma; private-duty nursing; maternity benefits provided during the first 240 days of membership; and for nongroup members treatment of preexisting conditions for the first twelve months of membership. Membership is not offered to people ages 65 and over.

CONSUMERISM

Until recently, consumers of health care have been a rather passive group of people who silently obeyed physicians' orders without knowing what was happening to them. Or perhaps they failed to obey orders because they did not understand and were too timid or too intimidated by the system to ask for an explanation. People have been generally loath to ask for a second opinion for fear of in-

sulting their physician and because it is expensive, and so a great deal of misdiagnosis and mistreatment has gone unchecked. A man who would unhesitatingly send an overdone steak back to a restaurant kitchen would not question an ''overdone'' bill for physicians' services. A woman who goes from dress shop to dress shop, spending an entire day looking for the just-right outfit, will accept the first gynecologist she tries just because of a referral by a friend, even if she does not like or trust the physician. A person who, when faced with a strange new vegetable at a friend's dinner table, will ask, ''What's that?'' will swallow, without question, a strange new medication in a hospital.

Slowly but surely this is changing. Consumers in general are becoming more aware of their rights in regard to the products and services they purchase, thanks in large measure to the consumer advocacy movement. Consumers of health care are beginning to scrutinize the products and services they are purchasing. The element of the purchase of service cannot be emphasized too strongly. Physicians, dentists, and other health professionals in private practice are hired by their clients. The health care provided is a service just as surely as window washing, catering, and business consultation are services provided by people who are *hired by* their clients. Americans are not accustomed to thinking of health care in this way (health professionals have encouraged us to think of them as "super people" who have so much esoteric knowledge and expertise that we dare not question it), but until we do, we will remain uninformed consumers who are prey to all kinds of unprofessional and unethical practices (Fig. 1-4).

There is no point in keeping our anger inside. The justifiable anger of consumers can be used in practical ways, exemplified by the following:

A professional woman went to an ophthalmologist for a routine biannual examination. He had a reputation of medical excellence *and* of keeping his clients waiting for long periods of time. Knowing this, she requested the first appointment in the morning. When she arrived on time, she found six or seven clients had been squeezed in ahead of her. She waited for over 3 hours, despite repeated pleas that she had to get to work. When she was finally seen by the physician, she voiced her displeasure at being kept waiting, but he was unimpressed. When the bill arrived ($50 for a routine examination), she enclosed it with a letter saying that as a professional woman she valued her time at $25 an hour and that she had waited 3 hours to see him. She gave him a half hour "free time" and enclosed a bill for $62.50 with her letter. He *owed her* money, she said. He never paid, but neither did he rebill her for the examination. She feels she can never return to that ophthalmologist, but there are dozens who are equally competent who do not waste her time, which is just as important to her as a physician's is to him.

Following is another example:

A man had abdominal surgery and was in the hospital for seven days. There were no major complications, but he proved to be a rather obstreperous client, very demanding and hostile and voicing his complaints about the hospital in a very loud and bitter way. His complaints were all justified, but his surgeon gave him a rather severe tongue lashing, threatened to remove himself from the client's care, and then prescribed 10 mg of diazepam (Valium) three times a day to "keep him quiet." When the client returned home, he experienced much pain, enough to frighten him, so he telephoned the surgeon's office. The call was never returned, and during the two weeks the client spent recuperating at home, he was able to speak with the office nurse once, but the surgeon never came to the phone. In due course the bill arrived with a charge of about $200 for services not covered by the client's health insurance. The client wrote a letter to the surgeon saying that the surgery was performed adequately and that he agreed with what the insurance company was willing to pay for the actual operation. As far as the other services were concerned, he felt there were none and went on to list the ways in which the surgeon had behaved in a cruel and unprofessional manner. The client said that since there was no service beyond the actual surgery, there would be no payment of the fee. He sent copies of the letter to the hospital administrator, the chief of surgery, the consumer reporter of the local television station, and to several people and agencies. He never heard from the surgeon again, *and* the bill was not resubmitted.

Both these examples involve nonpayment of medical bills, and it should not be assumed that "stiffing" physicians and dentists at every turn is recommended. However, refusal to pay a bill when services were either not rendered or rendered in a less than satisfactory manner is protesting in terms that can be readily understood. There are those who think this may be a drastic measure, and it may very well be, but there is no reason why consumers of health care should not be as militant as consumers of any other service. There is no service that is more important to one's survival, and there is no service that is more unethical to provide in a less than satisfactory manner. A person who complains bitterly to his auto mechanic for an improperly done valve job and then meekly accepts poor medical care from his physician is doing himself a grave injustice.

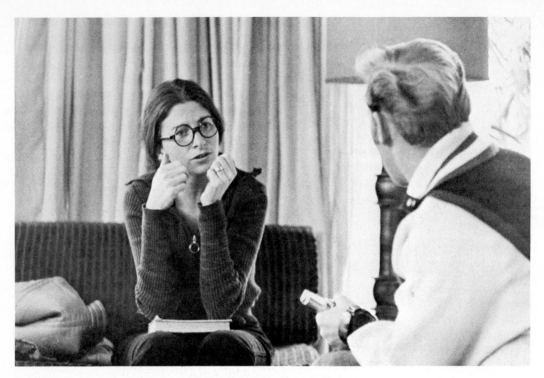

Fig. 1-4. It is essential that the consumer of health care have major input in the planning and implementation of that care. (Photograph by Eugene Luttenberg; courtesy Editorial Photocolor Archives, Inc., New York.)

There are reasons other than sheer personal satisfaction for the use of consumerism in health care delivery. Everyone's personal dignity depends in part on having a sense of meaning and control of one's life. Being buffeted about the system without having any input into that system creates a loss of control and a subsequent loss of self-esteem. The fewer the feelings of self-worth, the more passive the consumer will become, and the more he will be used by the system instead of his using it. Consumer involvement also helps to find ways in which health resources—facilities and personnel—can be applied to meet people's needs with greater effectiveness. Providers of health care are mostly well-intentioned people, but they are not mind readers, and, without some consumer feedback and input, they will not know where or how the service can be improved. Consumers can also let the provider

of health care know what their priorities are. If the community feels that money should be spent on a dental program for children rather than on another radioactive cobalt machine, then it should make its wishes known to the people who are the health care decision makers. Many states are beginning to develop legislation that will require an agency to have a certificate of need before making major purchases. It does no good to remain silent during the planning stages of any aspect of the system and then to complain that needs are not being met *after* the plans have been implemented. Health organizations and professional societies should solicit consumer input, if for no other reason, because it is good business practice. Spending money or providing services that are not needed is a waste of money because either the services will not be used and *more* money will have to be spent to provide what is really needed, or the services will be used whether they are needed or not simply because they were prescribed or ordered by a physician.

Consumer input can help in the recruitment of additional health workers, especially among young people. People are attracted to occupations and professions in which they sense humanity and an interest in meeting the needs of the people they serve. If people are reluctant to enter the health care system as clients, they most assuredly would not want to work in it. Involving consumers in the planning, implementation, and evaluation of health services may minimize the need for governmental intervention, but if the needs of the people are not met, the people, by way of Congress, will begin taking what they want in the form of more and more governmental controls.

"The greatest potential for improving the health of the American people is not to be found in increasing the numbers of physicians or in forcing them into groups, or even in increasing hospital productivity, but it is to be found in what people do . . . for themselves."[7] The uninformed consumer is a threat to and a drain on the health care system. The need for consumer education about all health matters is a necessity, not just so consumers can receive better health services, but so they can remain as healthy as possible. Thus they will spend less time, energy, and money as consumers.

Many of this country's major health problems such as automobile accidents, alcoholism, drug addiction, venereal disease, obesity, some premature births, certain kinds of cancer, and much heart disease are attributable not to the shortcomings of the system itself, but to the ignorance or irresponsibility of the individual consumer or of the community. A person who smokes two packs of cigarettes a day and eats red meat for dinner every night cannot blame the health care system for heart and lung disease. The person may be able to cast blame for not being warned about the dangers of smoking and eating quantities of cholesterol, but the complaint is becoming less and less justified in recent years. This nation has made a commitment to comprehensive high-quality health care for every person, and even though this commitment may still be more theoretical than practical, it assumes that people will accept rational responsibility for their own health, which includes knowing when to seek professional help. Individuals who cannot or will not take this responsibility endanger their own health and place a drain on the resources of the entire system. A community that permits its air and water to be polluted, refuses to punish drunken drivers, and permits the safety of its citizens to be threatened by unsafe streets makes a mockery of the commitment. The medical community itself (and this includes health professionals other than physicians), by remaining silent on such issues as environmental pollution, the overuse of drugs, highway and automobile safety, food additives, and birth control, are also contributing to the undermining and ineffectiveness of the national commitment.

Consumer participation in health services is advancing. It is now customary for governments to require a substantial number of consumers (sometimes a majority) on the advisory boards of programs and institutions. Third-party payers, neighborhood health centers, and even private hospitals solicit lay board members. Sometimes the lay participants do not know what is expected of them in the decision-making process; they are often resented by health professionals, and their timidity and lack of experience can result in intimidation by the professionals. But as time goes on, this is less of a problem, and consumer representatives are learning to speak up, to ask questions, and to have confidence in their ability to grasp the complexities of the decision-making process.

Health education is probably the greatest single contributory factor to intelligent and informed consumer participation in the health care system. Courses, both formal and informal, are popping up in the most unexpected places. I have taught a course called "Our Bodies: How They Work and How They're Used" to groups of laywomen from churches, synagogues, women's political organizations, and other groups. It is basic female anatomy and physiology, with some pathology, contraception, and abortion information, and there is a section on pregnancy and childbirth. I am constantly amazed about how little women know about their own bodies, how eager they are to learn, and how quickly they are able to assimilate the information and ask intelligent questions. From health education in high school to community smokers' clinics, consciousness raising groups on mental health problems, and first-aid courses in night school, consumers are attending classes in droves and urging their neighbors to join them. Americans want to be healthy; they simply need help in learning how to achieve their goal. The increase in sales of do-it-yourself health books and home medical encyclopedias, the burgeoning of health clubs and exercise spas, and the interest in the low-calorie "nouvelle cuisine" from France should certainly attest to the sincerity of the consumer.

Health professionals surely have a responsibility for contributing to the consumer's education, but so do business and other professional groups. The mass media are probably the most potent force. Although heroin is not advertised on television, the "drug culture" is clearly advertised and glamorized. Although cigarettes are no longer advertised, many popular television characters are still seen enjoying smoking and thus providing negative role models for children. Private insurance companies have not only a moral responsibility but a vested interest in keeping their policyholders healthy. If a company rewards safe drivers with lower auto insurance premiums, why could it not give the same privilege to nonsmokers or to people who maintain normal weight? Schools have a captive audience; reading, writing, and arithmetic mastery are required for graduation; why not require a passing grade in a series of courses in health education? The American Cancer Society and the American Heart Association, which have contributed greatly to the public knowledge about cancer and heart disease, are excellent examples of public responsibility. There is a foundation for practically every disease in the medical lexicon, and most of the organizations spend all their advertising dollars on fund raising. Why not, in the course of seeking

money, give a small lesson on the symptoms and the course of the disease? People might be willing to donate more money if they were faced with the reality of what the disease looks like. Some organizations do this to a small extent. For example, the American Cancer Society always lists the seven danger signs of cancer.

Somers[2] proposes a permanent high-level national council on health education, which would be responsible for formulation of national policy in such areas as the following:

1. National goals with respect to health education
2. Teacher training for formal health education courses
3. Curricula for schools and colleges
4. Programs for adult education and for the mass media
5. Health education in hospitals and other public institutions
6. Health education and the insurance industry
7. Consumer participation in health care programs as a technique of health education

Membership on the council should include all professional and nonprofessional people who have an interest in health care (theoretically everyone has such an interest), and it should be advisory to the Secretary of Health and Human Services. "In the first instance, it should undertake a thorough evaluation of existing efforts in health education and develop a new package that would add up to a meaningful national program. Thereafter, it would periodically evaluate ongoing programs and re-formulate policy to meet new needs."[2,p.85]

Consumer participation clarifies the health needs that should be met. The perception of needs will often vary between the provider and the consumer of service; because these perceptions are based on different values and different kinds of knowkledge and experience, there must be continuing dialogue. The professionals must avoid feeling that they know everything and can anticipate every need, and consumers must try not to feel that they are being hoodwinked and bamboozled at every turn. The difference between an irrational demand and a true need must be clarified and compromises worked out. For instance, there may be a need for a walk-in mental health clinic for emergency psychiatric problems, but the mental hospital is unwilling or unable to provide the service. The outreach mental health workers tell the community that there is no money available to build and staff such a clinic, but the community is adamant in its need. Perhaps an agreement can be worked out: a local church donates one of its public rooms; peer counselors instead of expensive psychiatrists are employed; a hot line is established between the walk-in clinic and the mental hospital so the peer counselors can call for professional advice. The needs of the community are met, at least partially, and there has not been an enormous outlay of money.

Lay participation can validate whether needs are being met. Sometimes it is only the consumer who can judge this, just as it is only the person with an itchy back who can tell when exactly the right spot has been scratched! Consumer participation can also bring new skills and knowledge into the health care system; the latent talents of lay people are often surprisingly beneficial. Welfare recipients may know the ins and outs of the system far better than a community nurse and can be employed very effectively as counselors to new welfare enrollees. Former military personnel can cut through red tape faster than any physician in private practice; they have had years of experience.

Committees

Public responsibility may be encouraged and recognized by the creation of elective or appointive boards, health councils, or advisory committees for various public and private health agencies. Key health administrative positions, on both state and local levels, could be elective instead of appointive; referendums on major public health issues should be on the ballot. The public must be aware of all the ramifications of the issues about which they are voting. Having the public vote on both issues and health officials entails some risk. An election can be, and often is, based on political party affiliation;

the public can be given insufficient or misinformation about the issues at hand; and the frequent changes in office of elected officials can cause health programs to lack continuity and effective leadership. And there is so much vested interest in our political system that graft and corruption might become even larger problems than they already are.

Communication between health professionals and the lay public is essential for effective consumerism. The community health administrator must make it known that health policies and services are geared toward the values and mores of the community, and public health policies must be reported to the people so there can be suggestions and feedback. Annual reports of both public and private health agencies should be made available to the people of the community and should include such information as what the agency set out to do, what it actually did, how what was done compares with what was intended, what still needs to be done, what problems were encountered in carrying out the programs, and what the plans are for the next reporting period.

If the public is to be involved in health work, it must perceive a need; it is up to health professionals to translate this need into reasons why the public should take action. Public apathy, more than a lack of desire to contribute to the public good, causes people to fail to exercise their right of participation. Not only must the public feel a need for participation, it must be convinced that things will *not* be the same without this participation, that there is a role for them to play, that their participation will be welcome, and that they are capable of doing what is asked. In short, the public often needs to be wheedled and cajoled into participation, and it is easy for health professionals to simply ignore the public, who frequently fade quietly out of sight.

Committee membership is one of the best ways of using public participation, and there are various types of committees:

1. Policy-making committees have the responsibility for setting the general directions of the agency and authorizing programs and budget expenditures.

2. Advisory committees represent the public or other interested groups and bring to the health agency the points of view of these groups or of the public. They study and advise but do not have any authority to control the actions of the agency.

3. Technical committees advise about certain specific aspects of the running of the agency. They have somewhat more authority than does an advisory committee because they are experts in an area, but they are also advising within a much narrower range and sometimes lose sight of the general goals of the agency.

4. Liaison committees exist for the purpose of exchanging information and planning activities and projects. They are also the link between the agency and the general public.

5. Special project committees recruit volunteers, arrange for publicity, and generally do the work involved with activities that are not part of the day-to-day work of the agency.

It is not always easy for health professionals to work with lay committees. There are problems involved, but there are also certain principles that can be followed to avoid many of the common roadblocks. Each committee should have a clear and written charge of its tasks and responsibilities and to whom it should report. The limits of authority should be well defined, and each committee member should be made aware of the organizational structure and functioning of the agency. Membership on permanent committees should be rotated, and the tenure of the chairman should be terminated after a period of time, usually two or three years. The membership of the committee should be heterogeneous, representing as many interest, ethnic, and sociopolitical groups as possible. It is also necessary to have a chairman who understands the goals of the agency and who can motivate committee members to work. Sometimes the workings of a health agency can be technical and esoteric, so it is up the the health professionals to see that committee members have sufficient knowledge and information to carry out their responsibilities. "Committees provide new sources of ideas and competence, they keep the public close

to the administrator, and in time of trouble, they represent a quickly available force to interpret the needs and the problems of the agency to the public.''[5,p.423]

Volunteer activities are another way for the consumer to participate in the delivery of health care. The value to the community cannot be measured only in terms of money and time; they are a most effective liaison between the agency and the public. Volunteers learn a tremendous amount about health care as they are going about their jobs, and this knowledge and information is passed to their family and friends who in turn learn about health. Volunteers also can translate the health needs of the community to the health professionals and to the agency administration. The volunteer should also be given information about the purposes and goals of the agency, and there should be a close working attachment between a volunteer and a professional health worker.

OMBUDSMAN CONCEPT

One of the most interesting and efficient ways of protecting the consumer is by the ombudsman concept. The institution of the ombudsman has been traced to a thirteenth century Norse edict: "With the law the land shall be built, not by lawlessness laid waste. And he who will not grant justice to others shall not himself enjoy the benefits of the law.''[8,p.9] An ombudsman in government is a high-level, independent, legally constituted officer who looks into citizens' dissatisfactions with their government. The fact that the ombudsman is independent of any government agency (or a private agency if that is where he performs his service) and legally constituted is central to his effective functioning. Without financial and organizational independence he is impotent to help the people he is trying to serve.

The ombudsman idea originated in Scandinavia, and the first one was appointed in Sweden under the constitution of 1809. His function was to receive complaints from the people and to protect them from injustice. In the beginning the ombudsman's duties were mostly concerned with the courts and police, but the increasing complexity of twentieth-century administration has shifted his emphasis to the bureaucracy. The ombudsman institutions in Sweden and Finland have some unusual features that make them workable. First, the ombudsman is appointed by the legislative rather than the executive branch of the government; he can report back to the legislature at any time; and he publishes an annual report in which he comments on unusual or important cases. The second feature is that he is an impartial investigator and is politically independent, even of the legislature. His office is established by the constitution, and legislators are not permitted to intervene in the investigation of a case. Third, he has no right to reverse a court decision and no direct control over the courts or the administration. His main power is the right to investigate and get the facts. His influence is based on objectivity, competence, superior knowledge and prestige, and, if all else fails, publicity. Fourth, he has the power to investigate on his own initiative; a case does not need to be initiated by a citizen complaint. An example of the way in which the Swedish ombudsman works is the Graveyard Case.

It happened a few years ago that a farmer was buried in a churchyard in the country. It was during the winter when the ground was covered with snow and it was difficult for the digger to find the family grave. A few weeks after the burial, the daughter of the farmer came to the rector of the parish and said that she was afraid that her father's coffin had been placed outside the family grave; and the rector went to the digger, but the digger said that he had not committed any fault; and then the daughter, who was a waitress, asked the municipal parish council for permission to investigate through digging, but the municipal council said "No."

Then she appealed in the ordinary way to the county board and there the governor of the county said "No." And then the Cabinet said "No." Then she quarrelled with all the authorities concerned for many years, but they always said "No."

Then she complained to the Ombudsman. I sent the complaint to the municipal parish council and asked for information, but they didn't have much to say. Then I ordered the police to ask all persons who could give information. When I had got this information, I couldn't

say with security whether the coffin had been placed outside the family grave or not. But the circumstances were such that the parish council ought to have ordered an investigation through digging. The Ombudsman has no power to order digging in a churchyard. So I couldn't do anything else than to criticize the parish council because they had not made a real investigation in this case. But, the waitress took my decision and she went straight to the Cabinet Minister and said "Look here, Mr. Minister, here you see that the Ombudsman says that there are reasons for investigation through digging," and so the Cabinet council had nothing else to do than to order an investigation through digging. When they dug, they found that the coffin had been placed outside the family grave.

You can say that this case is a very small one, and it doesn't matter where the coffin was placed. But for the daughter, the case was of great importance, and even for all Swedes, it is important to feel that they can get justice, even if the prestige of a Governor and a Bishop and a Cabinet Minister is involved.*

This case may seem funny or farfetched, but it is a perfect example of how citizens need help in dealing with the extremely frustrating government bureaucracy.

Alfred Bexelius, a Swedish *justitieombudsman*, in a report to a subcommittee of the United States Senate in March, 1966, summed up the advantages of the ombudsman system. He said that it is of great importance that unwarranted complaints are rejected to protect public officials from abuse. He also stated that it is essential that complaints or accusations made in the press be investigated by an impartial agency free from bureaucratic influence and that the results of the investigations be made available to the public. Bexelius also said that the office of ombudsman, by its mere existence, tends to counteract the tendencies of authority to abuse its power. It is also an expression of real democracy that a government sets up an agency whose sole purpose is to protect the citi-

*From Rowat, Donald C.: The spread of the ombudsmen idea. In The American Assembly, Columbia University: Ombudsmen for American Government? (edited by Anderson, Stanley V.), Englewood Cliffs, N.J., Prentice Hall, Inc., p. 13.

zens. Even the poorest and lowest person in society has the right to have a complaint investigated.[9]

After World War II the ombudsman idea spread to other Scandinavian countries, West Germany (where it was limited to the military), New Zealand, and some of the countries of the Commonwealth of Great Britain. In Canada in 1961 a private welfare organization called "Underdog" was founded by a former newspaperman to help mistreated and beleaguered citizens. The organization grew quickly, found that most of its complaints were about the federal and provincial governments, and by 1964 had expanded its operations to fifteen countries, including the Untied States. Several silly and counterproductive publicity stunts (throwing cow's blood on the floor of the House of Commons to protest the plight of a Royal Canadian Mounted Policeman accused of Communism) diluted the future credibility of the organization, but the ombudsman idea had been firmly planted, and dozens of daily newspapers in the United States and Canada have "ombudsman columns" (e.g., "The Action Line" in the *Philadelphia Inquirer*), which are deluged with complaints and requests.

In the Untied States, the ombudsman idea has become so popular that the word and concept are frequently misused. Complaint officers or employees of organizations such as private industry, hospitals, and universities have been mistakenly referred to as ombudsmen, and even so has the person handling customers' complaints in a San Francisco department store. None of these people are true ombudsmen because they are *employed by* the organization from which they are trying to protect people. A true ombudsman is *politically and financially independent*. To be otherwise is to end up in the vest pocket of an employer. The way an ombudsman office functions involves very precise and logical steps:

1. A complaint is received from an individual who feels he has been mistreated in some way; all it takes is one letter. The citizen is put to almost no bother or expense; he merely has to write the letter and buy the stamp.

2. If the complaint is obviously unfounded or beyond his jurisdiction, the ombudsman explains this in writing to the complainant and dismisses the case.

3. If the ombudsman believes the case has merit, he begins an investigation by speaking to public authorities, contacting witnesses, examining files, etc.

4. On his own initiative the ombudsman may investigate matters that have come to his attention through sources other than a formal complaint.

5. He may conduct investigations of any government or administrative agency.

6. After the investigation, although he is not permitted to order an administrator to do anything, the ombudsman may try to persuade an agency to reverse itself. If the complaint is groundless, he explains things to the complainant; if it is not, he can make suggestions to the agency to change its operation in order to prevent recurrences. The ombudsman must rely on persuasion, but he is very strongly supported by the press and public opinion. His suggestions carry much weight.

7. The ombudsman submits an annual report to the legislature.

The value of an ombudsman is the protection of the public. Government agencies tend to do more for citizens and are more careful not to tread on their rights than if there were no ombudsman. This improvement in government service stems partly from his recommendations and partly from his mere existence. The legislature more closely follows administrative practices and procedures as a result of the annual reports. The ombudsman becomes aware of overall patterns of function that would not be readily apparent with isolated complaints to separate agencies. In this way whole areas of functioning can be improved. The fact of the ombudsman's existence tends to give people greater faith in their government and public administration and consequently makes them more cooperative with civil servants. Public employees are also protected by being shielded from cranks and unwarranted complaints. A complaint that comes from the office of the ombudsman is much more likely to be heeded than one which comes from an irate citizen. There is also a learning process involved in the ombudsman system. Citizens learn to have more effective relationships with public employees, who in turn learn to be more responsive to the needs of the citizens. Fear of the powerful and impersonal bureaucracy is lessened if people know they have a dependable ally in the office of the ombudsman.

There are also unintended and undesirable consequences in having an ombudsman. It is possible that public officials could become so intimidated by the power of the ombudsman that their work effectiveness could be reduced. The feeling that the ombudsman is constantly looking over his shoulder could make the civil servant too nervous to do his job effectively. Another government agency (the office of the ombudsman), no matter how beneficent, leads to increased red tape and increased costs for which the citizens must pay. Occasionally, the ombudsman gets carried away with himself and attempts to overstep the bounds prescribed for him, and because he is so independent, it could be a long time before anyone realizes what is happening. It is possible that the activities of the ombudsman might adversely affect the support of the public administrators and civil servants. The latter, fearing exposure of incompetence or wrongdoing, could place innumerable obstacles in the path of the ombudsman's investigations. An inherent defect in the system is that the ombudsman is not engaged in the practice of administration, and his suggestions for operational reform may not be taken seriously. If the ombudsman is doing his job effectively, citizens have a tendency to become complacent about their government administration and take a less active interest in controlling the people they elected.

The American Bar Association on January 27, 1969, adopted a resolution urging cities and states to consider establishing an ombudsman system. The need for an ombudsman system in the United States is very evident. There are, however, some problems that would be encountered in transferring a Scandinavian political system to this country. Most people feel that the sheer size of the United States, both in territory and population, would be an obstacle. There is no reason why the system cannot be broken down into smaller, more manageable units: ombudsmen for local, state, and federal matters. If the court system can be run this way, there is no reason why the ombudsman system cannot. The introduction of the institution must not disrupt the desirable aspects of our present political system, and there is no reason why it should. The ombudsman system is as democratic as any conceived, and an amendment to the Constitution directing both the federal and state governments to set up the system would give the ombudsmen the political independence they need. If separate ombudsman systems were organized for local, state, and federal problems, there would be no impediment to the constitutionally guaranteed separation of power between federal and state government.

The method of appointment of the ombudsman is a problem. In our society, election would seem the most likely way to do it, but executive appointment (by the mayor, governor, or president) for *one* very long term of ten or twelve years might solve the problem of having to curry favor with the electorate. In a society that is as culturally and racially mixed as ours, it would be difficult to eliminate bias from the office of the ombudsman. There is much to be said for this argument, except that during the process of educating the American public about the ombudsman system itself, the citizens might come to realize what an essential service it is and that the appointment or election of someone who has a reputation for being as free from bias as is humanly possible is crucial.

If the ombudsman system is so desirable, why has it not been adopted in this country? There are several reasons, not the least of which is the reluctance of legislators who fear (for the most part for very good reason) a politically independent watchdog breathing down their necks. Legislators are elected to represent the people, and an ombudsman would certainly do his part to see to that. Public officials, most notably the police, have been insulated from criticism by the public at large, and it is thought that the ombudsman system would strip away this insulation, and some questionable practices would be open to public scrutiny. This fear is not always justified because an examination of the ombudsman system in Sweden shows clearly that the ombudsman does not automatically side with the complainant but is interested in effective administration and a sense of justice. It is often the public official or agency who "wins" the case. The fear that the ombudsman would take power away from public officials is completely unfounded, and setting up the small staff and minimal office space would not require much capital investment. A great block in the establishment of the ombudsman system is the fantasy that the ombudsman will singlehandedly, in one stroke, wipe out all the social injustice and unrest that plagues us today. When reality penetrates and people realize that he will not eliminate poverty, racial tension, hunger, pollution, and all the other scourges with which we live, there is the feeling that if he can't do that, why bother? Why not leave the system, imperfect as it is, alone and continue our inertia? Public apathy is a powerful—and negative—force. Another reason we do not have an ombudsman system is the lack of public knowledge and understanding of what he is empowered to do and how he functions. People are not likely to vote a system into effect if they don't know how it works.

The reader, by this point, might well be asking why there is such an involved discussion of the ombudsman system in government, and Scandinavian government at that, when this chapter is dealing with health care delivery systems. The *concept* of the ombudsman system is an excellent one and could be used to help and protect consumers of health care. Obviously a political system needs to be modified when it is transferred to private industry (remember, health care *is* an industry), but the essential ingredients of the system should remain as they are. Although the use of the term ombudsman is not technically accurate unless it refers to a system that is an independent part of a government, it will be used here in a loose rather than in a literal sense.

The most important aspect of the system, and

one that must be transferred intact, is the independence of the ombudsman. If he is employed by a hospital or other health care agency, he automatically has a vested interest in that organization and is vulnerable to its whims. If an agency hires, pays, and can fire an ombudsman, he becomes largely impotent in dealing with people's complaints about that very agency. In a short time he could become an apologist for incorrect procedure and a mere explainer of errors. It is essential that an ombudsman not be paid by any health care agency. However, this is not easily accomplished. Where will the funds and personnel come from?

Ombudsman, Inc.

One solution is the creation of a nonprofit company that is supported by mandated funds from all health care agencies. It would be required by law that *any* agency providing *any* kind of health care contribute to the support of this nonprofit company (perhaps "Ombudsman, Inc.," would be an appropriate name), and the agencies would also be required to cooperate fully in any investigation that Ombudsman, Inc., thought necessary. The public would be made aware, through heavy media campaigns, that Ombudsman, Inc., exists, and all agencies would be required to forward all phone calls and letters of complaint to Ombudsman, Inc. It would not have any administrative control over the agencies, but its power of persuasion to remedy injustices would be strong. If the system were successful, it would have the press and public opinion solidly behind it.

Skeptics will immediately point to the fact that employees of Ombudsman, Inc., can be "bought" and that the potential for graft and corruption is as enormous in this system as in any kind of "watchdog" organization, such as government building inspectors' or fire marshalls' offices or any type of agency that regulates the activities of any other agency. We have all been in places that are obvious firetraps or in buildings which have so many structural defects that they are unsafe. In many instances these places have not been closed down because the building inspector was bribed. So it could be with Ombudsman, Inc. A justified complaint (even one in which the health care has been proved to be downright dangerous) could be ignored or covered up if the Ombudsman, Inc., investigator were paid enough by the offending agency. This potential situation is perfectly possible, perhaps even probable, given the greedy nature of human beings. Paying excellent salaries to the ombudsmen would cut down but not completely eliminate this problem. No matter how much money people make, some still want more. The only solution would be to create an atmosphere, based on fact, of course, around Ombudsman, Inc., that portrays it as a totally trustworthy organization. Ombudsman, Inc., itself should immediately fire any employee found to be receiving graft. Although it would not be an agency of the government, Ombudsman, Inc., would be an agency of the people, and legislation could be passed to make the manipulation of complaints (either by employees of Ombudsman, Inc., or by employees of health care agencies) a criminal offense. Making something a crime does not necessarily prevent it from happening; it merely happens less frequently. If Ombudsman, Inc., were known to be incorruptible, people would try to corrupt it less frequently.

There are problems inherent in the creation of an agency such as Ombudsman, Inc. How would financial assessments for the participating agencies be arranged? Would the share be equally divided or be based on the number of people receiving care? What would be the qualifications for the Ombudsman, Inc., investigators? Where would they receive their training? What kind of person would head the agency, and what would be her function? Who would oversee the overseers? Would there be a government regulatory agency to whom Ombudsman, Inc., would be responsible? How would the media campaign be carried out? What resources would Ombudsman, Inc., have access to? The questions are endless, but *none* of the problems are insurmountable.

It is obvious that there is little consumerism in the health care delivery system. Those who have worked in the system, for even a short time, have seen so many instances of the flagrant disregard for human rights that there is no doubt that a consumer advocate agency is essential. Ombudsman, Inc., may not be the complete answer, but it could be a beginning. Perhaps if health care agencies knew that they were being policed by outsiders, they might reform their operations to such an extent that Ombudsman, Inc., investigators would spend more time drinking coffee at their desks than they would investigating complaints. It is, after all, consumers for whom the health care system exists. If we ignore their needs or trample on their rights, the whole concept of providing health care will become so perverted that it will cease to exist in the way we have come to expect.

PROFESSIONAL STANDARDS REVIEW ORGANIZATION

In October, 1972, Public Law 92-603 was passed. This legislation, which is an amendment to the Social Security Act, provided for creation of Professional Standards Review Organizations (PSRO) to review and evaluate services provided by Medicare, Medicaid, and the Maternal and Child Health Program. These organizations are based on the concept that health professionals are the persons best qualified to evaluate the quality and quantity of health care delivered. The concept is sound in theory, but it poses problems in practice. For example, in September, 1972, the Committee on Finance of the United States Senate heard testimony that many services provided under Medicare and Medicaid were medically unnecessary and therefore financially wasteful.[10] More than a decade later these practices continue, even in increased measure.

The federal PSRO program was to be administered by individual states or multiple areas within states and would affect several hundred thousand physicians and about 50 million clients (those eligible for the above-mentioned Social Security Act service programs). Each PSRO was to be comprised of physicians and osteopaths, and a mechanism was to be established whereby the general public could have input into the organization. Advisory groups for each PSRO were to be made up of nonphysicians. Major responsibilities of a PSRO are the following:

1. Review of health care provided under Medicare, Medicaid, and Maternal and Child Health Programs and judgment about the medical necessity and quality of care
2. Review of care provided in both long-term and short-term care institutions such as hositals, nursing homes, and the like
3. Performance of institutional review in the form of admissions certification, continued stay review, and medical care evaluation studies
4. Utilization of the findings of hospital review committees
5. Provision of evidence that nonphysician health care practitioners are involved in review procedures of their own and work to establish continuing education programs

This last responsibility is the one that relates directly to nursing, although the nursing profession should consider it less than desirable because the evaluation process is done at the direction of physicians. Nursing must continue to develop quality assurance standards of its own. The American Nurses Association (ANA) does publish standards of professional practice, and most community health nursing agencies adapt their own standards to those devised by the national organization. The federal PSRO legislation provides for nurses to be included on the governing board of the PSRO, but they are not eligible to vote on issues pertaining to medical practice. Nurses can participate in advisory groups, and they must demonstrate that they have established their own peer review system.

Nurses should be concerned about the establishment of PSROs because they are affected in the following ways:

1. Nursing may be subjected to physician review of professional nursing practice.
2. It is permissible, but unusual, for nurses to be included on PSRO governing boards.
3. Most hospital utilization review plans are written by physicians and nonnurse administrators.

Nursing has little, if any, input, and community health agencies often pattern their utilization review procedures on those of hospitals.

4. PSRO review procedures are generally divided into those that affect physicians and those that affect nonphysicians. Therefore nursing tends to be lumped in with all other nonphysician health workers and runs the risk of being "lost in the shuffle."

5. PSRO does not include discharge planning, an activity in which nurses are heavily involved.

Although nurses need to learn about PSRO law because they are directly affected as delineated above, they should be aware of the current conservative political movement in the Untied States that is causing drastic cutbacks in health services funding. The federal PSRO program was one of the first to be cut by the Reagan administration. Health care (both research and services) is certain to be drastically curtailed in this decade. This movement will have a tremendous impact on the practice of nursing, particularly in the community, and it would seem advantageous for nurses to be aware of current sociopolitical trends.

SUMMARY

When viewed as a multibillion dollar industry, the health care system, in its organization and functioning, is a shambles. The one who suffers is the one for whom the system was designed in the first place: the consumer.

The system is divided roughly into two unequal parts, the fee-for-service system and health maintenance organizations. The fee-for-service system is based on the fact that a fee is paid for health care services *after* the service is given. Fees are paid to a private health care practitioner or hospital, either by the individual who received the care or by a third party.

The fee-for-service system can be further divided into the public and private sectors. The private sector is based on the private physician in a one-to-one relationship with the client. It is primarily disease and cure oriented, and there is no provision for health maintenance unless it is paid for by the consumer. The public sector, while operated on a fee-for-service basis, encompasses various official and voluntary agencies that emphasize health promotion, health education, and disease prevention. There are screening programs for certain diseases, but there still is no provision for large-scale complete health maintenance for significant numbers of people.

It is difficult to change so large and complex a system. Costs of providing care are accelerating more rapidly every year, and there is no ceiling in sight. The burden of paying these costs is the consumer's, either directly by paying doctor and hospital bills or indirectly through insurance premiums and taxes. Medicare and Medicaid are a partial answer to the consumer burden. Through Social Security contributions and general taxation, Medicare provides health care to people over 65, and Medicaid picks up the tab for people who are indigent.

There are many inequities inherent in the fee-for-service system. The most obvious is that health care is available only to those who can afford it. There is also the uneven accessibility of health services. Personal power of the "medical elite" contributes to the status quo and consequent inequities in the system, and special interest groups also perpetuate the system.

There are several steps that can be taken to solve some of these problems. The supply of health personnel must be increased by recruiting more people and by altering the nature of professional education. The health care system needs to make increased use of paraprofessionals, including volunteers and physicians' assistants. The dehumanized and impersonal relationship between health care workers and consumers must be improved, and there should be more effective means of evaluating the delivery of health care. The "forced" redistribution of health care personnel by a draft system would alleviate one of the major problems, as would generous government loans for professional education.

The greatest innovation in the health care system in recent years is the health maintenance organization. The HMO concept is aimed primarily at health maintenance and prevention of disease; its basic ingredients include the following:

1. Prepayment for health care
2. Group practice by primary physicians and specialists
3. A unified center (and satellite clinics) that provides all health services
4. Voluntary enrollment
5. Salaries for all employees, including physicians
6. Coverage that includes all health care for a single fee

An HMO provides primary health care, that is the provision of accessible and equitable health care, including all support services. Nurses are an integral part of an HMO, and they function as primary care practitioners. All HMOs are organized along the same basic lines, and the preceding ingredients are a part of them all. Individual differences are based on the availability of services, geography, and the needs of the clients.

Consumerism in health care delivery is becoming a larger and larger issue. Because of the consumer movement in general, health care consumers are transforming themselves from a passive group of people into angry citizens who want to have a voice in the delivery of their own health care. There are good reasons for this. A sense of participation in one's own destiny creates feelings of self-worth and consequent activism. Consumer involvement can help find ways in which health resources can best be applied to meet people's needs. Consumer activism tends to lead to increased health education and consequent awareness of and prevention of disease. Lay participation in the health care delivery system can bring fresh ideas into the planning of health care, and volunteers can work tirelessly when they are well motivated. Public responsibility can be increased by placing major health care decisions into the hands of the public and out of those of the medical establishment. For consumerism to be effective, there must be good communication between health care workers and the lay public. Participation on the boards of health agencies is an excellent way to accomplish this, and many agencies are not eligible to receive federal funds unless they can prove there is consumer participation in policy making and operational decisions.

One of the best ways to encourage and promote consumerism is through the ombudsman concept. This is a system that originated in Scandinavia and is a way to deal with citizens' grievances and complaints about their government. The ombudsman is politically and financially independent from any branch of the government, and his sole function is to investigate complaints. If the complaint is justified, he may recommend changes and improvements to the appropriate agency, but he has no authority or control over them. There are, of course, advantages and disadvantages in the ombudsman system, but it works well in Sweden and several other countries because the people want it and because the ombudsman receives cooperation from public officials and civil servants. The power of public opinion and the fear of having incompetency exposed in the press may very well give impetus to this spirit of cooperation.

A form of the ombudsman concept could be used in the health care system. A nonprofit organization is proposed, financially supported by all health care agencies, to which all complaints would be directed. Ombudsman, Inc., would investigate the complaints and make appropriate recommendations to the offending agency. Again, public opinion and the press would go far to ensure the effective functioning of Ombudsman, Inc.

Consumerism is absolutely essential to health care delivery, and almost any method used to achieve it would be an improvement on what exists today.

NOTES

1. Time, June 13, 1977.
2. Somers, Anne R.: Health care in transition: directions for the future, Chicago, 1971, Hospital Research and Educational Trust.
3. Medicare will not make payments to clients unless the hospital in which they receive care has been accredited by the JCAH.
4. Benson, Rose, and McDevitt, Joan: Community health and nursing practice, Englewood Cliffs, N.J., 1976, Prentice-Hall, Inc.
5. Freeman, Ruth B., and Holmes, Edward M.: Administration of public health services, Philadelphia, 1960, W.B. Saunders Co.
6. Murray, Ruth, and Zentner, Judith: Nursing concepts for health promotion, Englewood Cliffs, N.J., 1975, Prentice-Hall, Inc.
7. Fuchs, Victor R.: Medical Economics, February 5, 1968.
8. Gellhorn, Walter: The ombudsman concept in the United States. In Levinson, Harold L., editor: Our kind of ombudsman, The Southeastern Assembly on the Ombudsman: a symposium, Gainesville, Fla., March 13-15, 1969, University of Florida.
9. Rowat, Donald C.: The spread of the ombudsman idea. In The American Assembly, Columbia University: Ombudsmen for American government? (edited by Anderson, Stanley V.), Englewood Cliffs, N.J., 1968, Prentice-Hall, Inc.
10. Davidson, Sharon Van Sell: PSRO: utilization and audit in patient care, St. Louis, 1976, The C.V. Mosby Co., p. 86.

BIBLIOGRAPHY

The American Assembly, Columbia University: Ombudsmen for American government? (edited by Anderson, Stanley V.), Englewood Cliffs, N.J., 1968, Prentice-Hall, Inc.

Analysis and planning for improved distribution of nursing personnel and service—WICHE, U.S. Department of Health, Education, and Welfare, Pub. No. (HRA)77-2, Washington, D.C., 1976, U.S. Government Printing Office.

Archer, Sarah, and Fleshman, Ruth: Community health nursing, ed. 2, N. Scituate, Mass., 1979, Duxbury Press.

Baum, Martin A., et al.: Planning health care delivery systems, American Journal of Public Health **65:**272-275, 1975.

Benson, Rose, and McDevitt, Joan: Community health and nursing practice, ed. 2, Englewood Cliffs, N.J., 1979, Prentice-Hall, Inc.

Cauffman, Joy G., et al.: A study of health referral patterns, American Journal of Public Health **64:**331-356, 1974.

Corey, Lawrence, Epstein, Michael F., and Saltman, Steven E.: Medicine in a changing society, ed. 2, St. Louis, 1977, The C.V. Mosby Co.

Crichton, Michael: Five patients, New York, 1970, Alfred A. Knopf, Inc.

Davidson, Sharon Van Sell: PSRO: utilization and audit in patient care, St. Louis, 1976, The C.V. Mosby Co.

Freeman, Ruth B.: Community health nursing practice, Philadelphia, 1970, W.B. Saunders Co.

Freeman, Ruth B., and Holmes, Edward M.: Administration of public health services, Philadelphia, 1960, W.B. Saunders Co.

French, Ruth M.: The dynamics of health care, New York, 1974, McGraw-Hill Book Co.

Gentry, John T., et al.: Attitudes and percpetions of health service providers, American Journal of Public Health **64:**1123-31, 1974.

Hanlon, John J., and Pickett, George E.: Public health: administration and practice, ed. 7, St. Louis, 1979, The C.V. Mosby Co.

Health maintenance organizations: questions and answers, Pamphlet No. M9868, Trenton, N.J., New Jersey State Department of Health.

Kelly, Lucy Y.: Dimensions of professional nursing, New York, 1975, The Macmillan Co.

Leahy, Kathleen M., et al.: Community health nursing, New York, 1972, McGraw-Hill Book Co.

Levinson, Harold L., editor: Our kind of ombudsman, The Southeastern Assembly on the Ombudsman: a symposium, Gainesville, Fla., March 13-15, 1969, University of Florida.

Lumi, Doman: The health maintenance original delivery system: a national study of attitudes of HMO project directors on HMO issues, American Journal of Public Health **65:**1192-1201, 1975.

Milio, Nancy: The care of health in communities, New York, 1975, The Macmillan Co.

Murray, Ruth, and Zentner, Judith: Nursing concepts for health promotion, Englewood Cliffs, N.J., 1975, Prentice-Hall, Inc.

Reinhardt, Adina M., and Quinn, Mildred D., editors: Current practice in family-centered community nursing, vol. 1, St. Louis, 1977, The C.V. Mosby Co.

Roemer, Milton I.: Rural health care, St. Louis, 1976, The C.V. Mosby Co.

Shonick, William: Elements of planning for area-wide personal health services, St. Louis, 1976, The C.V. Mosby Co.

Somers, Anne R.: Health care in transition: directions for the future, Chicago, 1971, Hospital Research and Educational Trust.

Tinkham, Catherine, and Voorhies, Eleanor F.: Community health nursing, New York, 1972, Appleton-Century-Crofts.

Twaddle, Andrew C., and Hessler, Richard M.: A sociology of health, St. Louis, 1977, The C.V. Mosby Co.

Weaver, Jerry L.: National health policy and the underserved: ethnic minorities, women, and the elderly, St. Louis, 1976, The C.V. Mosby Co.

Weeks, Kent M.: Ombudsmen around the world: a comparative chart, Berkeley, Calif., 1973, Berkeley Institute of Governmental Studies, University of California.

Weiler, Philip G.: Health manpower dialectic, American Journal of Public Health **65:**858-863, 1975.

Wyner, Alan J., editor: Executive ombudsmen in the United States, Berkeley, Calif., 1973, Berkeley Institute of Governmental Studies, University of California.

2

HISTORY OF THE HEALTH CARE SYSTEM

ANITA GOLDEN PEPPER

OVERVIEW

The United States derived its medical heritage from Europe but put its own stamp on the European model. It created new approaches, used the hospital system differently, resources more extravagantly, and imparted a more democratic cast to the system. Technology, scientific methods, and industrial skills overtook the medical care field more rapidly in this country, and specialization flourished quickly. The combination of greater technological development and larger numbers of medical specialists modified practice in the United States and made it more expensive and luxurious. The existence of a frontier and an open labor market made planned social intervention either in health or welfare services difficult.[1] As we outline the history of the health care system, it will become apparent that the crisis we are now facing is a result of our success. The art and science of health care are now more precise in diagnosis and intervention and more effective in their capacity to prevent disability from diseases they cannot cure and in their capacity to prevent certain diseases from occurring. The growth of the economy and industry and the increased capacity of the health care system has produced a healthier and more affluent population. Parts of the population are better educated, but education, like health care, is not equally available to all.[2] It is now conventional wisdom that the American health care system is in crisis.

The crisis may be defined in many ways. The United States spends a larger percent of its gross national product on health care than any other country in the world. Yet, when one looks at traditional health indicators such as infant mortality and longevity, statistics indicate that we are less healthy than many other countries. The steep rise in the number of malpractice suits and consequent rise in insurance rates for health professionals attests to increasing concern among the people who receive health care that they are not being adequately treated. Maldistribution of health professionals has been identified as a contributing cause of the crisis; fewer professionals are practicing in inner city and rural areas than are needed. Although the rate of growth of technical knowledge has increased enormously (itself a contribution to the crisis), it has not led to the equal dissemination of that knowledge throughout the system. A rapid rate of growth of knowledge has led to the fragmentation of services and specialization of care, creating difficulties in the availability, accessibility, and continuity of care. Increasing numbers of health care providers and changing patterns of practice have led to the sense of crisis as well.[1] Historically, the health care system is a loose confederation of many kinds of services, provided by many different practitioners and institutions, funded from a variety of sources, and separated into preventive and curative services, with different patterns and scope of service available to rich and poor. It is now coping with changing concepts of health care as well as rapidly rising expectations from the citizens who have become more knowledgeable about the benefits of health care. We have been a population accustomed to using unlimited resources and expenditures to solve problems. This can no longer be so.

The health care system is growing and changing rapidly, as are the boundaries of its responsibilities. It is easy to see why the sense of crisis is so urgent even if the solutions do not seem immediately apparent. This is a country in which social and cultural patterns are changing and that is facing a crisis of resource availability and allocation.

Perhaps it is easiest to understand the present crisis by looking at the past. A historical view often enables the practitioner to understand why incongruities and difficulties persist even though they do not seem necessary or logical.

The framers of the United States Constitution had long and serious debates about the structure of our government. The yoke of an oppressive government that was strongly centralized had just been thrown off, and there were intense debates as to the proper scope and extent of power the national government should have. The Hamilton-Jefferson debates are a fine distillation of the arguments for and against a strong central government. It was decided that in the Untied States a strong federal rather than national model should prevail. This structural decision has had a profound effect on the organization of health care services. Collection of vital statistics, establishment of educational facilities and standards, and laws that relate to the lives of citizens were left as residual rights to the several states. The federal government's responsibilities were severely curtailed in these areas, although it does have responsibilities for populations directly under its jurisdiction, such as the armed services.

Although the states had the major responsibility for health of their citizens, the care of the sick poor has been a local responsibility in this country from its earliest period. Precedents for local poor relief systems stem from England, with its small homogeneous communities and sharp sense of public responsibility for their membership. In 1662, the Rhode Island Assembly included the sick among those who should be maintained by the towns. The first important poor law in New England, dating from 1673 in Connecticut, established public responsibility for anyone who had lived in one of the towns in the colony for three months and who by "sickness, lameness, and the like comes to want."

Although the community obligation remains clear, practices to help the indigent sick and subsequent American welfare legislation still bear the stamp of the English poor laws in their assumption that poverty is due to personal irresponsibility. Under the Elizabethan poor law of 1601, debtors could be imprisoned; even today public charity carries a certain moral and social stigma.

Such traditions were continued as the colonies and later the states expanded westward. In 1790, the Northwest Territory poor law mentioned sickness along with poverty, accident, or "any other misfortune" that made persons "wretched and proper objects of public charity."

In 1809, a New York court ruled that if a pauper was sick, "medicine and attendants are as necessary as food"; the law should not be narrowly construed to leave the poor in the hands of either fate or of private compassion. In the same vein, a California court in 1917 ruled, "It has never been, nor will it ever be, questioned that among the first or primary duties evolving upon the state is that of providing suitable means and measures for the proper care and treatment, at the public expense, of the indigent sick, having no relatives legally liable for their care."[3]

Although they were extended throughout the rest of the young United States, the appropriateness of British and New England precedents for local poor relief systems has been questioned. In England, local responsibility for relief was qualified by national supervision; until very recently this has not been possible in the United States. Small homogeneous communities with an active sense of public responsibility for their members gradually gave way to large cities with transient populations and weakened community ties. Locally self-sufficient, predominantly agricultural economies and handicraft production rapidly yielded in nineteenth-century America to urban industrial economies, mass production, and wage labor.[4]

Although there is a long historical precedent for medical services for the indigent, recognition of health care as essential became widespread only in the 1930s. In the United States health care has been traditionally viewed as primarily an individual responsibility. Communities generally restricted their health activities to control of communicable diseases and sanitation. Neither the federal constitution nor those in most states contain references to governmental functions in health care. Two types of governmentally sponsored medicine developed in this country: the official public health services, including the prevention of disease, usually instituted in a health department, and medical care of the sick poor, increasingly provided by welfare departments. Though related, they were seldom considered together.[5]

Local authorities had responsibility for the care of the poor, both well and sick. For others who were sick, private care was available and rested in the physician who practiced as an individual entrepreneur. The United States, in its early years and until the mid-nineteenth century, was a country of small farmers and small businessmen, Protestant, white, and middle class in it orientation in the north, slave in the south. It was a small country, rich in resources, that was expanding westward. The Protestant ethic of rugged individualism and hard work permeated the institutional values in the country, and the poor were a class apart from and not equal to those who could make their own way financially. The private sector of medical care was separate and apart from the public system. Citizens who could afford to pay for medical care were attended by a physician who had relatively little knowledge about the pathophysiology of the disease he was treating and few drugs or other ther-

apeutic agents that could intervene and alter the course of the disease. He did, however, have time to spend with his patient, usually knew the family, and was able to provide whatever comfort might be given. It has often been said that until 1910, a patient being attended by a physician had a 50-50 chance that the doctor could intervene effectively in the course of the disease. Rarely did patients go to hospitals. They were cared for at home by a physician who learned his art usually by being apprenticed to another physician or who received his diploma by mail. There were no public standards for his education and no limitations on his practice; neither did he have to prove to anyone that he was competent to be a medical practitioner. Licensing laws and professional societies hardly existed in the first half of the nineteenth century. The sick poor, as has been mentioned before, were cared for in the local alms houses or country poorhouses, many of which became the models for public hospitals now run by cities or counties. A few physicians were educated in universities, and some even went abroad to study.

Private medical practitioners could hardly remain immune from the historic and economic forces producing social legislation. Like the circuit-riding frontier minister, mid-nineteenth-century physicians often brought their skills directly to the patient. Given the limitations of medical techniques and the ability to significantly change the course of disease, the traditional "family doctor" carried his tools with him and commonly delivered his services in the patient's home. As an independent professional who determined his own fees, the physician responded to and practiced the ideology of free competitive business. By using a sliding scale, he charged some patients substantially more than others. He could thus serve indigent patients without fee, and this practice became his entrée into municipal hospitals.

With the mid-nineteenth-century transition from apprenticeship to formal medical education, the physician's practice was increasingly centered in his office. There he could dispense services more conveniently and efficiently. He could also employ growing knowledge of bacteriology, immunology, and anesthesiology, together with equipment like the microscope, stethoscope, and ophthalmoscope to improve medical diagnosis and treatment.

Medical sophistication and burgeoning technical apparatus, together with the rise of specialization, the explosion of knowledge, dramatic advances in therapy, and the need to coordinate medical services, were to dramatize the importance of hospitals in medical practice in the twentieth century. Although only later would the hospital become known as the "doctor's workshop," the principle of private medical use of public hospital facilities was established early.[5]

During the last quarter of the nineteenth century and the first decade of the twentieth, there was increasing knowledge about health and disease, the integration of medical education into the university in Europe, and growing recognition that there needed to be public control over standards of practice. As a result of these forces, the American Medical Association was organized. Each of the states began to set standards for medical practice, and the Flexner report was issued. This study was commissioned as a result of the problems in American medical practice, especially when compared to the differences in European practice. Medical education was becoming increasingly a part of the university in Europe, scientific knowledge was exploding, and the interaction of the two led to a dramatic change in control of disease. Health care in the United States was exclusively the province of the physician at that time. Hospitals as we know them now hardly existed except for the care of the sick poor.

Nursing care was given in the home by either the female members of the family or servants, depending on the family's economic status. In the United States it was not until after Florence Nightingale and the beginnings of the practice of professional nursing that nurses began to be trained explicitly to attend the sick. Nursing education, such as it was, took place in hospitals, and nurses worked in the hospitals. Professional community health nursing did not become a part of nursing until the twentieth century, although the practice had its beginnings in the almoners of medieval

England. It should be remembered, too, that nursing practice had been carried on by women.

The social position of women has always had a great influence on nursing practice. In the United States, women generally were not expected to have a career or vocation apart from marriage and childbearing. While many women did work, they did so out of necessity, not because it was considered a legitimate role for women in our society. No woman was able to vote until 1928. They had little financial or social independence from men, and higher education for women evolved only in the last quarter of the nineteenth century and even then was available to only a very few.

As the country became increasingly industrialized after the Civil War, large immigrant populations came to the United States where there were economic opportunities as well as political and religious freedom. From 1820 to the end of that century, almost 20 million immigrants came to this country. Every decade from the 1870s to the outbreak of the First World War saw the stream of immigration increasing. During the first ten years of the twentieth century, the annual influx of Europeans averaged one million. The public domain was opened up for homesteading and for speculation. Great fortunes were built. American industry had an aggressive leadership, and productivity increased. The economy experienced booms and depressions. There was unrest among farmers and workers. Income inequities became more pronounced. Child labor became essential to aid in the support of the family. In short, during the last half of the nineteenth century, the United States changed from a primarily agricultural and mercantile country to an industrial giant. The frontier continually moved westward, immigrants came, blacks moved north, industrial wealth grew, monopolies and trusts developed, and natural resources were exploited. Cities grew, as did public education and private charities.

The country experienced a growing disparity in the economic well-being of its population. At one extreme there were industrialists growing rich, and at the other extreme there was the population that served American industry massed together in the tenements and slums of the growing cities. Housing was overcrowded, without running water and adequate sanitation. Workers fell under the exploitation of sweatshop proprietors. Cities grew rapidly in advance of public services. Infectious diseases swept through slum communities.

Alongside these rapid changes in the larger cities, millions of Americans still lived in towns and small cities, employed as skilled factory craftsmen. Public education increased during this period. In 1854 Massachusetts passed the first compulsory school attendance law, and by 1900 nearly all states and territories in the North and West had such legislation. In 1870 there were 7 million children enrolled in school; by 1900 their number had doubled. The public high school had emerged. In reaction to an increasingly literate population, newspapers developed during this time. The organization and distribution of philanthropic activities was expanded and modernized.

In the first decade of the new century there was much social ferment. Power of big business was growing, natural resources and labor were exploited, the frontier was closing, a transportation network developed, cities grew more rapidly than the services that could make them habitable, and local and state governments suffered bossism and corruption. Within the health care system, there was a great deal of quackery and poor practice: there were virtually no standards in the education and practice of physicians. Nursing as a profession was first beginning on the heels of the reforms of Florence Nightingale in England. There was a great deal of pressure for many reforms from a variety of groups, and their pressures began to have an effect. Regulatory commissions came into being, and welfare legislation began to make its appearance. Workmen's compensation laws, laws regulating maximum hours of work for children, women, men, and minimum wage laws, and safety and health codes were all passed. Mothers' assistance to furnish public aid to dependent children and old-age pension laws were all passed at the state level.[6]

State laws licensing physicians had been passed, outlawing quackery. The Pure Food and Drug Act set standards for products marketed across the country. The Flexner report recommended that medical education be solidly tied to university education and that diploma schools, independent medical colleges, and apprentice training of all physicians be abandoned. It also recommended that medicine should integrate into its practice the growing knowledge about causes and treatment of disease arising from the enormous growth in scientific knowledge.

It would be useful at this point to present the levels of intervention of the health care system, so that we can examine how the system evolved and why it has grown to be so complex. The interaction of all four levels should define the system of health care and should clarify the areas in which crisis persists. This in turn may emphasize the problems that will have to be confronted in order to assure the health of citizens, which is the primary goal of any health care system.

There are four levels of intervention:
1. Health promotion
2. Primary prevention
3. Secondary prevention
4. Tertiary prevention

Health promotion concerns itself with understanding the attributes of a society that enhance the health of its population. Pure water, clean air, occupational health and safety, and eradication of poverty or malnutrition are among its concerns. Primary prevention provides for the more specific prevention of specific diseases. It is concerned with communicable disease control, vaccinations and immunizations, good nutrition, and occupational safety. Secondary prevention is concerned in the main with curative medicine: curing the diseases it cannot prevent. Tertiary prevention intervenes in the course of chronic diseases or conditions, enabling the restoration of a person to a maximum level of function even when nothing can be done to cure the disease.

LEVELS OF INTERVENTION
Health promotion

Health promotion is the primary level of intervention. It preserves and protects the health of the population and is concerned with aspects of the environment that can enable human growth and development. Thus it includes environment, preservation of pure air and water, adequate shelter, and food for healthy growth. It is also concerned with attributes of society that promote personal growth and productivity, the availability of education and jobs, and freedom to develop one's own innate capacities to the maximum extent. As we know from studies in public health and epidemiology, the world into which citizens are born plays an essential part in creating healthy individuals. Thus we have had, since the beginning of this century, public policy translated into laws that protect citizens in the workplace, in the adequacy of their housing, and in preserving the purity of food and drugs available to them. Throughout this century we have become more highly industrialized, especially in the last twenty years as the petrochemical industry has dominated manufacturing. New health problems have cropped up in employment: those which were not solved by existing laws governing factory safety, child labor, hours of work, and the establishment of minimum wages.

Because industry has changed, workers are now exposed to a variety of substances that cause grave and mortal diseases over long periods of time. While this has been true for specific workers since the industrial revolution and before, it has now become true for larger groups of people. Miners have always been at risk for a variety of lung diseases, but now they are being joined by workers in asbestos and other industries. People working with polyvinyl compounds are also exposed to serious disease. Apart from occupational hazards, risks arising from impure air and water as a result of the industrial process are again growing concerns to the United States population. Standards had been set for pure air and water. However, new synthetic materials in fertilizers and pesticides are polluting the land (and some of the animals that graze on it). Toxic substances used in factories are released into the air and water, polluting them. In addition, because of accelerated technology and food production, more chemicals are being added to our food supply, either to enhance the supply itself, to preserve it, or to increase the yield. Some

of these synthetic substances or additives may have a disease-producing potential and need to be monitored over time. It would seem that the environment into which we are born, although safer in some respects than at the beginning of the century, may be more hazardous in others. Recognition of these problems in the environment has led to the establishment of the Environmental Protection Agency and to the Occupational Safety and Health Act, which gives the federal government the authority to research and monitor the effects of the environment and industry taken alone or in their interaction on the health of the public.[7]

In addition, health promotion is concerned with health education, the dissemination of knowledge that enables people to preserve and protect their own health. When associations have been made between cigarette smoking and the risk of lung cancer or the risk of thrombophlebitis to women taking contraceptive pills, it is the function of health education to disseminate this information so that people can make informed choices. One aspect of the crisis that has developed relates to the enforcing of laws with regard to certain industries to desist from pollution. Another problem seems apparent in the fact that the federal government spends more money each year to subsidize farmers who are growing tobacco than it spends on research about the effects of tobacco on the human organism or effective ways of educating the public about these effects. To properly assess the long-term effects of chemical contraceptives on the cardiovascular system in women becomes very difficult in a country where the drug industry is very large and where many physicians' postgraduate education with regard to new drugs comes from the representatives of the drug companies engaged in a competitive and highly profitable business.

It is apparent that many hazards to health, perhaps the most noxious ones, are intimately embedded in the society in which we live. Authority to enforce laws or to carry out public information programs or even to design clinical trials of new drugs or other medical practices becomes difficult to achieve when opposing interests in our society are powerful and are pursuing goals other than health. It is in part the complicated interrelationship between the factors which promote health and those which serve other interests that create major problems for the health of Americans today. Health promotion is a part of the health care system that requires intervention at many levels. Public laws and policies must be formulated and enforced. Problems must be addressed and understood in their varying complexity, and public information disseminated. In all of this the health care system and its practitioners should be held accountable. Consumers have in recent years played an increasingly active role in this aspect of the health care system. They have lobbied for seat belts in moving vehicles, safer products, testing of products that are used in the home, and more precise labeling practices in food, to mention but a few of their activities. Individual practitioners have responsibility to keep themselves informed, to counsel their clients and patients, to share information, and also to participate in collective activity on behalf of the public health and to continuously assess and research the health status of the population with which they are concerned.

Funding for health promotion comes largely from the public pocket. It is a much smaller part of the health care budget than that which is allocated for very complicated curative treatment. If funds for health promotion were increased, it is likely that we would have a healthier population and could save money by not having to treat so many acutely ill people. It could lessen human suffering and the social disorganization that occurs in the wake of crippling disease. Health promotion is frequently neglected in medical education (just the opposite is true in nursing education) and is sometimes thought to be beyond the scope of physicians' practice.

Allocation of funds for health care is a major ethical dilemma. The problem exists on several levels:

1. Should funds be used for prevention of disease and health promotion or for cure of disease?
2. Should funds be used for research or treatment?

3. Are there any health behaviors or practices that should be mandatory (e.g., screening for certain genetic diseases)?
4. Should persons be "punished" for certain behaviors (e.g., smoking or being overweight)?

Because there is, and will continue to be, a finite amount of money available for health care, the ethical dilemma is a serious one.

Primary prevention

Primary prevention is the component of the health care system that seeks to prevent disease by direct intervention. Traditional public health programs, sanitation reform, nutrition, health education, immunization and vaccination, and the control of infectious disease are all a part of this level of intervention. Ever since the last quarter of the nineteenth century when the germ theory of disease was discovered and health professionals were enabled to intervene in the course of disease, there has been remarkable improvement in the health of the population as a result of the control of infectious disease. One needs only to look at the shift in the major causes of death in this country during the course of this century to see the dramatic change. Control of infectious disease has also added to longevity, lowering of infant and maternal mortality, childhood mortality, and morbidity. While certain infectious diseases still exist, the progress made with regard to mortality, morbidity, and lifelong handicaps as a result of infectious disease is one of the major triumphs of public health and curative medicine in the twentieth century.

Secondary prevention

Most of the resources, both public and private, of the health care system have been spent on secondary prevention.

This has happened for many historical reasons. The rate of growth of knowledge about the causes and cure of disease has been phenomenal over the past hundred years. Knowledge about the human organism and the processes of life and growth has created highly specialized areas of scientific work. In addition to basic biology, there has also been an increase in knowledge about chemotherapeutics, providing an armamentarium of powerful drugs to assist in altering or curing a disease. New tools, such as the x ray, the electron microscope, and the laser beam, expand our capacity to understand and diminish disease. Modern health workers are armed with a curative capacity that grows, changes, and enlarges at a very rapid rate. They have the use of many different modalities, drugs, machines, and knowledge that constantly alter the effectiveness of intervention in a variety of very simple and complicated diseases. A wide range of pharmaceuticals can prevent and cure many diseases. Surgery has been improved by equipment, machines, and technology not available even fifteen years ago. Computers have given rise to a capacity for investigation, storing and retrieving data, monitoring a patient through a physical crisis, and even making certain therapeutic decisions. Diagnosis and treatment have become more precise because of the availability of new instruments and techniques. The capacity of curative medicine keeps growing, both in scope and in depth, and this growth has led to the diminution of certain diseases. It has also led to some of the consequences of greater longevity and survival. Within the system itself there is greater specialization and complexity that in turn has led to greater expense and fragmentation of service. This means more complicated facilities and greater manpower needs. Most public and private resources of the health care system have been placed at this third level of intervention (curative medicine). While much has been gained, the triumphs of curative medicine have also created problems that become increasingly obvious as we examine the fourth level of intervention.

Tertiary prevention

Tertiary prevention is the level of intervention that, although it cannot prevent or cure disease, attempts to promote the maximum function of people who are diseased. Tertiary prevention is concerned largely with chronic diseases, with the restoration and function of people who suffer them. Because curative medicine has been so successful in delaying death from infection, we are now facing problems of tertiary prevention, since more of the population at all ages are surviving with chronic disease. While the problem existed in the past, the magnitude of the problem of maintaining people with chronic illnesses at maximum levels of function has become greater. It involves problems not only of resource allocation and the consequences of increased knowledge, but also a health care system that was designed in the main to care for people with acute diseases. People with chronic disease require a variety of treatment modalities in and out of different institutions over long periods of time. The growing number of persons who need this level of care strains the health care system, adding another dimension to the "crisis." It causes the system that is largely concerned with acute care to cope with ever-increasing numbers of people who need continuing care over time in a variety of settings.

PROBLEMS

Having taken the historical view and having examined the changing population and its needs, the changing capacity of health care, and the changing system of care, one must examine the interrelationship of all these changes as they are reflected in the structure of the health care system and the problems currently associated with it.

In the United Stated at the present time we need to care for a continuously growing population. It is one with increasing numbers of dependent youngsters and elderly people. The population as a whole is healthier and living longer. Because of growth and changing industrial patterns, citizens are facing new problems in maintaining a healthy environment. Because of the factors in the health care system that have already been discussed, another kind of problem must be addressed. The health care system is largely designed to give acute episodic care. New problems arise as a result of previous successes in prevention and the need for continuous comprehensive care for the growing numbers of chronically ill people who are living longer. The emphasis on curative medicine and high technology has created problems with which the current system cannot easily cope. Perhaps an example or two will make the point. It has been estimated that the care of a 1,500-gram baby in a perinatal intensive care unit costs about $150,000 a case. We know from almost fifty years of epidemiological study that health promotion and primary prevention can sometimes avoid the necessity of the use of a perinatal intensive care unit.

We know that healthy, educated, economically advantaged women who do not give birth in their early teens or forties are likely to have full-term babies weighing more than 2,500 grams (a normal birth weight for a baby born at term). If the population of mothers does not meet those criteria, it is still possible, at the secondary level, to give comprehensive prenatal care early to a mother and positively affect the chances of her delivering a normal–birth weight baby. Furthermore, we know that babies born at low birth weights are subject to many more life-crippling conditons than babies born at normal birth weights.

Given the epidemiological information and the possibilities for intervention, it would seem that intervention should be possible at every level and that the birth of a low–birth weight baby might be seen as the failure of the first two levels of intervention. If one examines the allocation of resources, it is apparent that large amounts of resources in research, money, and manpower are put at the third level—in the perinatal care unit—with very little money or manpower and service available at any of the other levels. In fact the major thrust is at a level of care in which least can be done to ensure the development of a healthy adult, although it is the most expensive level to maintain. In addition, even this most costly intervention is not equally available to every citizen who might need it. This is archetypical of the success and failure of the health care system in the United States.

MATERNAL AND CHILD HEALTH CARE AS AN EXAMPLE OF THE DEVELOPMENT OF PUBLIC POLICY

If we look at the history of public policy with regard to maternal and child health in this country,

we can see how we as a nation responded to all of these developments and have created a health care system in our own image. Examining public policy with regard to maternal and child health services serves more than the purpose of seeing the development of services to a given population as a case history. It is also in the health policy of maternal and child health services that the major patterns of public health policy were elaborated and the intricate interrelationships and problems of the public and private health care systems were articulated. The growth of public policy in this area set patterns for the growth of public policy in many other areas of the health care system, and many important precedents were established, among which are the following:

1. The federal government's right to be involved in health care
2. The system of matching grants-in-aid to the states from the federal government
3. Setting of standards by the federal government within which state and local programs must be carried out
4. Provision of money for categorical programs (not only disease categories but those defined by geographical area and economic status as well)
5. Consumer influence on the exercise of public policy in health
6. Participation of consumers not only in formulation of policy but also in carrying out research and the formulation of programs
7. The role of the federal government in conducting research in health problems and the use of research findings for planning programs, services, and facilities
8. National collection of vital statistics pertaining to health
9. Integration of health and social services

In fact many of the hallmarks of public policy in health were conceived, experimented with, and worked out in the implementation of programs in maternal and child health. In addition, in the history of maternal and child health policy, we can clearly see the concern with and intervention in relation to the four levels of prevention, as well as the integration of research, knowledge, and service.

Establishment of Children's Bureau

The Children's Bureau was created in 1912. Its establishment was another aspect of the reform movement in the first decade of this century that was responding to abuses of child and female labor, growing infant and maternal mortality rates, living conditions in the city, and the growing movement for women's rights. On April 9, 1912, President Taft signed a bill passed by Congress creating in the federal government a children's bureau charged with investigating and reporting ''upon all matters pertaining to the welfare of children and child life among all classes of our people.'' This act was the fruition of a great deal of effort by many people and organizations springing from the great social reforms that grew from the 1880s on. In 1903 Lillian Wald had first suggested a federal children's bureau to Florence Kelley of the National Consumers League. Kelley, herself, as early as 1900, had proposed a United States Commission for Children which should make available and interpret facts ''concerning the mental and moral conditions and prospects of the children of the United States.'' She specified seven subjects of immediate urgency: (1) infant mortality, (2) birth registration, (3) orphanages, (4) child labor, (5) desertion, (6) illegitimacy, and (7) degeneracy. Later, Lillian Wald spoke to Theodore Roosevelt about the idea. The following years were spent in considering the intent and purpose of a federal children's bureau, and the National Child Labor Committee undertook the bureau as its major legislative goal.

In 1905, Kelley published a book that described why federal action on behalf of children was needed. Much of this material was used in legislative hearings and also gained support from women's organizations. Evidence from New Zealand, which had been monitoring its own experience in programs designed to lessen maternal and infant mortality, was also used in legislative hearings to bolster the arguments for a department in the federal government that would be concerned with women and children. Also in 1905, the National Child Labor Committee, at its second annual meeting, presented a proposed draft of the legislation. Bills were introduced proposing a federal children's bureau in 1906 and annually during the next six years. During this time organizations of parents, labor unions, health workers, social workers, and women came to actively support the legislation. In 1909 the first White House Conference on the Care for Dependent Children recommended that the bureau be established. President Roosevelt sent a special message to Congress urging passage of the measure.

The first appropriation for the Children's Bureau was $25,640. Fifteen positions were created in addition to a chief, the latter to be appointed by the president with the advice and consent of the Senate. The act establishing the Children's Bureau was an important precedent in legislative history because it institutionalized the notion that a function related to the welfare of children was an appropriate one for the federal government. The general welfare clause of the United States Constitution was cited as the base authority for the act. Originally placed in the Department of Commerce and Labor in 1912, the bureau was transferred to the newly created Department of Labor on March 4, 1913.

In 1913 the bureau conducted its first study on infant mortality. Investigations were carried out in nine representative studies. Their general results indicated that (1) death rates of babies declined as father's earnings went up; (2) breast-fed babies had a better chance to survive the first year than bottle-fed babies; (3) a baby whose mother was home during its first year survived better than a baby deprived of mother's care; (4) illegitimacy played an important role in infant mortality; (5) sanitary conditions were important; and (6) ''community action can remedy many conditions dangerous to infants.'' Between 1914 and 1922 the bureau published several reports on the kinds of prevention measures already instituted by public and private agencies in the Untied States, in several countries in Europe, and in New Zealand.

Most infant deaths were found to result from diarrhea, infectious diseases, premature birth, congenital disability, or birth injury. It was felt by people in the Children's Bureau that these factors were related to maternal care. Several studies of maternal deaths were conducted and inquiries made on how they might be reduced. Policy, laws, and finances pertaining to maternity care in other countries were reviewed. Between 1915 and 1921 infant mortality in this country fell 24%. The largest decrease took place among infants one to twelve months old, and the decrease was more marked in cities than in rural areas. In 1913 the Children's Bureau published a bulletin for parents that discussed prenatal care. "Infant Care" was published in 1914. In 1919 an advisory committee of pediatricians representing organized medical groups was set up to advise the bureau on its publications. Up until that time, physicians had not been directly involved in the bureau's activities.

Birth registration was a prime concern, since it was very difficult to conduct infant mortality studies without the necessary statistics. A pilot study to see how many births were registered was done in 1913 by the General Federation of Women's Clubs at the request of the bureau. In 1915 this study resulted in the establishment of birth registration in ten states and the District of Columbia and by 1933 included all states.

An outgrowth of the infant mortality studies was a nationwide observation of Baby Week in March, 1916, and May, 1917. Sponsored by the Children's Bureau and the General Federation of Women's Clubs, its purpose was to feed back to the public information from the investigations. Baby Week led to Children's Year in 1918. During this year, age, height, and weight standards for children were compiled from weighing and measuring thousands of youngsters. Another aspect of the activity was a "back to school" drive to decrease child labor in which 17,000 committees participated, composed of 11 million women. In 1919 the bureau started issuing its own bulletin. Children's Year culminated in the 1919 White House Conference on Standards of Child Welfare. A small meeting of specialists was held first, and then regional conferences were held on four main topics:

1. Protection of the health of mothers and children

2. The economic and social base for child welfare standards
3. Child labor
4. Children in need of special care

Sheppard-Towner Act, 1921 to 1929

In the 1917 report of the Children's Bureau, a plan was published for the "Public Protection of Maternity and Infancy." The program included the following recommendations:

1. Public health nurses should be available for inspection and service covering the field of hygiene for mothers and children.

2. Conference centers affording mothers a convenient opportunity to secure examination of well children and expert advice as to their best development should be provided.

3. Adequate confinement care should be provided.

4. Hospital facilities should be made available and accessible for mothers and children.

The campaign for this purpose, sponsored largely by groups of organized women, was long and hard. On November 19, 1921, the Maternity and Infancy Act, popularly known as the Sheppard-Towner Act, was passed by the House and Senate. As signed by President Harding on November 23, 1921, it included a five-year limit on authorization for appropriation. The act provided that the states should originate and carry out their own plans. The Federal Board of Maternity and Infant Hygiene, composed of the Children's Bureau, the Surgeon General of the Public Health Service, and the Commissioner of Education, was given authority to approve or disapprove of state plans, but the act specified that a plan must be approved by the board "if it was reasonable, appropriate, and adequate to carry out its purposes." In all but four of the forty-five states cooperating between 1921 and 1927, the administration was lodged in the state department of health. Following were some of the more important features of many of the state programs:

1. Conferences with mothers were held by specialists in maternity and child health.

2. Distribution of supplies to mothers unable to go to hospitals for confinement was made so that

adequate and sterile materials might be available at their homes.

3. More maternity care, infant and child care centers, nutrition classes, and dental hygiene care were provided for mothers and children.

4. More public health nurses and physicians, particularly in rural areas, were made available.

5. Education was given to mothers in the essentials of maternity and infant hygiene through correspondence courses and to young girls through classes for "little mothers."

The Sheppard-Towner Act was the initial step in a system of highly complicated and varied patterns among federal-state-local relationships. The suggestion that the federal government provide grants to states for "maternal and infant protection to be distributed in local areas where investigation showed need and contributions are duly authorized from State and county funds in such proportions to the Federal Fund as may be determined" came from Julia Lathrop, then chief of the bureau. The precedent for these grants-in-aid was based in the Smith-Level Act of 1914, which provided matching grants-in-aid for cooperative agricultural extension work between agricultural colleges and the several states.

Although the proposals were initially made at a time of deepening American involvement in the First World War, they were consonant with the administration's concern to protect the health and strength of the civilian population, and with Children's Year. Support for the act came from women's groups in the children's health and welfare fields.

The bill, first introduced in 1918 by Jeannette Rankin (the first woman member of Congress), was partly a result of the findings of the many investigations of infant and maternal mortality made by the Children's Bureau since its inception. Opposition to the act came only from ultraconservative organizations, antivivisectionist groups, and women's organizations opposed to women's suffrage. (The AMA expressed opposition in its journal but did not appear at the hearings.) By 1927, forty-five states and the territory of Hawaii had accepted provisions of the bill; Massachusetts, Connecticut,

and Illinois did not participate. In 1929, fifteen states and Hawaii appropriated funds equal in amount to the combined state and fedreal funds of the previous year.

Although the AMA had been mild in its criticism at the beginning, by 1926 it was outright in its opposition and actively organized the country's physicians and other groups against the act. Several other arguments were made against the act: objections were to the specialized nature of the health services, to the Children's Bureau administration rather than administration by the Public Health Service, and to the constitutionality of the act itself, which was challenged by the commonwealth of Massachusetts. To quote Schlesinger, "the Sheppard-Towner Act was clearly in advance of its time. Its seed was planted by a courageous individual; it was nurtured in the soil of war-time concern for the well-being of the civilian population; it grew in the favorable climate of the movement for women's rights; it flowered under the impact of universal suffrage, and it withered as a solitary plant often does, when the political and social climate changed. But the roots were sturdy, and when the environment was favorable again it sprang into full bloom."[8]

During the 1920s, while the Sheppard-Towner Act was in effect, the country's population growth was slowing down because of restriction of immigration, movement from the country to the cities, and wider use of birth control. By 1930, 49% of the population lived in communities of more than 8,000. The machine was becoming the hallmark of culture; industrial productivity accelerated. This was a period of increase in national wealth, income, and real wages, along with pockets of unemployment. However, there were many danger spots in the United States at the same time: agriculture was depressed, and land values, crop prices, and farm income had dropped. The problem of blacks coming north from the 1880s on, "last to be hired, first to be fired," was another grave portent. Excluded by trade unions, partly because they were often given work as strikebreakers, they lived in poverty and segregation. In 1915 to 1920 the second great black migration into northern cities took place. Signs of the depression appeared early in 1929. The building boom had ended, automobile and sheet metal production had dropped, and the unemployment that had been endemic throughout the 1920s rose sharply. The increasing difficulties of the rural areas were to become an area of special focus in Title V of the Social Security Act of 1935.

In 1927 and 1928 the bureau appointed an advisory committee of prominent obstetricians and did a large field study of the causes of maternal death and conditions associated with it. This study covered the deaths of 7,500 women attributed by the census to a puerperal cause. Some startling facts were revealed by the study: (1) a large proportion of women had little or no prenatal examination by a physician, and many others had little or poor care; (2) a large proportion of deaths was due to controllable causes: 40% resulted from sepsis, nearly one half of these caused by abortion; and (3) 30% of deaths resulted from some presumably toxic condition. At the same time this study was done, there were similar investigations by the New York Academy of Medicine and the Philadelphia Medical Society reporting similar results. About 65% of deaths of mothers in childbirth were assumed to be preventable.

At the 1930 White House Conference on Children, the Children's Charter was adopted by the conference as a statement of the rights of children. Articles IV, V, VII, and XIII relate specifically to the health needs of children and guarantee the following as rights for every child:

1. Full preparation for his birth, his mother receiving prenatal, natal, and postnatal care; and the establishment of such protective measures as will make childbearing safer.
2. Health protection from birth through adolescence, including: periodic health examinations and, where needed, care by specialists and hospital treatment; regular dental examinations and care of the teeth; protective and preventive measures against communicable diseases; the insuring of pure food, pure milk, and pure water.
3. A dwelling place, safe, sanitary, and wholesome.

4. For every child who is blind, deaf, crippled, or otherwise physically handicapped, and for the child who is mentally handicapped, such measures as will early discover and diagnose his handicap, provide care and treatment, and so train him that he may become an asset to society rather than a liability. Expenses of these services should be borne publicly when they cannot be privately met.
5. To make everywhere available these minimum protections of the health and welfare of children, there should be a district, county, or community organization for health, education, and welfare, with full-time officials, coordinating with a statewide program which will be responsive to a nationwide service of general information, statistics, and scientific research. This should include: a) trained, full-time public health officials, with public health nurses, sanitary inspection, and laboratory workers; b) available hospital beds; and c) full-time public welfare service for the relief, aid, and guidance of children in special need due to poverty, misfortune, or behavior difficulties, and for the protection of children from abuse, neglect, exploitation, or moral hazard.

Social Security Act, Title V

As part of the program of recovery from the depression that had begun in the second half of the 1920s, in 1934 the Committee on Economic Security asked the Children's Bureau to assemble facts and make proposals for federal legislation on children's programs. Partially on the basis of facts and proposals presented by the bureau, federal aid to the states for the development and expansion, especially in rural areas, of Maternal and Child Health Programs (among others) was incorporated into legislation. The Social Security Act was signed into law by President Roosevelt on August 14, 1935. Funds became available in February, 1936.

Title V of the act included federal aid for three types of programs in the states:
1. Maternal and child health
2. Medical care for crippled children
3. Child welfare services

All of these were to be administered through the Children's Bureau. Within nine months of the time when maternal and child health funds became available, all forty-eight states, Alaska, Hawaii, and the District of Columbia were cooperating. This prompt action was a result in part of the experience gained during the Sheppard-Towner Act.

The initial appropriation of funds granted to the states was used under the administration of the state health departments to pay for physicians, dentists, public health nurses, medical social workers, and nutritionists to help reach mothers and children (living for the most part in rural areas) through prenatal and child health clinics and through school health services. The emphasis on rurality stemmed from the relative under-development of health services outside the metropolitan areas and the difficultis in financing extension of services in rural areas without federal assistance. This act extended the scope of the already existing programs by support for (1) maternity and newborn services to include health services for children up to 21 years of age (this aspect of the program was intended primarily to develop preventive health measures) and (2) training for professional personnel, as distinguished from the provision of actual medical or hospital care.

Between 1936 and 1940 many changes in the program occurred. The scope of services widened to include demonstration projects showing how new knowledge could be put to work. There were progressive improvements in maternal and neonatal care. Special programs for the care of premature babies developed in training centers. All the states used some of their funds for the training of professional personnel to provide these services.

In 1938 a Conference on Better Care for Mothers and Babies was called. At the opening session, facts were presented that revealed the size and complexity of the problem:

1. One half to two thirds of maternal deaths were preventable.

2. Almost no progress had been made in saving infants who died in the first month of life.

3. No progress at all had been made in saving infants who died in the first day of life.

The conference concluded that preservation of the lives and health of mothers and babies was of such importance to all the people that it warranted immediate and concerted national consideration and action.

Emergency maternity and infant care, 1941 to 1949

In 1941 war broke out, although preparation for it had begun some time earlier. Because of the need for women workers, the Children's Bureau called its first conference on day care for children of working mothers. A year later a maternity policy for industry was worked out. Also in 1941 state health agencies requested and the Children's Bureau approved the use of federal maternal and child health funds for maternity care for wives of enlisted men in the armed forces. In wartime certain aspects of health and social services long fought for easily became instruments of social policy. Federally sponsored day-care centers became possible when women were needed in the labor force, and maternity care became available for the wives of men in the army.

Steady progress was made in the period 1940 to 1945 in safeguarding mothers and children. The maternal mortality rate for 1945, 21.7 per 10,000 live births, was the lowest recorded in the United States up to that time. It had decreased from 37.6 in 1940. The infant mortality rate declined from 47 per 1,000 in 1940 to 39.3 in 1945. However, despite the encouraging reduction in national rates beginning in the thirties, an analysis in 1944 showed that maternal mortality among nonwhite mothers lagged fifteen years behind the rest of the population.

In August, 1941, the commanding officer of Fort Lewis in the state of Washington requested funds from the state health department to pay for the maternity care given to wives of soldiers stationed there. The state health department in turn asked the Children's Bureau for permission to use maternal and child health funds available under the Social Security Act for these women. The Children's Bureau appealed for funds under the provisions of the Maternal and Child Health Program (Title V, Part I of the Social Security Act) to the

Bureau of the Budget in August and September, 1942. A deficiency bill was approved in March, 1943. Money appropriated was to cover the costs of medical, hospital, and nursing care for the wives and babies of men in the four lowest grades of the armed forces. This Emergency Maternity and Infant Care Act of 1943, popularly referred to as EMIC, made available without cost to wives of servicemen in the fourth through seventh grades of the armed forces medical, nursing, and hospital care throughout pregnancy, at childbirth, and for six weeks thereafter. Hospital care was paid for at ward rates. The babies of these servicemen were also eligible for medical, hospital, and nursing care if sick during any time the first year of life. From the beginning of the program to the end of June, 1949, 1.5 million maternity and infant cases were authorized for care. Most of the mothers were young and having their first babies. At the direction of Congress, 1947 to 1948 marked the beginning of the end of the program, which concluded in June, 1949.

The program ran up a record of 92% births in hospitals. At its height, 48,000 doctors and 4,000 hospitals cooperated. It was the biggest public maternity program ever undertaken in the United States and was a major force in promoting public understanding of and demand for a high standard of obstetrical and pediatric care. However, there was no money set aside to evaluate its effects on maternal and infant mortality rates or to examine in detail the kind, quality, and effects of services it gave. Although in the program's beginning only hospitalization was covered for maternity services, by the time the program was in full swing, complete care was covered, including services delivered in physicians' offices and clinics. This was a result of the recognition of the special character of maternity care and was also probably due to the precedents established under the Emergency Maternity and Infant Care Act itself. The name of the program was later changed to the Civilian Health and Medical Program of the Uniformed Services. Because the program required each state to develop a plan with priority given to areas most in need of hospital beds, it concentrated on places where delivery at home was still a common practice.

In the late 1950s there was a resurgence of interest in the broad health problems related to the pregnancy cycle and infancy. There emerged an awareness that the infant mortality rate for the country as a whole was not declining as rapidly as it had in earlier years. Infant mortality was rising in some areas, and there was not enough money to pay for needed services.

National Institute of Child Health and Human Development

In 1963 the National Institute of Child Health and Human Development was authorized as one of the National Institutes of Health. It unified the federal funding of research projects that were concerned with reproductive and perinatal biology, growth and development, aging, mental retardation, congenital malformations, developmental pharmacology, and communication.

Social Security amendments of 1963

In 1962 the report of the President's Panel on Mental Retardation noted the need for a preventive program for mental retardation. It recognized the lack of adequate maternity and infant care, particularly in inner cities. The report led to amendments to the Social Security Act in 1963 that dealt with the prevention of mental retardation. These amendments authorized a gradual increase in the annual appropriation for these grants from $25 million to $50 million by 1970. The amendments also established a new program of grants for maternity and infant care for high-risk groups in low-income families, starting with $5 million in 1964, increasing to $30 million a year during 1966 to 1968. These grants, covering 75% of the costs, were made to localities for special projects, either through or with the approval of the state department of health. A new program was authorized for the support of research aimed at the improvement of maternal and child health and crippled children's services. An appropriation of $4 million was made in 1966 covering such areas as (1) new approaches to provision

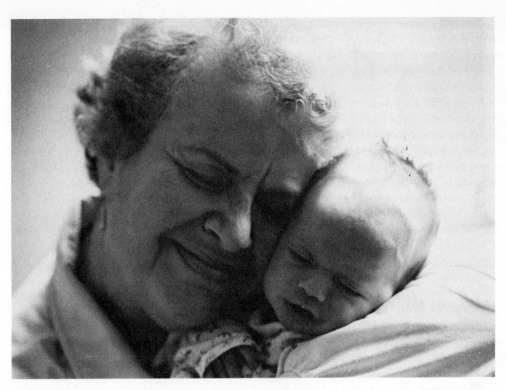

Fig. 2-1. Maternal and child health care has become an increasing concern of all health professionals. (Photograph by Arthur Sirdofsky; courtesy Editorial Photocolor Archives, Inc., New York.)

of maternal health services, (2) factors affecting use of community health resources, (3) evaluation of effectiveness of programs, and (4) family planning services (for the first time).

Economic Opportunity Act of 1964

The Economic Opportunity Act of 1964 provided the legal framework for the antipoverty program. It opened up new avenues for improvement of maternal and child health among segments of the population in greatest need by providing funds for the development of neighborhood health centers offering comprehensive health care, including maternal and child health services. Operation Head Start was begun under this legislation and incorporated into its education programs important health components such as health examinations, follow-up care for adverse health conditions, dental

treatment, lunches, and health education through parent participation. The most novel feature of the legislation was the provision of funds directly to local governments and community agencies.

Social Security amendments of 1965

The Social Security Act amendments of 1965 have probably comprised the most significant single measure in recent years affecting health services for mothers and children. These amendments strengthened further the traditional grants-in-aid to states for maternal and child health and crippled children's services by authorizing larger amounts for each type of grant to the annual ceiling of $60 million by fiscal 1970. At the same time, the states were required to show that they were extending their maternal and child health and crippled children's services to ensure statewide coverage by

1975. A new program of special project grants for comprehensive health services for children and youth was established. These projects seek to eliminate artificial barriers between preventive and treatment services. The projects provide screening, diagnosis, preventive service, treatment, aftercare (both medical and dental), and coordination of health care and services with other health, welfare, and educational programs for children. Project grants may be made directly to schools of medicine and to teaching hospitals affiliated with medical schools, as well as to state and local health agencies and to state crippled children's agencies. A major difference in this new federal health legislation was that it covered both preventive and curative services. This is reminiscent of the recommendations embodied in the Children's Charter of 1930.

Social Security Act, Title XIX (Medicaid)

The intent of Title XIX is to promote high-quality family-centered health care for all persons who cannot afford it entirely by themselves. Maternity service became more comprehensive, and in fact, some think that the current downward trend in infant mortality rates is related to the provision of services under this enactment. However, the evidence is not clear because at the same time women with different social and biological characteristics entered into the childbearing period.

Child Health Act of 1967

Under the Child Health Act of 1967 the various authorizations in Title V for formula and project grants were combined. This included formula grants for maternal and child health and crippled children's services, project grants for training of personnel for health care and related services for mothers and children, research in maternal and child health and crippled children's services, and a new program of project grants for dental health services. The combined authorization was for $250 million for fiscal 1969 and increases in stages of $25 million a year up to $350 million for 1973 and

thereafter. By July 1, 1968, each state was required to submit a single plan to cover all Title V child health programs. For four years ending on June 30, 1972, funds would be allocated with the added requirements that programs designed to reduce infant mortality be included as part of maternal and child health programs, and that a greater emphasis in crippled children's service programs be placed on periodic screening for the early identification of children in need of health care and services. In addition, 6% of funds appropriated must be earmarked for family planning services.

In July, 1972, responsibility for administering the grants was transferred to the states. Any agency within a state receiving child health grants was required to cooperate with the state agency administering medical assistance under Title XIX providing care and services for children eligible for medical assistance. The state agency, in turn, is responsible for providing early and periodic screening and diagnosis of children eligible under Title XIX for care and treatment to correct or ameliorate chronic conditions that are discovered and for the reimbursement of agencies providing such services under Title V.

A word should be said about family planning services. Prior to the 1960s only seven states, all in the South, were providing such services, mainly in rural areas through local health departments. Elsewhere, family planning services were provided by private physicians, hospital outpatient clinics, and voluntary agencies. By 1965, 119 counties in twenty-one states were providing such services. Since then, family planning services have been included in many federally funded maternal and infant care programs. The 1967 amendments of the Social Security Act require that family planning services must be offered to families receiving Aid to Dependent Children, which they are free to accept or reject. The services were mandatory as of July 1, 1969, and were given 75% matching funds. In 1971, under the Family Planning Services and Population Research Act (Public Law 91-572), $30 million each for research and services in family planning was authorized. Only $6 million was actually appropriated, however, and this only for service programs.

THE FEDERAL GOVERNMENT AND HEALTH

Because of the nature of our own history and constitution, the federal government has had to look for ways to become involved in the health of its population. This concern ordinarily belonged to state and local governments. There are many levels of federal responsibility for health, and this has resulted in a wide variety of health care programs. Financing, control, and implementation of public programs occur in many ways and are authorized in many different pieces of legislation that affect different agencies at many levels of government.

The amendments to the Social Security Act from 1963 to 1972, especially as they relate to Title V, have attempted to reduce the random patchwork of services available to mothers and children and to integrate the sources of funding, availability, and accessibility. Increasingly, single agencies at the regional and state levels will be authorizing funds for local services. Community mental health centers, OEO neighborhood health centers, neighborhood health centers funded under Section 314-e of Public Law 89-749, Maternal and Infant Care Centers, and Children and Youth Projects, as well as Head Start programs, are all delivering comprehensive care (i.e., preventive and curative services) in a geographically designated area to a defined population. Bills proposing welfare reform and health maintenance organizations are also designed to provide services for a defined population. The notion of community health services delivered in a defined geographical area to a defined population has now taken hold so that almost all the proposals now being advanced in Congress contain such provisions. Several of the national health insurance bills currently before Congress also address themselves to this issue.

Two outstanding problems remain, both dealing with the effective integration of services. One concerns the integration of the many different preventive and curative services now existing in local communities; the other concerns the integration of the separate services now existing that in effect constitute a dual system of medical care, one for the poor, the other for the rich. Both will be formidable tasks. An example of the latter problem, the duality of services available for the rich and poor, is the Hyde amendment to the Social Security Act, Title CIC (Medicaid). The Hyde amendment prohibits use of Medicaid funds to pay for abortion. Although abortion has been legal (in the first two trimesters) in the United States since January, 1973, it is in fact more available to rich women, who can pay for private abortions, than to poor women who are denied public funds for this purpose. The morality of abortion is not the issue here. The issue is denying health care to some women while providing it to others *solely* on the basis of ability to pay.

Following are health care programs sponsored by the federal government that affected the health of the entire population as well as mothers and children:

1. Establishment of National Institutes of Health (creating a national capacity for research)
2. Hill-Burton legislation (providing for construction of health care facilities in areas where they were lacking)
3. Mental Health and Mental Retardation Planning Act of 1963 (providing a model for community mental health services to defined populations in defined geographical areas)
4. Titles XVIII and XIX, Social Security Act of 1965 (providing medical care to the elderly and poor, also known as Medicare and Medicaid)
5. Health Manpower and Training Acts (providing health manpower through the use of federal money to educational institutions)
6. Professional Standards Review Organization, amendment to the Social Security Act of 1972 (providing for assessment by peers of quality and cost of care)

7. Comprehensive Health Planning Acts

As one looks at health legislation in this country over the last seventy-five years, certain patterns emerge. The federal government, because of its original constitutional limitations, has participated in health care policy mainly in indirect ways and only in ways that were allowed by the health care delivery system and the states. It has accomplished the following:

1. Provided a patchwork of preventive health services
2. Provided curative care only for patients who were not able to buy services in the private system
3. Filled gaps not met by the private sector
4. Provided national funding for public services traditionally funded at other levels of government
   a. The care of the mentally ill (formerly a state function)
   b. The care of the sick poor (formerly a city or county function)
5. Regulated certain costs where it is responsible for care (Medicare)
6. Encouraged assessment of care (PSRO)
7. Began to plan at regional and state levels for an organized system of care (National Health Planning Acts)

The national government of the United States has been the actor of last resort in the health care system, acting only to smooth over critical situations, meet unmet needs, and provide seed money for new directions. It has had to push and pull the private sector in a variety of ways, mostly with a carrot but sometimes with a club, to carry out its bidding. It has used money and public law to shape the health care system, working through the private system. Entrepreneurial medicine has had a profound and lasting effect on the health care system and still exercises great power. This historical tradition in the United States is different from most other countries in the world where there had been government regulation, intervention, or direct ownership or management of the health care system for quite some time. Even where a private system

exists alongside a public one in other countries, it is controlled more directly by the government than is the system in the United States.

The federal government has enacted three separate laws to introduce regional and state planning of health services. The legislation popularly known as "the Heart Disease, Cancer, and Stroke Legislation" (Public Law 89-239, passed in 1965) emphasizes coordination of existing institutions into regional medical programs without interfering with existing forms of medical practice, financing, or hospital administration. The grants for regional medical programs provided inducement for voluntary regional planning through cooperative arrangements between medical schools, hospitals, and other appropriate institutions for education and treatment of people with heart disease, stroke, cancer, and related diseases.

At the same time, there was an alternative and competing federally assisted program to help hospital and nonhospital services to plan for areawide health services. This effort culminated in the "Partnership for Health" legislation, the Comprehensive Health Planning and Service Act of 1965 (Public Law 89-749). This act consolidated preexisting project and formula grants to states through a new system of grants for comprehensive health services. It stipulated a program of federal, state, and local planning for comprehensive health services, with emphasis on local services. The intent of the new legislation was to broaden the base of state and local health programs. The comprehensive health planning agencies created in the act offered a focus for coordination of health institutions and personnel. Both the regional medical programs and the comprehensive health planning agencies have little clout in the form of available funding or facilities and services and little authority. In 1975 a new law superseding the other two attempted to integrate the two preceding efforts into one, modeling itself after Public Law 89-749, but carrying with it a little more authority: the power to determine whether federal monies can be allocated to recipients in the region based on assessments of need and regional planning.[9,10]

NATIONAL HEALTH INSURANCE

National health insurance has been in the legislative hopper in the Untied States since 1935 but has not yet been enacted. As a single act of public policy, it has the potential of extraordinary impact on the health care system. There has been a bill proposing national health insurance in every Congress since 1936. There was a proposal for national health insurance in the original Social Security Act. Title XX of the act was dropped for Title V when President Roosevelt was made aware that Congress might scuttle the entire Social Security program because of the pressures of the American Medical Association (opposed since 1919 to any system of compulsory national health insurance). There are many bills in Congress at the present time for various forms of national health insurance. Basically the plans are of three different kinds:

1. Catastrophic insurance, providing for the most expensive health care
2. Using the current private health insurance contracts as a model for a national one
3. Comprehensive coverage in a single system

The approach to catastrophic insurance is best seen in the Long-Ribicoff bill. The scope of services resembles the coverage of a major medical insurance contract. Its scope of service is the same as currently provided under Medicare but would not cover the first sixty days of hospitalization or the first $2,000 in family medical expenses. It would cover the cost of care to people suffering the end stage of disease or major traumatic illness. The number of people requiring this care is relatively small compared to the number of people receiving all health care in any one year.

Models of national health insurance based on current insurance contracts that feature limited scope of service, coinsurance, deductibles, and out-of-pocket payments are featured in four bills in the Congress (CHIP, Ullman, Fulton, Burleson-McIntyre). All are variations on the same theme. They provide the traditional insurance coverage for inpatient and outpatient services with deductibles, coinsurances, and copayment features. Employed people would be financed through a payroll tax on both employees and employers. Unemployed people would be paid for by the federal government. The federal government would allow fiscal intermediaries to administer the program as it does now under Medicare.

The third pattern for national health insurance is set in the Kennedy-Corman bill. It provides for an enlarged scope of services (preventive as well as curative) with no patient cost sharing. All services specified will be given without any copayment mechanism, and the plan will be administered directly by HHS through regional and local offices with no fiscal intermediary.

The passage of any health insurance bill would have a profound effect on the health care system. While one cannot predict all the consequences of such a law, some at least seem immediately apparent. If any catastrophic health insurance is passed, it will surely relieve a relatively small number of families of overwhelming debt when faced with catastrophic illness. It will also guarantee providers their costs for such care. Since it is a mechanism that will operate only after sixty days of hospitalization or after $2,000 has been spent by the family, it will do nothing about prevention or early detection. While it may relieve anxiety and great financial distress to people and families in dire trouble, by its very design it can do little to promote or preserve the health of the population.

The second set of plans will preserve in large measure the same system of services that many families have now. It cannot do a great deal to enhance the health of the population. It will provide care for many families that are not now covered. It will secure for them a legal entitlement to insurance and potentially do away with a "means test" to determine eligibility. (Means tests determine financial eligibility for care.) Qualifications for entitlement in this plan will be uniform, since they are national throughout the country and for every citizen. These bills will provide for payment for care for larger numbers of people and probably will add stress and strain in the beginning, since the plan not only will call on more services, but will reimburse providers as they are reimbursed now. In that sense it may add to the crisis and, by the same token, assure that some aspects of the crisis be remedied.

The Kennedy-Corman bill is the only truly comprehensive bill. Because of its lack of deductibles and coinsurance, it will pay a larger percentage of the cost to families for medical care. (It is estimated that the current health insurance plans cover approximately one third of the average family's medical cost per year.) It also has built into its administration some cost-containment features, quality assurance mechanisms, and a carrot for the organization of group practice units. It deliberately seeks to begin to change certain aspects of the health care system and to provide care at every level without financial barrier. As with the passage of Titles XVIII and XIX of the Social Security Act in 1965, the passage of any health insurance law will have profound effects on the health care system.

Of all health-related laws so far passed, it can safely be said that the passage of a national health insurance law will probably have the most profound effect on the system and eventually on the health of the people.[2] The impact on the health care system would be enormous, but the effects on the general economy would be even more noticeable. Some claim that passage of a national health insurance law would throw us into irreversible inflation and that it would create opportunities for provider fraud which would surpass anything that has occurred with Medicare and Medicaid.

It is evident that the mounting spirit of social conservatism has considerably dampened Congress' already shaky enthusiasm for national health insurance, and it seems unlikely that any of the plans described above will be enacted in this decade.

SUMMARY

Looking at the crisis now, we can see that it exists within and without the health care system. Some aspects of the crisis have been brought about by the great successes of the United States as a country and by the successes of science and the health care system. We have only to look at the rise of the gross national product and the rise in spendable income, even though differentially distributed throughout the population, to know that this affluence has had a positive effect on the health and nutrition of the population. In the main, people in the United States are now better nourished, better housed, better clothed, better educated, and healthier than ever before. However, the gap between white and black has not lessened, neither has the gap between rich and poor (both black and white) in many significant areas. The result of our affluence and increased technology has altered not only the population structure but also the capacity to intervene when disease occurs. Remarkable strides have been made in the reduction of certain diseases (diarrhea, infectious diseases, and deficiency diseases). By virtue of this success, we must now be concerned with more chronic diseases, requiring long-lasting and continuous care. The changing population structure, the changing technology, and the changing profile of incidence and prevalence of disease in the population all interacting with each other have been cause and result of a health care system as we know it. It is characterized by rapid change and increasing expense. It has less effect on the health of the people than one might like or expect, given its technical and financial capability and the general level of health of the population.

There has been an attempt to alter federal, state, and local policies and fiscal positions, and new methods of delivering service, which can increase accessibility of that service, have been demonstrated. We have taken steps to produce new manpower, use traditional manpower differently, and create new roles and new professionals. There has also been an attempt to broaden the base of decision making by designating the community a partner in some of the decision-making processes. An introduction of legislated planning and peer review to ensure quality and a national health insurance scheme may lessen the financial barrier to good health care for all. We have created formidable capability and have not yet found the way to use it most effectively.

NOTES

1. Silver, George A.: Ordering social objectives, presented at the Annual Meeting of the American Public Health Association, Washington, D.C., Nov. 1, 1977.
2. Falk, I.S.: Proposals for national health insurance in the USA: origins and evolution, and some perceptions for the future, Milbank Memorial Fund Quarterly; Health and Society **55**(2):161-191, 1977.
3. Pepper, Anita G., and Menke, W.: Maternal care: its receipt and value for a population of primiparous women, unpublished doctoral dissertation, New Haven, Conn., Yale University.
4. Stevens, Rosemary: American medicine and the public interest, New Haven, Conn., 1971, Yale University Press.
5. Rosen, George: From medical police to social medicine, New York, 1974, Science History Publications.
6. Hacker, Louis: The shaping of American tradition, New York, 1974, Columbia University Press.
7. Brodeur, Paul: Expendable Americans, New York, 1974, Viking Press.
8. Schlesinger, E.R.: The Sheppard-Towner era: a prototype case study in federal-state relationships, American Journal of Public Health **57:**1034-1040, 1967.
9. Stevens, R., and Stevens, R.: Welfare medicine in America, New York, 1974, The Free Press.
10. Titmuss, Richard M.: Essays on ''the welfare state,'' London, 1960, Unwin University Books.

BIBLIOGRAPHY

Abel-Smith, Brian: History of the nursing profession, London, 1960, William Heinemann Ltd.

Alcott, Louisa May: Hospital sketches, New York, 1957, Sagamore Press.

Altmeyer, A.V.: The foramtive years of Social Security, Madison, Wis., 1966, University of Wisconsin Press.

Bremmer, R.H., editor: The United States Children's Bureau, 1912-1972, New York, 1974, Arno Press, Inc.

Brodeur, Paul: Expendable Americans, New York, 1974, The Viking Press, Inc.

Children's Defense Fund: Doctors and dollars are not enough, research project, Washington, D.C., 1976.

Coll, Blanche D.: Perspectives in social welfare: A history, Department of Health, Education, and Welfare, Washington, D.C., 1970, U.S. Government Printing Office.

Committee for the Costs of Medical Care: Medical care for the American people, U.S. Department of Health, Education and Welfare, Washington, D.C., 1970, U.S. Government Printing Office.

Falk, I.S.: Proposals for national health insurance in the USA: origins and evolution, and some perceptions for the future, Milbank Memorial Fund Quarterly; Health and Society **55**(2):161-191, 1977.

Gruenberg, Ernest M.: The failures of success, Milbank Memorial Fund Quarterly; Health and Society **55**(1):3-24, 1977.

Hacker, Louis: The shaping of American tradition, New York, 1947, Columbia University Press.

Harris, Richard: A sacred trust, London, 1965, Penguin Books Ltd.

Hirschfeld, D.S.: The last reform, Cambridge, Mass., 1970, Harvard University Press.

Illich, Ivan: Medical nemesis: The expropriation of health, New York, 1976, Pantheon Books, Inc.

Keniston, Kenneth, and the Carnegie Council on Children: All our children; the American family under pressure, New York, 1977, Harcourt Brace Jovanovich, Inc.

Knowles, J., editor: Doing better and feeling worse, New York, 1977, W.W. Norton & Co., Inc.

Mechanic, David: Ideology, medical technology and health care organization in modern nations, American Journal of Public Health **65**:241-244, March, 1975

Pepper, Anita G.: Maternal care: its receipt and value for a population of primiparous women, unpublished doctoral dissertation, New Haven, Conn., 1972, Yale University.

Pepper, Anita G., and Menke, W.: Maternal and infant health services in the United States, unpublished paper.

Rosen, George: A history of public health, New York, 1959, MD Publications.

Rosen, George: From medical police to social medicine, New York, 1974, Science History Publications.

Schlesinger, E.R.: The Sheppard-Towner era: a prototype case study in federal-state relationships, Journal of American Public Health **57:**1034-1040, 1967.

Silver, George A.: A spy in the house of medicine, Rockville, Md., 1976, Silver, George A.: Ordering social objectives, presented at the Annual Aspen Systems Corp.

Silver, George A.: Ordering social objectives, presented at the Annual Meeting of the American Public Health Association, Washington, D.C., November 1, 1977.

Stevens, Rosemary: American medicine and the public interest, New Haven, Conn., 1971, Yale University Press.

Stevens, R., and Stevens, R.: Welfare medicine in America, New York, 1974, The Free Press.

Titmuss, Richard M.: Essays on ''the welfare state,'' London, 1960, Unwin University Books.

3

AGENCIES

LAURA J. REILLY

Much is said and written today regarding the complexity of health care services, duplication of agency efforts, and gaps in the provision of services. Yet the nurse must be able to work with and within these community health agencies to assist in the solution of individual and community health problems. Thus an understanding of community health agencies is a prerequisite to effective participation in community health care.

Although community health agencies have several forms with different structures providing a variety of services, one common denominator serves as the framework for understanding how community health agencies work: the fact that each agency is an organization, an entity which can be described and analyzed. Building on this framework, different types of agencies can be discussed, and the role of nurses in community health agencies put into perspective.

COMMUNITY HEALTH AGENCIES AS ORGANIZATIONS

An organization can be described in a number of ways. It has been defined as a group of people working together toward a common goal. These are goals that could not be achieved alone or that are more effectively accomplished together. In the case of a health care institution, the goal is the well-being of the individual client and the community. Working together, the group of people can pool resources to accomplish this goal in greater measure than could each health care practitioner alone.

Etzioni[1,p.3] says that such organizations are characterized by the following:

(1) divisions of labor, power, and communication responsibilities . . . deliberately planned to enhance the realization of specific goals;
(2) the presence of one or more power centers which control the concerted efforts of the organization and direct them toward its goals; these power centers also must continuously review the organization's performance and re-pattern its structure, where necessary, to increase its efficiency;
(3) substitution of personnel. . . .

The problem with defining organizations in terms of their goals is the difficulty in finding out the exact nature of these goals. The organization may have a written charter or philosophy but, in fact, may have been sidetracked from these goals as attention was focused on the means to obtain them. If the leaders of the organization are asked, the goals of this group will be ascertained unless the interests of the leaders are in fact identical with the organization.[2] Another problem with the goal-oriented approach is the often idealistic nature of the goals as stated by the organization. The organization thereby becomes difficult to evaluate in terms of its goals because it may be functioning very effectively, meeting the community's needs, and yet be very far from reaching its goals.[1] The "high-level wellness" of many community health agencies is one such idealistic goal.

Realistically, the organization is more fully described as part of a system. Under general systems theory, resources are "inputs" into the organization, which processes them into "outputs." This occurs in an environment or set of conditions that affects the *inputs,* the organization, and the *outputs*. The resources, or inputs, of a health care organization include money, staff, clients, and equipment. An organization *processes* these into the service or product output, which in this instance is health care. The environment includes the technology that is available to the health care organization at any given time, the legislative or public commitment to health care that is translated to dollar commitment to the organization, the health care personnel pool from which the organization can select its members, and social demand for or acceptance of the organization's output: health care.[3]

Such a system is an open rather than a closed one because it interacts with the total environment context rather than insulating itself from the environmental situation or needs. Such an open system encourages ongoing exchange with the environment.

The system can be visualized as shown in Fig. 3-1. This diagram illustrates the reciprocal effects of the total system and provides the basis for the emphasis of the systems concept that (1) the organization needs to adapt to its environment in order to survive and (2) the focus of attention must be on the total cycle of inputs, processes, and outputs.[4]

An organization can also be described in terms of its components, remembering, of course, that it exists within the larger system. Any organization has structure, behavior, and processes. Structure is the component most often associated with organizations and refers to the stable, consistent, relatively constant relationships among jobs within the organization. The behavior within organizations includes individual, group, and leadership behavior. Processes occurring within an organization are communication and decision making. These components make up an internal system within the organization existing in reciprocating relationships.

Organizational structure

An organizational structure, created through an organizational design process, facilitates achievement of the organization's goals. This design process establishes the division of work into functions that can be designated by a job description. The process then groups jobs that can best be performed together into departmental units. Then it must be decided what leaders will control the departments as well as how many departments each will control. Finally, authority must be delegated to the various jobs, departments, and leaders. These components must be used in designing an effective organization.

JOB DESCRIPTION

The process of job description is ultimately one of division of work, or who will be accountable for what tasks. Division of the work among the organization's members allows them to concentrate on one type of function and thereby become proficient. Additionally, the division of labor permits specialization that facilitates rotation among those with the same specialization. The rotation of nurses through a position in community health well-child clinics is one such example. The process of describing a particular job requires analysis of what and how many functions and tasks the individual will be responsible to perform. This is commonly designated as the *range* of a job. A job description also requires thought as to the degree to which the individual will be allowed to alter the performance of the functions and tasks. This is referred to as the *depth* of a job. In other words, will the jobholder have any room for exercising decision making? This issue has often been raised by nurses when they are not given authority commensurate with the responsibilities entailed by the job. When

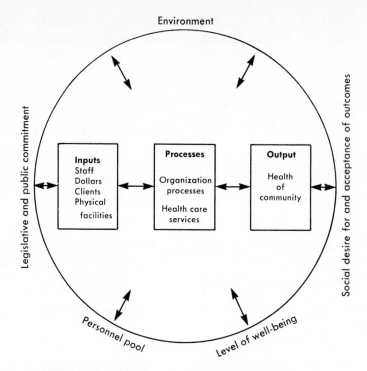

Fig. 3-1. Systems view of a community health organization.

analyzing the range, depth, functions, and tasks of a job, the following questions are relevant:

1. What are the philosophy and goals of the organization?
2. What level of training or education will be required for performance of the job?
3. What attitude does the organization have toward the staff members? Are they encouraged to be creative, innovative, and contribute to the organization's achievement of goals?
4. Are staff members given authority commensurate with their education and level of responsibility? Are their actions and decisions supported by their leaders?

Some staff members in an organization will have a few tasks to perform in a routine prescribed manner. These are the positions with the least depth and range. The position of a home health aide in a community health agency would be so limited. The aide would be given specific tasks to perform in a prescribed manner. Although the range or number of tasks might not be severely restricted, the aide would have no authority to deviate from the routine. The community health nurse, on the other hand, would usually be expected to perform a very broad number of functions such as community health assessments, well-child assessments, and home nursing care. The depth of the nurse's job, however, will vary from organization to organization, depending on its philosophy and leadership practices. It should be recalled, of course, that the job description of many health care professionals will be a function to some extent of the state licensure laws. The community health nurse cannot perform duties outside the scope of the nurse practice act.

DEPARTMENTALIZATION

Departments are organized by a number of different methods. One of the most traditional methods is by functional units. For example, a community health agency may have departments organized according to the functions of medicine, nursing, sanitary engineering, nutrition, and dentistry. Thus specialists are grouped together who can, theoretically, pool their common expertise to the advantage of the organization and of the community served. One of the problems with such units, however, is the lack of communication between departments and the development of loyalty to the department rather than to the total organization and its goals.

A type of department that alleviates some of the problems of functional units is the mixed department. This type consists of experts from the several specialties who work together to serve a given population. One section of a city might be served by a mixed department that is composed of one or more community health nurses, a nutritionist, a sanitary engineer, a social worker, and a health educator. This type of department, while perhaps losing the benefits of pooling the expertise of those in the same specialty, enhances cross-specialty communication. Working together, the experts can share their different perspectives when assessing community health problems, discussing alternative solutions, implementing a plan, and evaluating its effectiveness. This type of department also tends to avoid the duplication of efforts that occurs when specialists whose work may overlap are separated into different departments. This type of mixed department may also be referred to as a territorial department if it serves a specific area of a city, county, state, or country. An example might be a substation of a large, metropolitan health department that serves a defined section of the city. A territorial department could be organized as a functional department, described previously, if it is a large unit.

Another type of unit is a project department that is organized to accomplish a specific objective, such as controlling venereal disease. Usually such a department contains all personnel necessary for the project, although outside consultants may occasionally be required.

A mixed department or a department composed of functional units may be organized to meet the needs of one particular group. A community health agency with a maternal-child department would be such a unit, which may also be referred to as a client-oriented department.

These are the major types of departments. Perhaps the more important consideration is the criteria for determining this departmentalization. Following are some questions that can evoke information basic to such a determination[5]:

1. What are the philosophy and goals of the organization?
2. How can all expertise available to the organization be fully utilized?
3. How can duplication of effort be avoided?
4. How can communication within the organization be enhanced?
5. What jobs are similar or complementary?
6. Can control of the organization's service or product be enhanced by separation of the evaluation activities from those who are evaluated?
7. Can a better balance be achieved by the combination of formerly ''competitive'' jobs into the same department?
8. How will individual motivation be affected by the chosen style of departmentalization?

Another component of structure design is the number of departmental units that one person will control, including leader-subordinate interactions.[6] Several factors are involved in these interactions: the complexity of jobs, the amount of direction and control required, and the amount of personal contact necessary.[4] Community health nurses, for example, may be able to work relatively independently after their initial orientation; weekly conferences with a supervisor to discuss progress, any problems, and new ideas may be sufficient. Home health aides, on the other hand, will require a personal orientation to each new situation, an instance that decreases the number of staff members a supervisor could manage effectively.

AUTHORITY

The final component of an organization's structural design is the matter of authority. There are several types of authority: legitimate authority,

authority of competence, personal authority, and authority of position. Legitimate authority is derived from the employment relationship itself; that is, those who are subordinate have a duty to obey their superiors. The authority of competence is derived from a person's own technical knowledge and experience. The authority of position is the concern when establishing the design of the organization. It is the authority inherent in a particular position that may be altered according to the desires of the organization. This authority is delegated to the given position by the organization. The issue becomes one of centralization of authority. Should lower-level employees have the authority to make decisions without the approval of their superiors? Decentralization, or delegation of authority to lower levels of the structure, offers the following advantages[7]:

1. The increased speed at which a decision is made
2. A feeling of equality and a sense of fairness
3. The motivation and increased creativity of the decision makers as they become more autonomous
4. The increased pool of staff available to assume supervisory or other leadership roles.

However, decentralization has its problems. Those entrusted with decision-making power may need formal training. Those who must give up some authority when it is delegated may resist the delegation vigorously in an overt or covert fashion. Also the subordinate may resist the delegated authority because of an existing overload of work or as a result of low self-confidence.

ORGANIZATIONAL DESIGN

Thus the building blocks for structuring an organization are job descriptions, departmentalization, establishing span of control, and delegating authority. The larger issue then becomes how these are employed to design an effective, efficient structure for a specific organization. How does an organization go about structuring or restructuring to achieve the most efficient, effective entity possible? The traditional structures, most often found

in organization, are based on the classical or bureaucratic design theories. The classical design assumes that the more effective organization is characterized by division of work into specialized jobs, homogenous departments, narrow spans of control, and a fairly centralized seat of authority. There is a graded chain of superiors through whom all communications flow. According to the classical design theory, the desirable characteristics of any organization are order, stability, initiative, and esprit de corps. The bureaucratic design theory, similar in form, is intended to assure predictability of the behavior of the staff or employees of an organization.[4]

A simplified organizational chart for the traditional structure set up according to the classical or bureaucratic design is shown in Fig. 3-2. This demonstrates the hierarchy of superiors that continues down through the departments. Department 1 might be structured as shown in Fig. 3-3.

These two design theories have several inherent problems according to research. The rules and procedures necessary to procure such order, stability, or predictability of behavior may become more important than the organization's goals. Decisions become a routine matter of applying the appropriate policy, rule, or procedure.[8] The departmental goals

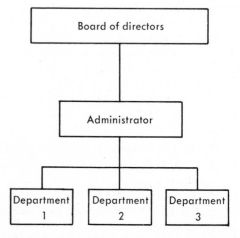

Fig. 3-2. Organizational chart for the traditional organization.

often become more important than the organization's overall goals when the minimal authority necessary is delegated. Competition arises between the departments in order to ensure the preservation of that authority and the department itself.[9] Finally, employees define acceptable work as the minimal level stated in the rules and procedures.[10]

Research has shown that *effective* organizations or subunits of organizations focus attention on endeavoring to create effective work groups with high performance goals. *Ineffective* organizations, in comparison, focus attention on the following[11]:

1. Breaking the total operation into simple component parts or tasks
2. Developing the best way to carry out these tasks
3. Hiring people with the appropriate skills to perform the tasks
4. Training people to perform the tasks according to the procedure book
5. Providing supervision to see that the tasks are performed according to procedure
6. Using monetary or bonus incentives

It is clear that the focus of the less effective organization is quite similar to that of the classical or bureaucratic organization.

Alternative design theories are available to assist the organization to achieve an effective, efficient structure. One was derived by Likert[11] from his research, which distinguished the effective organization from the less effective one. He states that there is an effectiveness continuum with a Systems 1, the classical design organization, at one extreme and a Systems 4, the effective organization, at the other extreme. The Systems 4 reflects the demands of its changing environment for greater recognition of the human potential of all employees. Some of these environmental conditions include a trend toward greater individual freedom and initiative; a trend toward higher education, resulting in higher expectations of job incumbents regarding responsibility, authority, and income; an emphasis on the growth of individuals into healthy, emotionally mature adults; and the development of diverse, complex technologies and highly specialized skills and professions.

The structure of a Systems 4 organization is based on the following principle[11,p.103]

The leadership and other processes of the organization must be such as to ensure a maximum probability that in all interactions and all relationships with the organization, each member will, in the light of his background, values, and expectations, view the experience as supportive and one which builds and maintains his sense of personal worth and importance.

This principle of supportive relationships leads Likert to the conclusion that management will fully

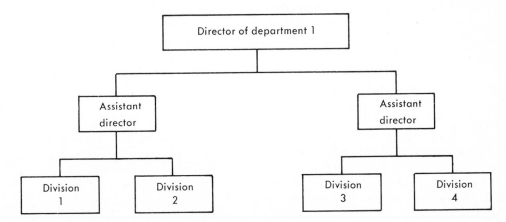

Fig. 3-3. Structure of department 1.

utilize the human potential of employees only when each employee is a member of one or more effectively functioning work *groups* that demonstrate group loyalty, effective interaction skills, and high performance goals. The emphasis in the structure of such an organization then becomes groups and overlapping groups.

While it could be argued that such a structure remains hierarchical in nature, the structural diagram attempts to illustrate the organization's emphasis on work groups rather than the chain of command with its span of control and authority concepts. Rigid hierarchical definitions are broken down so that communication, decision making, and control flow throughout the organization. The diagram also attempts to illustrate the impact of influence vertically and laterally within the organizational structure, conceptualizing different levels within the organization, not in terms of amount of authority, but rather in terms of coordinating or linking larger or smaller numbers of work groups.[11] The groups are still departments or sections of departments, and individual jobs are defined, but the structure is responsive to the changing environment noted before. One small group or section with expertise in a given area, for example, may be able to exert more influence on a decision than the department head. It is logical in an environment of highly specialized employees and professionals who are mature adults accustomed to thinking and acting on their own initiative that the structure which facilitates this will be more effective than one which thwarts such abilities.

Another form of organizational structure is called a *collegial design*. It would seem to be an extension of the group supportive relationship developed by Likert. The exception to Likert's model is the absence of a formal leader from the group. Such an organization or subunit of an organization would be diagrammed as shown in Fig. 3-4.

A collegial design is used with professional or scientific employees, since it depends on mutual contribution, self-direction, and control by the organization's members. They must work cooperatively to coordinate their activities to achieve the

organization's objectives. Such a design has limited uses.

The current trend in design of organization structures is toward contingency designs. That is, rather than one best way to design an organization, the structure must fit the situation.[4] *Either* a bureaucratic/classical or a Systems 4 design should be adopted, depending on the situation of the organization or of subunits within the organization. The environment of the organization is one of the most important factors to consider, as was suggested under the Systems theory description of an organization. If the environment is changing rapidly, if there is a great deal of resulting uncertainty about environmental conditions, and if the feedback to employees on the results of their decisions is prolonged, a Systems 4 type of structure is appropriate for the organization. If the converse situation is present, a bureaucratic structure is appropriate. Two departments within the same organization may have different environments requiring different structures. The personnel department of a large public health agency exists within a relatively stable environment. Technology and knowledge regarding selection and placement of personnel are not changing rapidly, and feedback to staff members regarding their decisions is relatively fast. Therefore, a classical/bureaucratic structure may be appropriate in such a task-oriented department. Regarding health care delivery, technology and knowledge are changing rapidly, while feedback to the staff regarding their decisions and actions is much longer. Therefore, a project department charged with delivery of certain health care services to the public would be an appropriate place for a Systems 4 structure.[4]

Of course, where there is more than one department, the work of all departments must be coordinated to achieve unity of effort for the overall organizatonal goals. Under contingency design theory, this varies with the situation. Integration of the departments should be, according to rules and procedures of a classical/bureaucratic nature, in a very stable environment. As it becomes less stable, plans are required; as it becomes highly unstable,

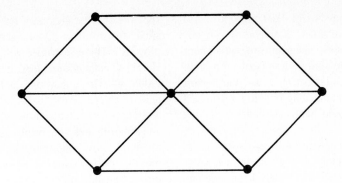

Fig. 3-4. Collegial organizational structure.

coordination by mutual adjustment is necessary.[4] In a community health department, integration of departments through the use of plans would usually be appropriate in recognition of the changing needs and demands of the community. However, in a disaster or epidemic situation, coordination by mutual adjustment would be necessary, requiring open communication throughout the organization.[4] Without it, the health agency could not respond adequately to the situation. A health care organization should recognize the potential for such situations and begin facilitation of communication between departments before the disaster occurs or it will risk the danger of responding too slowly.

Organizational behavior

Organizational behavior is somewhat a misnomer because it is not the behavior of the organization itself but of the people within the organization that is considered. Individual, group, and leadership behavior affects and is affected by the organization. Sometimes conflict exists between the goals of the organization and the needs of the individuals within that organization. For example, it occurs in hospitals that nurses want to provide quality care for the clients, which entails a certain number of nurses to provide that care. Hospital administration wants to keep its operating costs as low as possible, which implies hiring as few nurses as it can while still maintaining a margin of safety. A conflict thus exists between the nurses and hospital administration regarding the number of nurses required to provide quality client care—a concept that might also be disputed.

INDIVIDUAL BEHAVIOR

The individual is the basic component of the organization. Attitudes, needs, perceptions, and personality all affect the behavior pattern of any individual who becomes an organization member. Depending on how the organization perceives and influences the attributes, the performance of the individual can be altered toward a greater contribution to the organizational effort. These personal attributes and characteristics are relatively fixed behavior patterns in an adult. However, principles of learning can be employed to make behavioral characteristics work *for* a group of employees or an organization.

The concept of reinforcement maintains that when a positive reinforcement or reward is made contingent on the performance of a desired behavior, the probability of the appropriate behavior occurring or being repeated is increased. It is not an exact relationship between the reinforcement and the desired behavior because of other possible variables in the situation, peer pressure, for example. Of course, it is necessary that the reward follow the behavior closely in time. Positive reinforcement can also be used to extinguish undesirable behavior by failing to reward it and, at the same time, reinforcing the more desirable behavior. Negative reinforcement or punishment used to control undesirable behavior or cause it to extinguish has some serious drawbacks. The results of punishment are not as predictable and are less permanent than those of positive reinforcement. Also, the person receiving the punishment may develop a poor attitude or dislike for the person(s) and system administering it.[4]

Another important learning concept is feedback. In order for the person who wants to learn the desired behavior to know whether he is accomplishing his objective, the learner needs immediate and accurate feedback regarding his performance. Is it approximating the desired behavior? If not, why not, or how can the learner improve? Feedback allows the learner to correct any errors in performance; at the same time, it can be used to reinforce the desirable aspects of that performance.

Motivation is one of the central concepts in learning and, indeed, one of the most influential factors for determining anyone's behavior. Motivation is the driving force resulting from a person's desire to satisfy needs. These needs cause a physical or psychological tension, resulting in a search for ways of reducing the tension. If human needs are recognized, the appropriate motivators can be used by an organization to increase the individual's performance within the organization. That which motivates human behavior varies from individual to individual and from one period to another. Effective organizational motivators will be those which enable the employee to satisfy needs while at the same time contributing to the organization's achievement. The motivators will be rewards for a socially acceptable, indeed encouraged, mode of behavior that will reduce the tension accompanying unmet needs.

Human needs have been classified in several ways. Maslow arranged needs in a hierarchical order.[12] The reader is referred to the chapter on high risk families and situations for a description of Maslow's theory of needs.

Another theorist, Herzberg, looks at motivation of the organizational worker from a different perspective.[14] What factors, if not present in the work situation, result in dissatisfaction among the employees? These extrinsic job conditions, which Herzberg calls *dissatisfiers,* include salary, job security, working conditions, status, company policy and procedures, expertise of technical supervision, and quality of relationships with peers, superiors, and subordinates. According to Herzberg, there is a second set of conditions, *satisfiers,* which, if not present, do not cause great dissatisfaction but, if present, result in satisfaction and good performance by employees. These intrinsic conditions include achievement; recognition; responsiblity; advancement; interesting, challenging work; and the potential for growth. While this two-factor theory has been criticized for being a simplified view of the working person, it has implications for organizations. The dissatisfiers are conditions that are necessary to meet the primary needs of human beings and a few of the secondary needs as set forth by Maslow. The satisfiers allow people to meet their needs for self-actualization. Another writer has put this into a needs-path-goals framework that shows their relationship[15] (Table 3-1).

The organization must match appropriate goals, which can be used as positive reinforcers, to the individual's needs to influence the employee toward the desired behavior. Too often, however, employees, especially those in lower levels of an organizational hierarchy, are stereotyped and perceived as needing, wanting, and responsive to only one reward: money. The primary needs are, in fact, satisfied by economic remuneration, and, to some extent, it provides recognition and status. Most of the secondary needs, however, are satisfied from psychic and social experiences. These experiences can also be referred to as intrinsic motivators, which occur while the person is performing the work and motivate continuing good performance by the satisfaction they give. In contrast, extrinsic motivators occur after and/or away from work so that the person is motivated to get through the work in order to leave it and enjoy an extrinsic reward such as a retirement plan or a paid vacation.[16]

Table 3-1. Framework of motivation within an organization*

NEEDS	PATH USED BY EMPLOYEE TO OBTAIN GOAL	GOALS OF WORKER
Self-actualization Esteem and status	Excellent performance within organization	Job with potential for growth Responsibility Achievement Recognition
Social	Determined by group norms to be high or low performance	Good relationship with peers
Safety and security Basic physiological needs	Minimally acceptable performance	Salary, job security, working conditions, avoiding censure from superiors

*Modified from Miles, Raymond: Theories of management: implications for organizational behavior and development, New York, 1975, McGraw-Hill Book Co.

One company vice president[17] described how he convinced other company officials of this distinction:

I once refuted two of my "money solves everything" associates in a nasty but effective way. I asked them to pick up their checks at my office. As they took them, I remarked, "I want to tell you that you've been falling down in your work lately." In the shocked pause that followed, their own feelings were worth a thousand discussions.

The organization's leaders, therefore, must first have a goal or objective for the employee's behavior. Motivated behavior is directed toward some goal. The leader must also be empathetic in order to determine the employee's needs. Only then will the organizational interests be truly integrated with the workers's interests to gain a mutually satisfactory relationship.[12]

GROUP BEHAVIOR

Individuals work together in groups within any organization (Fig. 3-5). A group is defined as two or more individuals who interact in such a manner that the behavior or performance of one or more individuals is influenced by that of other members.[18] This influence occurs because of the roles, status, and structure of the group. These guide and control the behavior of the group members and

become an important element of an organization's achievements.

Two types of groups arise within organizations, formal and informal. The formal groups are made up of individuals who occupy certain positions within the organization. These groups may be either command groups or task groups. A command group is composed of a group of subordinates who are under the leadership of one individual. This type of group is specified on the organizational chart. The task group is composed of individuals who work together on a given task or project.

The informal groups are formed within organizations by individuals because of social needs. Interest groups that are task oriented are composed of individuals who attempt to accomplish a mutual objective that does not have to be related to organizational goals. Another type of informal group, the friendship group, forms because of the need to socialize.

Organizational members join or form groups to satisfy their needs. Social interaction, esteem, and security needs are satisfied by groups. Other factors also enter into the formation of groups. Physical proximity and the opportunities for contact between individuals are important factors, allowing members to exchange ideas and attitudes about the organization and other activities. Individuals who perceive themselves to be similar to others in

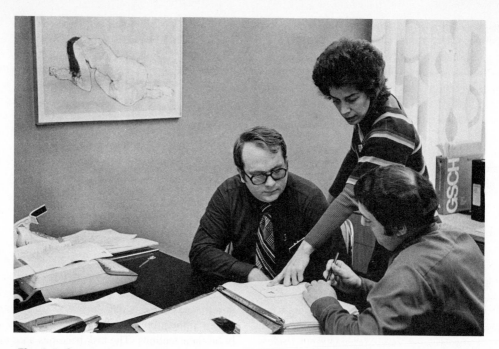

Fig. 3-5. Group process is the keystone of a community health agency. (Photograph by Jim Smith; courtesy Editorial Photocolor Archives, Inc., New York.)

perceptions, attitudes, performance abilities, and motivation are also encouraged to join that group. An individual may also be attracted to a group because of the group's goals and activities.

Groups have definite characteristics that assist the organization or staff member in understanding the behavior of the group.[4] Each group has a definite *structure* consisting of a pattern of relationships between members. Each group member occupies a position within the group depending on such factors as expertise, power, aggressiveness, and status. The positions vary in their importance to the group and their consequent status. Recall the neighborhood group of childhood and the important position occupied by one who was the best athlete. This member was assured status in this informal group because of the member's expertise in an area of interest to the group. Status may be ascribed to a person because of achievement, age, task assignment, or seniority. The status attached to a group member influences relationships and com-

munication within the group. Communication and attention is more often directed toward one who has a high status position within the group.

Groups also have norms that are standards of conduct or performance shared by group members. The norms are established for activities that are important to the group, for example, standards of poor performance of a group of nurses who are resistant to the policies of an organization against overtime. They may, however, apply to only a part of the group or may not be accepted by all group members to the same degree. Acceptance of the norms and conformity to the norms are influenced by group members' personalities. The more intelligent, nonauthoritarians are less likely to conform to a group norm. Relationships within the group also affect conformity to norms. This includes pressure exerted by the group, success of the group in achieving group goals, and the member's degree of identity with the group. Although conformity can result in a loss of individuality, it is necessary to sustain the group. Another possible side effect of conformity by group members is the establishment of poor or mediocre levels of performance so that one individual in the group does not outperform the others, forcing them to work harder or explain their poorer performances.

Group cohesiveness is another characteristic that may affect performance. Cohesiveness is the force that pulls on members to keep them within the group. It is a result of the group's attraction to the individual, which in turn depends on the extent to which the group satisfies an individual's needs. When a group member is attracted to the group, the member is motivated to conform to the group norms. Some possible positive effects of membership within a cohesive group include a lower nervous tension among cohesive group members, a feeling of supportiveness, and less anxiety about rules, procedures, and policies. If the group's cohesiveness has resulted in conformity to low standards of performance, the organizational leaders may need to consider modifying the group by replacing members of the group with other personnel or by emphasizing the group's task through use of incentives.[4]

Groups develop in definite patterns.[19] A problem-solving group, whether formal or informal, such as a project group in a community health agency, begins with a phase of mutual acceptance. During this phase, the group members experience a reluctance to communicate with each other. Once they become oriented to one another and achieve mutual acceptance, they communicate freely and move on to the phase of communication and decision making. During this phase, the group focuses on the problem-solving activity and the development of different strategies. The third phase is motivation and productivity designed to achieve the group's goals through cooperative efforts. Finally, the phase of control and organization is reached. The group membership is valued for itself, and controls or sanctions are applied to regulate the members.

Other groups, including those called sensitivity training groups, have two aspects of develop-

ment.[20] The first is the total pattern of interactions or development of group structure. This begins with a stage of testing and dependence. Group members attempt to define acceptable interactions. The group member is dependent on the group for guidance. The second stage is one of conflict within the group. There is little unified effort at this point. The group members then develop group cohesion and accept each other and their differences. Finally group members begin to take on functional roles within the group that enhance group achievements.

The second aspect of the small group interactions is task activity development, which is based on the assumption that any group, even if originally designed only to help people become aware or sensitive to each other's feelings, will ultimately become concerned with the accomplishment of a task.[20] One hypothesis on the concern of a small group with a task is the stress and frustration experienced by group members when they focus solely on their feelings. The task becomes an outlet or focal point for the group's activity around which they can examine feelings with less intensity. The four phases of task activity development begin with (1) orientation to the task as the group members attempt to identify the task and determine what is needed to accomplish it. Then the group members make (2) an emotional response to the demands of the task as a form of resistance. The emotional response is followed by (3) an exchange of relevant interpretation of the task including beliefs, attitudes, and opinions. These two phases offer the group an excellent opportunity to examine each other's ideas and feelings. Finally, (4) solutions begin to emerge as the group begins constructive activities to complete the task. When the organization is aware of the stage of development of a group, it can facilitate the group's completion of that phase. Orientation of members to each other in a newly formed project group could be catalyzed in a meeting or social situation prior to the introduction of the task to the group.

Groups within organizations are bound to come into conflict. Although it may be possible to ignore the problem for a while in hope that it resolves itself, the probability of such an occurrence is unlikely. Rather, use of a confrontation to minimize the conflict is more likely to be effective. Confrontation may take the form of negotiation between the groups. Of course, this requires compromise on the part of both groups. Confrontation may be used to find appropriate goals to which both groups can adhere. These goals must supersede the conflict between the groups.

Another form of confrontation is the interchange of personnel where possible in an effort to exchange viewpoints and thereby increase understanding and communication. The most frequent form and common interpretation of confrontation is the confrontation meeting. The conflicting groups are brought together to discuss their differences and opinions. This is intended to enhance intergroup understanding.[4] Confrontation, if it is to be productive and not hurtful to the individuals involved, requires a great deal of skill and practice in group dynamics. The organizational group that finds itself in conflict with another group would be well advised to seek the services of a professional experienced in helping groups resolve conflict.

Groups, in summary, attract new members for two reasons: (1) satisfaction of needs and (2) achievement of a task or goal. It is to the organization's benefit that the group member's satisfaction as a participant in the group is facilitated and the group's task or goal achieved. Task achievement is influenced by the individuals involved in the group; the environmental conditions of the group such as the organization, social context, location, and relationship with other groups; and the purpose for which the group is formed.

LEADERSHIP BEHAVIOR

Leadership is a role often assumed by or thrust on nurses. Effective leadership is necessary for the organization to accomplish its goals. Leadership is the ability to influence others to accomplish the desired objective "full speed ahead." Nurses should understand the elements of effective leadership rather than fear its burdens.

Leadership has been defined as an attempt to influence others through the communication process in order to accomplish some goal.[21] This requires power and acceptance by the "others." Power may stem from the leader's position and/or from the leader's personal attributes. Personal power is normative; it is based on manipulation of symbols of prestige and esteem and induces the greatest amount of commitment from followers. Positional power may be either normative, coercive, or utilitarian. Coercive power is control based on the application of physical means or means that ultimately threaten the person. Utilitarian power stems from material rewards granted to followers.[1]

The elements of successful leadership have been studied in a number of ways. Original studies focused on the traits of a leader.[22] Physical appearance, intelligence, and personality characteristics such as self-confidence, originality, and integrity were assumed to have a positive correlation with effective leadership. The studies showed, however, that there was no predictable pattern of traits from which one could identify a potentially effective leader.

Studies then began focusing on the interplay of personality and behavioral styles of leaders, that is, patterns that are consistently found with effective leadership. The White and Lippitt studies focused on the relationship between three styles of leadership and group behavior: authoritarian, democratic, and laissez-faire.[23] An authoritarian style of leadership is fairly self-explanatory. The leader insists, either benevolently or not, that subordinates behave as the leader wishes them to behave. A democratic leader, while still providing direction and coordination, permits and encourages subordinates to contribute to the running of the organization. Decisions are not solely in the hands of the leader. A laissez-faire leadership style implies that the leader leaves all operational and policy decisions to subordinates, functioning mainly as a consultant. White and Lippitt found that groups with authoritarian leadership were more aggressive and more passive. This took the form of scapegoating, aggressive outbursts, dependency or submissive behavior, and attention-getting behavior. The authoritarian groups were slightly more productive than the democratic groups in terms of task accomplishment. However, the democratic groups were more original, and a friendly atmosphere prevailed. The laissez-faire groups had very poor production as well as very poor membership satisfaction.

The personal behavior studies that followed revealed two distinct styles of leaders: (1) the job-, production-, or task-centered style and (2) the employee-centered, people-centered, or consideration style. The University of Michigan studies with Likert[11] were directed toward identifying characteristics of leadership of departments in an organization that are the most and least effective. These studies also showed two distinct styles of leadership existing that are called job-centered and employee-centered. The job-centered leader closely supervises subordinates, relying on coercive, legitimate, and utilitarian power. The employee-centered leader delegates decision making and attempts to assist subordinates in satisfying their needs and creating a supportive work environment. These studies could not show conclusively a causal relationship between leadership and productivity or satisfaction of employees, but did tend to show generally the following:

1. Supervisors who do more nonsupervisory tasks are less effective.
2. Having concern for a subordinate as a human being increases performance.
3. Delegating tasks to subordinates enhances their performance of these tasks.
4. The supervisor must assume an active rather than a passive role.[24]

The Ohio State studies, another personal-behavioral approach, examined two factors involved in leadership: initiating structure and consideration.[22] Initiating structure is the degree to which leaders will structure their roles and those of their subordinates toward achievement of a goal. Such leaders establish well-defined patterns of communication, set schedules, and make other plans toward goal accomplishment. Consideration is the extent to which a leader will establish job relationships that are characterized by mutual trust, warmth, rapport, respect, and open communication. Although this research can be criticized for its simplicity and

failure to control variables, it shows positive relationships between initiating structure and satisfaction among employees.[4]

Thus, these and other personal-behavioral studies tend to show that the job- or task-centered approach will work in a short-term situation. In fact, it is necessary to some degree to accomplish the organization's goals. However, if the employees of the organization and their needs for esteem, growth, recognition, belonging, and self-actualization are ignored over a long period, the result may be employee dissatisfaction that may be manifested by absenteeism, lowered productivity, and a high turnover rate.

Some critics of the personal-behavioral approach pointed out that these studies did not account for the situational variable such as the organization, task of the employees, and characteristics of the leaders themselves. This led to development of other theories to answer these criticisms, including the life-cycle theory of leadership and the contingency leadership model.

The life-cycle theory focuses on the level of maturity of the employee.[25] Maturity is defined in terms of motivation to achieve, education, experience, and willingness to accept responsibility. Those who are below average in maturity require more task-oriented leadership to direct their activities toward accomplishment according to the desired methods. The employee exhibiting an average level of maturity requires that the leader exhibit a balance of task-orientation and supportive relationships with the employee. As this employee becomes more mature, the leader must shift the balance toward an emphasis on relationships. Finally, as the employee exhibits above-average maturity, the leader can both implement a very low level of relationship and task-oriented behaviors and still be effective as a leader as the employee becomes self-directed and requires few controls.

The contingency leadership model developed by Fiedler[26] brings the work situational or organizational variables into the determination of what characterizes an effective leader. The results of Fiedler's studies suggest that the effectiveness of a given leadership style depends on the favorableness of the situation for the leader. Fiedler defined the following favorableness variables:

1. Affective leader-member relations. The relationship between leaders and group members determines to some extent the ability of the leader to influence the group toward the desired goal and the circumstances under which this can be done. This reflects the group's confidence, trust, and respect for the leader. A favorable situation exists, of course, when the leader is accepted by the group.

2. Task structure. An unstructured task situation with a leader who does not have any more knowledge than group members regarding how to accomplish the task results in a very unfavorable situation for the leader. The degree to which the task is structured is determined by the following:

    a. Goal clarity: the degree to which tasks and duties of a job are stated and clearly understood by the workers

    b. Goal-path multiplicity: the extent to which more than one procedure can be used to accomplish a goal

    c. Solution specificity: the degree to which there is more than one solution to a problem

3. Power inherent in the leadership position. The more power a leader has, the more favorable the situation is for the leader. Of course, the position power of a leader is determined to a large extent by the leader's ability to distribute rewards and punishments such as bonuses or promotions without the approval or consent of the leader's own boss. That is, does the leader have authority commensurate with the responsibilities?

If the sum total of these situational variables indicates either a very favorable situation for the leader or a very unfavorable one, a task- or job-oriented style of leadership is appropriate. If the situation favorableness is a medium or average one, the employee- or relationship-oriented style of leadership is more effective, according to Fiedler. Fiedler's theory adds an additional dimension or consideration to the problem of leadership effectiveness. That is, altering the situation by giving the leader more authority may be a better answer to increasing the effectiveness of leadership than

attempting to alter a leader's personality, behavior, or skills.

Thus leadership research offers no certain answer to "What is an effective leadership style?" Theorists do offer the two basic styles, job or task centered and employee or relationship centered, with acknowledgement by some that a situational variable exists.

Organizational processes

The structure of organizations and the behavior within organizations are influenced by, and, in turn, affect the ongoing processes of communication and decision making within an organization. Communication and decision making will be done by certain people depending on their position within the organizational structure and will be done in a certain way depending on the types of behavior that are encouraged within the organization. For example, according to traditional decision-making theory, those who occupy a position high in the organizational hierarchy will make broader policy decisions, whereas lower level–position occupants make more detailed decisions to implement the policy. Communication downward or upward within a traditional organization's hierarchy may be quite free, while horizontal communication is frustrated by the organizational structure. In designing an organization's structure, these processes must be considered in order to accommodate the most effective means of communicating and making decisions.

COMMUNICATION

Effective communication enables those involved to have a common understanding of a message. The childhood game "rumor" or "telephone" exemplifies all the errors that can and do occur if a message is not understood. Unfortunately, it is not always so amusing when it occurs in an organizational setting. Misunderstood policies or directives, a confused staff, and/or delayed work are just a few examples of the effects of poor communication.

Communication encounters certain barriers that

are common to many organizations. The organizational design often interferes with effective communication by increasing the route and number of people through which a message must pass. The efficiency of the communication is thus decreased substantially, as is possibly its effectiveness. This may be true in either upward or downward communication through many hierarchical levels, but it is also true of messages sent to another through horizontal communication. If a person must go through two, three, or four hierarchical levels before the message is sifted back downward to others in another department at the same horizontal level in the organization, the message usually loses its impact as well as increasing the time involved to produce a response and increasing the probability of garbling or even losing the message (Fig. 3-6). This barrier to horizontal communication created by organizations that are so highly structured is one impetus for the mixed department structural design.

Filtering and communication overload are other organizational barriers to effective, efficient communication. Filtering refers to a manipulation of information that is sent upward in a hierarchy so that it is perceived in a positive light. The subordinate who sends it does not want to be associated with negative messages. Communication overload occurs in most organizations because of the amount of information being constantly generated, both internally and externally. As a result, much of it is ignored.[4]

Messages are more acceptable and more likely to be accurately perceived if the receiver and the sender trust and respect each other.

Another cause of misunderstanding or garbled communication is the language symbols of the receiver and sender. If the language is highly technical, the receiver may not understand it. If the receiver does not understand it, rather than ask for clarification, the receiver may respond in any manner that the sender thinks is appropriate. The reasons for not asking for clarification are usually related to fears of appearing uneducated or incompetent. This is true whether the receiver is a subordinate or superior within the organization or is an outsider seeking assistance or information from the organization.[4]

Therefore, it is imperative that communication is recognized as an important process and is facilitated by the organization. It is important to ascertain that the message received is understood as the sender intended it. This can be done by employing a feedback mechanism. This may be difficult to establish, especially on an upward basis

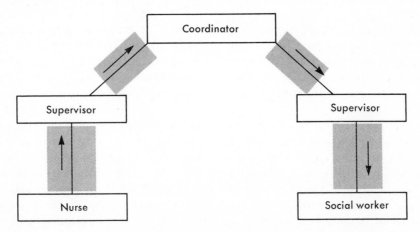

Fig. 3-6. Horizontal communication is forced to pass through five hierarchical levels in going from the nurse to the social worker. Shaded areas represent possibilities of losing or garbling the message.

in the hierarchy. Some suggestions to facilitate upward feedback (from subordinate to supervisor) include suggestion boxes, group meetings, and prescribed grievance procedures. Another useful device is planned supervisory conferences based on the issues and problems. The sender of any message should also attempt to empathize with the receiver. That is, how will the receiver interpret the message in light of the receiver's education, experience, values, and beliefs? An empathetic sender can attempt to structure any communication so it will be received and understood in the desired manner. Development of a trusting relationship with others, repetitive messages, and appropriate timing are other means to enhance communication.[4]

DECISION MAKING

The making of decisions is the process that enables the organization to attempt to achieve its desired goals. It is the means by which organizations solve problems and select from among several alternatives the solution they will implement. Some decisions are routine and repetitive; that is, every time a given situation occurs, the same decision is made and applied. Such decisions are codified in policy rules and procedure manuals. Other decisions are more unique or involve complex or technical matters and therefore cannot be made before the situation arises.

Nurses are familiar with decision making through the problem-solving process. Decision making first requires the identification of a problem. The problem must be distinguished from symptoms of the problem. In the instance of an organization, the symptom of a problem could be a high turnover rate among employees. The problem itself could be salaries, a supervisor, or the working environment, for example. The identification of the actual problem is an important step, since it will determine what type of alternatives will be considered as a possible solution.

Alternatives should be developed in light of the total system within which the organization operates. In a time of pressure from taxpayers to curb all government spending, for example, how realistic is it to develop an expensive new program for health education? Whether health education is carried on within existing programs with a minimal amount of additional expenses should be investigated as a possible alternative. Each alternative should be evaluated in light of *all* the goals and objectives of the organization to ensure that one goal is not being met at the expense of another. Additionally, as each alternative is discussed, it should be examined for the probability that the intended outcome will occur. That is, what is the *risk* that if a given alternative is implemented, it will not solve the problem but, rather, will result in another outcome?

Organizational decision making has another dimension that requires consideration. Should a given decision be made by an individual or by a group? In comparing the quality of group decision making to individual decision making, the following has been demonstrated:

1. Groups are generally superior in establishing objectives because of the collective knowledge available to them.
2. Groups are generally superior in the evaluation of alternatives, since their collective judgment incorporates a wider range of viewpoints.
3. A group is usually willing to accept more risk in making a decision than is an individual.[27]

There is an additional factor encouraging the use of group decision making: those who are involved in making a decision are usually more motivated in implementing it. Of course, group processes considerably increase the amount of time involved in reaching a decision. Also, group members are subject to peer pressures and position influences that affect their decision-making processes. Therefore, a balancing must be done between the variables that affect which style of decision-making process, group or individual, will be selected. These variables include (1) the quality of decision that is desired, (2) the extent to which subordinates or members of the group are or will be committed to a decision during its implementation, and (3) the amount of time in which a decision must be made.[28]

Vroom and Yetton[29] have developed a model to determine whether an individual leader, a group decision-making process, or a combination thereof should be selected based on the first two variables. The situation of a given problem or decision is considered in making this selection of the group or individual decision-making style. The Vroom and Yetton model employs seven rules to govern selection of the decision style. One or several of these rules might be applicable to a particular situation:

1. Information rule. If the quality of the decision is very important and the leader does not have enough information or expertise to make the decision alone, the individual or authoritarian style of decision making is eliminated as an alternative, since it could result in a low-quality decision. A group must provide input at least in the information-gathering stage.

2. Goal congruence rule. If the quality of a decision is important and the group members or the leader's subordinates are not motivated to attain organizational goals, then the group should not have the final determination of a solution. This prerogative should be reserved for the group leader to ensure that the organization's goals are adhered to, thereby enhancing the quality of the decision. This would be true in a more immature group.

3. Unstructured problem rule. If the quality of the decision is important but the leader cannot make the decision alone because it is not clear as to exactly what information is needed, where it is to be located, or how it can be found, the group method in which all work together to generate a solution is clearly indicated. It provides for collection of information in the most efficient manner. Of course, depending on other factors, leaders may or may not reserve the final determination of a solution to themselves. An example of such a problem might be the possibility of a new project for a community health agency. Although the agency's leaders may have some information such as the cost of any materials and staffing required, they would clearly benefit from the input of staff members regarding the agency's clients and the community's need for the project.

4. Acceptance rule. If acceptance of a decision and its implementation is of great importance, then any decision-making process by an individual is eliminated from the possible styles. The subordinates or group must participate to some extent in the decision. An example would be the determination of who from the current staff would be selected for permanent assignment to a new neighborhood health center.

5. Conflict rule. If acceptance of a decision is critical and there is likely to be some conflict over the final determination, then the group method is a necessity. Additionally, not only must all information be given to each group member so that he can contribute, but it must be done in a group setting to allow for interaction of all group members. Again, the final determination can be reserved for the group leader.

6. Fairness rule. If the quality of decision is not important at all, as in a staffing problem where all are equally qualified, and acceptance of the decision is very important, then the group is allowed to make the final selection of a solution.

7. Acceptance priority rule. If acceptance of a solution is the critical factor and subordinates are trusted, they are allowed to make the final determination of the solution to the problem.[29]

Of course, if time enters the organizational decision-making setting as a variable, the decision-making style may necessarily have to be altered to accommodate it.

Some methods have been used to enhance the group process in its decision-making capacity. The nominal group technique[30] is one such method in which a group meeting is structured so that the group members write their ideas on paper without speaking to each other. After a specified time (e.g., 5 minutes), each person in turn presents one idea, proceeding around the table enough times so that all ideas are presented. As each idea is related, it is not discussed, but rather, recorded. A discussion period follows during which each idea receives attention. Voting by the group members, individually in private, takes place to rank or choose an idea. The group decision thus becomes the idea receiving the greatest support.

NURSES AS ORGANIZATIONAL CHANGE AGENTS

The nurse as a change agent has been an overworked phrase in recent years, often without adequate definition of what is meant or what activity is to be engendered by the nurse. The change agent is used here with reference to facilitation of the processes of organizational development. Although organizational development is defined as a process of prepared management of change, this does not result in a circular definition of change agent. A measure of the success of the managerial process is found in the effectiveness of the organization's ability to facilitate the achievement and integration of organizational and individual goals and objectives.[4] The nurse as a staff member or in a leadership role will have many opportunities to contribute to or initiate organizational development, for example, as a staff member, as supervisor of a small group of workers, as a member or leader of a department, as director of a project or organization, or in a consulting capacity. It is important for the nurse to recognize opportunities to enhance the organization's effectiveness.

Before looking at organizational development, some attention should be given to the general concept of change. Change is difficult at best; it engenders a considerable amount of anxiety in those who experience it. Resistance to change is common and must be overcome. Unless the individuals involved have experienced a need for the change, it is not likely that they will be committed to the change processes or the desired outcome. The change agent must sell the proposed change. This means, initially, a knowledgeable change agent may have done considerable work to document the value of the proposed change. Organizational members need a mental picture of how the proposed change would improve their condition or the organizational function. The objectives for change

need to be specific, with small steps of tasks outlined that can be accomplished successfully to achieve the tasks.

The methods employed by the change agent are essentially those of problem solving: diagnosis, development of alternative methods of changing the organization, deciding on one alternative and implimenting it, and evaluating the impact of the alternatives on organizational effectiveness. The following list of organizational problems may help in clarification:

1. Inadequate programs for recruitment and selection of personnel.
2. A confused organizational structure results in waste and inefficient use of staff, time, and resources.
3. Inadequate control of personnel, money, resources, activities, etc. There can be too little control within an organization as well as too much.
4. Orientation or training too frequently limited by time and inappropriate methods. It should be planned carefully so as to meet the new employees' needs.
5. Low motivation of the staff results in a lack of committment to achievement of the goals and objectives of the organization.
6. Low creativity among all levels of the organization's staff. Good ideas of staff members must be encouraged and implemented to prevent stagnation.
7. Poor relationships among staff members prevent the staff from working together on a task or project as a team.
8. An unrealistic or inhumane philosophy.
9. Poor planning and management by the organization to adapt to the changing environment, whether technological, social, or legislative.
10. Unfair rewards for the staff members, such as lack of personal and monetary recognition, or punitive attitudes and practices toward staff members.
11. Unclear aims of the organization prevent staff members from becoming committed to the organization and from achieving the tasks nec-

essary to the accomplishment of these aims.[31]

The methods that can be considered as alternatives in making changes within the organization to solve the problem include those which concentrate on the formal structure of the organization and those which concentrate on the behavior and processes of an organization.

Structural methods affect in some way the formally designated relationships within the organizations, such as job definitions, departmentalization, or span of control. Management by objectives is one such method that has received considerable attention.[32] According to this method, objectives should be established by all those involved, supervisors and all staff members. Those involved should meet and discuss the goals of the organization and what objectives their department(s) can formulate to contribute to these goals, which are feasible, and then decide on those which will be implemented. This same group should meet at a later date to evaluate the objectives.

Another method for organizational development of the structural components is job enrichment. Job enrichment calls for the development of attitudes, skills, and behavior so that members begin to manage their own jobs and concomitantly satisfy their needs for achievement, recognition, and growth. Job enrichment may include an assessment of the job description and tasks assigned to each position to ascertain whether a change in the depth of the job is indicated to make the job more interesting and meaningful. Recall that job depth refers to the amount of authority or the amount of control over their jobs that job incumbents have. The intended outcome is enhancement of employee satisfaction, employee acceptance of responsibility for their jobs, and increased employee commitment to the goals of the organization.

Other methods that may be selected for organizational development are designed to develop the organizational processes, communication, and decision making through improvement of the employees' knowledge, skills, and attitudes. These methods include training of the organizational members for their own jobs, and familiarizing them with other organizational goals and objectives. This may be done on the job, as in orientation of a newly employed nurse to the policies and procedures of a program or clinic. Another on-the-job training method is rotation of staff through each other's positions. This facilitates understanding of others' roles, enhances communication, and facilitates replacement of a staff member who is absent from work.

Still other methods of organizational development are directed at changing individual, group, or leadership behaviors. Sensitivity training is the methodology in vogue, especially during the late 1960s and early 1970s. This method is intended to enable participants to become sensitized to their own feelings, their relationships with others, and to others feelings. Such a group requires a skilled leader who is very knowledgeable in this type of group activity. One of the major problems with sensitivity groups is that, although the organizational member who attends is sensitized, the organization is not and does not reinforce or, in some instances, even permit such behaviors.

Organizational development can be implemented by unilateral fiat from the agency or unit head, or through an entirely delegated approach with the entire organization (or unit thereof in which the change is planned) involved, or by employing an implementation plan that is somewhere between these two extremes. This might be thought of as coerced change, even though subordinates had given permission to superiors to institute this change.

At the other extreme, the delegated approach, the organization lacks control over proposed changes. Organizational involvement is necessary to control adherence to the goals and aims of the organization. Of course, methods such as sensitivity group training, wherein only group behaviors and attitudes are changed, are effective delegated styles.

The in-between approach, or the participative mode of implementation of organizational development requires hard work, staff and supervisors who are secure enough to listen to others and accept suggestions, and a sincere utilization of the method. For example, a group of home health aides may believe that the nursing director is merely trying to manipulate them into "more work" by presenting them with an opportunity to plan for change. They might believe that the change has already been planned and the participative approach is designed to get them to accept it. In an atmosphere of such distrust, the participative approach will never work effectively even if the correct motions are made.[4]

COMMUNITY HEALTH AGENCIES

The nurse, whether working in a hospital setting or in another type of health care setting, will have the opportunity to use the resources of innumerable community health agencies (Fig. 3-7). The nurse on a community health agency staff will also need to be aware of the availability of other agencies to which a client family may be referred. Agencies vary from one community to the next, but general types can be described. The effectiveness of any particular agency cannot be assessed in a vacuum. While some guidelines will be proffered, the nurse will have to analyze the particular agency with which she is working in light of nursing and organizational principles.

Community health agencies are usually categorized as official (governmental) and voluntary. This refers to the funding source for the agency, the official agency's source being a governmental body, and that of the voluntary agency coming from private sources such as subscriptions

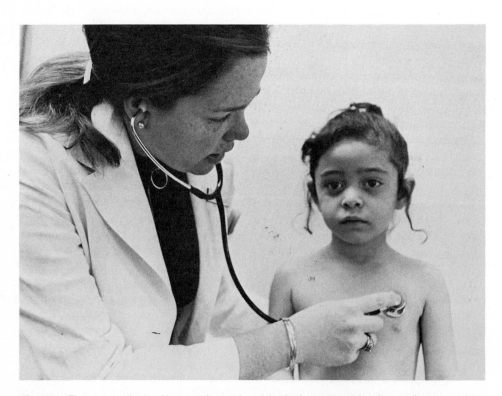

Fig. 3-7. The community health nurse is employed by both state and local agencies to provide nursing service to the client. Here a pediatric nurse practitioner gives primary care at a well-child conference. (Photograph by Eugene Luttenberg; courtesy Editorial Photocolor Archives, Inc., New York.)

of public contributions or grants from private groups.

Official community health agencies

Although the United States Constitution did not mention public health as an area of governmental concern or responsibility, the police power of the Constitution has been interpreted to allow federal and state legislation to protect the public health and safety. The development of the government's interest in public health has been from an economic standpoint as well as concern for the welfare of the citizenry.

The police power of both the Constitution and that of individual states has been interpreted such that various laws can be enacted to protect the public's health and safety. In one sense, official agencies were established to help enforce those laws, but as the country's social consciousness developed and changed, the focus of official agencies was enlarged to become beneficent as well as paternalistic.

LOCAL HEALTH DEPARTMENTS

The early nineteenth century ushered in a trend toward employment of a health officer that was attributable to the growing demand of an urbanizing population and governmental recognition of the relationship between strong industrial development and a healthy labor force. It was not until the late nineteenth and early twentieth century that working local health departments emerged. By 1966 there were 1,712 full-time official health agencies at the local level serving municipalities, counties, or some combination thereof. Only 4.6% of the U.S. population, or 9 million people, were not being served by a local health department.[33]

The American Public Health Association[34] has issued policy statements setting forth the fundamental responsibilities of a local health department as determining the health status and health needs of the people within its jurisdiction. Specific functions have been outlined by Hanlon[35]:

1. Recording and analysis of vital statistics such as morbidity records

2. Health education and information provided to the public individually, in groups, or en masse

3. Supervision and regulation of sources of illness or accidents such as protection of food supplies, regulation of housing, and regulation of water and sewage disposal

4. Provision of environmental services such as monitoring of air pollution or provision of rodent control

5. Administration of personal health services whether of a preventive, maintenance, or restorative nature

6. Operation of health clinics and other health facilities

7. Coordination of activities and resources of health care

The actual services offered by a local health department must be responsive to the needs of the population, those which are perceived and those which are not. In a suburban area this may mean more emphasis on maternal and child health programs, whereas emphasis on the needs of the elderly may be more appropriate in a particular rural area. The preventive, restorative, and maintenance services for tuberculosis were major programs for health departments in the past; epidemiological reality of today requires more emphasis on prevention and cure of venereal disease. The health implications of our environment are also receiving increased attention. These changing needs must be assessed and met with the appropriate services by a health department.

The organizational structure for local boards varies, usually according to the size of the population served, the fiscal commitment of local government to public health, and the philosophy of the agency's leaders. In a rural or small urban area the local health department is small and the structure correspondingly simple. The most simple organizational structure usually involves a board of health appointed by the governmental unit (mayor, city council, county board of supervisors, etc.) that employs a health officer qualified according to local and/or state standards. The health officer may in turn employ a staff of public health workers. Nurses are found in almost all local health departments. Other staff members who may be found in the smaller department are environmental health engineers, nutritionists, and a laboratory worker.

In the smaller local health department the simple organization allows for establishment of an easy flow of communication and a small group atmosphere (Fig. 3-8). The larger the health department, the more complex the resulting organizational structure. The department may be structured according to functions, projects, specialties, geographical distribution, or some combination thereof.

Limited evaluation efforts have been undertaken that substantiate the existence of some problems in local health departments as currently organized. One study, using a system analysis approach, showed that the more centralized health departments (i.e., organized along classical design structure or highly bureaucratic structure) were less productive, had higher costs per unit, were less innovative, and had a narrower program range.[36] It has also been shown in studies of health departments that the more reliance that is placed on for-

malized work procedures and on records of personnel performance, the lower the productivity and innovation of the department.[37] Much of the time, 54.46% in one study, is spent in local health departments strictly in administration, information processing, and transportation.[38] Local health departments should not exempt themselves from evaluation and necessary changes. Some of the problems facing health departments, other than organization structural matters, are the scarcity of qualified personnel; inadequate fiscal support for salaries, building, and equipment; duplication of services by other governmental health departments; and government health workers' failure to strike a leadership role in community health.[39] Today's fiscal exigencies and the heightened awareness of people as to the variety and quality of health services they should receive mandates evaluation of each department's effectiveness.

STATE HEALTH ORGANIZATIONS

Although all fifty states have a health department within the state government, they come in a variety of forms. Frequently part of the health care func-

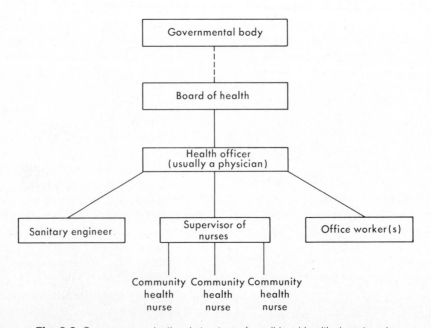

Fig. 3-8. Common organizational structure of small local health departments.

tion is provided by more than one department. According to Hanlon,[35] this variation is due to two principal factors: (1) the complexity of state government organization and (2) the extent of health services provided by the state.

The principal state health agency is usually charged with assisting local health agencies in the provision of services. This usually does not entail the provision of personal services, with a few noteworthy exceptions: the provision of diagnostic and rehabilitative crippled children's services, the equipping and staffing of mobile clinics for services to areas without local health departments that can provide them, and the provision of health education services. The activities of state health departments usually fall within administration, preventive health services, environmental health, local health services, and laboratories. In a report of the organizational charts of forty-nine states and the District of Columbia,[35] the following were the most frequent activities engaged in:

1. Maternal and child health (50)
2. Nursing (50)
3. Environmental health (50)
4. Health education (50)
5. Vital statistics (49)
6. Laboratories (47)
7. Dental health (46)
8. Communicable disease (45)
9. Tuberculosis control (43)
10. Local health services (42)

The organizational structure of state health departments varies widely, with some being strongly centralized, while others tend toward decentralization. The span of control of the state health department director tends to be limited to six or seven units.

Federal health programs

In 1953 Congress established the cabinet-level Department of Health, Education, and Welfare (DHEW). The department brought together a myriad of agencies that were intended to benefit the health of the nation, educational opportunity and development, and economic well-being. The health-supportive agencies ranged from the Public Health Service to the Maternal and Child Health Service (formerly the Children's Bureau). The extensive range of activities and programs had culminated in a complex and frequently revised organizational structure.[40] One of the organizational administrative problems had been the agencies that are within the DHEW yet were strongly independent by history, congressional and public support, and administration.[35]

Because of the organizational administrative problems, in 1980 the DHEW was divided into two cabinet-level departments: the Department of Education and the Department of Health and Human Services (DHHS). The latter department includes all those services formerly under the auspices of DHEW except those specific to education. The Public Health Service, which is directed by the Assistant Secretary of Health, is now within the DHHS. The following are in the Public Health Service:

1. The Health Services Administration (HSA), which provides community health services, Indian health services, and emergency medical services and is generally concerned with the quality of health service. The HSA also funds and administers grants to state and local health agencies, as well as private health organizations.
2. The Health Resources Administration (HRA), which is concerned with collection of vital statistics and the research and development of health services and manpower (including nursing).
3. The Food and Drug Administration (FDA), which is concerned with regulation of product safety, veterinary medicine, radiologic health, and biologics, in addition to promotion of purity in and accuracy of labeling of food and drugs.
4. The Centers for Disease Control (CDC), which is concerned with the epidemiology of disease, providing training programs and tropical disease programs, directing the National Institute for Occupational Safety and Health (NIOSH), and serving a clearinghouse for smoking and health.

5. The National Institutes of Health (NIH), which are responsible for biomedical research, housing the National Library of Medicine, and establishing biologic standards.
6. The Alcoholism, Drug Abuse, and Mental Health Administration (ADAMHA), which is responsible for research, public education, and training of professional personnel.

Aside from the DHHS, federal health programs are found in the Department of Agriculture through such activities as meat inspection and administration of the Insecticide Act. The Department of Agriculture also makes funds available for medical and dental care to low-income farm workers. The Department of the Interior regulates the safety and health aspects of mining.[35] The American Red Cross, while usually thought of as a voluntary agency, is a quasifederal program. The President of the United States serves as the president of the Red Cross, and it is the official disaster relief organization. In addition to the functions specified above, almost all federal agencies concerned with health operate information clearinghouses. These are tax-supported programs whose services are available free of charge to anyone. They will provide computer printouts of research and other literature pertinent to that agency's specific field.

Voluntary community health agencies

Voluntary community health agencies are abundant in the United States despite the financial recession of the early 1970s and some negative attitudes engendered by a few disclosures of excessive administrative costs that utilized a large percentage of contributions. However, the private sector continues to support a confusing complex of voluntary agencies. Hanlon[35] has categorized them into three groups: (1) those supported by public donations; (2) foundations financed by private philanthropy, such as the Carnegie Foundation or the Johnson Foundation; and (3) professional associations such as the American Nurses Association. The agencies of the first category are by far the most numerous. They include those which are concerned with the eradication of the causes and effects of specific diseases (e.g., the National Multiple Sclerosis Society), organizations that are concerned with the protection or preservation of certain organs of the body (e.g., the American Heart Association), agencies that are concerned with the health of a particular group (e.g., the National Health Association), and those which are concerned with a particular aspect of health (e.g., the Planned Parenthood Association).

The major voluntary community health agencies have a national organization that establishes national objectives, distributes funds, and supervises and guides the programs and activities of the state organizations. These offices, in turn, work with the local units in establishing objectives and programs. The unit organization chart of the American Cancer Society (Fig. 3-9) is an example of the type of local organization that may be established. Most communities have a directory of local health and welfare organizations available that will indicate the agencies' services.

The general categories of services provided by these agencies include the following[41]:
1. Education, both of the general public and professional training
2. Supplementation of individual and community services provided by official agencies, an excellent example being the Visiting Nurses Associations
3. Lobbying activities in local, state, and national legislative bodies on matters of health
4. Demonstration of the need for a particular service to induce the government to begin providing the service
5. Financial assistance to individuals or groups with health-related needs or projects
6. Research regarding preventive, restorative, and rehabilitative aspects of health problems
7. Analysis of community health needs
8. Coordination of community health services

In a study[42] conducted by a citizens' committee, the following problem areas among voluntary community health agencies were identified:
1. The need for stronger voluntary agency leadership requiring the establishment of person-

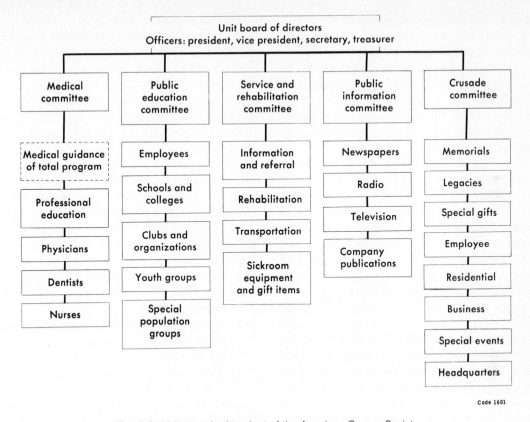

Fig. 3-9. Unit organization chart of the American Cancer Society.

nel standards, the recruitment and training of personnel, the provision of adequate salaries to retain qualified personnel, emphasis on development and evaluation of the agency program, and the setting of realistic agency goals

2. The need for higher standards for the local affiliates of national voluntary organizations requiring personnel standards, provision of advisory and consultative services, and coordination of public education and distribution of research funds at the national level

3. The need for increased participation in organized planning among agencies within a community to avoid wasteful duplication of effort and to fill existing gaps in services

4. The need for better reporting of programs and agency accomplishments to the public

5. The need for greater emphasis on research and the application of new knowledge

In evaluating the effectiveness of any agency, the citizens' committee suggested review of the following aspects of a voluntary organization in order to develop measurable criteria of effectiveness:

1. Are the organization's objectives stated in a pamphlet available to the public? Are these objectives reviewed and updated periodically?

2. Does the program agree with these objectives, serve a real need within the community, not duplicate services of other agencies, and measure up to accepted national standards?

3. Is the board membership representative of the community, the professionals, and any client population involved? Are the board members kept

informed about the agency activities?

4. Are the physical facilities accessible, adequate, and fiscally responsible?

5. Is the organizational structure clearly defined? Is it appropriate to the functions and goals of the agency? Are the job descriptions of staff and volunteers written? Is the size of the staff, professional and clerical, and staff case load within established guidelines?

6. Are the professional staff members qualified? Is staff performance evaluated according to objective criteria?

7. Is the budget available to the public in an accounting form that can be compared to similar agencies? Does the agency undergo annual audits?

8. In the area of community relationships, does the agency coordinate its efforts with those of other agencies, both official and voluntary?

Many voluntary agencies already conduct ongoing evaluation of themselves, especially since community councils and United Fund organizations require accountability of member agencies. These organizations enable the local voluntary organizations to conduct fund drives together in order to share the costs of such appeals. However, each agency must make available an accounting of its finances and services to the community. While this may establish quantity of services, it does not ensure quality, efficiency, or effectiveness. The agency must continue to develop effectiveness criteria to measure the organizational structure, behavior, and processes.

International health organizations

The World Health Organization (WHO) was established in 1948 in response to the need for coordination of health activities among nations. This was a continuation of previous global attempts to coordinate health-related activities in past generations. The atmosphere of cooperation after World War II and during the establishment of the United Nations facilitated the development of the WHO. It is a special organization within the United Nations and has a membership of 139 nations. The member nations contribute funds to the WHO,

which also receives funds from the United Nations Technical Assistance Board. The headquarters of the WHO are in Geneva, Switzerland, with several regional offices around the world (e.g., the American Health Organization in Washington, D.C.). The assembly, consisting of representatives of member nations, convenes each year to decide the direction of the WHO. The executive board, elected by the assembly, implements the programs and policies of the assembly and carries out the day-to-day activities of the WHO. In addition, programs are formulated and carried out by the regional offices appropriate for their particular areas.

Following are the functions of the World Health Organization[43]:

1. Direction and coordination of authority on international health work
2. Provision of technical assistance to member organizations
3. Assistance for nations to strengthen and improve their health services through advisory and consultative efforts

The major world health problems have been listed by member nations as (1) environmental deficiencies, (2) malaria, (3) tuberculosis, (4) malnutrition, (5) helminthiasis (caused by worm infections), (6) other communicable diseases, (7) chronic degenerative diseases, (8) accidents, (9) venereal diseases, and (10) mental illness.[44]

International health-related activities are also carried on by various governments in the form of training and financial and technical assistance. In addition, nongovernmental organizations, principally church related, carry out health-related activities throughout the world, rendering invaluable services.

SUMMARY

The community health nurse has a myriad of organizations on which to draw for assistance in solving the health problems of a population, group, or family. The services offered by these organizations vary widely, making a local directory of agencies or the agency itself the best resource as to types and availability of services within any given community. However, no directory will indicate the effectiveness of the agency as a community health organization. As a leader in community health or as a staff member of such an organization, the nurse should be able to evaluate organizational effectiveness and act as a change agent for development of the organization.

NOTES

1. Etzioni, Amitai: Modern organizations, Englewood Cliffs, N.J., 1964, Prentice-Hall, Inc.
2. Silverman, David: The theory of organizations, New York, 1971, Basic Books, Inc., Publishers.
3. Churchman, C. West: The systems approach, New York, 1968, Dell Publishing Co., Inc.
4. Gibson, James, et al.: Organizations: behavior, structure, processes, Dallas, 1976, Business Publications, Inc.
5. Dale, Ernest: The division of basic company activities. In Litterer, Joseph A., editor: Organizations: structure and behavior, New York, 1969, John Wiley & Sons, Inc.
6. Ouchi, William G., and Dowling, John B.: Defining the span of control, Administrative Science Quarterly, pp. 357-365, September, 1974.
7. Drucker, Peter: Decentralization. In Litterer, Joseph A., editor: Organizations, vol. 1. Structure and behavior, ed. 2, New York, 1969, John Wiley & Sons, Inc.
8. Merton, Robert K.: Bureaucratic structure and personality, Social Forces, pp. 560-568, 1940.
9. Selznick, Philip: TVA and the grass roots, Berkeley, 1949, University of California Press.
10. Gouldner, Alvin W.: Patterns of industrial bureaucracy, New York, 1954, The Free Press of Glencoe.
11. Likert, Rensis: New patterns of management, New York, 1961, McGraw-Hill Book Co.
12. Maslow, A.H.: A theory of human motivation, Psychological Review **50:**370-396, 1943.
13. Maslow, A.H.: Motivation and personality, ed. 2, New York, 1970, Harper & Row, Publishers.
14. Herzberg, Frederick, Mausner, B., and Synderman, B.: The motivation to work, New York, 1959, John Wiley & Sons, Inc.
15. Miles, Raymond: Theories of management: implications for organizational behavior and development, New York, 1975, McGraw-Hill Book Co.
16. Davis, Keith: Human relations at work: the dynamics of organizational behavior, New York, 1967, McGraw-Hill Book Co.
17. Krakauer, Daniel: Worker psychology: a formula that works, Factory Management and Maintenance, p. 226, August, 1953.
18. Shaw, Marvin E.: Group dynamics, New York, 1971, McGraw-Hill Book Co.
19. Bass, Bernard: Organizational psychology, Boston, 1965, Allyn & Bacon, Inc.
20. Tuckman, Bruce W.: Developmental sequence in small groups, Psychological Bulletin, pp. 384-399, June, 1965.
21. Fleishman, Edwin A.: Twenty years of consideration and structure. In Fleishman, Edwin A., and Hunt, James G., editors: Current developments in the study of leadership, Carbondale, Ill., 1973, Southern Illinois University Press.
22. Stogdell, Ralph M.: Handbook of leadership, New York, 1974, The Free Press.
23. White, Ralph, and Lippett, Ronald: Leader behavior and member reaction in three "social climates." In Dorwin, Cartwright, and Zanders, Alvin, editors: Group dynamics: research and theory, ed. 3, New York, 1968, Harper & Row, Publishers.
24. Miner, J.B.: The management of ineffective performance, NewYork, 1963, McGraw-Hill Book Co.
25. Hershey, Paul, and Blunehard, Kenneth: Management of organizational behavior, Englewood Cliffs, N.J., 1972, Prentice-Hall, Inc.
26. Fiedler, Fred: A theory of leadership effectiveness, New York, 1967, McGraw-Hill Book Co.
27. Harrison, E. Frank: The managerial decision making process, Boston, 1975, Houghton Mifflin Co.
28. Finch, Frederic, Jones, H., and Litterer, J.: Managing for organizational effectiveness: an experiential approach, New York, 1976, McGraw-Hill Book Co.
29. Vroom, Victor H.: A new look at managerial decision making, Organizational Dynamics **1**(4):66-80, 1973; and Vroom, Victor, and Yetton, Phillip: Leadership and decision making, Pittsburgh, 1973, University of Pittsburgh Press.
30. Delbecq, Andre L., Vande Ven, Andrew H., and Gustafson, David H.: Group techniques for program planning, Glenview, Ill., 1975, Scott, Foresman & Co.
31. Frances, Dave, and Woodcock, Mike: People at work, La Jolla, Calif., 1975, University Associates, Inc.
32. Drucker, Peter: The practice of management, New York, 1954, Harper & Brothers. Cited in Gibson, James, et al.: Organizations: behavior, structure, processes, Dallas, 1976, Business Publications, Inc.
33. Public Health Service: Organization and staffing for local health services, U.S. Department of Health, Education, and Welfare, Pub. No. 582, Washington, D.C., 1966, U.S. Government Printing Office.
34. The local health department—services and responsibilities, Washington, D.C., 1963, American Public Health Association. Cited In Hanlon, John J., and Pickett, George E.: Public health: Administration and practice, ed. 7, St. Louis, 1979, The C.V. Mosby Co.
35. Hanlon, John J., and Pickett, George E.: Public health : administration and practice, ed. 7, St. Louis. 1979, The C.V. Mosby Co.

36. Palumbo, D.J., et al.: A system analysis of local public health departments, American Journal of Public Health **59:**673-679, 1969.

37. Walker, B.: Environmental quality and the local health agency—a re-examination, American Journal of Public Health **63:**352-353, 1973.

38. McCandless, L.A.: Urban government and politics, New York, 1970, McGraw-Hill Book Co.

39. Smolensky, Jack, and Haar, Franklin: Principles of community health, Philadelphia, 1967, W.B. Saunders Co.

40. U.S. Department of Health, Education, and Welfare: A common thread of service—an historical guide to HEW, DHEW Pub. No. 73-45, Washington, D.C., 1973, U.S. Government Printing Office.

41. Gunn, S.M., and Platt, R.S.: Voluntary health agencies: an interpretative study, New York, 1945, The Ronald Press Co.

42. Hamlin, Robert: Voluntary health and welfare agencies in the United States, New York, 1961, The Schoolmaster's Press.

43. Division of Information: The World Health Organization, Geneva, 1967, The World Health Organization. Cited in Hanlon, John J. and Pickett, George E.: Public health: administration and practice, ed. 7, St. Louis, 1979, The C.V. Mosby Co.

44. The world health situation: major problems, WHO Chronicle **22:**11, January, 1968.

BIBLIOGRAPHY

Bass, Bernard: Organizational psychology, Boston, 1965, Allyn & Bacon, Inc.

Churchman, C. West: The systems approach, New York, 1968, Dell Publishing Co., Inc.

Dale, Ernest: The division of basic company activities. In Litterer, Joseph A., editor: Organizations, vol. 1. Structure and behavior, ed. 2, New York, 1969, John Wiley & Sons, Inc.

Davis, Keith: Human relations at work: the dynamics of organizational behavior, New York, 1967, McGraw-Hill Book Co.

Delbecq, Andre L., et al.: Group techniques for program planning, Glenview, Ill., 1975, Scott, Foresman & Co.

Etzioni, Amitai: Modern organizations, Englewood Cliffs, N.J., 1964, Prentice-Hall, Inc.

Fiedler, Fred: A theory of leadership effectiveness, New York, 1967, McGraw-Hill Book Co.

Finch, Frederic, et al.: Managing for organizational effectiveness: an experiential approach, New York, 1976, McGraw-Hill Book Co.

Fleishman, Edwin A.: Twenty years of consideration and structure. In Fleishman, Edwin A., and Hunt, James G., editors: Current developments in the study of leadership, Carbondale, Ill., 1973, Southern Illinois Univerisity Press.

Frances, Dave, and Woodcock, Mike: People at work, La Jolla, Calif., 1975, University Associates, Inc.

Gibson, James, et al.: Organizations: behavior, structure, processes, Dallas, 1976, Business Publications, Inc.

Gouldner, Alvin W.: Patterns of industrial bureaucracy, New York, 1954, The Free Press of Glencoe.

Gunn, S.M., and Platt, R.S.: Voluntary health agencies: an interpretative study, New York, 1945, The Ronald Press Co.

Hamlin, Robert: Voluntary health and welfare agencies in the United States, New York, 1961, The Schoolmaster's Press.

Hanlon, John J., and Pickett, George E.: Public health: administration and practice, ed. 7, St. Louis, 1979, The C.V. Mosby Co.

Harrison, E. Frank: The managerial decision making process, Boston, 1975, Houghton Mifflin Co.

Hershey, Paul, and Blunehard, Kenneth: Management of organizational behavior, Englewood Cliffs, N.J., 1972, Prentice-Hall, Inc.

Herzberg, Frederick, et al.: The motivation to work, New York, 1959, John Wiley & Sons, Inc.

Krakauer, Daniel: Worker psychology: a formula that works, Factory Management and Maintenance, p. 226, August, 1953.

Likert, Rensis: New patterns of management, New York, 1961, McGraw-Hill Book Co.

Maslow, Abraham H.: A theory of human motivation, Psychological review **50:**370-396, 1943.

McCandless, L.A.: Urban government and politics, New York, 1970, McGraw-Hill Book Co.

Merton, Robert K.: Bureaucratic structure and personality, Social Forces, 1940.

Miles, Raymond: Theories of management: implications for organizational behavior and development, New York, 1967, McGraw-Hill Book Co.

Miner, J.B.: The management of ineffective performance, New York, 1963, McGraw-Hill Book Co.

Ouchi, William G., and Dowling, John B.: Defining the span of control, Administrative Science Quarterly, pp. 357-365, September, 1974.

Palumbo, D.J., et al.: A system analysis of local public health departments, American Journal of Public Health **59:**63,1969.

Public Health Services: Organization and staffing for local health services, U.S. Department of Health, Education, and Welfare, Pub. No. 682, Washington, D.C., 1966, U.S. Government Printing Office.

Selznick, Philip: TVA and the grass roots, Berkeley, 1949, University of California Press.

Shaw, Marvin E.: Group dynamics, New York, 1971, McGraw-Hill Book Co.

Silverman, David: The theory of organizations, New York, 1971, Basic Books, Inc., Publishers.

Smolensky, Jack, and Haar, Franklin: Principles of community health, Philadelphia, 1967, W.B. Saunders Co.

Stogdell, Ralph M.: Handbook of leadership, New York, 1974, The Free Press.

Tuckman, Bruce W.: Developmental sequence in small groups, Psychological Bulletin, pp.384-399, June, 1965.

U.S. Department of Health, Education, and Welfare: A common thread of service—an historical guide to HEW, DHEW Pub. No. 73-45, Washington, D.C., 1973, U.S. Government Printing Office.

Vroom, Victor H.: A new look at managerial decision making, Organizational Dynamics 1(4):66-80, 1973.

Vroom, Victor H., and Vetton, Phillip: Leadership and decision making, Pittsburgh, 1973, University of Pittsburgh Press.

Walker, B.: Environmental quality and the local health agency—a re-examination, American Journal of Public Health 63:352-353, 1973.

White, Ralph, and Lippett, Ronald: Leader behavior and member reaction in three "social climates." In Dorwin, Cartwright, and Zanders, Alvin, editors: Group dynamics: research and theory, ed. 3, New York, 1968, Harper & Row, Publishers.

The world health situation: major problems, WHO Chronical 22:11, January, 1968.

4

MEMBERS OF THE COMMUNITY HEALTH TEAM

CONCEPT OF THE TEAM

Would it not be wonderful if the community health team were a well-defined entity? The fantasy comes to mind of a group of people, perhaps dressed in very official-looking blazers with emblems on the pockets, meeting each morning in an office with a coach handing out assigned duties, giving a short pep talk, and then the team members dispersing to stamp out poverty, illness, and misery in their own specialized and highly effective ways. What a pity real life is not like this.

There are few instances in which the community health team actually functions as a cohesive unit with all members under the direction of and responsible to the same person. In associating community health concepts with the word *team,* perhaps the dictionary definition ("a number of persons associated in some joint action, especially one of the sides in a game or contest"[1]) should not be taken too literally. Theoretically all those who are concerned with the community's health are engaged in a joint action to improve and maintain that health, but in reality there is often so much political squabbling, duplication of services, power struggling, buck passing, and "ego tripping" that it is a wonder that anything at all is accomplished. If one stands back far enough from the everyday machinery of the organizations involved in community health work, one *can* see a grand scheme: one can see the theoretical concepts being put into practice, and one can see the development of new concepts and ideas. It is just that we are so busy with the day-to-day activities of our jobs (and frequently complaining about other people not doing theirs!) that we don't take the time to stand back and look at what is happening.

If the team approach to community health is to work, there must be some basic factors operating. First, there must be a common goal, although it is understood that each group of health workers will have its own subgoals. The goal of the community health team should be the achievement of optimum health for all members of the community, and for methods to achieve that goal, the reader is referred to Chapter 3 on agencies. Second, the presence of professional people who have the skills necessary to achieve the goals is essential. Third, there must be a process of communication to plan and to evaluate the goals. These three necessary ingredients have separate functions, but they are all interdependent (Fig. 4-1), and none can exist without the other two. The professional health workers plan, implement, and evaluate the goals; without their skills there would be no way to achieve them. The communication process is the means by which the goals are formulated in the first place; without the process there would be no way to determine whether or not the plans had been implemented.

Discussion of the community health team is very

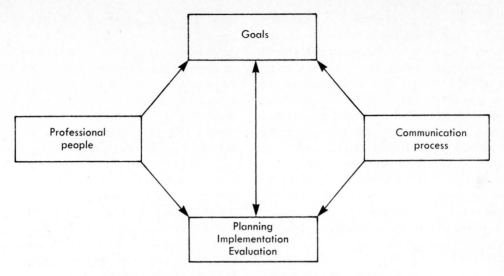

Fig. 4-1. Conceptual framework of the community health team.

much like the discussion of x-rays or airwaves. They exist; we see the results of their existence by looking at a radiograph or listening to the radio; we may even understand the physical principles of how they work. But they cannot be *seen* in action, so they seem amorphous and elusive, and we tend to dismiss them as some vague force in our lives that cannot be dealt with in a concrete way. So it is often with the community health team. We see the results of its action and know it exists in theory, but we do not see these people in their blazers ''doing their thing'' in a well-defined and precise manner. So the team concept tends to be dismissed by saying that it does not work, that bureaucratic red tape will prevent its ever working, or that whatever is done will not make it less elusive. This chapter will try to dispel some of these notions by discussing the community health team from a pragmatic view and by describing the functions of various team members, both in terms of their own professional skills and of how they function on the team and interact with other members.

Communication

There is a great deal of confusion on the part of all professional groups about the roles and func-tions of other professionals, and this has frequently led to decreased communication, lack of under-standing, jealousy, overlapping of service, gaps in service, and feelings of insecurity and threat, all with the result that the goals are not being met as completely or as efficiently as they should.

Rarely is there congruence between the way that a profession defines its functions and the way teammates perceive them. The interprofessional team has some-times been plagued by the false assumption that merely bringing members of different professions into proximity would enable them to work together. On the contrary, layers of ignorance and misunderstandings first need to be peeled away. Sometimes education into the attributes of another professional group dispels the difficulty, and sometimes a subtle difference of value or emphasis is responsible.[2,p.321]

It is very difficult to peel away these layers, and the sophistication of communicative ability needed is elusive indeed. It is the same kind of ability needed to make any human relationship work: a marriage, a friendship, or a professional relation-ship. It is really not the nature of the relationship that matters, it is the way in which it is approached. Probably the most important ingredient in effective communication with other team members is the ability to listen and to understand what the other person is trying to achieve *without* automatically becoming threatened by what we misinterpret to be our own goals and efforts. If we look at the multitude of health problems with which we are faced, it is easy to see that there is more than enough work to be done, but this does not seem to prevent us from being perpetually afraid that the next person's stated functions or goals will put us out of a job. This, quite naturally, creates resentment and jealousy and even the deliberate thwarting of other people's goals. Not only is this counterproductive, it is unprofessional and unethical. Creative listening, however, can be an antidote, and it can make one's daily functioning more pleasant and satisfying, although by itself it cannot solve health problems or create solutions to the factors that cause the problems. To make a conscious effort to clear one's mind and to really hear what another person is saying can lead to real learning. By learning about someone else's job function, the fear of threat to one's own job can be lessened, resulting in greater cooperation.

DEVELOPMENT OF THE TEAM

It is easier to discuss the *function* of a community health team than it is to discuss its *definition* because the former is definitive, palpable, and results in actual consequences. The latter exists only in the abstract except in very rare and isolated circumstances; therefore I shall let the reader extrapolate a definition of a community health team by assimilating and understanding its function. Community health teams are always interprofessional, and there are several trends in their development and function. The integrative approach means that there is shared responsibility for decision making, the leadership changes, and roles are flexible and interchangeable. Sometimes even role titles are nondescriptive; that is, all professionals are called community health workers and drop their titles of doctor, nurse, social worker, etc. Functions and roles are so flexible that it may be uncomfortable for many team members. Involvement of the client as a member of the team is a rather recent inno-

vation and will be discussed in detail later in the chapter. Teams are also beginning to evaluate themselves in terms of professional effectiveness and cost control. Many community health teams are experimenting with flexible leadership arrangements in which the team leader changes in response to differing needs of clients.

Kane[2] has listed several ingredients of competent teamwork, which are summarized here:

1. An understanding of group processes and the way they are used to achieve team goals. These processes include problem solving and principles of measurement and research design.

2. A knowledge of the nature of the various professions involved in the team, including the concepts of status, role identification, and power. Realizing the difference between the realities and expectations of role functions is essential.

3. Skills, both in one's own professional function and in the management of the group process, and the ability to participate in the setting, clarification, and meeting of goals set by the group.

4. The ability to communicate clearly and to be sensitive to the feelings and needs of others. This implies the ability to speak without the use of professional jargon and to be able to communicate effectively in writing.

5. Confidence in one's own professional ability and in the ability to function as a contributing member of the team. There must also be respect for other team members and for the fact that there is more than one way to reach a goal.

6. Acceptance of shared tasks *and* acceptance of the knowledge that there will be conflict. There must be willingness to participate in the working out of that conflict.

7. An attitude of research-mindedness and the desire to constantly search for new ways to solve problems and to meet clients' needs.

Administration of a community health team is a formidable task, and it is the function of the administrator (on many teams the person filling the role of administrator may change) to see that the goals of the team are met. This involves each member's merging with others while at the same time maintaining individuality in terms of talents and functions. Whether leadership responsibility shifts—and there is much controversy about the desirability of changing leadership—there *must* be a team leader. The leader's role may be more or less authoritarian, but there needs to be someone who can direct and coordinate the task at hand. Even on the most socially and functionally democratic teams, there needs to be one person who knows what everyone else is doing. In order to function effectively, a community health team must develop a sense of unity and cohesiveness, and this cannot be achieved and maintained without an effective, strong leader. A strong leader does not mean one with dictatorial power. It frequently takes greater strength of character to permit each team member to function in his most effective way than it does to directly control the activities of an individual. The administrator can also be the communications coordinator to promote dialogue among the team members.

A discussion of an interdisciplinary or interprofessional community health team with an administrator and several members functioning as a cohesive unit may be purely theoretical to most community health nurses. Their experience has likely been in a community nursing agency that functions autonomously but in friendly cooperation with other community health workers. Many community health nurses work mostly with other nurses (this has been expanded to include home health aides who are considered to be "nursing" personnel) and have little opportunity to practice the interprofessional team approach. This is not true for nurses who work in big city official health departments where there are many kinds of professional workers.

There are, however, increasing numbers of organizations in which the nurse can function as a member of an interprofessional community health team. Probably the best opportunity for the nurse is in a health maintenance organization, which was described in Chapter 1, because of its emphasis on primary health care, health maintenance, and the independent functioning of nursing. Community mental health centers are also an excellent opportunity for the nurse to function as an independent practitioner and to be part of an interprofessional team. Community mental health centers usually employ psychiatrists, psychologists, and psychiatric social workers, as well as nurse practitioners. There is usually emphasis on case discussion and the communication process among team members. They also usually work closely with other health agencies. The nurse who finds herself working for a *nursing* agency can still function as a member of a team and employ all the concepts of the team approach. The only difference will be a smaller variety of professionals with whom to work.

One of the most important concepts of the community health team is health education. It is important to acknowledge this function, but it often seems that the various members of the team become so involved with the specifics of their own function that they lose sight of the broader goal of health education for individuals, families, and communities. It is ironic to note that all professions concerned with the provision of health care and social services have education of clients as a professional goal and function, yet there is still a group of health professionals who devote themselves entirely to health education. The Committee on Professional Education of the American Public Health Association has listed the functions of a public health educator,[3] a short summary of which is presented here:

1. Determination of community health needs and analysis of factors that affect health action
2. Promotion and coordination of the health education activities of an agency and development of an overall plan for health education that is compatible with the general goals of the agency
3. Service as a technical consultant to staff and community groups; advice on education methodology
4. Liaison with other community groups that have health education programs

5. Organizing community groups for impending health services
6. Development and use of mass media for communication

Until recently the role and functions of a health educator were rather nebulous and differed little from profesisonal nurses and some social workers. In the past few years, however, health education has taken its place in the vastly increasing number of health occupations, and several universities offer baccalaureate and higher degrees in health education. Although education is still a vital part of the professional nurse's function, she can work in conjunction with the health educator to meet the health needs of the clients. Health education draws heavily on the principles of cultural anthropology, behavioral psychology, and sociology. Without a working knowledge of these social sciences, the health educator, nurse, or any other health worker will not be able to understand why different people have different needs and why they react in the variety of ways that they do when faced with health problems. Sociologists, psychologists, and anthropologists are frequently called in as consultants to health agencies when there is a problem that may require their expertise.

The concept of the community health team is still confused and confusing. With the proliferation of all kinds of new allied health professions and occupations, nursing is not certain exactly where it is going and what its place is in the general area of community health.

Indeed the concept of the health team remains, by and large, a figure of speech. The health professions resemble more a hierarchy than a team. Most doctors, and even nurses, are individual entrepreneurs, in work habits, even if not financially. The irony is that this individualism, instead of improving the patient-professional relationship, frequently makes a sound relationship impossible.*

It seems that some basic research needs to be done to assess the future of the community health

*Reprinted with permission from Health care in transition: directions for the future (p. 95), by Anne R. Somers, copyright 1971 by the Hospital and Educational Trust, 840 North Lake Shore Dr., Chicago, Ill. 60611.

team, and some questions need to be answered:
1. In what way shall the team be organized in order to achieve stated goals?
2. Under whose aegis will the team be? How will it be funded, and how will present lines of organization be shifted (or should they be changed at all?) to accommodate the various team members?
3. How will government and private agencies work together to achieve common goals?
4. What legislation will be necessary to achieve the goals?

MEMBERS OF THE TEAM
Clients and families

Clients[4] are the *most important* members of the health care team (Fig. 4-2). Without them there would be no reason for the team to exist. And without their active participation on the team, health care goals cannot be fully met. The concept of consumerism in the delivery of health care has been discussed in Chapter 1, and for all those reasons clients must participate in every decision regarding their care. All other members of the health team function for the sole purpose of serving these most important members, and teams that do not include the clients cannot possibly function effectively. It is ironic that of all the members of the team, the clients are the ones who do not know they are members. They probably have no idea that there is such a concept, and, if they did, they could not imagine themselves as the hub around which all the other members revolve (Fig. 4-3). It is the responsibility of the other members to inform clients of their importance, to explain the concept of the team and their function on it, and to help them take a position of active responsibility in their own behalf.

Clients may have to be taught behaviors so they can function as team members. They need essential knowledge about their own bodies so they can recognize malfunction, and they need to be made aware of various resources and facilities so they can do something about the malfunction. Just as the professional members of the health care team

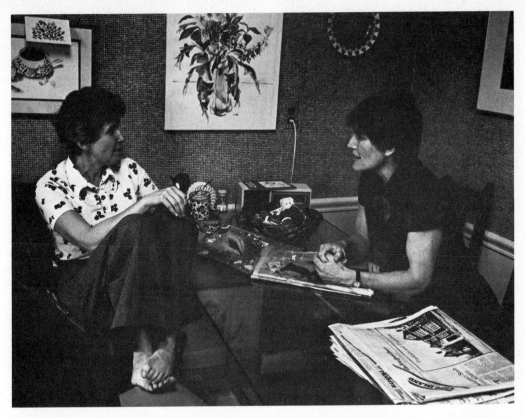

Fig. 4-2. The client is the most important member of the community health team and must be included in all phases of the nursing process. (Photograph by Ann Chwatsky; courtesy Editorial Photocolor Archives, Inc., New York.)

need to understand each other's roles and functions, so do the clients, perhaps more than any other members. They are usually the ones who are least likely to have a working knowledge of everyone else's functions and are consequently the most likely to have misinformation and misunderstandings. Clients must be encouraged to participate in dialogue with other team members, and, although it may sometimes not be practical or even desirable, to participate in team conferences and discussions. They should be encouraged to ask questions and to satisfy their curiosity about health matters. Above all, clients should participate in all the decisions that directly or indirectly affect their own health. This may include deciding what drugs they

will take, how many times a week they have physical therapy, which nurse will make home visits, or whether or not a grandmother will be placed in a nursing home. Without the client's participation in the decision-making process, the decision itself becomes professionally and ethically invalid.

Some people deliberately refuse to be considered as part of the orthodox health care team and turn to quackery for a variety of reasons. Cornacchia[5] lists some reasons for this:

1. People tend to underestimate the degree of illness or believe that they cannot afford health care.

2. Religious and spiritual beliefs may lead to

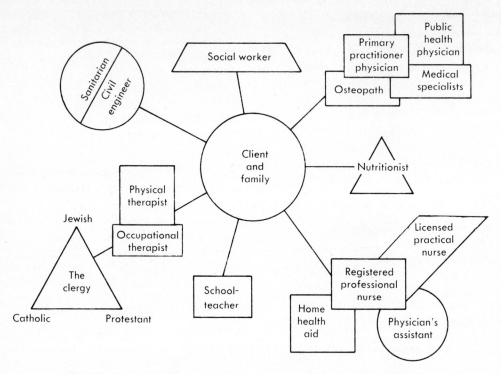

Fig. 4-3. The health care team showing the client and family as the focal point.

dependence on faith healers, magic, or sorcery.

3. There may be a language barrier.
4. People may distrust physicians and feel alienated from the health care system because of its depersonalization.
5. Pride and modesty or the fear of embarrassment about undressing in front of a physician may lead to fear of discussing problems that are perceived as being shameful.
6. People fear being told that they are very ill or may die.
7. The desire for easy, quick, or miraculous cures cannot be filled within the orthodox health care system.
8. Physicians are unable to relieve psychological problems, which comprise about 60% of all visits to general practitioners.
9. There is just plain ignorance about health matters.

Some of these people are known, in a peripheral way, to members of the health care team. They may be relatives of clients or they may even be former clients who have left the team for one reason or another. When a member of the health team sees a client or a potential client who refuses to join the team, he should be encouraged to do so. However, a dilemma is then created. Persons have the legal and moral right to refuse any and all health care, even if that refusal will eventually lead to their death. On the other hand, without the client there is no reason for the existence of other members of the health care team. Case finding is the responsibility of all health professionals, but they must also constantly guard against coercing the client to become a member of the team.

Physicians

It might seem superfluous to define the roles and functions of a physician to nurses and nursing students, but on the community health team the physician is not necessarily the leader, the administrator, or always the decision maker. The qualities that go into making excellent physicians or surgeons in private practice are not necessarily the same qualities that would make them function well as members of the community health team. In order for physicians to be happy, and consequently effective, on a community health team, they must be able to relinquish their notions of autonomy and authoritarianism. Physicians need the same empathetic and communicative skills as their fellow team members, and they must see themselves as peers in relation to the others. This is difficult for many physicians and is not the way they have been accustomed to practice. Physicians should be concerned primarily with health maintenance and primary health care. Those who cannot give up their disease-oriented philosophy might be happier in private practice with an occasional consultation on the community health team. They must have a dedication to the concepts of community health and in most instances must work for a fixed salary rather than the unlimited income of private practice.

Most of the physicians on the community health team are specialists in family practice or pediatrics, but all the medical specialities are represented at one time or another through consultation. Even as consultants, physicians should be chosen because they have a community-oriented approach to medical care and because they understand and applaud the goals of the community health team.

OSTEOPATHS

Osteopathy is becoming an increasingly recognized form of medical care; there are about 1,500 practitioners and seven schools of osteopathy in the United States.

Osteopathy originally expressed the theory that diseases were caused by interference with or malfunctioning of the nerves and the blood supply due to dislocation of small bones of the spine, called subluxations of the vertebrae. The pressure on the nerves and the blood vessels prevented the body from manufacturing its own curative agents, and, therefore the osteopath had to locate the subluxations and adjust them. Drugs, serums, vaccinations, electricity, hydrotherapy, and other practices were not recommended. Modern osteopaths still cling to the use of spinal adjustments but also utilize practically all the features of modern medicine. They attempt to use electrical treatment, water treatment, massage, anesthesia, drugs, and even surgery. In fact, osteopathy functions in terms of diagnosis and treatment much the same way physicians function with the exception of the spinal adjustments.[5,p.57]

Osteopaths are recognized and licensed in all states, and in many communities, particularly those near schools of osteopathy, they are almost fully integrated into the medical community. Many osteopaths, because of their emphasis on the holistic approach, seem to be inclined toward community health and would probably function well as members of the community health team.

PUBLIC HEALTH PRACTITIONERS

The physician who specializes in public health, occupational health, or preventive medicine occupies an important place on the team. Public health practice was established as an approved medical specialty in 1949 by the AMA through creation of the American Board of Preventive Medicine. Directors or principal officers in public health departments are traditionally physicians, even though many of their functions are administrative and not medical. The physician on the community health team is usually responsible for devising and enforcing sanitary laws and regulations, providing medical supervision and requesting specialist consultation services for the team, coordinating care with physicians in private practice, and often organizing and directing the various research projects being carried out by the team. The public health practitioner provides consultation in epidemiology and communicable disease control and is generally the person who decides whether a public health emergency exists. The physician shares responsibility with other team members for interpreting various health policies in the community and is frequently called to testify as an expert witness for legislative bodies.

Probably more important than the sum of the activities of the public health physician serving as the principal administrator of the health department is the impact of his acceptance as a leader on the public health team. Habit and the status conferred upon the physician make his philosophy, his breadth of vision, his capacity to work with and through others as well as his practical know-how in medical matters a tremendous force for community betterment.[6,p.118]

In many large organizations the public health physician may also be an epidemiologist (although an epidemiologist may more than likely have a doctorate in philosophy rather than one in medicine) who organizes and participates in epidemiological studies. But the public health physician does establish all medical policy for the team and may also serve as a medical consultant to public, private, and parochial schools.

Registered and licensed practical nurses
PROFESSIONAL NURSES

The functions of the professional nurse on the community health team are detailed in Chapter 6. The term professional nurse in this chapter and throughout the book indicates a nurse who practices in a professional manner (Fig. 4-4). Although most nurses working on a community health team are required to have or to be working on a baccalaureate degree, the professionalism of the nurse has more to do with the manner in which she practices than with the degrees she holds. There is great controversy and debate raging over who is a technical nurse and who is a professional nurse, what the responsibilities of each are, and in what areas each should be permitted to practice. It has been almost thirty years since Mildred Montag published *The Education of Nursing Technicians* in which the concept of the technical nurse was first detailed. Since then hundreds of associate-degree nursing programs in community colleges have graduated thousands of ''technical'' nurses, many of whom function in an exceptionally professional manner without having had any further formal nursing education. The American Nurses Association (ANA) has made an attempt to differentiate professional from technical nursing practice, and in 1965 they

published a position paper on the subject that sparked an even hotter debate. A summary[7] of the ANA's position on the function of a technical nurse follows:

1. Carries out nursing measures and medically delegated techniques with a high degree of skill using principles of physical and behavioral sciences
2. Evaluates the patient's immediate physical and emotional reactions to therapy and takes measures to alleviate distress; knows when to act and when to seek more expert guidance
3. Works with professional nurses in planning day-to-day care of patients; supervises other workers in the technical aspects of care
4. Practices in a manner that is unlimited in depth but limited in scope; must render care under the direction of professional nurses; education for technical practice requires attention to scientific laws and principles with emphasis on skill; the education is technically oriented and scientifically founded but not primarily concerned with evolving theory

Although this chapter will not concern itself with a refutation of the ANA's position, it seems that all the functions of a technical nurse can be carried out in such a manner as to give her practice of nursing the same professional integrity that a baccalaureate-prepared nurse brings to *her* practice. The educational preparation of a nurse does indeed make a difference in the scope and depth of nursing practice; the *manner* in which nursing is practiced should be the same, however, for all types of nurses. By ''manner of practice'' is meant the technical expertise and philosophical attitude that attends the performance of functions. If a nurse with a doctoral degree in nursing behaves in an automatic, unthinking, uncaring, and unintelligent manner, she cannot be said to be engaged in professional practice. If a technical nurse uses *all* her physical, intellectual, and emotional skills in the practice of nursing, it might be said that she is functioning in a professional manner.

Education is designed to prepare nurses on two distinct levels: technical and professional. This may or may not be as it should be; it surely is the

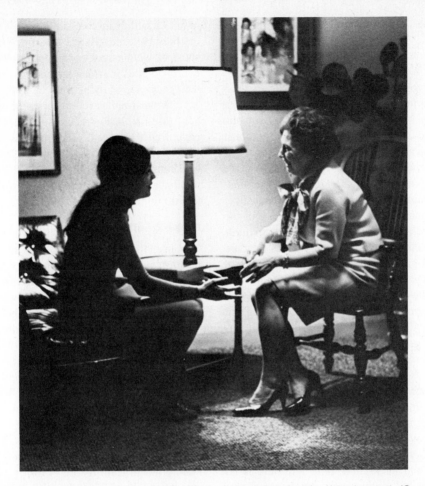

Fig. 4-4. Professional nursing function is a behavior, not an educational background. (Courtesy Editorial Photocolor Archives, Inc., New York.)

cause of much of the divisiveness in nursing education and nursing administration. It is not within the scope of this chapter to discuss the direction in which nursing education should be headed; however, all teachers of nursing have met students who are in the "wrong" program and most likely will not function in the role for which they were educated. For instance, some students in community colleges demonstrate an ability to do *professional* nursing and will practice as professionals, even though their job description and education label them as "technical." The converse is also true; some baccalaureate students will never develop be-

yond the task-oriented approach of technical nursing, no matter how much education they obtain. There *is* a difference in the amount and kind of knowledge held by various practitioners, just as there is a difference between the amount and kind of knowledge held by nurses and physicians, but this does not mean that physicians are professionals and nurses are technicians (although many physicians cannot be convinced of this!). The difference between technical and professional practice can be discussed and debated endlessly, but the purpose of this chapter is to distinguish between professional and licensed *practical* or vocational nurses in their roles and functions on the community health team.

PRACTICAL NURSES

Practical/vocational nurses (LPNs) are increasingly able to find a place on the community health team. Many health problems do not require the expertise and depth of knowledge of a professional nurse. Practical nurses have been trained for a year in a program that is licensed by the state and are then eligible to take the state licensing examination. The training combines theory and practice, and the emphasis is on direct physical care of the client. There are few treatments and procedures that LPNs cannot do, and in many states they are permitted to give medications. The LPN may not have the range of knowledge in the behavioral sciences that the RN does, neither does she have a strong background in the physical sciences. But she is as much a thinking, feeling, and caring human being as an RN and thus is as qualified to relate to clients on a humanistic level. So many clients have health needs requiring a home visit from someone who can perform physical tasks while providing human companionship, a warm hand to hold, a person to share a cup of tea with, and some conversation in an otherwise lonely day. Not every client needs the sophisticated talents of the professional nurse, and, although there is no such thing as a "routine case," there are clients whose needs are less complex than others.

An example might be an elderly person living alone who has severe arthritis and who needs a visit three or four times a week to help with bathing and meal preparation and perhaps an injection of vitamin B_{12}. This is an ideal client for the LPN to work with. She can be a source of physical assistance and good company, and she can make an ongoing assessment of the client's situation and discuss it with the professional nurse who might want to visit the client herself every other month or so for a professional evaluation. Most nursing service agencies who have hired LPNs find them to be an important and valuable addition to the team, and they have a definite role on the community health team that is not nearly as limited as has been believed. Many LPNs are mature women, some of whom were born and raised in the same neighborhoods in which they now work, who have the experience of living that can never be matched by a 23-year-old professional nurse whose entire adult life has been spent on a college campus. I have seen so many health problems solved, or at least alleviated, by the application of a combination of common sense and life experiences that there is no doubt that the practical nurse is essential to the functioning of the community health team.

Home health aides

Many home health aides on the community health team are recruited from the neighborhoods in which they live and work. They are almost all women, many with grown or growing children, and many have known for years the clients they are serving. They can serve as a link between the client and the health establishment, making it seem more familiar and less fearful. Sometimes the home health aide knows more about a client's or a family's problems than anyone else on the team. This could be because she knows the family or because she has encountered the same problem before in her own or her friends' experiences. It sometimes happens that the professional members of the community health team ignore or disregard the observations or suggestions of the home health aide. It may be that the aide is not able to discuss the problem in as "professional" or abstract a manner as other people, but to ignore her years of experience is not only unprofessional, it is silly and self-defeating. A professional often looks at a health problem in terms of what the ideal should be and is not. An aide, who has been there herself, often looks at the same problem in terms of why things are the way they are. Because of this, it is frequently the aide who comes up with the most practical suggestions for solving the problem.

Training for the home health aide has usually been on the job and is geared toward the particular agency in which she is employed. There has recently been a move to train aides in various manpower development training programs and vocational schools. The training programs take about two months, and a certificate is given on successful completion. There are various commercial "schools" in large cities that charge tuition for home and hospital aide programs and then often do not follow through on promises to guarantee the graduate a job. Home health aide courses often include, although in a very superficial way, such topics as concepts of wellness and illness, community health resources, emotional aspects of illness, the functions of other members of the health team, responsibilities, ethical and legal aspects of the job, nutrition, how to deal with emergencies and routine first aid, religious needs of the client, communication techniques, and recording and reporting. There is, of course, a practicum in which the health aide learns such tasks as measuring vital signs, bed making, general home care (not housecleaning) of "sickroom" supplies, bed baths, enemas, and the use of body mechanics in the transfer of clients to bed, chair, and back again.

The home health aide works under the leadership and supervision of the nurse but not necessarily under her constant surveillance. The primary function of the home health aide is to make home visits and perform needed physical nursing tasks. Her actual function, however, goes far beyond this. She is often a source of companionship for people living alone and sometimes is their only human connection with the outside world. Human warmth and compassion are characteristics essential to the successful functioning of a home health aide.[8]

Homemakers are becoming an increasingly important part of the health care team; they are on the staffs of many voluntary and proprietary home health agencies. The homemaker performs no physical nursing tasks but rather helps the client with maintenance of the home; this includes many housekeeping tasks as well as cooking. As with the home health aide, one of the most important functions the homemaker performs is a psychoemotional one: just being there is often the greatest comfort of all.

The clergy

The role and function of members of the clergy on the community health team may not be obvious at first. They often seem far removed from community health problems, and most people picture priests, ministers, and rabbis as being either concerned with exalted matters of theology or with mundane problems of church/synagogue administration. The clergy become part of the community health team as it relates to clients on an individual basis, and the clergyman can become an essential and integral part of healt care. In this time of rapidly dwindling church/synagogue attendance and growing cynicism about the tenets and functions of organized religion, many clients hesitate to admit that they have religious needs. Perhaps they feel the admission will be met with derision, or, if not, there is nothing that will or can be done to meet their needs. This is, of course, not true, but clients will not know unless they ask. Very often also, the nurse or other member of the community health team will not think to ask clients whether there are religious or spiritual needs they would like met. If religion does not play a central role in one's own life, it can be difficult to understand how it can be important to another person. And because religion is so personal, it is often not discussed. There are thousands of people who will freely discuss their sex lives but who will blanch at the prospect of sharing their religious beliefs with others.

Although clergymen are considered to be part of the community health team, their function is more consultative than full time. Their service probably can be used on a continuing basis, and it is likely that they could be of even greater service than they already are.

The functions of the clergy have changed since biblical days when religious leaders were not expected to do much more than to keep their human flock from straying off the path of moral righteousness. The roles and function of most clergymen do not vary much from religion to religion. Administrative headaches remain the same whether the sanctuary is graced by a cross, a crucifix, or a Star of David. Budgets need to be balanced whether the money comes from Rome, Sunday collection plates, or Rosh Hashanah pledge cards. A clergyman's function can be divided roughly into four categories:

1. *Religious.* He is responsible for setting religious, moral, and ethical policies for his congregation or for carrying out such directions from his church superiors. He is usually the final arbitrator of religious dilemmas, and it is to him that the congregants go for answers to questions of a religious nature. In most religions it is the clergyman who explains and interprets God's will to the rest of us. He is also responsible for organizing and officiating at religious ceremonies: regular prayer services, weddings, funerals, and special services.

2. *Administrative.* The clergyman is responsible for running the physical aspect of the church/synagogue, although he usually has secular help in this area. He must keep the congregation fiscally sound, keep the physical plant maintained and operative, administer the religious school and adult education department, and organize or give approval to the many social activities that are so much a part of organized religion.

3. *Psychological.* The clergyman is a counselor, listening to the problems of his congregants, some of which are very involved. Most schools of theology require a strong base in the behavioral sciences, especially psychology, and have special courses in marriage counseling and even rudimentary psychotherapy. Some congregations even have discussion groups for problems that have no basis in religion and that are led by the clergyman. Visiting the sick, either in hospital or at home, is also an important function.

4. *Public relations.* The clergyman has the task of explaining his religion's beliefs to the rest of the world. In some religions this includes proselytizing. It is the clergyman who must participate in Brotherhood Week activities, interfaith conferences, and the like. He is the spokesman for his religion and for his congregation.

The clergyman's function on the community health team has to do primarily with his counseling skills. Many people, especially older ones, feel more comfortable discussing their problems with a clergyman rather than with a psychiatrist or a psychologist. Somehow the negative aura of mental illness is not present. People who are confined to their home or to the hospital often take great comfort in being visited by the clergy, and those who have a terminal illness frequently find their interest in religion either rekindled or sparked for the first time and need to talk to a clergyman about their feelings and fears.

Many health professionals feel uncomfortable in the presence of the clergy. Perhaps we fantasize that they have the answers to questions that have been plaguing us for so long. Perhaps it is the old religion-versus-science issue. Perhaps we feel that religion no longer has much of a place in modern life. Perhaps we are reminded of uncomfortable or unpleasant childhood experiences. Perhaps we see the clergy as authority figures who are closer than we are to God, the ultimate authority figure. But whatever our discomfort, we must put it aside because the clergyman has a definite and useful function on the community health team.

Schoolteachers

The role of teachers, in both elementary and secondary schools, is primarily twofold. They are sources of referral to other members of the team and providers of health information to their students.

Information about health problems among schoolchildren usually come to the attention of the community health team from teachers through the parents. Children are often sent home from school ill and then are brought in for treatment, or the teacher recognized or sensed some health problem and requested a conference with the parent. Teachers, if they are observant and if they know what to look for, can spot all kinds of health problems: hearing and visual impairments, musculoskeletal dysfunction, emotional disturbances, and various communicable diseases. The critical element, however, is for the teachers to know what they are looking for. Teachers usually have no formal training in recognizing health problems and may not consider themselves to be a part of the community health team; in fact they may not even know that the concept exists. It is up to other members of the team to draw the teachers into their circle and to introduce them to the principles of health maintenance and primary prevention. The school nurse is in the best position to do this, but many schools do not have a nurse at all or are forced to share nursing time with a number of other schools. So the community nurse is probably the next person most likely to recruit the teacher for community health team activities. If a health problem has been referred to the team by a parent by way of the teacher, the community nurse should go back to the original referring source to gather data; it is in this way that initial contact is made. Teacher can also become part of the community health team through their association with school physicians.

Once teachers are part of the team, it is not difficult for them to learn how to recognize health problems and to take appropriate action. They can also learn to incorporate health concepts into the subjects they teach. Health maintenance may not be very applicable to algebra or geometry, but studying the health care system is certainly very pertinent to social studies, civics, history, and high school economics. Biology eventually emerges from the realm of amoebas and frogs to human biological systems; the maintenance of these systems is the next logical step. All teachers are required to devote a certain portion of their time to curriculum development and planning. Health-oriented teachers will do their best to integrate as many health concepts as they can into the general curriculum. Schoolchildren, particularly younger ones, are often impressionable, and sometimes they look up to their teachers as sources of wisdom and knowledge. Teachers can capitalize on these attitudes by inculcating as many positive health habits as they can.

The nature of teachers' relationship with parents is very different from that of other members of the health team. They are authority figures, it is true, but not about health matters, and for this reason parents may be more likely to accept suggestions from teachers than they would be from other members of the team whom they may see as more threatening.

Social workers

Almost no one will argue the fact that social workers have a definite function on the community health team, but many people do not know what social workers do. Judging from social work literature itself, even social workers cannot seem to agree on what their function is. (In this regard they are much like nurses, so we can perhaps understand each other better.)

Social workers are employed in almost every kind of agency that deals with human problems, including schools, hospitals, welfare departments, prisons, residential treatment facilities of various kinds, adoption agencies, the military, nursing homes, and children's bureaus. The functions they perform are as various as the settings in which they work.

What is it that binds together all these people doing such different jobs in varied settings? The link is that they are all members of a practice field. Social work by its very nature is operational. It has a pragmatic and specific function: the provision of service to people who need service. While there are many differences as to how and to whom the service should be provided, the basic purpose of the field and the justification for its entire being lie in the delivery of services to the people who are in need of help. If people's needs are not being met, then the "welfare of mankind" is not being promoted and social work is not fulfilling its stated purpose. This is a simple but usually overlooked fact about the nature of the profession.*

This is a well-stated *philosophy* of social work, but it still does not spell out exactly *what* social workers do and *how* they do it.

Social work practice is divided into three major areas:

*From Social work: the unloved profession (p. 21), copyright © 1973 by Willard C. Richan and Allan R. Mendelsohn, used by permission of the publisher, Franklin Watts, Inc.

1. Casework focuses on the individual or the family and consists mainly of a one-to-one relationship in which social workers consult with clients to solve some of their living problems. This can include crisis intervention or longer-term psychiatric care, helping clients to live with medical problems (here is where some of the conflict with the functions of the community nurse can arise), and working with foster children and their foster or natural parents. Casework can also arise out of school problems. There are few areas not open to casework, which is mainly individual.

2. Group work involves several clients at the same time and includes group therapy for a variety of problems: prison parolees, alcoholics, abusive parents or husbands, or any group of people who have similar needs. Group work is usually done under the aegis of some social agency, and the roles and functions of group workers are expanding rapidly.

3. Community organization is growing by leaps and bounds. Many urban planners have a social work background, and the advent of community and ethnic group cohesiveness in the past twenty years has provided much fertile territory for community organizers. The social unrest of the 1960s and the minority rights movements of the 1970s have shown that community planning needs the help of professional social workers.

Social workers are employed by a variety of agencies, but more and more of them are in private practice, either by themselves or in partnership with other members of the community health team. One of the most popular areas is the community mental health center in which the psychiatric social worker carries a client case load, as does the psychologist, psychiatrist, and psychiatric nurse practitioner. All provide therapy in their own ways, and all contribute their professional opinions to the periodic team conferences. In this setting the social worker is practicing psychotherapy, as are the other three professionals. The function is essentially the same; the salary scale differs drastically.

To understand social work—its strengths and its weaknesses—it is necessary to grasp its essentially ideo-

logical character. More than most professions that claim a scientific technology, social work is as much a set of ends as it is a means for achieving them. So social workers tell themselves and each other and the world of their lofty sentiments, and the layman begins to suspect that there is not much more to the field. Social workers do, in fact, have a technology; perhaps it is more accurate to say technologies because of the diverse specialties that come under the social work rubric. But it is true that the more persistent and enduring elements are ideological, and the shared value system provides virtually the only core around which the diverse elements can unite and claim to be a profession.*

This rather amorphous but honest definition of social work still leaves other members of the community health team scratching their heads in puzzlement about the exact nature of the social worker's function. Let us accept the fact that there is no exact nature, and let us see that the social worker fills whatever human needs that do not fall under the expertise of any other health profession. This, of course, leaves much room for overlap, and every community health nurse has experienced some degree of conflict over "territorial rights" in meeting the needs of clients. If an elderly person needs to be placed in a nursing home, who makes the arrangements, the nurse or the social worker? If there is child abuse in the family, who coordinates the group therapy and the foster home care, the nurse or the social worker? The debate can go on forever, and the conflicts can become so serious that the job satisfaction of both the nurse and the social worker is in jeopardy. Of all the members of the community health team, these are the two whose professional functions overlap the most. For this reason these are the two who should work in closest harmony, eat lunch together the most frequently, and be constantly aware of the way in which they communicate with each other. If they work for the same agency, they should take particular care to

*From Social work: the unloved profession (p. 37), copyright © 1973 by Willard C. Richan and Allan R. Mendelsohn, used by permission of the publisher, Franklin Watts, Inc.

discuss and eventually agree on roles, functions, and responsibilities.

Sanitarians

A sanitarian is a person who has the skills to "qualify him to engage in the promotion and protection of the public health. He applies technical knowledge to solve problems of a sanitary nature and develops methods and carries out procedures for the control of those factors of man's environment which affect his health, safety, and well being."[9] Sanitarians, like community nurses and social workers, work closely with the consumer of health care. Their functions are woven into the fields of epidemiology, city planning, engineering, occupational and home safety, and school health.

The sanitarian is concerned mainly with environmental threats to the public health, but there are so many ways in which the public health is threatened that the sanitarian is everywhere: at the airport studying the effects of noise from jets, at the reservoir to see if the drinking water is safe, at chemical plants to see what the factory workers are inhaling as they work, and at the beach to see how much oil we are swimming in and how many pollutants the fish we eat are ingesting. There is no aspect of our environment that should be immune from the sanitarian's investigations. According to Freeman and Holmes,[6] the sanitarian's functions include the following:

1. Investigation of sanitary conditions in hotels, restaurants, recreational facilities, domestic water supplies and sewage systems, and in all other places where people congregate
2. Education of the public in matters relating to environmental sanitation such as pest control and accident prevention, including organization of community groups and dissemination of information through mass media
3. Participation in surveys, epidemiological studies, and public health research
4. Help in formulation, interpretation, and enforcement of public health regulations
5. Support and promotion of all phases of the public health program; encouragement of the public to understand and use public health services, particularly in the areas of civil defense, accident prevention, and home, school, and industrial safety

Sanitarians are usually employed by a government agency, and their educational backgrounds are usually in engineering. The more complex our environmental technology becomes, the more rigorous the sanitarian's training, and there is a greater diversity of job opportunities.

Civil engineers can also be considered members of the community health team in that they design and are responsible for the maintenance of the physical structures that affect the public's health. Civil engineers build water supply and sewage systems, and, as they design highways, they must take into account the pollution from vehicle exhausts. They are consultants to city planners who must consider the safety of housing and recreational sites and the placement of factories in relation to residential areas. All the facilities that we use for work, recreation, and living space contribute directly to the state of our health, and the sanitarian and civil engineer have much to say about how these facilities will be built, used, and maintained. Consequently they have a tremendous impact on our environment and on our health.

Nutritionists

The function of the nutritionist on the community health team is not very different from what it is in any other health area, which is basically to improve and maintain people's health by improving (or helping them to improve) their diets. There are a number of ways of doing this:

1. The provision of direct services to families or community groups. This can include conferences, in clinics or even during home visits, and demonstrations to groups of people as they sit in the waiting room of the health center.

2. Educational services, either directly to the client or to other members of the community health team for them to pass along to the client, about nutrition, meal planning, budgeting, and food preparation. Teaching people how to shop and cook

economically is as much a needed service as is giving them information about the nutritional content of food. Safety lessons about home canning or freezing are also important.

3. Consultation with and training of other members of the community health team. Health professionals in general (although they dislike admitting it) are woefully ignorant about nutrition and have only the vaguest notion about the content of most foods. The nutritionist can also provide valuable insights about the psychological, social, and cultural attitudes toward food and eating.

4. Coordination and planning of the nutritional aspects of all the continuing health programs. For example, prenatal care is incomplete without attention to correct diet, and it is up to the nutritionist to devise correct ways in which pregnant women can be taught about nutrition and to see that the programs are not only implemented but are carried out on a permanent basis.

5. Service as a liaison worker with other health teams, schools, welfare programs, and the nutrition departments of health agencies such as hospitals and nursing homes.

Many of the nutritional problems faced by families are outlined in Chapter 11, and there is no aspect of all these problems that could not be well served by nutritionists. They have the knowledge and expertise to give direct service to families. They can also serve as consultants to other members of the community health team who have direct contact with the clients. Nutritionists can single out groups of individuals who require special nutritional attention—for example, the elderly, pregnant women and lactating mothers, people who have prescribed diets, diabetics, vegetarians, fruitarians, infants and children, people who are overweight or underweight, adolescents, and people who have heart disease—and can devise special programs for them, which might include group discussions, films, lectures, or other kinds of educational activity. Their recognition of people's nutritional needs and problems and their ability to do something about them, either themselves or through others, is the nutritionist's function on the community health team.

Physical therapists

The function of physical therapists is to restore and/or maintain the physical abilities of clients through various active and passive exercises and other physical activities. Physical therapy is one of the most essential aspects of any kind of rehabilitation, and physical therapists have a definite place on the community health team. They are valuable members of the team as practitioners, consultants, and teachers of clients and of other team members. The reader is referred to an appropriate text for the specific activities of physical therapists.

As practitioners they make home visits to help the clients exercise and to teach the family to do the exercises. They also make periodic progress evaluations to the physicians and nurses and assess the client's physical abilities. They may also participate in outpatient services for clients who are not restricted to their homes. As consultants they evaluate clients in terms of what exercises or other activities they need and either carry them through themselves or delegate them to other health team members. They may also consult with the rest of the team about the kind of physical therapy programs that might be needed. Physical therapists can act as liaisons with other health agencies and hospitals about therapy programs. They are particularly valuable as teachers. There are all kinds of exercise therapies that can be done or supervised by nurses or even home health aides; since physical therapists cannot see all the clients, they must teach the exercises to others. Close family members are the logical ones to be taught because they are present most frequently and usually have the strongest interest in helping the client to regain physical abilities. Nursing personnel—professional and practical nurses and home health aides—can do exercises with the client after they have been taught by the physical therapist, although it is still the responsibility of the therapist to periodically assess the client's progress and to suggest changes in the therapy program.

Occupational therapists

Occupational therapy (OT) goes beyond simply giving the client something to do while he is institutionalized. Most nurses have a rather vague idea that clients "make things" in the OT room and that the purpose of the therapy is to maintain and improve range of motion, particularly in the hands and arms. These concepts are true, but occupational therapy also includes teaching the ability to perform tasks of daily living to clients in their own homes. The occupational therapist most often works with clients who have (had) a cerebrovascular accident, neuromuscular disease, amputation, and diminution of sensory acuity.

Occupational therapy differs from physical therapy in that the latter is concerned with muscle restoration and increase in function, whereas the former translates that increased mobility and function into meaningful activities, especially when the upper extremities are involved.

The OT is educated at the baccalaureate level and provides both direct and indirect care. Direct care usually consists of the following activities: evaluation of functional level and ability; collaboration with other members of the health care team to establish a course of therapy; guidance of the client through therapeutic activities; provision of prosthetic training; selection and teaching of various adaptive techniques to help clients accomplish daily living tasks; selection and construction of splints to prevent deformities; coordination with the speech therapist for various exercises; and assessment of the client's home with suggestions for modifications.

Indirect care consists of working with other members of the health care team to integrate occupational therapy in a total plan of care; suggesting, as a result of observation of clients, potential areas of need; communicating with members of the health care team who make home visits to alert them to specific areas of need; and referring new clients to other members of the team.

The number of home health agencies that offer OT services is increasing, and all indicators point to even greater numbers in the future.

It is only natural that occupational therapy make the transition from institution to home, since its purpose is to assist clients to make the adaptations necessary for them to live in and participate in their communities. Occupational therapy does so by enabling clients to become self-reliant in their performance of meaningful daily living activities. Occupational therapists through staff consultation, evaluation, and direct client care, assure that home care clients are seen not in terms of their disabilities but their existing abilities and how these can be improved to achieve maximum client independence.*

Medicare will sometimes pay for occupational therapy, but the regulations state quite explicitly who is and is not eligible. In general, the client must demonstrate potential for the restoration of function or must demonstrate a need for help in carrying out a self-treatment regimen. Occupational therapy cannot, however, be provided alone, that is, when it is not provided in connection with physical therapy, speech therapy, or home nursing care. The Medicare regulations use phrases such as "significant," "reasonable period of time," "practical improvement," and the like when making determinations about eligibility for occupational therapy. This is highly imprecise language and leaves almost unlimited room for arbitrariness in approving or denying requests for OT. Medicaid regulations are essentially the same with the added proviso that the state is not obligated to provide OT services; it does so at its own discretion.

Physician's assistants

Nathan Hershey has defined a physician's assistant (PA) as

an individual, not a physician, providing health services as an employee of a physician, or a health care institution such as a hospital or health center, who, under medical supervision and direction, engages in a range of activities and decision-making that does not fall completely within the scope of activities of any of the traditional, currently licensed health professions or occupations, and whose range of health care activity includes some tasks and functions now reserved to physicians, and not recognized by laws as within the area of

*Stewart, Jane E.: Home health care, St. Louis, 1979, The C.V. Mosby Co., pp. 76-7.

practice of any other health profession or occupation.*

Physician's assistants always practice under the supervision of a physician, although the quality and nature of their training may vary considerably. Most receive their education in a baccalaureate program, but there are many on-the-job training programs, and some receive informal instruction from the physician himself. In general, the physician's assistant performs only those tasks that are specific to the employing physician's specialty. For example, an assistant to a surgeon may cleanse a wound, prepare the skin, and drape the area in preparation for the physician's suturing.

A physician's assistant will also take a history so the physician can better visualize the medical problem. An assistant can perform certain tasks while under the surveillance of the physician, but the degree of professional independence permitted is limited.

Following is a sample of what PAs do while working for a primary care physician:
1. Take a history and perform a physical examination
2. Perform or assist in laboratory procedures
3. Give injections and immunizations
4. Suture and care for wounds
5. Provide counseling service and refer clients to other health services
6. Respond to emergencies within their range of skills and expertise

There is a role and function for the PA on the community health team, but there is also conflict with practitioners of nursing. Some people see the functions of the PA and the nurse practitioner to be the same or similar, and indeed there *are* many similarities. Nursing, of course, is not the performance of delegated medical activities, but some of the functions that involve counseling, referral, and other kinds of independent judgment do overlap.

There are also conflicts in legal and ethical relationships among nurses, physicians, and PAs. In many situations PAs earn higher salaries than nurses, and this is naturally a source of resentment for the nurse practitioner. The fact that the majority of PAs are men and the majority of nurses are women has a great deal to do with this salary discrepancy.

Although nurse practitioners can offer services to the public beyond any that the PA can offer, frequently nurse and PA may be competing for the same job. For a number of reasons the PA may not only be the one employed, but will also receive a higher salary than would be offered to the nurse practitioner. Despite the fact that most physicians tend to say that they prefer nurses to PAs, the truth is that too often doctors have inadequate or no knowledge about the nurse practitioner's capabilities. What they are talking about is a nurse as a physician's assistant. A number of nurses have made this choice, which is certainly theirs to make, although it has caused some negative reaction from other nurses and nursing associations. It is possible that the situation will clarify as more nurse practitioners are prepared in standardized educational programs. Unfortunately, at the moment such programs are as varied as those of the PA and it is not as easy to pinpoint the nurse practitioner's functions and responsibilities in reality as it is in theory.*

PAs on the community health team can be used in two different ways: as assistants in clinics and various other outpatient facilities and on home visits performing tasks ordered by the physician. On home visits PAs would function very much as would practical nurses, and in the clinic they could perform routine tasks, thus freeing the professional to engage in more sophisticated and complex nursing functions. Just as it is the responsibility of the nurse and the social worker to keep effective lines of communication open in order to avoid professional conflict, so it is also the responsibility of the nurse and the PA.

---

*From Kelly, Lucy Y.: Dimensions of professional nursing, ed. 3, New York, © 1975, Thomas M. Kelly, Macmillan, Inc., p. 142.

*From Kelly, Lucy Y.: Dimensions of professional nursing, ed. 3, New York, © 1975, Thomas M. Kelly, Macmillan, Inc., p.103.

NONTRADITIONAL HEALTH PRACTITIONERS

The following health practitioners are considered to be nontraditional because they do not follow accepted scientific principles and operate outside the medical establishment (Fig. 4-5). Some of the practitioners, such as acupuncturists, are being grudgingly accepted; some may be considered to be cultists, practitioners of a system for curing disease based on dogma invented by the cultist himself, with no basis in scientific fact. Some are religious or spiritual in nature, some call on psychic powers, some use chemicals or herbs that may or may not have curative or healing value, and some are out-and-out crooks. The latter abound in large cities, particularly in neighborhoods where poverty, ignorance, and fear are rampant.

We tend to think that most of these nontraditional practitioners disappeared during the last century when the last bottle of "snake oil medicine" was sold from the back of an itinerant's wagon. Or we think they exist only in the form of medicine men on Indian reservations or in the jungles of Africa. This is untrue. We are surrounded by these practitioners; many of *our* clients are also theirs, al-

though the clients frequently choose not to mention the fact. It is necessary that we know and recognize these nontraditional practitioners, what they believe, and what they do. They are frequently the "competition," and they often do irreparable harm to clients who should be receiving orthodox and accepted health care.

Acupuncture

Acupuncture has been used in the Orient for 5,000 years as a medical treatment for the whole body, not just a specific disease, by restoring the balance of yin and yang that flow through the body along fourteen meridians.[10] The process is accomplished by inserting needles into the body along the meridians, according to a complex chart, and manipulating or twirling them in a specific manner. Acupuncture *is* effective in some instances, notably the control of pain. The reason *why* it works and exactly *how* it works is a subject of great controversy, but respected Western physicians and scientists have reported success in achieving total anesthesia by acupuncture. There are various theories about why acupuncture works:

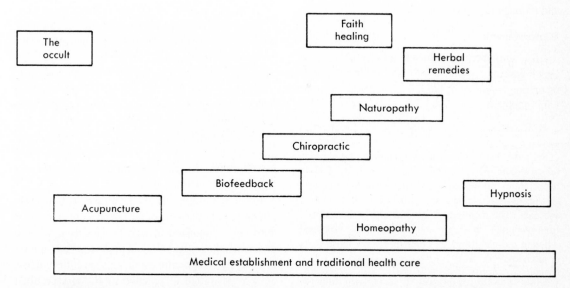

Fig. 4-5. Various nontraditional health practices and their relation to the medical establishment.

1. Sensory nerves block pain impulses to the spinal cord and brain.
2. There is some unspecified relationship between the central nervous system and the autonomic nervous system.
3. The power of suggestion by the practitioner may exert a hypnotic effect on the client.
4. External suggestion, autosuggestion, and cultural conditioning are potent forces.

In the United States a number of orthodox health institutions are conducting research (much of it funded by federal grants) in acupuncture, and there are four areas in which it has been used with some degree of success: deafness, narcotics withdrawal, relief of chronic pain, and removal of the death risk and postoperative nausea in surgery. Acupuncture as a treatment modality is still very experimental and should be used only by people licensed to practice medicine. There has been much publicity lately about acupuncture, and, as a result, all kinds of quacks are opening acupuncture parlors, and some even do grave physical harm to their clients. Great expertise is needed in the placement and twirling of the needles, and the technique improperly done can cause needle breakage, pneumothorax, hematomas, cardiac stabbing, infection, and damage to the spinal cord.

Biofeedback

Like acupuncture, biofeedback is an area in which fascinating and legitimate medical experimentation is going on, but it is also heavily infused with unethical practitioners.

Biofeedback is a process whereby one can learn to voluntarily produce changes in the involuntary functions of the body through visual and aural monitoring of physiological data. These changes include altering of body temperature, raising and lowering of blood pressure, slowing of heart rate, and controlling of the flow of blood and pain. The monitoring provides one with feedback from the brain, the heart, the circulatory system, and different muscle groups in order to control those parts of the body.[5,p.31]

All this is done by the use of machinery that records the electrical impulses produced by body parts; the individual learns to recognize undesired impulses and then to modify them. The reasons that some people are able to do this is not known, but biofeedback has been very successful in the management of such health problems as anxiety, migraine and tension headaches, hypertension, muscular tics and spasms, ulcers, and even epilepsy. The two most commonly used machines are the electroencephalograph and the temperature feedback machine, both of which can be purchased by charlatans who use them to bilk people out of huge sums of money. Like acupuncture, biofeedback is being seriously investigated by reputable scientists, but the amount of actual known fact is still small.

Chiropractic

"Chiropractic practice is the specific adjustment and manipulation of the articulation and adjacent tissues of the body, particularly of the spinal column, for the correction of nerve interferences . . . designed to restore or maintain normal nerve function."[11]

Chiropractic was founded in 1894 by D.D. Palmer, who refused to believe the germ theory of disease and disregarded the need for medicine and surgery. A "school" was founded by his son, B.J. Palmer, in Davenport, Iowa, and the practitioners were little more than manipulative (in both the literal and figurative senses of the word) quacks. Today there are two types of chiropractors, the "straights" and the "mixers." The former still believe that all disease can be eliminated by correcting subluxated vertebrae. The latter combine spinal manipulation with other procedures that include light, air, water, exercise, diet, and electricity. Chiropractors are licensed in all states except Mississippi and Louisiana.

Education in schools of chiropractic is four years after high school (none of the schools are associated with any recognized university) and is a mixture of science theory and clinical practice. The training is basically an apprenticeship because chiropractors are not permitted to practice in JCAH-accredited hospitals, and they are not authorized to perform surgery, prescribe drugs, or practice obstetrics. Following are services usually provided by chiropractors:

1. Adjustment therapy to achieve normal nerve function
2. Nutritional counseling to return clinical balance to the body
3. Physical therapy
4. Psychosomatic counseling
5. Regulated exercise and the use of herbs and colonic irrigations

Chiropractic is recognized as having some therapeutic benefit, but there are drawbacks as well. Improper or rough manipulation can cause dislocations and even fractures; the sudden twisting of the neck or joints can cause nerve and blood vessel damage; arthritis is often exacerbated. Perhaps the greatest danger lies in the belief by clients that chiropractic can cure whatever ails them; thus they fail to seek traditional treatment. Many chiropractors engage in deceptive advertising and exceed the bounds of what they are licensed to practice.

There is sometimes confusion between a chiropractor and an osteopath because both are called "doctor" and both are associated with bones. The major difference is that the former is not a medical practitioner whereas the latter is. There are differences in the scope and depth of education and practice in chiropractic and osteopathy as well as a difference in orientation toward physical illness.

Faith healing

The definition of faith healing is as amorphous as the definition of faith itself. There are two general ways in which faith healing operates. The first is that the healer himself has the power to cause cure of or recovery from illness and that God's will gave the healer his power. The second is that the healer does not have actual power but is a conduit from God to the person to be healed in much the same way as a Catholic priest hearing confession is a conduit from the confessor to God. The believer's faith goes beyond that which most people consider ordinary, and of course he is not fazed by the lack of a rational explanation for any phenomenon. Orthodox medical practitioners have long recognized the power of the mind to alter a physical course, and there have been so many instances of remissions in a disease thought to be hopeless that the occurrence is no longer uncommon. But the client's *belief* that the remission or cure was caused by another *person* through the will of God characterizes faith healing.

Faith healing has been around almost since the beginning of recorded history; the most famous practitioner was Jesus Christ. The techniques vary and include the laying on of hands, inducing trances, and asking the believer to concentrate on a specific object. Of all the unorthodox forms of health practice, faith healing leads in the number of crooks and charlatans who hoodwink the hopeful and unsuspecting. Almost everyone is a potential victim, although the elderly, poor, and uneducated are "taken" most frequently.

Christian Science, an organized religion, has faith healing as one of its basic tenets. Its founder, Mary Baker Eddy, in 1875 published her experiences of being healed by "truth in Christ" through the hands of Phineas Parkhurst Quimby, who used the hypnotic philosophy of the great Mesmer. Mary Baker Eddy regarded herself as a healer and as infallible as Christ and demanded absolute obedience from her followers. Her dogmatism brooked no argument, no criticism, and no challenges.

Christian Science contends that people are spiritual beings and therefore cannot be sick. The belief of illness is an illusion that is so powerful that it causes individuals to suffer. Therefore, all disease is in the mind. Bad health is equated with bad thoughts. By correcting the error, the cause is destroyed and the effect will cease. The system rests on faith in knowing and altering a false material view to a true spiritual understanding.[5,p.38]

The system claims to cure illness and prevent disease. Prayer is the only technique used because there is no recognition of illness in the first place. The only thing necessary is prayer that the illusion of illness will pass. Christian Science practitioners, who have a few weeks' training in Mary Baker

Eddy's philosophy, will consult with clients—for a fee—and help them to reaffirm their belief in God. They do not believe in or use drugs, surgery, or any other medical aid, and, of course, hospitalization is a taboo.

There is much evidence that people have been healed by a faith in Christian Science, and there is much evidence that people have died as a result of this belief and a resultant refusal to seek orthodox medical help.

Herbal remedies

Herbs, roots, bark, spices, and all kinds of other flora have been ascribed with curative and restorative powers over the years. Many of today's established drugs, such as quinine, digitalis, rauwolfia, and belladonna, are all based in naturally occurring vegetation. Herbs are rarely harmful (and sometimes even helpful if provided by an experienced herbalist), except when people depend on them to cure disease that requires something more. Catnip is fine for amusing one's feline friends, and some people even enjoy it brewed as a tea, but it is *not* a cure for cancer, kidney problems, arthritis, or any other known ailment.

Homeopathy

This philosophy, founded by Samuel Hahnemann, is based on the principle that a variety of herbs, drugs, and chemicals, when introduced into the body in infinitesimal doses, could cure or prevent a disease that was caused by a larger dose of the same substance. "Similarly, a clinical symptom could be treated by administering a very small amount of the substance that in larger amounts would produce the same or similar symptoms."[5,p.41] Hahnemann's treatise, the *Organon of the Art of Healing,* written in 1810, describes three main tenets[5]:

1. Diseases or symptoms of diseases are curable by particular drugs that produce similar pathological effects in the healthy body.
2. The dynamic force of the drug is increased by giving it in a small dose.
3. Chronic diseases are a manifestation of a suppressed itch or "psora" and are a matter of

the spirit. The psora was an evil spirit that manifested itself on the surface of the body by a sore of some type.

Homeopathy reached its pinnacle of popularity in this country in the 1880s and then gradually declined, but its use is still flourishing in Britain, Europe, and parts of Latin America. The Hahnemann Medical College in Philadelphia, although traditional in all other respects, still teaches one course in the theory and principles of homeopathy. The homeopathic theory is alive in the principles of desensitization to allergens, and the concept of acquired immunity is substantially related to homeopathy.

Hypnosis

Hypnosis is a state of altered consciousness produced by repetitious and rhythmical stimuli during which the person has an increased suggestibility. It is a trancelike state of intense concentration in which the person is both relaxed and aware at the same time. It has become a valuable medical tool for the relief of pain, particularly in childbirth and dentistry, but it is also frequently exploited by charlatans. It has become a popular form of entertainment on television talk shows and in nightclubs, and unscrupulous practitioners make all kinds of false claims about curing various diseases. Posthypnotic suggestions have been used, with some degree of success, in changing unwanted behavior patterns, such as smoking, drinking, and overeating. There is much legitimate experimentation going on in these areas, but there are also an enormous number of con artists.

Naturopathy

As the name implies, this is a method of healing that relies solely on "nature," for example, massage, good diet, exercise, sun, vibration, light, and water. No chemicals or drugs are used, although x-ray films are permitted for diagnosis only. Naturopathy does not accept the germ theory or bacterial causes of disease, and naturopaths are rather moralistic in their belief that diseases are caused by errors in behavior, thinking, and moral, social, and sexual conduct. The removal of poisons from the body, the purification of the bloodstream, and correction of modes of behavior can cure all diseases, according to naturopaths. John H. Kellogg of cornflakes fame was a pioneer of naturopathy. There is, of course, nothing wrong with exercise, diet, massage, and good moral thinking. Our lives would probably benefit from an increased amount of all of them. What is harmful, and what makes a warning about naturopathy essential, is that they should not be used when there is existence of actual disease. The danger is that reliance solely on a naturopath as a primary care practitioner precludes the diagnosis and treatment of whatever disease exists. Naturopaths simply will not use orthodox methods of treatment and thus contribute to the continuing illness of people who are persuaded not to seek proper medical attention. If an obvious infection is treated with a vegetarian diet instead of a course of antibiotics, serious further damage could ensue.

The occult

Occult means hidden, and occult beliefs and practices, which have become increasingly popular in the last decade, are those involving mystery, magic, incantations, the reading of tea leaves, and all kinds of other phenomena. All recognized religions involve some mystical or magical qualities, and many people see no *real* difference between the practice of the occult and practice of any religion that is familiar to us. Many cults promise all manner of good things, such as inner peace, transport to higher spiritual planes, cure of illness, and a variety of consciousness-expanding experiences. There are many variations of occult philosophies and many fascinating rituals and practices. Most of them are unusual, but not essentially harmful: chanting, the casting of "spells," wearing of specific garments, reading tarot cards, or throwing the I Ching coins. Seances rarely hurt anyone, except in the wallet, neither does meditation with a mantra every day. These practices may bring a kind of psychic fulfillment if one believes in them. What is dangerous is the belief that any or all of these practices can cure illness or solve life's problems. As in naturopathy, chiropractic, or any of the other

nontraditional forms of practice, it is not the practice, the philosophy, or even the theory that does harm; it is the refusal to seek proper medical care.

SUMMARY

The concept of the community health team is an amorphous one. A variety of health workers, professional and nonprofessional, work together with some kind of organization and communication to improve and maintain the community's health. The workers all may be employed by the same agency, or they may be connected by professional or occupational ties. The ultimate goal of all team members is the same, but the means to achieve this goal vary greatly. Several factors must be operant if the community health team is to be successful:

1. There must be a common goal that has been identified by the client, although each group of health workers may have different subgoals.
2. The team members must have the talents and skills necessary to achieve the goals.
3. There must be a well-developed communication process to set goals and then to implement and evaluate them.

These three factors are all separate, but they are interdependent. Without goals there is no reason for the community health team to exist. Without human talents and skills there is no way for the goals to be achieved, and without effective communication each team member will not know what the others are doing, and the whole concept can easily fall apart. In addition to these three factors, the members of the community health team must have a working understanding of group process and be willing to use the concepts in practice. Each one must know everyone else's function and how it relates to his own. The desire and willingness to work as part of a team is an essential ingredient of the team concept; perhaps it is the most elusive one. Cooperative working arrangements are difficult to achieve, and they require constant attention and effort from all those involved.

Most community health teams have a leader or administrator who is responsible for the coordination and guidance of the day-to-day activities and who tries to keep all members communicating with each other. The task of administering an inter-professional community health team is the most difficult of all.

The concept of the community health team is confused and confusing. There is much controversy about what the team is, who belongs on it, and what its functions and purposes are. The idea is often ephemeral, and the philosophies espoused in texts are rarely put into practice. The following health workers are generally considered to be an integral part of the community health team: the client, who is the most important member and without whom there would be no reason for the team to exist; the physicians, including the primary care practitioner, the specialist, and the public health physician (the specialty is sometimes called oc-cupational or preventive medicine); registered and licensed practical nurses; the clergy; schoolteach-ers; social workers, whose roles and functions are frequently confused with those of the professional nurse; sanitarians and civil engineers; nutritionists; physical and occupational therapists; physician's assistants, whose functions are also sometimes con-fused with those of nursing; and home health aides.

There are also a number of nontraditional health practitioners who abound on the fringes of main-stream health care. They include, but are not lim-ited to, practitioners of acupuncture, biofeedback, chiropractic, faith healing, herbalism, homeopa-thy, hypnosis, naturopathy, and the occult. The danger lies not so much in the actual practice of these forms of health care but in the fact that while the clients are being convinced of the efficacy of these unorthodox forms of treatment, they are not receiving the kind of care that could be of some benefit to them. The longer they delay, of course, the more likely it is that their illnesses will increase in severity. Some of these practitioners are well meaning and truly believe in the worth of what they are doing. Others, however, are out-and-out charlatans and are deliberately cheating and mis-leading their clients. P.T. Barnum said, ''There's a sucker born every minute,'' and these charlatans are making millions of dollars by preying on the fear and ignorance of people who do not know any better.

NOTES

1. Random House dictionary of the English language, New York, 1966, Random House, Inc.
2. Kane, Rosalie A.: Competency for collaboration. In Rein-hardt, Adina M., and Quinn, Mildred D., editors: Current practice in family-centered community nursing, vol. 1, St. Louis, 1977, The C.V. Mosby Co.
3. American Public Health Association: Educational qualifi-cations and functions of Public Health Educators, 1957, American Public Health Association.
4. To avoid redundancy, whenever the client is mentioned as part of the health care team, it is automatically implied that the client's family is included.
5. Cornacchia, Harold J., and Barrett, Stephen: Consumer health, ed. 2, St. Louis, 1980, The C.V. Mosby Co.
6. Freeman, Ruth B., and Holmes, Edward M.: Administra-tion of public health services, Philadelphia, 1960, W.B. Saunders Co.
7. American Nurses Association: Preparation for nurse prac-titioners and assistants to nursing: a position paper, New York, 1965, American Nurses Association.
8. Human warmth and compassion are essential for the suc-cessful functioning of any professional or nonprofessional health worker, but many employing agencies seem so con-cerned with academic preparation and past experience that they ignore the personality characteristics of the health workers.
9. Committee on Professional Education: Educational and other qualifications of public health sanitarians, Washing-ton, D.C., 1956, American Public Health Service.
10. According to Chinese philosophy and religion, two prin-ciples, one negative, dark, and feminine (yin) and one positive, bright, and masculine (yang), interact to influence the destinies of all creatures and things.
11. Sare, Rauson L.: Chiropractic educational evolution, term paper for the course Health Frauds, Fads, and Fallacies, San Francisco, 1965, San Francisco State University.

BIBLIOGRAPHY

Blackham, H.J.: Religion in a modern society, New York, 1966, Frederick Ungar Publishing Co., Inc.

Brown, Barbara B.: New mind, new body: bio-feedback: new directions for the mind, New York, 1974, Harper & Row, Publishers.

Chamberlain, Leo M., and Kindred, Leslie W.: The teacher and school organization, New York, 1949, Prentice-Hall, Inc.

Collins, Mattie: Communication in health care: understanding and implementing effective human relations, St. Louis, 1977, The C.V. Mosby Co.

Cornacchia, Harold J., and Barrett, Stephen: Consumer health, ed. 2, St. Louis, 1980, The C.V. Mosby Co.

Fleming, Mary C., and Benson, Marion C.: Home nursing handbook, Boston, 1961, D.C. Heath & Co.

Freeman, Ruth B., and Holmes, Edward M.: Administration of public health services, Philadelphia, 1960, W.B. Saunders Co.

Fromer, Margot J.: A course for the preparation of home health aides, prepared for Community College of Delaware County, Media, Pa., 1973, unpublished.

Greeley, Andrew M.: The Catholic priest in the United States, Washington, D.C., 1972, U.S. Catholic Conference.

Kelly, Lucy Y.: Dimensions of professional nursing, New York, 1975, Macmillan, Inc.

Leahy, Kathleen M., et al.: Community health nursing, New York, 1977, McGraw-Hill Book Co.

Merwick, Donna: Boston priests, Cambridge, Mass., 1973, Harvard University Press.

Milio, Nancy: The care of health in communities, New York, 1975, The Macmillan Co.

Miller, Samuel H.: Religion in a technical age, Cambridge, Mass., 1968, Harvard University Press.

Neusner, Jacob, editor: Understanding American Judaism, New York, 1975, KTAV Publishing House.

Rasmussen, Sandra: Foundations of practical and vocational nursing, New York, 1967, The Macmillan Co.

Reinhardt, Adina M., and Quinn, Mildred D., editors: Current practice in family-centered community nursing, vol. 1, St. Louis, 1977, The C.V. Mosby Co.

Richan, Willard C., and Mendelsohn, Allen R.: Social work: the unloved profession, New York, 1973, New Viewpoints.

Sloane, Robert M., and Sloane, Beverly L.: A guide to health facilities: personnel and management, ed. 2, St. Louis, 1977, The C.V. Mosby Co.

Somers, Anne R.: Health care in transition: directions for the future, Chicago, 1971, Hospital Research and Educational Trust.

Spears, Harold: Curriculum planning through in-service programs, Englewood Cliffs, N.J., 1957, Prentice-Hall, Inc.

Stewart, Jane E.: Home health care, St. Louis, 1979, The C.V. Mosby Co.

Toren, Nina: Social work: the case of a semi-profession, Beverly Hills, Calif., 1972, Sage Publications, Inc.

5

ETHICS RELATED TO HEALTH CARE

Ethics is a system of moral principles, rules of conduct recognized in respect to a particular class of human actions or to a particular group of people. It is also the branch of philosophy dealing with human conduct with respect to the rightness and wrongness of certain actions and to the goodness and badness of the motives and ends of such actions. Bioethics are principles and rules of conduct applied to living things; biomedical ethics is the system applied to the area of human endeavor in which health care is given. In this chapter the term biomedical ethics will refer to the ethics of providing care to the people who enter the health care system. Because all people have, at one time or another, been a part of the health care system, the scope of the ethical system dealt with applies to all human beings.

To define ethics, one must define the term human being. At first glance it seems simple; we see a person walking on the street, going through the checkout line in the supermarket, or even unconscious on an operating table, and we have no problem recognizing the person as a human being. But life is no longer so simple. Medical technology has complicated our lives, making the line between a human being and a nonhuman being less finite than it was. The person on the operating table is a human being, even though all his muscles are paralyzed by curare, he cannot breathe on his own, his reflexes are so depressed that he would surely die if he were left unattended, he is totally oblivious to his surroundings and cannot communicate even his

most basic needs, and he is a hair away from death. But it is an incontrovertible fact that he is a human being. What about the person in an intensive care unit (ICU) who is ''dead'' but who is being kept alive by artificial means such as drugs, respirators, or intra-aortic balloon pumps? This person, too, is uncommunicative, unable to respond, has no reflexes, no brain waves, cannot communicate even his most basic needs, and is in a coma of oblivion. Not everyone recognizes this person as a human being, even though he may look and appear exactly like the person on the operating table. The differences are important to understand; therefore we must define the term human being. There is, of course, no single sentence that can be used—only a set of criteria. A problem arises when one must decide what *kind* of criteria to use: biological, psychological, spiritual, emotional, cultural, or a myriad of others. It is not my intent to write a rule or even a guideline of what the community nurse should assume constitutes a human being. Rather, the thoughts and experiences of people who are experts in the field of ethics will be explored, and the reader can decide what constitutes humanness or the humanity of a person: what makes one individual a human being and another individual not a human being.

CRITERIA FOR HUMANNESS

Travelbee[1] defines a human being as a unique, irreplaceable individual who is unlike any person who has ever lived or who will ever live. This individual has certain characteristics that are unique to him alone; he is, according to Travelbee, affected, influenced, and changed by all his experiences, his heredity, and his culture. He assimilates and incorporates everything that happens to him in both material and nonmaterial ways. A human being is constantly faced with choices and conflicts, and he has the capacity to make decisions, to weigh alternatives, to predict possible outcomes, and to be responsible for the outcome of a particular choice. A human being is capable of rational thought, of intellectual and psychic growth; he is able to communicate some of his thoughts and feelings to others, although "each individual possesses a basic core of individuality and alone-ness that is elusive and cannot be grasped or understood by another."[1,p.26] A human being is capable of socialization, of responding to the needs, thoughts, and feelings of others; people interact and form relationships on a variety of levels, from the most superficial business association to a deep and abiding commitment of love. Human beings are aware of, but sometimes do not fully believe in, the fact of their own future death.

Each human being on earth is different from every other human being on earth. Differences in physical characteristics are obvious and accepted. What are not so obvious and what are crucial to the topic of biomedical ethics are other, less tangible differences. Every human experience leaves a permanent impression on the psyche of every person. The collection of these impressions affects every thought and every action, and each one of these thoughts and actions forms part of the permanent collection, thus creating an impenetrable jungle of constantly fluctuating thoughts, feelings, and emotions.

It has been stated that human nature is the same the world over—that all individuals have the same basic needs and hence that people are more alike than they are different. This has resulted in the unfortunate tendency to assume that everyone is alike when the opposite is probably more valid. It is true, as far as we know today, that all human beings have the same basic needs. However, their needs may be modified by the culture of the person. Although all individuals have the same basic needs, the strength and intensity of these needs vary and they are expressed differently. . . . A guiding supposition to use in relationships with others is to assume and act on the assumption that *human beings are more different than they are alike.* Using this assumption will help one avoid the common error of assuming or supposing that others are like himself when they aren't and judging others according to what one would or would not do.*

There is not a single nurse in the country who has not been taught this premise. It is one of the primary foundations of a human health care system, but in many areas of our lives humanity is no longer a guiding factor. Health care is no exception. Everyone has made decisions and judgments for clients, based on what we ourselves would want to have done. "That gallbladder in room 312 can't possibly be in so much pain; it's his third postop day. He can wait a few minutes." "Stop crying, little girl. It doesn't hurt that much." "You can lead a perfectly normal life with a colostomy, there's no need to be embarrassed about the stoma." "You'll get over your grieving for your lover; you're still young and attractive, and there are lots of people to love." How do we *know* how much pain a person is having? How do we *know* what will or will not affect a person's life? How do we *know* what is happening in the mind of a grieving person? Because we as human beings can never feel another person's feelings, either physical or psychic, we can never, ethically, make a decision for another person. But as providers of health care, we make these kinds of decisions all the time. Does this mean we are all unethical and unprincipled, deciding the course of people's lives with no input from them? Of course not. But it does present interesting questions and complex moral dilemmas. As providers of health care, we are in a position of power; we possess certain kinds of knowledge, and we have the tools to apply that knowledge. This chapter will explore some of the

*From Travelbee, Joyce: Interpersonal aspects of nursing, Philadelphia, 1971, F.A. Davis Co., p. 28.

moral and ethical problems inherent in the provision of health care.

Advances in medical research and constantly expanding technology create new moral dilemmas as well as variations on old ones. The morals and ethics of society in general are changing; biomedical ethics merely reflects and absorbs this change. Ethics can no longer be assumed to be a set of codes of behavior, a kind of moral etiquette. Simple following "accepted procedures" will not suffice. Students are no longer content to follow the ethical precepts of their teachers. It is not enough to say, "This is right for me; it will be right for you." Philosophical, moral, and ethical questions, when debated by rational and humane people, rarely lead to answers. Instead, new kinds of questions are asked, and new problems are presented. A reader looking for easy answers, or even specific guidelines for behavior, in this chapter will be disappointed. I know none of the answers, but the questions need to be raised and pondered. It is not sufficient for nurses to place all moral and ethical responsibility in the hands of physicians who have traditionally held it. What will be discussed in this chapter is *human* responsibility, the moral and ethical questions that affect every person. All our roles in life are temporary; today we are the providers of health care, in a position to make a decision that will affect a person's very life. Tomorrow we may be in an ICU, lying helpless, unable to speak, listening to others debate the course and even the existence of our future. It cannot be stressed strongly enough that we are "all in this together," that physicians do not necessarily have a more sensitive ethical outlook than nurses, that social workers are any more moral than their clients, that philosophy professors are any closer to the solution of moral dilemmas than are assembly line workers. Productive ethical discussion and inquiry can take place only when there is disagreement about what ought to be done. Total agreement with what has always been done never leads to advancement of thought.

Fletcher[2] believes that "a profile of man" is essential to the discussion of biomedical ethics. Medicine and the nature of human beings cannot be questioned until one defines that nature. Following is a set of criteria, in no rank order, of what Fletcher thinks humans are and what they are not.

Positive human criteria

1. Minimal intelligence. An IQ of 40 on the Stanford-Binet scale is questionably indicative of a person; a human being with an IQ of 20 or below is definitely not a person. Mere biological life, if there is no intelligence, does not constitute personhood.

2. Self-awareness. Being conscious of the self is a characteristic of a person. Unconsciousness, when it is incorrigible, is indicative of irreversible damage to the brain neocortex and would also be indicative of intelligence that falls below the minimum.

3. Self-control. An individual must not only be not controllable by others (except by force), but he must be able to control himself. This does not include short periods of lack of control that can be medically rectified. There must be evidence of "means-ends" behavior for an individual to be considered a person. "Means-ends" behavior is that which is under control. A certain kind of behavior leads to certain consequences, and unless an individual is conscious of the results of his behavior, he cannot be considered a person.[3]

4. A sense of time. This is meant to be clock time, not time in a philosophical sense. A person must be aware of the passage of time.

5. A sense of futurity. Human beings are the only life forms who realize that there is time yet to come. An individual who is totally unaware of the fact of the future is not a person. A sense of purpose has often been equated with a sense of humanness, and one cannot have purpose without a sense of the future.

6. A sense of the past. Conscious recall or memory is a unique neurological development of the neocortex of the cerebrum. An individual without a sense of the past is an instinctive rather than a cultural creature and consequently not a person.

7. The capability to relate to others. Interpersonal relationships on a variety of levels are es-

sential for personhood. Various species of animals function in social systems, but theirs is based on instinct and is not characterisitc of humanity.

8. Concern for others. This is not necessarily meant in a traditional altruistic sense but more in the sense of the awareness of the personhood of others.

9. Communication. Total alienation or disconnection from others is dehumanization. This criterion must be applied only to individuals who do not communicate only because they have no choice. A hermit who prefers the solitude of the forest is certainly still to be considered a person.

10. Control of existence. A person is not a helpless subject of the forces of physical and psychological nature. He can, to some degree, control his own destiny. His knowledge, freedom, and initiative are limited, but they do exist, and a person can set his own course within these bounds.

11. Curiosity. Indifference is inhuman. The nature of a person is to learn, to know, and to explore.

12. Changeability. Biological and physiological change go on as long as life exists, but the capacity to change one's mind and behavior is what characterizes a person. All human existence is on a continuum; it is a process of always becoming. The inability to become is the inability to change.

13. A balance between rationality and feeling. A person is rational and cerebral as well as a creature of intuition and feeling. To be only one or the other is not to be a person.

14. Idiosyncrasy. To be a person is to have an identity, to be recognized by others.

15. Neocortical functioning. Without this indicator, none of the others is possible. Personal reality depends on cerebration, and to be ''humanly dead'' is to be excerebral, no matter how many other body functions remain.

Negative human criteria

1. A person is not nonartificial or antiartificial. A ''test tube baby,'' although conceived and gestated outside the human body, is nonetheless humanly reproduced and is therefore a potential person.

2. A person is not essentially parental. Reproduction is not necessary for personhood.

3. A person is not essentially sexual.

4. There is no such thing as human nature, and there is no such thing as human rights, except what is artificially granted by a social system.

5. A person is not a worshiper. Faith in supernatural realities is not essential to being a person.

Fletcher presents these criteria for testing. The comparisons and combinations of questions resulting from a discussion of the criteria are endless. Applications of results will lead to other questions and new moral problems. It is the *way* in which these and other criteria are tested that will most profoundly affect our lives.

ISSUES TO BE EXPLORED

This chapter will deal with a few specific areas in which biomedical ethics are playing a larger and larger role: genetic counseling and chromosomal manipulation; death and the prolongation of life by artificial means, euthanasia, and organ transplantation; human subjects for research; fetal research; psychopharmacology, psychosurgery, and behavior control; and abortion. Inherent in and essential to the discussion of these topics will be several primary issues. These issues are human and ethical ones and remain the same in whatever area of human endeavor they are applied.

Responsibility for health care

The first area is what a person ought to be who is responsible for the administration of health care on any level. We shall assume that this person is not merely a technician and dispenser of ''things.'' But what kind of person should he be, and how should he relate to the client as a person? How much of his being is he required to invest in the role of provider of health care? The relationship between client and giver of health care is an important issue in biomedical ethics. This relationship has traditionally been a superior/inferior one with the client meekly acceding to decisions of the person providing care. The ''stick-with-me-kid'' syndrome is still very much in evidence; the providers of health care have traditionally assumed that they have the right, because of their knowledge and expertise, to make decisions about the minds and bodies of the people who seek their help. In matters of health care, the prevailing attitude has been that all clients are dependent on the advice of health professionals. Most health care clients would like not to be dependent, and they should be viewed as people consulting other people about specific problems in their lives. Travelbee describes this phenomenon:

It requires little thought, effort, or emotional involvement on the part of "the nurse" to view human beings as "patients." The "patient" is an abstraction, a set of expectations personified by tasks to be performed, treatments to carry out, an illness, or a room number. No one likes or feels warm toward a patient but towards a human being whose personality and uniqueness is perceived and experienced. It therefore matters a great deal whether an individual is perceived as "a patient" or as a unique human being. A nurse never sympathizes, understands, or has compassion for a patient but for a particular human being. It is probably that once an individual is designated "a patient" that a dehumanizing begins if ever so subtly. It well may be that once an individual assumes the role of "nurse" or the role of "patient" a wall goes up between these two human beings until, unless this process is interfered with, both perceive the other as an abstraction or a set of abstractions.*

Defining biomedical ethics

The second issue is what biomedical ethics is all about and how decisions should be made. Some see ethics as a code of behavior, a set of rules to be followed, always allowing for various interpretations of any given situation. This is not ethics. Codes of behavior (as in ones established by various professional organizations) are merely guidelines for suggested actions, how the profession wishes its members to behave. Although most codes make a concerted effort to include only behavior that is ethical, one must never accept these

codes at face value. They are not *necessarily* ethically correct. Ethics is a process of search and discovery rather than a behavioral indoctrination. This search involves analysis of the facts, a determination of the values involved, and a vindication of the judgments made. Health care professionals need to continually develop a sensitivity to issues and moral questions so that ethics are always in the front of their minds. One must constantly question and reevaluate one's outlook on the meaning of life, death, suffering, and eternity. Without this constant introspection, ethics cannot be a part of one's life.

"Values clarification" is a phrase that has become popular in nursing in the past several years. Most people use it synonymously with the study of ethics and see it as a process to determine ethically correct behavior. This is a serious mistake. Values clarification is *only* what its name implies: it seeks to help people understand what their values are and how they came to hold a particular set of values. It is nonjudgmental and *cannot* determine whether values or actions based on values are morally correct or incorrect. Values clarification is only a beginning; it may be used as a foundation for the study of ethics, but it is not the same as ethics.

Health care delivery

Although the structure and nature of the health care delivery system has been explored in Chapter 1, it is always an issue when dealing with ethical problems. One cannot debate the problem of whether to terminate a life-support system unless one considers the social, financial, and logistical ramifications. When Karen Quinlan was removed from her respirator as the result of a decision by the New Jersey Supreme Court in 1976, she continued to live. She was comatose (and certainly not a person by any of Fletcher's criteria), but a decision had to be made about what part of the health care system would support her, both medically and financially, for the rest of her life.[4]

Ethical sensitivity

A fourth issue is the general level of ethical sensitivity in our culture. The dominant values of

*From Travelbee, Joyce: Interpersonal aspects of nursing, Philadelphia, 1971, F.A. Davis Co., p. 33.

life in the United States today appear to be vastly different than they were fifty or even thirty years ago. Great emphasis is placed on money, youth, beauty, creature comforts, efficiency, leisure, immediate gratification of desire, affluence, and technological progress. None of these values is bad or negative, in and of itself. It does seem, however, the more important they become, the more blind people become to ethical sensitivity and personal integrity. It has become more important for a man to buy his family a microwave oven than it is to spend an afternoon reading a novel or rolling on the lawn and giggling with his children. Health care workers are a part of this changing sense of values, and it cannot help but influence us as we make bioethical decisions. Who shall receive the very precious donated kidney? What is the quality of the life we are empowered to save or not to save? Whose life is worth what? Is it the productivity of the client, his ''goodness,'' his contributions to the lives of others, the amount of money he has? What shall be the criteria? It is impossible for our own values not to play a crucial role when we make these kinds of decisions. And our own values are very much influenced by the values of the society in which we live.

The sanctity of life

Another issue is the sancitity of life itself. This is the most basic and fundamental value to be considered. Not everyone values life for its own sake. To be (or to once have been) a human being does not necessarily mean that the human being is a person. Life itself has not been defined to every-

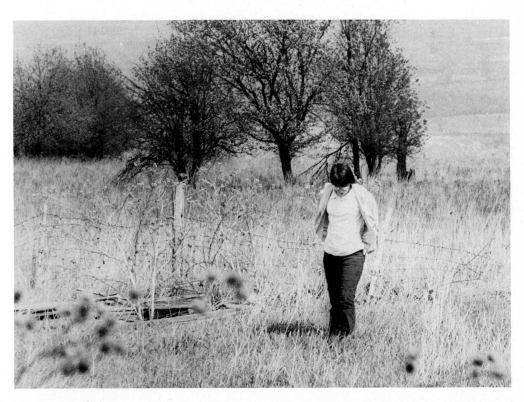

Fig. 5-1. The concept of ethics, morality, and behavior is a personal one that is developed as a result of years of introspection and contemplation of all the issues. (Photograph by Susan McKinney; courtesy Editorial Photocolor Archives, Inc., New York.)

one's satisfaction, neither has death. There are times when sacrificing "life" may be a greater good than preserving it. There are times when we are called on to make the impossible decision about the quality of another human being's life. ". . . contemporary medicine has propelled to center stage the sanctity of life in a new guise: the quality of life. It asks us to view life *also* in terms of its quality, to admit that there comes a time when living is no longer *human* life—and to take the consequences of this admission."[2,p.106] When we discuss life, the series of questions raised is endless. Who decides what quality of life is tolerable and what is not? Who has the right to make that decision? If a decision must be made, what are the criteria to be used? What kind of intervention is to be employed, and who employs it? What is the moral difference between active and passive euthanasia? Is there a value to suffering? How much pain is enough? The questions go on and on. Intelligent and humane people ponder the answers, think they have arrived at a conclusion, and then discover aspects of the question they had not considered, so the process continues. The important thing is that the process continues.

Health professionals espouse the concept of the "worth" of human life and the dignity of every human being. This concept, in theory, is part of the fabric of American society. But we have only to look around to see that we do not practice what we preach. Some life is worth more than others; some people are accorded greater dignity than others, which is immoral, unprincipled, and unethical. But it is a fact of life, and we must deal with it. The purpose of this chapter is not to give the reader a step-by-step method of righting the wrongs of the world (or at least of the health care system) but to present the questions for deliberation.

Sexuality and the family

The sixth issue is the meaning of sexuality and the family. The quality of our lives is very much determined by the meaning we give to the expression of our sexuality. Everyone somehow expresses sexuality. Some people are heterosexual; some are homosexual. Some make love only to themselves, and some make love only in their minds. We have entered an era where sexuality is openly discussed; laws concerning our sexual and reproductive lives are being questioned. Homosexuals are demanding that their civil rights not be impinged on because of what they choose to do in the privacy of their own lives. Women are demanding the right not to bear children should they so choose. Voluntary and involuntary sterilization is a hotly debated issue. Women are now able to bear children that were conceived outside their own bodies, either in the body of another woman or in vitro. What are the moral and ethical considerations inherent in this technology? Sexuality, pregnancy, procreation, abortion, sterilization, and contraception are all issues that are deeply involved in the entire framework of biomedical ethics.

HUMANITY, EXISTENCE, AND ETHICS

When we deal with moral and ethical problems, we deal with human existence at its most basic level. All the ethical questions that will be explored in this chapter are concerned with human beings as they experience pain—physical and psychic—suffering, hope, and hopelessness. Pain and suffering are an intrinsic part of life; no one escapes. We all live with the pain we have already experienced and with the knowledge that we again will be in pain. Death is the only escape. Most people, when they are in pain, wish it to be alleviated and will seek help to relieve suffering.[5] Suffering is caused by so many things: physical and mental pain, loss of love, loss of material possessions, wounding of pride or ego, violation of one's integrity, loneliness and alienation from others, transgression of one's religious or moral convictions. No human being can feel another human being's pain; the understanding of the existence of pain must be on a purely cognitive level. Every single day, sometimes countless numbers of times a day, health workers come in contact with people in pain. Empathy with other people's pain plays a large role in the kind of ethics espoused and the kinds of decisions made. It is impossible to make an ethical decision unless the decision maker demonstrates some degree of compassion, which can be achieved only by sensitivity to the pain and suffering of others. Some people seem to achieve this sensitivity merely by living; others need to consciously work to develop it. Although there is no way to take "sensitivity development lessons," there are a few mental and emotional exercises that the reader might consider while thinking about the ethics of pain and suffering.

1. As you are on your way to an appointment, hurrying along the street, imagine yourself immobilized in some way, either by being confined to a wheelchair or to bed or even imprisoned. Think how you would feel if you could not get to that appointment under your own power.

2. Listen to a symphony or go to a woods and sit absolutely silent, then consider deafness. Consider blindness as you are walking through a museum or art gallery. The next time you chat on the telephone, imagine being mute.

3. What is the most important thing in your life? What was the most important thing five years ago? Consider your priorities, how they have changed, and, most essential, how you would rearrange them if you were faced with a terminal illness.

4. What do you fear most? Think about the times you have been afraid, what feelings were evoked, how you went about calming the fear, and what your needs were at the time.

5. Consider the person you love best in all the world and then pretend this person has just died. Let the feelings come through and permit yourself to experience the pain.

6. The next time you are ill and confined to bed with the flu or are in the hospital for surgery, imagine what it would be like if you always felt that sick, if tomorrow and the day after you would feel exactly the same as you do today. Consider never getting better.

7. The next time you experience a severe tension headache, do not immediately reach for the aspirin. Let the pain build up and permit your head to throb for as long as you can tolerate it. Then when you finally swallow the aspirin, consider what it would be like if you could not have relieved the pain.

8. Lie in bed alone at night, with the room as dark as possible, close your eyes, and imagine your own death. What were the circumstances surrounding your death? How did you die? Were you in much pain? Who was with you when you died? How do you feel? How do you think everyone else feels? Where are you now?

The consideration of ethics is also the consideration of hope. Hope is one of the major factors that motivate all human behavior. Scientists devote their lives to the hope that they may discover a cure for cancer. People give up the pleasure of eating cholesterol-laden foods in the hope of avoiding heart disease. Time, energy, and money are invested in learning a profession in the hope of helping someone and achieving self-satisfaction. Without hope there is little reason to get up in the morning because there is no prospect for a change or improvement in life. As health workers we are confronted by people who exhibit varying degrees of hope and, all too often, varying degrees of hopelessness. We have been trained that it is our professional responsibility to motivate people to have hope. But what if there is none? What if death is inevitable? What if the client's blindness is truly permanent? What if the plastic surgery can never repair the disfiguring facial scars? We must consider the ethics involved in dealing with clients in these kinds of situations. One can say that there is always hope in any situation, that death may be inevitable but that it need not be painful, that blindness is a handicap which can be successfully overcome, that a disfigured face is not a disfigured soul, and worthwhile human relationships are not based on physical beauty. How far do health workers go to instill hope in the hopeless client? How morally obligated are health workers to concern themselves with the pain and suffering of others? How much pain must they subject themselves to in order to alleviate the pain of others?

GENETIC MANIPULATION AND COUNSELING
Cloning

Two single cells, merged, form the basis of every human being. It has always been that way, and it always will. Or will it? In recent years hundreds of experiments have been done to unlock the mysteries of reproduction, all the way from single-celled viruses to humans. Cell nucleus transplantation, or cloning, is the isolating of a single cell and placing it in a specialized nutrient medium so that it begins to grow in an organized manner and eventually reaches the maturity of the organism from which it was taken. Cloning experiments have led to two fundamental facts: mature organisms can be *asexually* grown from single cells, and all the organisms will have exactly the same genetic makeup of the "parent" organism.

Change in the way the human race is propagated cannot help but have a profound effect on the meaning of human identity and existence. Consider meeting hundreds of your cloned "self" every day. Consider the possible outcome of the "battle between the sexes" if asexual reproduction becomes a practical possibility. Perhaps the very nature of femaleness and maleness would be altered, if neither sex needed the other for reproduction. Why bother having two separate sexes? Consider the possibility of having yourself cloned before death: serial immortality. The implications for every known religion, all of which acknowledge the inevitability of death, would be enormous. What would the absence of sexual reproduction mean to the expression of our sexuality? Cell fusion and cloning are probably one of the most controversial topics of our time, and as technology advances, the debate will grow hotter. There are reasons to favor and reasons to oppose continuing these experiments. Those in favor say that the direct copying of a superior person would create genetic immortality of these superior people, and the sex of offspring could be controlled. This could eradicate the existence of sex-linked genetic disorders. Many clones from the same "parent" would produce a pool of "spare parts" for organ transplantation, and rejection problems would be avoided because of the identical genetic makeup. A number of genetically identical clones could be raised in totally different environments and cultures to investigate environmental influences on child rearing. A new species could be created, or humanoid intelligence

could be "cloned" into primates so they could be used for routine or dangerous work.

Those opposed to the continued investigation of cloning say that by ceasing to mix genes through random mating and sexual reproduction, the human race will eventually be weakened by eliminating the process of natural selection. There is a great possibility that the cell nucleus chosen for transplantation will not be perfect and that a grossly malformed or malfunctioning clone will be produced. They also maintain that sexual reproduction is the nature of human beings and that cloning is a violation of this natural method. A greater than average number of clones (as seen now in frogs and other lower animals) are sterile, so the genetic pool could get smaller and smaller, and the proportion of harmful genes could grow larger. Clones, as they matured, would be subjected to strong psychological problems as they reflected on their origins. This would be particularly true if some individuals were cloned and some were reproduced naturally.

There are also many other forms of genetic manipulation, such as enzyme replacement, transformation of DNA from one individual to another, cell fusion for hybridization, recombinant DNA, four parent individuals, and others. Space precludes a discussion of these technologies, and the ethical issues involved go far beyond that of cloning. But cloning can be used as a paradigm for a discussion of the ethics of genetic manipulation.

ETHICS

There are myriad ethical, moral, and cultural ramifications involved in cloning. The possibility exists, because the concept of cloning is so foreign to our present way of thinking, that an entirely new set of ethics will have to be devised in order to provide a rationalization for new modes of behavior. There is also the thought that humankind should never do some things, no matter what the provocation and possible beneficial outcome. The nature of humanity would be irrevocably changed. The question arises of whether human beings have the wisdom necessary to take on the responsibility of being their own creators. Sexual reproduction is almost completely random, and "mistakes" can be ascribed to fate, to God, or to some other mysterious force. With cloning this would not be possible. Blame could be clearly established, and punishment could be inflicted. The entire cultural, sociological, and psychological meaning of parenthood would be changed, and there could no longer be any necessity for the family. The entire fabric of society would be unrecognizable.

In literary, social, cultural, and political areas, outstanding achievements have always been the result of individual human endeavor. What will cloning do to our sense of uniqueness? If there were a thousand Michelangelos chipping away at marble, what aesthetic value would be placed on those many statues of David? What would happen to the uniqueness and beauty of the "Trout" Quintet if a thousand Franz Schuberts could have written it? If we have the capability of not only creating ourselves but also of creating everything we will ever need, what need would we have of God? If we put the creator out of a job, how will we react, and, perhaps even more important, how will God react?

If sexual intercourse is no longer necessary for reproduction, it may eventually no longer be the primary form of sexual activity. Many people today believe that human beings by nature are bisexual, and it is only a strong social and cultural bias that keeps 90% of the people heterosexual. Cloning could relieve the need to conform to society's sexual expectations, and everyone might be free to relate sexually to whomever they choose.

How will a world of perfect people be managed? If a society were developed in which some individuals were to be cloned and some were to be reproduced sexually, what would be the social and political ramifications? Will cloning experiments be begun, and should they be? Who will make that decision, and should they be empowered to make it? Most scientific work of this magnitude is funded by either governments or large foundations. Individual citizens have no voice in the *kind* of sci-entific experiments that are done, but they are much affected by the *results* of the work. Engaging in human cloning will irrevocably change the form and function of humanity, and the people who will be affected by the decision should be the ones to make it.

It is in the nature of humankind to have an unquenchable thirst for knowledge and experimentation. If cloning will change the very nature of an individual, might it not distort or destroy the need to know and eventually be self-destructive? If the decision were to be made to begin human cloning, controls and guidelines would have to be established. Who would control the experiments, and who would control the controller?

Eugenics

Eugenics, or good breeding, has been practiced for years, for both good and ill, and in subtle and not-so-subtle ways. Hitler practiced his brand of eugenics by slaughtering people he considered to be non-Aryan. Animal breeders follow the practice in order to produce animals with certain desired characteristics. People practice eugenics in a social rather than in a purely biological sense. Intelligent people tend to be attracted to each other, to marry, and to reproduce. Similarly, nonintelligent people tend to mate. Because of the lack of scientific controls, human eugenics is haphazard, but it may not be for long.

Work is currently being done to induce genetic change. DNA extracted from one strain of a species can be injected into a genetically different strain of the same species, and the offspring will be genetically different from either of the parents. Recombinant DNA is also possible. The molecule can be cut in a variety of ways by x-ray or laser beams to be anastomosed with other DNA molecules to totally alter the genetic information of each molecule, or certain kinds of genetic information can be simply removed. The possibilities of recombinant DNA are endless. Given sufficient knowledge about any genetic code, it will one day be possible to build a DNA molecule from scratch. We might be able to have "people to order" the way we now can have our ice cream with chocolate chips or without.

The moral and ethical considerations in genetic manipulation are as enormous as they are in cloning. One advantage would seem to be the possible eradication of all genetic disease. But in the process of "snipping out" hemophilia from a DNA molecule, might we not substitute an unknown and possibly greater harm? Would it be possible for a child, who is the result of genetic manipulation, to have some legal recourse against the parents who knowingly changed his nature? There have already been several lawsuits in which children have sued their parents for "wrongful life"; that is, these children have claimed that because their severe genetic defects were known to exist during fetal life, they should have been aborted to prevent the suffering involved in living with serious handicaps. These kinds of suits are now rare, but they would surely increase in the wake of widespread genetic manipulation.

GENETIC COUNSELING

The process of eugenics has begun. Genetic counseling centers are being set up to discuss with prospective parents the advisability of having children. Tay-Sachs disease screening centers are an excellent example. Tay-Sachs disease is uncommon in the general population, but it has a high incidence (a hundred times more common) among Jews of eastern European origin. It is caused by a recessive genetic trait, and the children who are born with it always die by the age of 3 or 4. A marriage where both partners carry the Tay-Sachs gene is a marriage at risk, and the statistical implications are discussed. The husband and wife can then make an informed decision about whether to have children. Pregnant women can receive a definitive diagnosis in the fetus by amniocentesis. Thus the woman has the option of having an abortion rather than giving birth to a child who is doomed to die in early childhood. Other genetic disorders, such as Down's syndrome, cystic fibrosis, phenylketonuria, and sickle cell anemia, lend themselves to genetic screening programs. Al-

though most cannot be diagnosed by amniocentesis, all predictable genetic diseases can be discussed with the future parents. In addition to the genetic considerations of screening programs, much human pain and suffering can be avoided.

There are people, presumably many, who maintain that we should not, for a variety of ethical, religious, and physical reasons, tamper with natural methods of reproduction. The fact remains, however, that since the beginning of time, and particularly in the past fifty years, we have been tampering with our own reproductive capabilities. The taboo against incest to prevent the proliferation of recessive genetic diseases is one of the strongest we have. In most Western cultures marriage between close blood relatives is prohibited by law. Safe and accessible abortion has altered the available gene pool, as has the availability of reliable contraceptives. Genetically defective people are now living longer and are more likely to reproduce and alter the gene pool. The amount of chemicals that enter our bodies every day from drugs consciously taken or from food additives or chemicals used to pollute the air and water is prodigious. No one knows what the continuing and ultimate effect all this will have on our genetic makeup. Radiation released into the atmosphere from a thousand sources cannot help but have a profound effect.

Genetic manipulation and society

If we are able to alter genetic structures to produce the kinds of individuals we desire, and if we can clone our very selves, what will happen to one of the central themes in Judeo-Christian thinking: the dignity and worth of every individual human being? From this basically religious notion comes the democratic political tradition of individual liberty and equality. If there is no genetic distinctiveness, there might not be a need for individual dignity, and the whole concept of human rights would be open to destruction. One's unique appearance is symbolic of one's individual self and is a strong motivating factor in human endeavor. If we all looked alike and thought alike, there would be little need to do anything. There would be no need for achievement and creativity, and it is not too much to suggest that we might all be reduced to a rather bovine existence.

There are several ways in which society can protect itself from the misuses of genetic experimentation. One of the most practical is the establishment of a commission on genetics. It could be composed of scientists, theologians, lay people, economists, philosophers, and anyone else who has an interest. The most powerful influence on the direction of scientific research is the funding policy of government and large foundations. Although foundations are theoretically privately controlled, the philosophies of the people who run them are often similar to the philosophies of the people who run the government. So in actual practice the money comes from a similar source: those in power who run our lives, the "establishment." The challenge of citizen control of genetic research will be great. If citizens as a group are unable to reach an accord on a topic such as the legal restriction of abortion, how can they (we) be expected to agree on a topic as fundamental, and at the same time as complicated, as genetic research?

Public education and discussion are essential for the making of decisions. An uniformed populace is in danger of succumbing to its own apathy. True, the subject is far too complex for everyone to grasp entirely, but there is no reason why public ignorance should remain at its current level. If we are essentially responsible for own physical health, then we should be essentially responsible for our own genetic future. There is also no reason why everyone must avail himself of whatever technology exists. In a free society, one may make the choice of having one's genes manipulated, of being cloned, or of being frozen after death. Just as today individuals may refuse chemotherapy or surgery, so may they refuse whatever the technological future has to offer. Individuals must not be manipulated to do what they do not wish to do.

RESEARCH ON HUMAN SUBJECTS

Many ethical issues are involved in the topic of human experimentation: the relationship of the re-searcher and the subject; confidentiality; informed consent; coercion, no matter how subtle; the uncertainty of the results of the experiment; the interests of society in relation to the research process itself and in relation to the individual subject; the use of human beings as a means to an end rather than an end itself; the perceptions of the research subject, which may be different from those of the researcher; the formulation of research policy; the conduct and supervision of the research; the consequences of the research (the use to which the results are put); and on and on.

Abuses of human beings

In 1932 in Tuskegee, Alabama, 400 black men began receiving a series of "shots" because they had been diagnosed as having "bad blood" and would need treatment for an indefinite period of time. At the end of twenty-five years of "treatment" each man received $25 and a certificate of appreciation from the United States Public Health Service. Forty years later, even while the study continued, the story of the "Tuskegee syphilis study" began to emerge. No one had ever charted the course of untreated syphilis over a long period of time with both subjective and objective data. Some of the 400 men were given genuine treatment, and some were given placebos. The differences were pronounced. After twenty years 40% of the untreated men were dead, compared with only 20% of those treated. There is no mention of what treatment was used, but it must be remembered that penicillin was not discovered when the study began and did not come into general use until the late 1940s, when the study was well on its way. In 1972, after a series of articles in the Associated Press, an advisory committee appointed by the Department of Health, Education, and Welfare began to investigate the study. There had been no written protocols; in fact, very little was written down at all except some occasional progress notes. From these it seemed that the primary purpose of the study was to chart the course of untreated syphilis by *deliberately withholding treatment*. "None of the participants was informed of the nature of their disease or given the opportunity to choose or not to choose treatment. The U.S. Public Health Service from the onset of the study maintained a continuous policy of withholding treatment for syphilis from the infected subjects. . . ."[6,p.113] As it turned out, very little medical knowledge was gained from the study, but there was never a formal decision to terminate it. There was only an ambiguous statement that the remaining survivors should no longer be treated. Tuskegee is not an isolated example, and research on uninformed and nonconsenting human subjects did not stop.

One of the most famous examples of the abuse of human research subjects is the Willowbrook experiment in 1956.[6] Willowbrook is a large complex on Staten Island, New York, which houses about 5,000 mentally retarded children between the ages of 3 and 10. In 1949 the incidence of hepatitis began to climb drastically, and many of the children suffered severe liver damage. Overcrowding and the very primitive sanitary conditions undoubtedly led to the rapid spread of the infection. In 1956 the Armed Forces Epidemiological Board, with the endorsement of the New York University School of Medicine, began to develop a hepatitis vaccine. Live hepatitis virus was administered to some of the retarded children at Willowbrook, and, of course, they became ill. The justification for doing this was that the children would most likely contract hepatitis anyway sometime during their stay at Willowbrook, and in deliberately giving the virus, the infection would be extremely mild, it would be diagnosed early, and it would be well treated. The study produced the most definitive documentation of two different forms of hepatitis ever accomplished, and by scientific standards it was a huge success.

The arguments used to justify the study revolved around social rather than medical conditions. If hepatitis was rampant at Willowbrook because of its crowded and unsanitary conditions, was the development of a new vaccine an appropriate solution? Why not clean up and clear out Willowbrook? Perhaps what was called for was a full-scale revision of the prevailing attitudes at the time about the care of the mentally retarded. To make things

worse, all existing medical measures to eliminate hepatitis at Willowbrook had not yet been exhausted. . . . In summary, a situation existed where a potentially lethal virus was deliberately introduced to retarded children and an acceptable medical treatment was withheld in the interest of the experiment.[6,p.115]

Practicing physicians are primarily concerned with the treatment of individual people, and, no matter how remote or indifferent their contact with the client is, the relationship is still essentially one-to-one, and the physicians see the direct result of their treatment. This is not so with research physicians or scientists. They are dealing with large numbers of people, and their minds may not be so much on the treatment of an individual human being as they are on the eventual development of whatever it is they are working on. This is not to say that all researchers are heartless fiends, giving no thought to individuals. Most researchers are by nature no more or no less humane than the rest of the population; it is the effect of their work that can cause them to lose sight of the methods they use to achieve their goals. Most often researchers do not deal with their subjects on an individual face-to-face basis, and human interaction is missing from the relationship. The subjects become statistics in progress reports, so it is no wonder that it would be easy to lose sight of the fact that the subject is a human being.

During World War II one of the *least* horrendous experiments the Germans did was to place captured American pilots in the icy waters of the North Sea until they had almost frozen to death. Then the pilots would be removed and their bodies warmed in various ways while their temperatures were constantly monitored. Of all the warming methods tried, such as hot water soaks, piles of blankets, and exposure to room temperature air, it was found that lying naked next to the body of a naked woman was the fastest and least damaging way to warm the nearly frozen pilots. Some of the pilots froze to death in the sea, and some who were eventually revived suffered permanent damage from exposure. The women, who were all inmates of concentrations camps (actually they were favored prisoners because this ''duty'' did not involve the kind of harsh manual labor to which they were usually subjected, and they were saved from the gas chambers for at least another short while), were frequently raped by the pilots as they awoke from unconsciousness to find themselves in bed with a warm woman. Sexual activity was encouraged by the Germans because it served to raise the body temperature even more efficiently.

Today many pharmaceutical companies use prisoners for the clinical trials of a new drug. Clinical trials, which are required by the Food and Drug Administration, are the testing of a new drug on human subjects after a safe and therapeutic dose has been established for laboratory animals. The prisoners participate in the trials willingly; that is, they are given a choice by prison authorities to become subjects or not. It would be impossible, however, to eliminate coercion, no matter how subtle, from this method of recruiting research subjects. The fact that the prisoners are where they are is a coercive factor. Rewards are often given for participation in the trials: extra food or cigarettes, protection from the physical abuse by guards and other prisoners, marijuana and other drugs, and even time taken off a sentence.

Why has a comparison been made between the atrocities of the Germans forty years ago and the medical research that is going on today at the behest of a branch of the United States government? Because in ethical terms there is little difference. It is true that in both instances humankind was probably the ultimate beneficiary. But in both instances human beings were used as a means to an end without their absolutely free consent. There is no denying that most women would rather participate in the experiments described previously than be used as a communal prostitute for the Gestapo or even be put to death. And there is no denying that a shorter prison sentence with participation in clinical trials is more tempting than a longer sentence without participation. Giving people the choice between the lesser of two evils is *not* the same as requesting voluntary cooperation. There is also no

denying that it is difficult to recruit human research subjects. People mistrust having their bodies tampered with, even in the most controlled and routine circumstances, so it is little wonder that there is a dearth of volunteers. A little incentive goes a long way in persuading people to become research subjects, particularly if the person is in some degree of desperation—poor, ignorant, imprisoned, or even mentally unbalanced. The question of whether it is morally and ethically correct to coerce people for the eventual greater good of humanity is a major one. One may even debate the issue of whether human subjects should be used at all for scientific research. But whatever one's view, the central issue should be the presence of lack of informed consent and voluntary participation. To say that the men of Tuskegee participated voluntarily in the syphilis study because no one *forced* them to take the ''shots'' would be self-delusion of the worst kind. Consider the circumstances: black men in Alabama in 1936 are told that they have ''bad blood.'' White men from the government in Washington, wearing their officialdom as they probably wore their stethoscopes, kindly treat them with medicine. The black men are a hair removed from slavery; their fear and intimidation are so complete that they do not even consider questioning the procedure. This is coercion as surely as the American pilots were coerced by the Germans. The forms are different, but the act remains the same.

The Nuremberg trials in Germany were conducted in response to information gathered about Nazi physicians in concentration camps and elsewhere having conducted medical experiments without any regard for human life. The reader is referred to general history books for details about the trials, which have had an enormous impact on the medical and scientific communities. In 1947 as a result of the trials, the Military Tribunal of Nuremberg drew up the Nuremberg Code, which was the first attempt in modern science to codify what is and what is not allowable in human experimentation. Following are the principles of the code:[6]

1. Voluntary consent of the human subject is absolutely essential.

2. The experiment should be such as to yield fruitful results for the good of society that are not procurable by other methods, and it should not be random or unnecessary in nature.
3. The experiment should be based on the results of animal experimentation and on the knowledge of the natural history of the disease. The anticipated results should justify the performance of the experiment.
4. All unnecessary mental and physical suffering and injury should be avoided.
5. No experiment should be conducted where there is a prior reason to believe that death or disabling injury will occur, except perhaps in experiments where the experimental physicians also serve as subjects.
6. The degree of risk to be taken should never exceed the humanitarian importance of the problem to be solved.
7. Experimental subjects should be protected against even the remote possibility of injury, disability, or death.
8. The experiment should be conducted only by scientifically qualified persons. The highest degree of skill and care should be required through all stages of the experiment.
9. During the course of the experiment the human subjects should be at liberty to discontinue participation in the experiment if they wish to.
10. During the course of the experiment the scientist in charge must be prepared to terminate the experiment at any stage if he has probable cause to believe that a continuation of the experiment is likely to harm or kill a subject.

The Nuremberg Code was an important first step in the protection of human subjects, but its tenets are rudimentary and do not sufficiently protect subjects. The Code's major flaw is that all control remains in the hands of the researcher, and self-regulation in the conduct of the research is still voluntary.

Informed consent is a subject about which there is, surprisingly, great controversy. Jay Katz[6] of the Yale University Law School maintains that informed consent must include all the following:

1. A full explanation of the procedures to be followed, including identification of those which are experimental
2. A description of the attendant discomforts and risks
3. A description of the benefits to be expected
4. A disclosure of appropriate alternative procedures that would be advantageous for the subject
5. An offer to answer any inquiries about the procedure
6. An instruction that the subject is free to withdraw his consent and to discontinue participation in the project at any time

Informed consent is sometimes difficult to obtain. Often prospective subjects have irrational reasons for participating in research. They can be so enthusiastic that they do not listen to whatever explanation is given. The consent then is not truly informed, but blame cannot be laid on the researchers. Sometimes the nature of the study affects the kinds of people who volunteer. For example, when psychotropic drugs are tested, a higher percentage of psychopathology is found in the prospective subjects than is found in the general population. Again, informed consent is questionable. It is not sufficient to simply explain procedures to research volunteers. The subject must truly understand what is said, and there must be some proof of this understanding. If there is no certainty of this, there is no informed consent. The almost unlimited trust placed in the medical and scientific community is easily misplaced, and it is the researchers' obligation to dampen the volunteers' eagerness to ''sign up'' without full understanding of the research consequences.

Two different legal proposals have been offered as protection for human subjects of scientific experimentation. The first, sponsored by Senator Edward Kennedy, established a commission composed of people from the general public and from certain specialized fields to investigate and study "the development of basic ethical principles which should underlie the conduct of biomedical and behavioral research involving human subjects and develop and implement policies and regulations to insure that such research is carried out in accordance with the ethical principles established by the commission."[6,p.150] The intentions of the bill are praiseworthy, but it really does not say much. There are several serious weaknesses. One is that the commission's regulatory power is limited only to projects funded by the DHHS. It has no control over research funded by private money or even other branches of the government (most notably, the military). The second major weakness is that the commission has no real power to enforce compliance with whatever guidelines it devises. If researchers choose to ignore the commission, nothing can be done about it.

The second regulatory proposal sponsored by Katz and Alexander Capron of the University of Pennsylvania Law School calls for a national human investigation board. The proposed NHIB would investigate a wide area of subjects relating to research on human beings. So far the NHIB has not progressed beyond the planning stage.

FETAL RESEARCH

Fetology is the science that concerns itself with the study of the fetus, both inside and outside the uterus. Just as technology has given us new tools to study outer space and the depths of the ocean, so the passenger inside a woman's body, formerly considered just as inaccessible as the heavens or the seas, can now be examined in great detail. Color photographs and even color television pictures can be taken, and the amniotic fluid can be withdrawn in small amounts to study the cells left by the fetus. Thermography and ultrasonics can define fetal shape and detect some abnormalities. The fetus can even be removed from the uterus, while still attached to the mother by the umbilical cord, and can be observed and studied while birth defects are being repaired. After the surgery the fetus is replaced in the uterus to continue its development until delivery by cesarean section.

Geneticists have always been interested in the "improvement" of the human race. So are fetologists, but they study one individual at a time.

Kinds of fetal research

There are basically three classifications of fetal studies: (1) fetuses in utero in the case of planned abortion in which the risk of injury or pain to the fetus is definitely less than the planned abortion, (2) fetuses still connected by umbilical cord to the placenta and to the mother's support system as in the case of abortion by hysterotomy, and (3) intact, still-living abortuses after they are detached from the placenta and the mother's support system.

At the outset of this discussion it might be well to make a statement about the legal status of the fetus. According to Frank P. Grad of Columbia University Law School:

As a matter of law—whether immediately after insemination or in the ninth month—a fetus is *not* a person, the killing of a fetus, whether by abortion or otherwise, is *not* homicide, and the fetus as such does *not* have any legal rights. A fetus is not a person—at most it is an inchoate person with inchoate rights that do not become legally significant until birth makes it into a person. A fetus has no claim to its father's estate, though birth may give the child such a claim. A fetus has no claim for accidental injury while *in utero,* though the child will have such a claim once it is born. A fetus, some recent lawsuits have suggested, may indeed have an inchoate right *not* to be born, a right that may be asserted by the child after its birth, if the child must suffer a predictable deformity if the mother's request for abortion was denied.*

Because the fetus has no legal rights and because it is obviously impossible to obtain informed consent from a fetus, there is no *legal* protection for the fetus during experimentation. This fact will be upsetting to many, perhaps because the fetus is so totally at the mercy of the experimenter. A child

*From Hamilton, Michael P.: The new genetics and the future of man, Grand Rapids, Mich., 1972, Wm. B. Eerdmans Publishing Co., pp. 66-67. Used by permission.

has his parents' protection, and an adult has his own knowledge and common sense (although admittedly it is frequently not used) to deal with researchers, but the fetus has nothing. Many moral and ethical issues are involved here.

There has been some effort to protect the fetus from harm. The Peel Report from Britain in 1972 (the result of an advisory committee appointed by Parliament) stated that a fetus of twenty weeks' gestational age would be viable for research purposes. That is, no research could be done on a fetus after it had reached this age of viability unless the research was considered essential to preserve its life. In the United States the Advisory Council on Human Embryology of the National Institute of Child Health and Human Development in 1972 proposed regulations concerning fetal research. The proposal merely stated that the research must go on under acceptable scientific and ethical guidelines, although it did not at the time formulate any of those guidelines. It required informed consent of the appropriate party (presumably the mother), and it required that the researcher not be determined to terminate the pregnancy. The document is bland and almost totally unenforceable.

Congress in July, 1974, passed the National Research Act, which provides for a national commission to study, among other things, the ethical issues of fetal research. "Until that process is completed, the Secretary [of HEW] is forbidden to conduct or support research or experimentation in the United States or abroad on a living human fetus, whether before or after induced abortion, unless such research is done for the purpose of assuring the survival of that fetus."[7,p.18] The ban on fetal research was lifted in 1979, and there are now ethical guidelines to control research supported by DHHS funds.

Ethical issues

Several basic issues are central to any discussion of the ethics of fetal research. First it must be decided whether it is human research. Since a fetus is not legally a person, it may be argued that experiments involving fetuses are more akin to animal

research than human. If the research is to be considered human rather than "animal," then what ethical standards should apply? Should the rights of the fetus be protected as though it were a child, since that is what the fetus most closely resembles? The fetus can also be compared with an unconscious person, in terms of cortical functioning, ability to communicate, and others of Fletcher's criteria for personhood. In the case of the spontaneous abortion of a previable fetus (prior to twenty weeks' gestation), the characteristics are those of a dying person. What ethical criteria would apply? If research is to be done on the dying fetus, then the decision must be made as to whether the work is directly relevant to its current health status. Is there even a remote hope of successfully treating that particular individual, or is the work simply to be used to add to a general store of knowledge? It would seem that even a previable fetus, if it is born alive and is surviving without its mother's support system, must be considered a human being, if not necessarily a person, and must fall within the realm of the treatment of all human beings.

The question arises of consent for fetal research. At first glance it seems that there is no moral dilemma at all. The woman who is carrying the fetus "owns" it, and she should be the one who makes all the decisions about its fate. It is, however, not so simple. Although the fetus is inside the mother's body, it is genetically also part of the father; in fact, it is half his. Should he not then have equal determination in whether fetal research is to be done? Then there is the problem of whether a woman, by the act of making a decision to abort the fetus, abdicates all rights to and responsibility for it.

The question . . . is whether women undergoing elective abortion have or do not have a remaining claim to perform actions which care for the abortus and protect it from further indignity, neglect, pain, or harm. A strong case can be made that a woman—at least in many instances of abortion—has no standing to claim social endorsement of her moral authority to decide in cases of fetus or abortus research.[7,p.94]

Ramsey advocates that all previable abortuses be routinely used for research unless the woman expressly and of her own volition dissents. That would eliminate the problem of consent, but other problems would arise. If the hospital (or, even more likely, outpatient clinic) has no research projects going on, and most hospitals do not, then what would be done with the fetuses? A rather gruesome specter presents itself: stacks of abortuses, packed in dry ice or perhaps frozen, arriving in the morning mail of major research centers and being stored until a practical use could be found. Capron proposes "selection by guardian" for these decisions. This would preserve some of the intent of informed consent and would lend some protection to the fetus. It also assumes, perhaps mistakenly, that the selected guardian is better qualified, that is, has more moral authority, to make the decision than the woman undergoing the abortion.

Unresolved moral issues lead to an atmosphere of unfairness and injustice. What is acceptable and ethical at one institution may not be permitted at another. A woman who is asked for her decision about her abortus in one town may be totally ignored in a neighboring community. There will never be total agreement about so ephemeral an issue, but some standards should be established to not only protect the "rights" of the fetus but also, and perhaps more important, to ease the decision-making process for the mother, the father, and the researcher.

PSYCHOPHARMACOLOGY, PSYCHOSURGERY, AND BEHAVIOR CONTROL

Loss of control over one's mind or the irrevocable change in one's modes of behavior is greatly feared by most people. The ancients saw this phenomenon as possession by a dybbuk or by a variety of other demons. The Age of Enlightenment has generally eradicated these fears from the minds of "civilized" people. But should we rest so easily? Possession of one's mind can take many forms and can be accomplished in many ways. The surgeon's knife can easily cut out portions of our brain that

control certain kinds of behavior. Electroconvulsive therapy, used routinely for many years, has been thought to permanently alter some neural synapses. And the ever-proliferating variety of psychotropic drugs can change a person's way of behaving, even of thinking, long after the course of therapy has been terminated. "A second general source of concern regarding advances in behavior control stem from the increasing centralization of authority within all governments coupled with vastly more effective methods of surveillance. It is apparent that, should the decision be made to implement new techniques of behavior control, resistance would be difficult and there would be few places to hide."[2, pp.129-130] There is growing distrust of the wisdom of scientists and greater reluctance of larger numbers of people to blindly entrust their minds and bodies to another person. In the United States today behavioral freedom is more and more appreciated. One comes in contact with the live-and-let-live philosophy more frequently, and out of this feeling have come newer and freer lifestyles. Out of this has also come the civil rights movement, women's liberation, gay (homosexual) liberation, and all the various countercultures that one observes. This new behavioral freedom can be threatened by the permanent changes brought about by surgery, chemicals, or electric current.

Behavior control

We have all read about and are accustomed to some "benign" forms of behavior control: brainwashing by enemy governments, education, advertising, totalitarian forms of government, and total institutionalization. They are termed benign, not because they cause no pain, suffering, or anguish, since they do, but because we have lived with them for so long and are familiar with the ways in which they work. They are, for the most part, not permanent. What we should fear is the kind of research that leads to irreversible biological control. These kinds of research projects fall basically into four major categories: (1) devising new methods of treatment for mental illness, especially schizophrenia; (2) the control of recidivist criminal behavior; (3) the control of sexual orientation and drug usage; and (4) the modification of natural traits such as affection, aggression, or intelligence to arbitrarily established boundaries.

There are, of course, gradations in the desirability of finding solutions to any of these "problems." For example, the person who would gladly accept the fact of a chemical cure for schizophrenia might balk at a surgical procedure that would prevent a person from expressing homosexuality. As another example, one may wish to see the social and legal control of drug abuse, but one might not wish to see drug addicts subjected to such tremendous bursts of electricity that their need for drugs is "jolted out" of them. But whatever the gradations of desirability, the ethical issues are similar. By what moral authority is research undertaken to change the nature and essence of human beings? If effective behavior control becomes possible, who will make the decisions? There may be no solutions to the problems and no answers to the questions, but without extensive and vociferous public debate, we may one day soon not be *able* to debate.

Of great interest are the ethical issues involved in the deliberate planning of the alteration of someone's mind by the use of mind-altering, or psychotropic, drugs. If this sounds ominous, it is meant to. The moral dilemma ranges all the way from the general practitioner who prescribes tranquilizers for the client who is "always complaining about something or other" to the administrators of mental hospitals who keep clients so heavily sedated with phenothiazine tranquilizers that they are completely unable to function or even to think. They are as truly restrained as though they were in straitjackets. Chemicals today can be developed to exact specifications. The issue is whether anyone should have the control to specify that another human being's mind be altered in so drastic a way. It can be argued that severely mentally ill people do damage to themselves and to others and that they need to be controlled and protected. True. It can be argued that we have come a long way in the humane treatment of the mentally ill. True. It

can be argued that the giving of a pill to an insane person is less cruel than shackling him in irons to a damp cement floor. True. But it can also be argued that we have changed only the method of controlling people, not the fact that we do it at all. Also true. Then how far have we really progressed?

This is not to say that psychotropic drugs are intrinsically evil. There is no question that they will continue to be used, and in many instances they should be used. The issue is *how* and *by whom* they should be used. There are many reasons to favor the use of such drugs: relief of anxiety and depression, improvement of mood, enhancement of motivation for short periods, and, under controlled circumstances, gaining of new insights into one's psyche by the use of hallucinogenic drugs. There are also reasons to oppose their use: physical and/or psychological dependence is a very real possibility, the ultimate effect on the personality is unknown, there is a paradoxical (opposite from the intended) effect, and there are possible teratogenic[8] and chromosomal effects.

Humankind is confronted with new and enlarging dangers in the sphere of mind or behavior control. If a person's brain can be electrically stimulated by implanted electrodes, how much more sophisticated does the technology have to be to do it by telemetry (remote control)? What is to prevent a government, or even a group of private citizens, from substituting drugs or adding a drug to the syringe during public inoculations? Preposterous science fiction? Not at all.

Psychosurgery is a form of behavior control that has come out of the realm of science fiction and into everyday reality. The definition of psychosurgery might differ from scientist to scientist (and from lawyer to lawyer), but it is basically the surgical destruction of certain portions of the brain for the purpose of treating psychiatric conditions and modifying experience or behavior. In the past twenty years many forms of psychosurgery have been introduced. The most commonly treated person is the one who demonstrates intractably aggressive or violent behavior. Surgical removal of the amygdala of the brain tends to have a sedative effect. It is thought that violently antisocial behavior is frequently caused by disease of the limbic system, although there is no conclusive evidence of this. Temporal lobe epilepsy also is believed to cause violent behavior and is treated by an anterior temporal lobectomy. Intractable pain can be controlled by a lesion in the neural pathways that are the pain receptors in the brain.

Electrical stimulation of the brain (ESB) is receiving attention from researchers. All kinds of behavior modification can be elicited by applying electric current to various areas of the brain. Almost any one of the naturally occurring human emotions can be artificially induced by simply changing the placement of electrodes. There are three major categories of the effect of ESB: (1) the production of changes in feeling or mood to serve as positive or negative reinforcers of behavior (the sites are primarily in the limbic system); (2) activation of sensory and motor regions to produce experiences or movements, which are in the cortical and subcortical regions; and (3) suppression or inhibition of behavior or experience by the activation or disruption of ongoing brain mechanisms. These three areas comprise a great deal of human mental and emotional energy, and it is easy to see the possibilities of benevolent or malevolent uses of brain control by ESB.

The discussion of behavior control must include a discussion of values and ethics. If behavior is to be controlled for social living, then this control will reflect the values of the controllers and their view of humankind. Differing political and economic systems place differing values on freedom of behavior, the rights of individuals versus the welfare of the state, and all kinds of attitudes about the way people live. There is *no* way to make medical decisions about behavior control without confronting value judgments and ethical issues. The kinds of dilemmas involved are limitless, but some of the major issues can be defined.

Ethical issues

Informed consent is of primary importance when behavior and personality may be unalterably changed as a result of a psychosurgical procedure. Two major problems arise: the nature of the procedure may be so inexact that is is impossible to predict the outcome. The client must be made absolutely aware of this fact and be given sufficient time to consult with others and to think alone. The other problem is that the client may be in no condition, mentally or physically, to give consent. In this case the legally accepted procedure is proxy consent. The proxy is a person, usually the next of kin, who has responsibility for making the kinds of consent decisions that are in the best interest of the client, the kinds of decisions the client would most likely make for himself. The major problem in proxy consent, however, is that the proxy may or may not have the best interests of the client at heart.

Another ethical issue is the distinction between experimental and therapeutic procedures. There is no clearly drawn line; an experimental technique may be highly therapeutic for one client and not at all for another. A technique tried on a human being as a ''last-ditch'' therapy may still be in its experimental stage but is used in a therapeutic way on a particular person. The separation between the experimental and the therapeutic is particularly muddled in psychosurgery.

There is the issue of whether certain kinds of behavior, most particularly severe aggression and violence, are organic or nonorganic in nature. Antisocial behavior may be caused by some chemical imbalance, by a structural defect in the brain, or by any one of the myriad amorphous ''causes'' of mental illness. The ethical issue centers around the permissibility of destroying a part of the brain that may indeed be perfectly healthy. The decision to remove a brain tumor that is causing personality changes can be made easily. One knows the tumor exists. One cannot see a diseased limbic system or even know for certain that it *is* diseased. No woman would consent to the removal of a healthy breast simply to prevent cancer. Why should a person consent to the destruction of a part of his brain in the hope that his behavior will improve? On the other hand, many drugs are successfully used to treat nonorganic conditions. Tranquilizers and antidepressants are an excellent example of organic therapy for a condition without a clearly defined organic base. Why then should surgery not be used for the same reason? Aspirin relieves a headache, whether it is organically or psychically caused, and we do not even know how it works. Because its pharmacological action is unknown does not mean that it has no value.

A fourth issue is the distinction between therapy and social control and social engineering. The difference between an intrapersonal disease is the people who are affected by it and the way in which it is treated. An intrapersonal disease is one such as depression or anxiety in which only the person suffering is affected. The person alone suffers both the illness and the cure. An interpersonal disease is one that affects others, such as temporal lobe epilepsy in which the violence can have a direct effect on other people. The cure also affects others in that it can protect them from violent outbursts. Psychosurgery can be the institution of a means of social control. It is essential that control and therapy not be confused, and this is no simple matter. Who can say that control of behavior is not therapeutic? Would not a person who suffers from temporal lobe epilepsy be therapeutically benefited from the cessation of his violent behavior? However, "the incidence of violent behavior directly linked to brain changes seems so low as to raise the question whether the ultimate uses of the extensive research being suggested are to cure illness or to seek controls of violence for social purposes."[9,p.18]

Social control leads to social engineering. A crucial issue is the meaning of the concept of normalcy. In physical terms it is fairly easy to define. In psychic terms it is almost impossible. What are "normal" attitudes toward any aspect of life? How are the parameters of normalcy defined, and *who* does the defining? If it could be done, how much deviation from the norm would be acceptable, and what procedures would be used to bring the deviants back to the norm? We are familiar with the kinds of punishments that are today being meted out to "social deviants": the employee who dis-

agrees with company policy is fired; the black who chooses to live in a white neighborhood has his house firebombed: the homosexual is frequently not employable as a fireman, policeman, or teacher. Consider the social pressure alone on these "deviants" and then consider the possibilities of surgical, chemical, or electrical mind control.

A fifth issue is the question of human autonomy and the relative importance of freedom and dignity. Before mass behavior control for the purpose of social engineering could be initiated in any effective way, it would have to be proved that the concepts of individual freedom and dignity are false and even dangerous. There are those who think we are slowly moving in this direction. They point to the increased mechanization and dehumanization of so many aspects of our lives, to the rapidly increasing divorce rate and the failure of so many interpersonal relationships, and to the crumbling of so many of our social and moral values.

ORGAN TRANSPLANTATION

New technology creates new ethical problems. Not too long ago death was death, and that is all there was to it. When the kidneys failed, the entire body failed. When the heart valves became too clogged with plaque, the pump simply stopped. When skin was so badly burned that there was no barrier to invading microorganisms, massive infection led to death. There was no need to debate the issues of who should or who should not receive a donor kidney or be attached to an artificial one. There was no question about grafting various parts of the body, and there was no question about whether a person was really dead so his heart could be transplanted to another.[10] People have always died in parts, but it is now possible to replace some worn-out body parts with "previously owned" ones.

Logistical problems, as well as ethical ones, have arisen with the advent of "spare part surgery." The major problem is that there are not enough available donors for the number of recipients. Longmore, in his book, *Spare Part Surgery,* has suggested the establishment of a worldwide organ and tissue bank. Living donors and potential recipients would register at a local health center, and various kinds of biological data would be stored in a computer. When an emergency arose, the donor (or recipient) would be identified by his fingerprints, and if he died the organs that he chose to donate could be flown to an appropriate recipient. Another solution to the shortage of donors is the development of artificial organs to replace living tissue.

Ethical issues

The ethical and moral issues surrounding organ transplantation have created a swirl of public controversy. It heightened when Christiaan Barnard performed the first heart transplant in South Africa more than fifteen years ago. Corneal transplants or bone grafts do not provide much of interest for newspapers, but a heart is a different story. Ethicists, however, have been debating the issue far longer than has the public.

One of the most interesting questions is to whom the organs of a dead person belong. A dead person has no further interest in his own body, and because legally a corpse is not ''property,'' it belongs to no one. Within this frame of reference no family opposition should be allowed to stand in the way of removing any organs for transplant. In practice, however, this theory does not work. Even though a person is not owned in life and is not owned after death, there are certain social and humanistic attitudes to be taken into consideration. A high, but not absolute, value is placed on the integrity of the human body, and there is a strong tradition not to mutilate it in any way, even after death. There are also financial considerations. If a woman is paying for the disposal of the body of her husband, it has been her traditional right to say which parts of his body will or will not be buried with him. The decision whether to volunteer another human being's organs for transplant can be a most distressing one, made even more painful by the anguish of new grief.

Another ethical issue is money. Should human tissues and organs be obtained by purchase or by voluntary gift? If a person did not pay for his kidney in the first place, why should he receive money for it when he voluntarily gives it up? That seems logical enough, but then the question of motivation arises, especially in the matter of the most commonly donated organ, the blood. It is common practice in this country for people to sell a unit of blood to a private laboratory, which in turns sells it, at a profit, to a hospital. The hospital then passes on its expense to the client. It is easy to dismiss the practice of selling blood as immoral and unethical, and the temptation to do so is great. What if the donor, however, needs the money to feed himself or his children? What if it is a medical or nursing student who uses the money to buy textbooks? What if the money is given to charity? The issues are no longer so clear-cut. There is also the matter of the reluctance of people to donate their blood and the perpetual shortage of it. If people can be motivated by money to donate, there will most likely be a greater supply of blood. There is little likelihood that organs other than blood will be sold. How could one establish a fair price? What is to prevent people with enough money from contracting with donors or physicians on a private basis to receive preferential treatment for transplants? That could lead to the horrendous practice of murder for organs.

The free and informed consent of the donor is a special moral issue. All principles of informed consent previously discussed in regard to research on human subjects also apply here. There are some others, particularly if the donor is alive and expects to remain so. This occurs most frequently during kidney transplants. Donors must be made fully aware of the risks they are taking, both during the actual surgery and for the rest of their lives. The consent must be truly free. Most often the donor is a close relative of the recipient, and there may be all kinds of psychological factors operating. Guilt perhaps is the strongest. The power to save the life of a person dearly loved can cause guilt if that power is withheld. To give a kidney to avoid guilt can have serious psychological ramifications later. The recipient may also be exercising psychological power over the donor, and free consent may not be as free as it seems. Family pressure to give up a kidney to save a life can be tremendous, and it is a rare person who can handle the burden of guilt of refusal. There should be mandatory psychological screening for every donor. This may not totally alleviate the problem, but it would give donors an opportunity to explore and discuss their feelings.

Moral theologians have had some difficulty in justifying organ transplants from living donors. The question is a person's stewardship over his own body. Is a person justified in sacrificing part of his healthy self, thus mutilating himself, for the ultimate good of another person? Before organ transplantation became a reality, Christian moralists had come to agreement that healthy parts of a body may be sacrificed for the good of that particular body, as in removing the healthy tissue that surrounds a cancer. But then the question arose as to whether the parts of a human body exist only for the exclusive use of that individual, or do they also have a wider finality?

There is less resistance to the use of cadavers for organ transplantation, but it is not totally absent. There are various superstitious religious beliefs, and there is an exaggerated reverence for the physical body, perhaps a misinterpretation of the Christian doctrine of resurrection. People are frightened of the idea of rising from their graves and finding some vital organ missing. Resistance also comes from funeral directors who feel that they cannot do a neat embalming job if all the organs are not intact. And they cannot do an embalming job at all if the entire body has been donated.

Public opinion is very much in favor of organ donation after death. A 1968 Gallup poll showed that 70% of American adults would be willing to do so, but very few actually make the necessary arrangements. Some proposals have been made to increase the supply of donated organs. It has been suggested that a law be passed so that everyone is presumed to be a donor unless there are explicit instructions in writing to the contrary. This pas-

sive form of donation would surely yield a greater supply than our current active form. A proposal enacted into law in 1968 and now effective in all fifty states is the Uniform Anatomical Gift Act, which affirms the right of any adult to donate organs after death, and it denies the right of any relative to rescind or override this decision. Both of these proposals are practical in form but of highly different ethical nature. One is the societal *taking* of organs, and the other is the free *giving* of them. One is an act of medical practicality, and the other is an act of human charity.

The problem of the distribution of organs has been with us from the beginning and will be with us until the supply is equal to the demand. What criteria should be used in deciding who shall receive organs, who shall be chosen to live and who shall be allowed to die? An initial screening could be done on a strictly medical basis. If there were no hope at all for recovery, even with a new organ, then it would be wasteful and wrong to choose that person if there is another who has a better chance to live. There is always another person. But after the medical selection has been done, the moral issues are there in full force. Should the selection be on the basis of social worth, or should it be on a first-come-first-served basis? Should people whose lives are judged to be the most essential for the common good be chosen first? How can social worth and usefulness be realistically measured? Americans do not have agreed-on common social goals, so it is impossible to compare the worth of the lives of people. Hospital committees who make these decisions tend to reflect the mores and values of the community in which they live. These values differ drastically from one part of the country to another. It is difficult to see how a poet and philosopher could "win" over a mother of four in the Midwest or parts of the South. And the mother might be doomed in San Francisco or New York. An effort to make these decisions on the basis of social worth might seem practical at the time, but in an ethical or moral sense it can never be successful. The only other alternative is random selection: drawing lots. This may seem grossly unfair when a janitor draws a higher number than a Supreme Court Justice, but if we truly believe that we are a society in which every individual has the same worth as every other individual, then it is the *only* fair way of deciding. There is also legal precedent in the principle of random selection when some lives must be sacrificed in order to save others. "In the *United States vs. Holmes* it was ruled that in the desperate situation of an overloaded lifeboat, the decision of who should be saved and who abandoned must be made by lot. It was argued that a lottery is the only means of selection which avoids arbitrariness and shows respect for equal rights to life."[11,p.45]

ABORTION

Abortion has been discussed a good deal in the past two decades or so, both in the professional and public press, and community health nurses routinely come across women who are pregnant and who do not wish to be. Probably most nurses, except those who are morally opposed to abortion, have helped women make arrangements to obtain an abortion or have at least referred them to the community agency or hospital that performs them.

Abortion is a highly emotional subject, and most people have an opinion about it one way or the other. The trouble with these opinions is that many of them are uninformed and based on emotionalism and personal preference. Although this short discussion will make no attempt to dictate a correct ethical position on abortion, it will attempt to separate logical ethical arguments from emotional ones. Nurses should be able to do this; they ought to know how to argue logically about abortion and how to rationally defend a viewpoint. There are two basic ways to argue about abortion: on the basis of the ontologic status of the fetus and on that of the conflict between fetal and maternal rights.

The ontologic status of the fetus means the extent to which it can be considered a person *and* the extent to which it is owed moral responsibility. There are several criteria that can be applied to this determination of status. The first is the group of criteria established by Joseph Fletcher described in the opening pages of this chapter. It becomes evident, on even the most cursory examination of those criteria, that Fletcher would not consider the fetus a person. However, the matter of ensoulment is not so readily apparent. Ensoulment is the point at which the soul (if indeed there is such a concept or entity) enters the body and the point at which the being in question becomes a person to whom full moral obligations are owed, including the right to life. The Catholic Church, in an arbitrary move by Pope Clement XI in 1708 to establish the date of the ensoulment of the Blessed Virgin, considers the fetus ensouled at the moment of conception. This is the major reason why the Catholic Church and other Western and non-Western religions oppose abortion. Judaism and some other religions believe that ensoulment occurs at birth.

Another consideration in the ontologic status of the fetus is its distinction in regard to death; that is, philosophers have made a distinction between a person who is fully human and one who is irreversibly comatose although not quite dead because certain life processes are being kept alive artificially. Although an individual in such a coma cannot be compared biologically or rationally to a fetus, an ontologic comparison can be drawn. If the essence of humanity has departed the comatose individual, it could be said that it has not yet appeared in the fetus; thus because the fetus has no characteristics of personhood, no moral obligation is owed it. Those who speak of the fetus as a human being do so because of its potentiality, not because of its actuality. It is so obviously not *not* human (that is, it is not any other living thing) that to label it human seems the only reasonable course of action.

The potentiality of the fetus brings us to the second basis on which to argue logically about abortion: the conflict of fetal and maternal rights. We should, at the outset, be clear about the nature of the rights under discussion; I refer here to moral rights only, not to legal rights. If one chooses to grant any moral rights to a fetus, the problem of which ones to grant arises. Conservatives believe that a fetus has the same rights as a person who has already been born, and liberals believe that a fetus has no moral status. To some it might seem useless to argue about rights accruing to a being that has no developed sense of morality, but the debate is important insofar as rights are inextricably connected to obligations. If one assigns no moral rights to a fetus, then no corresponding obligations are assigned, and one may do with it as one pleases. However, if it is assigned full moral rights, then one is obligated to protect and care for it as for any other human being. It is easy, then, to determine one's moral position on abortion on the basis of one of these two divergent views. The ethical issue arises when it must be decided which rights exist and when they take effect. A moderate view is that a line is drawn during fetal life between the time when a fetus is genetically human but not a member of the moral human community and the time when it should be granted full moral rights. Viability is the most popular point at which this line is drawn.

The moral battle of abortion is often fought on the "right to life" field; the issue at stake is whether the pregnant woman's right to legitimately rid herself of the fetus ever overrides the fetus's right to life and, if so, under what circumstances. Is abortion justifiable homicide, is it murder in the first degree, or can it be considered killing in self-defense?

Even if the conservative theory is construed so that it entails that human fetuses have equal rights because of their moral status, nothing in the theory requires that these moral rights always override all other moral rights. Here a defender of the conservative theory confronts the problem of the morality of abortion on the level of conflicting rights: the unborn possesses some rights (including a right to life) and pregnant women also possess rights (including a right to life). Those who possess the rights have a (prima facie) moral claim to be treated in accordance with their rights.*

*Beauchamp, Tom L., and Walters, LeRoy: Contemporary issues in bioethics, Belmont, Calif., 1978, Wadsworth Publishing Co., Inc., p. 193.

When these rights conflict, a moral dilemma is created. Many moderates feel that the fetus has some claim to protection against the arbitrary actions of others, but they do not grant the fetus the same moral rights to life as possessed by a person already born. The ultimate justification for the morality of abortion lies in the determination of which rights and obligations take precedence over which others.

DEATH AND DYING
Definitions

At the outset of this discussion of death and dying, some terms and concepts are defined that will be used in this chapter and that have come into common use among health care professionals. The basic standard of the definition of death is the one devised by the Ad Hoc Committee of the Harvard Medical School.[12] The definition includes all organs, but we will be concerned only with the brain. The absence of cerebral functioning has occurred when the following are present:

1. Unreceptivity and unresponsivity. There is total unawareness to external stimuli and inner need (irreversible coma). Even the most intensely painful stimuli evoke *no* response whatsoever, no matter how fleeting.
2. No movements or breathing. Observation of at least one hour should confirm that there is no spontaneous movement or response to any stimuli. If the client is on a respirator, it should be turned off for 3 minutes to see if there is any spontaneous effort on the part of the client to breathe.
3. No reflexes. The pupils will be fixed and dilated, and there is no response to any of the usual eliciting of muscle or tendon reflexes.
4. Flat electroencephalogram. At least 10 full minutes of recording is essential for an accurate diagnosis, and the test must be repeated at least 24 hours later with no change. There must be no evidence whatsoever of any electrical activity in the brain.

Euthanasia is literally defined as "good death" and is sometimes called mercy killing by laypersons, a phrase that is neither accurate nor appropriate. Active, or positive, euthanasia is the conscious and deliberate act of one person toward another to spare the other an intolerable life. In blunt terms, it is the killing of a person with the intention of doing a positive service for the person killed. Passive, or negative, euthanasia is the act of refraining from any measure that would artificially prolong a person's life. It is the act of letting a person die. The difference between voluntary and involuntary euthanasia is whether the person has knowledge of and participation in the decision to administer euthanasia. There are four distinct kinds of euthanasia:

1. Voluntary positive in which the person is killed with his own knowledge and consent
2. Voluntary negative in which the person is permitted to die with his own knowledge and consent
3. Involuntary positive in which the person does not know he is being killed
4. Involuntary negative in which the person does not know he is being permitted to die

It is interesting to note here a synopsis of a euthanasia bill introduced in Britain in 1969,[12] the salient points of which are the following:

1. It shall be lawful for a physician to administer euthanasia to a qualified person who has made a declaration that is still in force. A qualified person is one who is over the age of majority and who has been certified in writing by two qualified physicians to be suffering from an irremedial condition.
2. The declaration of intent shall be made by the person. It shall take effect thirty days after it is made and shall be in force for three years. It can be revoked at any time.
3. As long as the physician prescribes the euthanasia treatment, it can be administered by a nurse, but no person may be required to participate in euthanasia treatment.

4. The physician or nurse cannot be held in breach of any professional code or affirmation.
5. The euthanitized person's insurance cannot be revoked simply because of the euthanasia.
6. A person suffering from an irremedial disease may have any and all drugs that he wishes to keep him free of pain even if the drugs will keep him unconscious.

Ethical issues

Birth and death are the central events in the life of every human being. There is no longer anything to be done about births, but there is much that can possibly be done about death (Fig. 5-2). The social, cultural, humanistic, moral, and ethical issues in death and dying are so complex that it is impossible to think about them all, much less write about them. As with the other issues already discussed, there will be no attempt to answer questions or to solve problems. There will merely be a setting forth of the issues and questions as many people see them.

The prolongation of life is a problem that nurses frequently encounter. During the terminal phase of an illness when the client is suffering pain and anguish that seems unendurable, would we serve him better to stop the pain by euthanasia, or should we permit (even help) him to live for every possible moment? We as health workers are so often unable to cope with death, either our own or other people's, that perhaps we deliberately, although unconsciously, torture our clients because of our own psychological inadequacies. We also have trouble dealing with the client's own expressed desire to die. He may have very different ethical and moral beliefs than our own. As in other forms of human activity, we have difficulty looking at moral and ethical issues from someone else's perspective. Physicians and nurses have been trained to treat and cure people at all costs, and their entire professional lives are devoted to this end. So it is no small wonder that the death of a client is viewed as a professional failure. As human beings we are

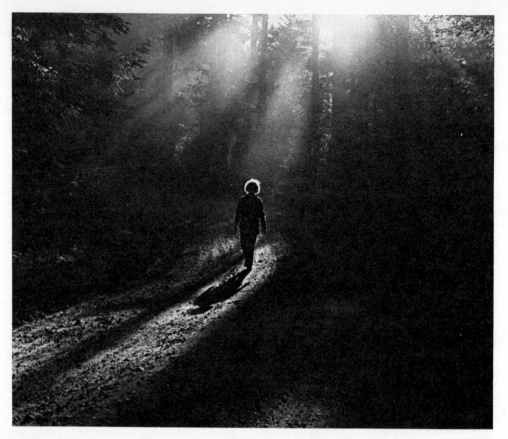

Fig. 5-2. We are all alone when we die, but it is one of the functions of professional nursing to help prepare the client for a peaceful death. (Photograph by Samuel Uretsky; courtesy Editorial Photocolor Archives, Inc., New York.)

trained to avoid failure, so again we torture clients because of our own inabilities to deal with the realities of life.

There are those who advocate that the prolongation of life by artificial means is not natural. They say that when one's time comes, it is an affront to God and to nature to stave off the inevitable. There are those who counter this argument by saying that it is also ''natural'' to die of plague, scurvy, or diphtheria. We have tampered with nature so that we can now prevent and cure many diseases; why not prevent death for as long as possible?

EUTHANASIA

In discussing euthanasia we must come again to that amorphous issue of the quality of life. How many times have we asked ourselves about the quality of life of a quadriplegic, who is able to move his face, blink his eyes, and think—and little else. What is the quality of life of a person who is in the last throes of agonizing illness, thrashing about the bed in what seems to be an effort to physically escape the pain? What quality of life is there in a human being who lies in a vegetative state attached to a respirator and a tangle of plastic tubes? Or a fireman who has been burned beyond recognition and waits only to die from the inevitable infection? The answer is that there is no answer. No one can judge the quality of another's life. In writing about the quality of life Marya Mannes says:

The inference here might be that those who opt for life on any terms have never known life in its fullest terms. One of the many alarming facts of our current society is the steady erosion of quality in the face of quantity. Too many people, surrounded by too many things, have too little. Not in terms of worldly goods but in the conscious savoring of the hours and days of their lives. Millions have never lived to their fullest capacities. And because of this, they would rather settle for a minimal life than no life at all. Their dread of death supersedes all else.*

Mannes believes that the will to die is a direct reflection of the quality of life and that by a mysterious mechanism of will we can somehow hasten our own deaths. Because of this she feels it is wrong for such people to be thwarted in their desire or need to die. There are many who would disagree. They argue that the sanctity of life itself is God given, and it must be only God who takes it away. By using this line of logic, are not the physicians who attach the client to the respirator to prevent an inevitable death then thwarting the will of God? But then, if God wanted death to occur in such a way, we would not have been given the intelligence and ingenuity to invent respirators in the first place. So the argument goes on and on and round and round.

Advocates for euthanasia are becoming larger in number and more vociferous in their demands to permit people to die with peace and dignity. The need for euthanasia would not be so great if we did not have such advanced technology. A treatment that was considered extraordinary ten years

*Reprinted from Nancy C. Ostheimer and John M. Ostheimer: Life or death—who controls? p. 232. Copyright © 1976 by Springer Publishing Co., Inc. Used by permission.

ago, for example, coronary artery bypass surgery, is considered ordinary and routine today. Circumstances change, but must ethics also change? People can always refuse treatment for themselves, but can others refuse it for them? Physicians are morally obligated to do whatever they can to cure the client, but they are also morally obligated to alleviate suffering. If the only end to suffering is death, are physicians obligated to help the person die? There are some central questions in the ethical issue:

1. Does a person have a constitutional right to die, and if so, is that right always in his best interest?
2. Does death by choice represent medicine's best answer to the question of incurable and/ or terminal illness?
3. Does society have an investment in the sacredness of human life that overrides the individual? Conversely, does the notion of easy death give society a weapon to regulate population in a world burdened with too many people?
4. Does the right to die sanction unconscious self-destructive impulses in people?

Until these questions can be answered once and for all to everyone's satisfaction, the moral dilemma of euthanasia will never be solved.

The legalization of positive euthanasia, which is advocated by many, is fraught with danger. It is true that euthanasia often is merciful, kind, and good. It is also true that it could empower physicians to kill all clients whom they could not cure, whom they thought they could not cure, whom they did not try to cure, or whom they did not choose to cure. Is this too extreme? Perhaps, but even the most far-fetched ramifications of any ethical issue must be considered. Legalizing euthanasia would be giving one human being, or even a committee of human beings, an enormous and dangerous amount of power. "If voluntary euthanasia were legal, there would be a standing risk of a person consenting to his extinction or an erroneous calculation of his prospects. If it were to become an acknowledged function of the medical profession to end life prematurely, could patients place themselves with complete trust in the care of physicians?''[13,p.248]

There can be a solution to the agony and indignity of a cold and impersonal death. St. Christopher's Hospice[14] in London is a haven for the dying. There is no attempt to prolong death, and there is no chemical or mechanical resuscitation when death has occurred. The only medications given are for the relief of pain and general discomfort. If a client contracts pneumonia or some other secondary infection, it probably would not be treated except for measures that would permit the client to rest more easily. Comfort, rather than cure, is the major criterion in the care of clients. Each person knows his diagnosis and prognosis, and admission to the hospice is purely voluntary. Death is discussed, and the clients are encouraged and actively helped to accept death. Cicely Saunders, the founder and medical director, believes that the acceptance of death is neither resignation nor defeat; it is the opposite of doing nothing. She says, ''Let us be *with* [those who are dying] so we can learn what their real needs are. We don't run from them, for the more you run, the worse death appears. Like most things, the closer you get, the less difficult it is.''[12,p.154]

No client is in pain all the time, and about 98% have total relief of pain, mainly through the use of heroin, although morphine is also used. The medication is given *before* the pain returns, so the client need not be put into the degrading position of a supplicant begging for relief. Heroin's psychic effect is a sense of peace and relaxation; there is a warm euphoria with a concomitant loss of fear. St. Christopher's philosophy is that there is no reason why a person should be expected to face death with apprehension, fear, depression, and anger, and if heroin can remove these feelings, there is no reason not to use it.[15]

The most important thing at St. Christopher's is that the client not be alone, that he knows he is with tender, caring, and loving people who will listen to him, help him give vent to his feelings, or who will simply hold his hand in silence for as long as he needs it. The client's family is an integral part of the care at St. Christopher's because they often need as much or more support than the dying client. There are no restrictions on visiting; the family is encouraged to take part in the support activities of the staff, and they are not abandoned after the death.

The hospice does everything possible to bring family and patient together. Inability to cope with someone who is dying and in pain often separates loved ones. When the patient is physically comfortable and the family has relaxed somewhat, the family sees the ''return'' of the person they had known before. Frequently, families divided by the illness come together and allow the patient to see his family ''whole again'' around his bedside before he dies.[12,p.161]

Because clients are in four- or six-bed rooms, there is a sense of community, and if one client has no family, he is ''adopted'' by another. The physical closeness of clients also promotes the sharing of their thoughts and feelings and removes some of the isolation of impending death. The hospice also has an outpatient service. Four nurses care for about seventy clients at home who are not yet ready to enter the hospice. But they know they may be admitted at any time they choose. If there is enough medical and nursing support, clients can be very well managed at home even up to the time of death.

There are about 800 hospice programs in the United States. Some are free-standing hospices, some are home care programs, and some are only a group of beds in a general hospital. Although the hospice concept has ''caught on'' to some extent in this country, most Americans still die in loneliness, terror, and isolation, and we do not even reach out our hands to them.

DEFECTIVE INFANTS

The moral and ethical issues involved in the involuntary euthanasia of defective infants are not only among the thorniest we face, but they are also ones that are receiving wider public attention. Certain conditions with which children are born would surely kill them if it were not for immediate and continuing medical care. Even with treatment, many of these infants are most likely doomed to profound handicaps and severe mental and physical retardation for the rest of their lives. It is with these kinds of hopeless individuals that this discussion will be based. Should these infants be treated or should they not?

Nontreatment has occurred commonly throughout history, first because nothing *could* be done and then because many thought that nothing *should* be done. The conscious decision not to treat these children happens countless times a day in the United States, but few know about it. In 1973 Raymond Duff and A.G.M. Campbell at Yale-New Haven Hospital[16] documented forty-three cases of withholding treatment from defective infants, thus exposing the issue to public debate. Since then other cases have been brought to light, and there are frequent articles in medical journals about the subject. Nontreatment of defective infants seems to be gaining status as good medical care.

This development is significant because it represents the only large-scale instance of involuntary euthanasia now being practiced by the medical profession, at a time when most physicians and the public retain strong opposition to involuntary euthanasia in other circumstances. This does not imply that the decision to withhold care is lightly made. The clash between the norms of preventing suffering and preserving life is too great to ignore and has engendered much soul-searching and ethical analysis on the part of parents, physicians and nursing staffs.*

Many conflicting claims and needs are involved. The child will very likely be doomed to a life of abnormalcy. There will be emotional and psychological anguish and perhaps even physical pain. The child will grow up knowing that he will *never* be like everyone else. His parents will have to

*From Robertson, John A.: Involuntary euthanasia of defective infants: a legal analysis. In Schwartz, Jane L., and Schwartz, Lawrence H., editors: Vulnerable infants, p. 336. Copyright 1977 by McGraw-Hill, Inc. Used with permission of McGraw-Hill Book Co.

watch his suffering, pay for all the treatment and special schooling, and always be prepared to devote their lives to the child. The child might never be independent, and the parents will need to find someone to care for him after they die. Or there is the anguish of knowing that the child will not live long, watching him die, and feeling helpless and useless.

But what of the child? Like any other human being, he, too, has a right to live. No one can say whether this day-old infant who is struggling to survive will have a satisfying life. Every day we hear about people who survive and blossom under the most incredible handicaps. They lead lives, no matter how short or how physically restricted, that are satisfying to themselves and to others. If the physician and parents agree not to treat the defective infant, who remains to speak for the child? And if the physicians and parents have conflicting interests, no matter what the morality of the ultimate choice, it seems unfair to subject the life of the child to the perhaps misguided discretion of the adults involved. In other circumstances (e.g., withholding insulin from a diabetic child) the right of parents to injure their child, even if done benevolently or unintentionally, is severely restricted, but in the matter of refusing treatment for a defective infant, the parent seems to have moral, if not legal, carte blanche. Parents and physicians who choose not to treat these infants run the risk of prosecution for homicide, but in reality the chance of their ever standing trial is small.

There are two questions that are at the core of the defective infant dilemma, and they are at the same time both ethical and legal. The first is whether there should be a definable class of human beings, including but not limited to defective newborns, from whom medical care can be withheld without their consent. The second question is who among us is best equipped to decide what the criteria are for inclusion in this classification of human beings and when care is to be withheld.

There are arguments for the legal and moral permission to withhold treatment from defective infants. Some say that severely deformed infants are not persons and cannot conform to many of Fletcher's criteria. The counter-argument is that the questioning of someone's humanity or personhood is the first step to genocide or other forms of inhumane suffering.

The second argument for nontreatment is that there is no obligation to treat when the costs of maintaining life greatly outweigh the benefits. Many think that the care of these infants does more harm than good, both to the parents and to the infant himself in the long run. In this view the suffering is not worth whatever pleasure is derived from that care. The largest loophole in this argument is that pain, pleasure, satisfaction, and the relative worth of people's lives cannot be measured, so no comparisons can be made. If six months of treatment in a newborn intensive care unit costs $500,000, how much of this is offset by the pleasure the parents take in holding, rocking, and singing to their baby? How much of the debt is canceled? This is not to say that we cannot possibly make a decision on this basis; it is simply that the argument is not a logical one. It goes back to the quality of life issue that has been discussed previously.

A third argument is that the suffering of others is not worth the life saved; consequently, treatment should be withheld. There is no doubt that the parents and other family members suffer tremendous anguish at the birth of a defective infant, and, in fact, it is not uncommon for the marriage to collapse under the strain. Health professionals suffer in concrete ways. Their sense of frustration and failure is strong, and the effects of their feelings can influence the quality of care given to the infant. Society suffers, even if in a purely monetary way. It is not only a matter of the dollars and cents spent on the care of the particular infant but on the energy that is diverted from the care of other children with better prognoses. How morally justified is anyone in killing someone else because of psychic or financial pain felt by the killer? By the same token, how morally justified is anyone to knowingly condemn another human being to life of pain, humil-

iation, and emptiness when there is a merciful and painless solution?

CLIENT'S KNOWLEDGE OF IMPENDING DEATH

Another ethical issue involved in death and dying is whether the person should be told he is dying. The general trend in the past several years tends to be toward greater frankness and honesty in dealing with the realities of illness. But there are still many people who feel it is kinder and more humane to protect the client from the truth, and there are many people who expressly wish not to be told.

There are, in the health community, various beliefs about whether a client should be told he has a fatal illness. Some think that the physician is the one who is best capable of knowing whether the client can cope with the news and that the decision to tell o not to tell should be entirely the physician's. It does not seem to matter how well the physician knows the client. There is the belief that under no circumstances should the client be told that he is dying. The feeling seems to be that the physical suffering should not be compounded by mental suffering, which would ensue if the client were told the truth. If everyone around the client pretends that everything will turn out fine, then he will be spared the gloom of impending death. At first glance this may seem like a humane attitude, but it does not meet the needs of the client. Kübler-Ross and others have done much research on death and dying, and they have found that one of the greatest needs is for the client to be able to talk about his own death and then prepare to accept it. Some believe that a person has a right to know, and should know, exactly what his condition is and how long he has to live. The dying person needs to make arrangements for the care of his family and perhaps conclude business or professional matters. There are certain decisions that no one else can make for him. There are those who think it should be the family's decision to tell or not to tell. They know the client better than anyone else;

they have seen his reactions to a lifetime of good and bad news; they know his values and his psychic makeup. Some believe that the decision to be told is only the client's, and it is up to the health worker, who, by skillful interviewing, finds out whether the client really wants to know.

These points of view all have merit, but they often turn out to be totally irrelevant because dying people usually know they are dying even though they have not been told in so many words. They are then faced with the burden of "protecting" their family and friends while at the same time *they* are being protected. The energy involved in the holding back of feeling is tremendous, and it seems that the energy would be much better spent recognizing, acknowledging, and talking about reality.

It has usually been assumed that if a client is to be told, then it is the physician who will do the telling. This is an assumption that has always existed, but there is no professional or human reason for it. Physicians have taken the prerogative of imparting news of a fatal illness, and they do not seem about to give it up. There is no reason why a nurse could not break the news. She is the one who spends the most time with the client, and it is to the nurse that the client is very likely to go if he cannot receive information from the physician. This kind of news must be given with the utmost gentleness and sensitivity, and physicians have not demonstrated any greater ability in this area than nurses. It can be argued that physicians are the ones who have all the details about the nature and the course of the disease and what kinds of physical problems can be anticipated along the way. This, however, is not the kind of information the client wants or needs at first. He wants to know only whether he is going to die, and if so, how long he has left to live. He is not interested, at that time, in the meaning of his reticulocyte count or how many bone marrow biopsies there will have to be. He wants only the essential facts, and the nurse has these. There is no reason why nurses should be required to break the news, but there is also no reason why they should be prohibited from

doing so. There is also no reason why physicians should always be burdened with this grim and emotionally draining responsibility. They have no greater or fewer emotional resources than anyone else and might even be willing or grateful to relinquish the responsibility. It does not, in the end, really matter *who* tells the client. It is the manner in which the discussion is conducted that is so vitally important. The way the health professional relates to the client can make the situation supportive and loving or cold and cruel.

BIOMEDICAL ETHICS AND THE PRACTICE OF NURSING

Many people, having read this far, may think, "All right, this is all very interesting, but what does it have to do with me as a practitioner of nursing?" It is highly unlikely that nurses will ever be cloning carrots or frogs or engaging in any of the other technological practices discussed. They certainly will not be permitted to make a decision of whether to terminate the life-support system of a person in an irreversible coma. Why then should a chapter on ethics be included in a community health nursing text? For two very great and very basic reasons: nurses are human beings and will be directly affected as *people* by the issues discussed, and, as professional health care workers, they will be caring for clients who are affected by the ethical issues. So nurses have a dual responsibility: to themselves and others as human beings and to themselves and others as nurses.

As people we are faced so many times with ethical choices. The poet James Russell Lowell said, "New occasions teach new duties," and they also teach new ideas. Any thinking, growing person constantly reevaluates the way he would behave in any situation. As new experiences accumulate in a person's life, there is a learning process that contributes to change, to the opening up of new choices and new ways of dealing with situations. Our codes of ethics change, and there is no immutability of our moral rules. We are always in conflict, and we are always faced with choices.

The kinds of ethical or moral choices we make are indicative of the kinds of people we are at any given time.

Morality and ethics are our culture's way of dealing with conflicts. If we had no moral or ethical code, we would be perpetually caught in a morass of indecision at every turn. Morality regulates conduct so we have some sense of stability and can count on that sense of stability in others. When we say, "Jane wouldn't lie about whether she saw that client," we are saying we know Jane well enough to predict certain of her behaviors based on her code of ethics. We have all known people who are so immoral (or worse, totally amoral) that we cannot predict any of their behavior or count on what they say to be true. The feeling of unease and discomfort that results from dealing with these kinds of people is the result of a poorly or incompletely structured ethical code. "The basic categories of moral life are conflict, choice, and conscience. These three Cs of morals logically involve each other. Whenever a moral conflict arises, a person is faced with a choice between conflicting possibilities of things to be or do. . . ."[17] Neither conflict nor choice can function independently of each other, and the moral process is the product of the interdependence of the two. Without this struggle, life would disintegrate from the lack of stimulation and direction. We would be truly automatons. "Man, as the only free moral agent in the organic world, is capable of deliberating among possible alternatives of action and choosing between conflicting courses of conduct. All of which are subject to being judged from an ethical point of view."[17]

As professional nurses we have a vested interest in the issues discussed. Although we will not personally be manipulating genes and chromosomes, we are working in genetic counseling centers where we need the information about the issues in order to discuss them with clients. Although we may not be personally responsible for terminating a life-support system, we as community nurses will care for clients who are facing terminal illness. They will want—and need—to talk about their feelings and their futures, and we need to know what they are facing and what their alternatives are. If we did not know that St. Christopher's Hospice exists, how could we refer a client there? How could we work to have professional nursing input in the formation of an organization like Hospice, Inc.? Although it is not we who will be transplanting an organ from one human being to another, it is we who make the home visits day after day to clients on portable artificial kidneys. It is we to whom they talk as they lie hooked up to the machine three or four times a week and wonder if there will be a donor before they die. It is our hands they hold, not the transplant surgeon's. Most nurses do not design chemical or biological research projects in which human subjects are used, and although it is not we who discovered the chemical to be tested, it is the community nurse who more and more finds herself participating in various kinds of research projects. Before we realize it, we find ourselves involved in research areas in which dubious ethical practices are used.

There is conflict and choice. We see things done to human subjects that we may know and feel are immoral or unethical. We can ignore what is happening and hope things work out well for the subjects; we can physically remove ourselves from the project by saying that we do not wish to participate; or we can stay and do what we can to protect the rights of the subjects. We can talk to them and make certain that the consent they have given is truly informed, and we can explain each step as the research progresses. We can act as intermediaries between the scientists and the subjects and can generally act as a moralizing and humanizing influence. Although we may not be doing the actual fetal research, we as community nurses most assuredly come in contact with thousands of pregnant women who are contemplating abortion. If a woman's fetus has been requested for research, we can amplify the explanation already given. The woman will have fears about what the fetus might feel and what is to be done with it after the research. As nurses we can listen to her feelings and help her to clarify her thoughts about what course of action she really wants to take.

Although we may not be engaging in psychosurgery or chemical or electrical behavior control, we are in daily communication with psychiatric clients who have been released from mental hospitals or who are being treated as outpatients. These are some of the most frightened and confused people of all and are the most likely to fall prey to unethical practices. We know what their treatment is and are obligated to explain it to the clients and their families, to talk about their fears, to find out how much they know about what is being done to them, and to help them to have the courage to refuse treatment if that is what they choose.

If aggressive defense of one's own value system creates conflict with nursing care needs, then ignorance and indifference to moral issues are even more alarming. The possibility that there is a certain dignity to be found in being criticized rather than being utterly ignored raises moral questions of its own, but there is little doubt that the dehumanizing so deplored in today's care system is based on the view of the individual as an object rather than a person.*

If nursing wishes to be considered a true profession, not only by its own members but by other people, then it had best get on with the process of critical self-evaluation in terms of ethical and moral issues. Will we continue to be paralyzed and not be able to do what we know to be ethically correct because a physician, or even a fellow nurse in a superior position, disagrees with us? Are we going to be so tied to one particular job that we will refuse to take an ethical position because we are afraid of being fired? What value do we place on being employed by people who conduct business in a way we know to be morally wrong? How long will we continue to keep our mouths closed? When shall we start being true to ourselves? When will we begin to see that there is no professional competence without human compassion and that compassion does not flow from a moral and ethical vacuum?

*From Levine, Myra E.: Nursing ethics and the ethical nurse, American Journal of Nursing, p. 845, May, 1977. Copyright 1977, the American Journal of Nursing Co.

APPENDIX A

CODE FOR NURSES[18]

1. The nurse provides services with respect for the dignity of man, unrestricted by considerations of nationality, race, creed, color or status.

2. The nurse safeguards the individual's right to privacy by judiciously protecting information of a confidential nature, sharing only information relevant to the client's care.

3. The nurse maintains individual competence in nursing practice, recognizing and accepting responsibility for individual actions and judgments.

4. The nurse acts to safeguard clients when their care and safety are affected by incompetent, unethical, or illegal conduct of any person.

5. The nurse uses individual competence as a criterion in accepting delegated responsibility and assigning nursing activity to others.

6. The nurse participates in research activities when assured that the rights of individual subjects are protected.

7. The nurse participates in the efforts of the profession to define and upgrade standards of nursing practice and education.

8. The nurse, acting through the professional organization, participates in establishing and maintaining conditions of employment conducive to high-quality nursing care.

9. The nurse works with members of health professions and other citizens in promoting efforts to meet the health needs of the public.

10. The nurse refuses to give or imply endorsement to advertising, promotion, or sales for commercial products, services, or enterprises.

APPENDIX B

A LIVING WILL[19]

Death is as much a reality as birth, growth, maturity, and old age; it is the one certainty of life. If the time comes when I, _____ , can no longer take part in decisions for my own future, let this statement stand as an expression of my wishes, while I am still of sound mind.

If the situation should arise in which there is no reasonable expectation of my recovery from physical or mental disability, I request that I be allowed to die and not be kept alive by artificial means or "heroic measures." I do not fear death itself as much as the indignities of deteriorating dependence and hopeless pain. I, therefore, ask that medication be mercifully administered to me to alleviate suffering even though this may hasten the moment of my death.

This request is made after careful consideration. I hope you who care for me will feel morally bound to follow its mandate. I recognize that this appears to place a heavy responsibility on you, but it is with the intention of relieving you of such responsibility and placing it on myself in accordance with my own strong convictions that this statement is made.

Signed _____

APPENDIX C

PRINCIPLES OF MEDICAL ETHICS*

PREAMBLE. These principles are intended to aid physicians individually and collectively in maintaining a high level of ethical conduct. They are not laws but standards by which a physician may determine the propriety of his conduct in his relationship with patients, with colleagues, with members of allied professions, and with the public.

1. The principal objective of the medical profession is to render service to humanity with full respect for the dignity of man. Physicians should merit the confidence of patients entrusted to their care, rendering to each a full measure of service and devotion.

2. Physicians should strive continually to improve medical knowledge and skill and should make available to their patients and colleagues the benefits of their professional attainments.

3. Physicians should practice a method of healing founded on a scientific basis; and he should not voluntarily associate professionally with anyone who violates this principle.

4. The medical profession should safeguard the public and itself against physicians deficient in moral character or professional competence. Physicians should observe all laws, uphold the dignity and honor of the profession, and accept its self-imposed disciplines. They should expose, without hesitation, illegal or unethical conduct of fellow members of the profession.

5. A physician may choose whom he will serve. In an emergency, however, he should render service to the best of his ability. Having undertaken the care of a patient, he may not neglect him; and unless he has been discharged, he may discontinue his services only after giving adequate notice. He should not solicit patients.

6. A physician should not dispose of his services under terms or conditions that tend to interfere with or impair the free and complete exercise of his medical judgment and skill or tend to cause a deterioration of the quality of medical care.

7. In the practice of medicine a physician should limit the source of his professional income to medical services actually rendered by him, or under his supervision, to his patients. His fees should be commensurate with the services rendered and the patient's ability to pay. He should neither pay nor receive a commission for referral of patients. Drugs, remedies, or appliances may be dispensed or supplied by the physician provided it is in the best interests of the patient.

8. A physician should seek consultation upon request, in doubtful or difficult cases, or whenever it appears that the quality of medical services may be enhanced thereby.

9. A physician may not reveal the confidences entrusted to him in the course of medical attendance, or the deficiencies he may observe in the character of patients, unless he is required to do so by law or unless it becomes necessary in order to protect the welfare of the individual or of the community.

10. The honored ideals of the medical profession imply that the responsibilities of the physician extend not only to the individual, but also to society, where these responsibilities deserve his interest and participation in activities which have the purpose of improving both the health and the well-being of the individual and the community.

*From American Medical Association, Chicago, 1967.

APPENDIX D

A PATIENT'S BILL OF RIGHTS*

The American Hospital Association presents a Patient's Bill of Rights with the expectation that observance of these rights will contribute to more effective patient care and greater satisfaction for the patient, his physician, and the hospital organization. Further, the Association presents these rights in the expectation that they will be supported by the hospital on behalf of its patients, as an integral part of the healing process. It is recognized that a personal relationship between the physician and the patient is essential for the provision of proper medical care. The traditional physician-patient relationship takes on a new dimension when care is rendered within an organizational structure. Legal precedent has established that the institution itself also has a responsibility to the patient. It is in recognition of these factors that these rights are affirmed.

1. The patient has the right to considerate and respectful care.

2. The patient has the right to obtain from his physician complete current information concerning his diagnosis, treatment, and prognosis in terms the patient can be reasonably expected to understand. When it is not medically advisable to give such information to the patient, the information should be made available to an appropriate person in his behalf. The patient has the right to know, by name, the physician responsible for coordinating his care.

3. The patient has the right to receive from his physician information necessary to give informed consent prior to the start of any procedure and/or treatment. Except in emergencies, such information for informed consent should include but not necessarily be limited to the specific procedure and/or treatment, the medically significant risks in-

volved, and the probable duration of incapacitation. Where medically significant alternatives for care or treatment exist, or when the patient requests information concerning medical alternatives, the patient has the right to such information. The patient also has the right to know the name of the person responsible for the procedures and/or treatment.

4. The patient has the right to refuse treatment to the extent permitted by law and to be informed of the medical consequences of his actions.

5. The patient has the right to every consideration of his privacy concerning his own medical care program. Case discussion, consultation, examination, and treatment are confidential and should be conducted discreetly. Those not directly involved in his care must have the permission of the patient to be present.

6. The patient has the right to expect that all communications and records pertaining to his care should be treated as confidential.

7. The patient has the right to expect that within its capacity a hospital must make reasonable response to the request of a patient for services. The hospital must provide evaluation, service, and/or referral as indicated by the urgency of the case. When medically permissible, a patient may be transferred to another facility only after he has received complete information and explanation concerning the needs for and alternatives to such a transfer. The institution to which the patient is to be transferred must first have accepted the patient for transfer.

8. The patient has the right to obtain information as to any relationship of his hospital to other health care and educational institutions insofar as his care is concerned. The patient has the right to obtain information as to the existence of any professional relationships among individuals, by name, who are treating him.

*From American Hospital Association: A patient's bill of rights, Chicago, 1975. Reprinted with the permission of the American Hospital Association.

9. The patient has the right to be advised if the hospital proposes to engage in or perform human experimentation affecting his care or treatment. The patient has the right to refuse to participate in such research projects.

10. The patient has the right to expect reasonable continuity of care. He has the right to know in advance what appointment times and physicians are available and where. The patient has the right to expect that the hospital will provide a mechanism whereby he is informed by his physician or a delegate of his physician of the patient's continuing health care requirements following discharge.

11. The patient has the right to examine and receive an explanation of his bill regardless of source of payment.

12. The patient has the right to know what hospital rules and regulations apply to his conduct as a patient.

No catalog of rights can guarantee for the patient the kind of treatment he has a right to expect. A hospital has many functions to perform, including the prevention and treatment of disease, the education of both health professionals and patients, and the conduct of clinical research. All these activities must be conducted with an overriding concern for the patient, and, above all, the recognition of his dignity as a human being. Success in achieving this recognition assures success in the defense of the rights of the patient.

NOTES

1. Travelbee, Joyce: Interpersonal aspects of nursing, Philadelphia, 1971, F.A. Davis Co.
2. Veatch, Robert M., et al., editors: The teaching of medical ethics, proceedings of a conference sponsored by the Institute of Society, Ethics, and the Life Sciences and Columbia University College of Physicians and Surgeons, Hastings-on-Hudson, N.Y., 1973.
3. This criterion is held up to serious question by many people. It could be successfully argued that babies and small children would not be considered people. They are not, and should not be expected to be, aware of the results of their behavior, neither can they control it.
4. At this writing Karen Quinlan is in a nursing home receiving only custodial care. The only life support she receives is food. The state of New Jersey is paying for her care.
5. Suffering is the endurance or the submission to pain, injury, or loss.
6. Restak, Richard M.: Pre-meditated man, New York, 1975, The Viking Press, Inc.
7. Ramsey, Paul: The ethics of fetal research, New Haven, Conn., 1975, Yale University Press.
8. A teratogenic effect is the effect on the fetus of a drug taken by a woman while she is pregnant.
9. Gaylin, Willard M.: Operating on the mind: the psychosurgery conflict, New York, 1975, Basic Books, Inc., Publishers.
10. The issue of death will be discussed in the following section.
11. Dedek, John F.: Contemporary medical ethics, New York, 1975, Sheed & Ward, Inc.
12. Heifetz, Milton D.: The right to die, New York, 1975, G.P. Putnam's Sons.
13. Ostheimer, Nancy C., and Ostheimer, John M.: Life or death—who controls? New York, 1976, Springer Publishing Co., Inc.
14. Hospice is a medieval word meaning a wayside station for travelers on a journey.
15. Heroin was used extensively in the United States in the past for the control of severe pain and was very effective. It was also used because it was thought to be a nonaddicting substitute for those people who were addicted to morphine. This did not work out to be true, as is happening today with methadone, which is proving to be just as addictive as heroin.
16. Robertson, John A.: Involuntary euthanasia of defective newborns: a legal analysis. In Schwartz, Jane L., and Schwartz, Lawrence H., editors: Vulnerable infants, New York, 1977, McGraw-Hill Book Co.
17. Romanell, Patrick: Ethics, moral conflicts and choice, American Journal of Nursing **17:**850-855, 1977.
18. American Journal of Nursing **17:**876, 1977.
19. Euthanasia Educational Council, 250 West 57th Street, New York, N.Y., 10019.

BIBLIOGRAPHY

Barber, Bernard, et al.: Research on human subjects: problems of social control in medical experimentation, New York, 1973, Russell Sage Foundation.

Beauchamp, Tom L., and Walters, LeRoy: Contemporary issues in bioethics, Belmont, Calif., 1978, Wadsworth Publishing Co.

Dedek, John F.: Contemporary medical ethics, New York, 1975, Sheed & Ward, Inc.

Epstein, Charlotte: Nursing the dying patient, Reston, Va., 1975, Reston Publishing Co.

Ethics, American Journal of Nursing, special section, May, 1977.

Fagothey, Austin: Right and reason: ethics in theory and practice, ed. 6, St. Louis, 1976, The C.V. Mosby Co.

Fletcher, Joseph: Morals and medicine, Boston, 1954, Beacon Press.

Fromer, Margot J.: Ethical issues in health care, St. Louis, 1981, The C.V. Mosby Co.

Gaylin, Willard M.: Operating on the mind: the psychosurgery conflict, New York, 1975, Basic Books, Inc., Publishers.

Hamilton, Michael P.: The new genetics and the future of man, Grand Rapids, Mich., 1972, Wm. B. Eerdmans Publishing Co.

Haring, Bernard: Medical ethics, Notre Dame, Ind., 1973, Fides Publishers, Inc.

Heifetz, Milton D.: The right to die, New York, 1975, G.P. Putnam's Sons.

Jacker, Corinne: The biological revolution, New York, 1971, Parents' Magazine Press.

Jones, Alun, and Bodmer, Walter F.: Our future inheritance: choice or chance? London, 1974, Oxford University Press.

Kastenbaum, Robert J.: Death, society and human experience, ed. 2, St. Louis, 1981, The C.V. Mosby Co.

Kübler-Ross , Elisabeth: Questions and answers on death and dying, New York, 1974, Macmillan, Inc.

Kübler-Ross, Elisabeth: Death: the final stage of growth, Englewood Cliffs, N.J., 1975, Prentice-Hall, Inc.

Ostheimer, Nancy C., and Ostheimer, John M.: Life or death—who controls? New York, 1976, Springer Publishing Co., Inc.

Ramsey, Paul: The patient as person: explorations in medical ethics, New Haven, Conn., 1970, Yale University Press.

Ramsey, Paul: The ethics of fetal research, New Haven, Conn., 1975, Yale University Press.

Reich, Warren T., editor-in-chief: Encyclopedia of bioethics, vol. 1-4, New York, 1978, The Free Press.

Restak, Richard M.: Pre-meditated man, New York, 1975, The Viking Press, Inc.

Roberts, Florence: Perinatal nursing, New York, 1977, McGraw-Hill Book Co.

Robertson, John A.: Involuntary euthanasia of defective newborns: a legal analysis. In Schwartz, Jane L., and Schwartz, Lawrence H., editors: Vulnerable infants, New York, 1977, McGraw-Hill Book Co.

Shills, Edward, et al.: Life or death: ethics and options, Seattle, 1968, University of Washington Press.

Smith, Harmon L.: Ethics and the new medicine, Nashville, 1970, Abingdon Press.

Travelbee, Joyce: What's wrong with sympathy? American Journal of Nursing **64**:71, 1964.

Travelbee, Joyce: Interpersonal aspects of nursing, Philadelphia, 1971, F.A. Davis Co.

Vaux, Kenneth: Biomedical ethics, New York, 1974, Harper & Row, Publishers.

Veatch, Robert M., et al., editors: The teaching of medical ethics, proceedings of a conference sponsored by the Institute of Society, Ethics, and the Life Sciences and Columbia University College of Physicians and Surgeons, Hastings-on-Hudson, N.Y., 1973.

Wertz, Richard W.: Readings on ethical and social issues in biomedicine, Englewood Cliffs, N.J., 1973, Prentice-Hall, Inc.

Young, David P.: A new world in the morning, Philadelphia, 1972, The Westminster Press.

6

FUNCTIONS OF THE COMMUNITY HEALTH NURSE

The first three chapters of this book dealt mainly with the structure and functioning of the health care system in general and in particular with the nature of agencies delivering that health care. All the agencies and systems in the world are useless without competent and caring people to make them work. This chapter about the community health nurse is divided into two major parts. The first discusses the purposes and goals of community health nursing; the second examines the means by which the nurse accomplishes these purposes and goals.

In any text of this type it is customary to define nursing so the reader will have some idea of the framework within which the nurse's professional responsibilities are discussed. The following definitions are the ones most applicable to this text and to the concepts of community health care. According to Rines and Montag[1,p.9]:

Nursing is a service designed to assist man within any age group, socioeconomic level, and social setting to perform those activities contributing to health or its recovery or to a peaceful death. Man, the consumer of nursing service, enters the nurse-client relationship directly or indirectly, when he lacks the necessary strength, will, or knowledge to perform those activities which are required to attain, maintain, or restore his maximum health potential.

Following is Henderson's classic definition[2] of the function of nursing:

To assist the individual, sick or well, in the performance of those activities contributing to health or its recovery (or to peaceful death) that he would perform if he had the necessary strength, will, or knowledge. And to do this in such a way as to help him gain independence as rapidly as possible.

Professional nursing has begun to evolve, and should continue to do so, from a rather task-oriented occupation into a profession whose practitioners function as advocates of their clients. All individuals, with varying ability to adapt on the health-illness continuum, are unique in their own being and have the right to health care and to an active role in determining and meeting their health needs. They also need health information whereby they can be as autonomous as possible in determining what their health needs are and what actions they will take to meet those needs.

The health-illness continuum is the abstract horizontal line along which an individual's health moves during his lifetime; one end of the continuum is optimum health functioning; the other end is death or total disability. Most professional caregivers believe that optimum health is a right of all people. Professional nurses have been taking a more responsible position in the health care system, and, as time goes on, their level of functioning will most likely become more and more independent.

Through continuing development of nursing theory, research activity, and application of the findings, professional nurses are prepared to be providers of primary care. Because of the needs of the people they serve, it is necessary to preserve and use the creativity of the individual nurse as well as to develop her potential for critical thinking and decision making. This should be accomplished through the use of the nursing process and in partnership with the consumer of health care and with other members of the community health team. Nursing process is defined as the systematic method of applying problem-solving techniques to the practice of professional nursing. The five steps are (1) data collection, (2) analysis or assessment of the client's health needs, (3) planning for nursing care, (4) implementation of the planned care, and (5) evaluation. Application of the nursing process to community nursing will be discussed in detail in Chapter 13.

The role of nurses today is wider and much more comprehensive than ever before. They are more independent, place greater emphasis on the prevention of illness and the maximizing of wellness, and are more than ever morally and legally accountable for their professional behavior. Today's nurses are assuming leadership responsibilities: planning and directing health care services, directing and supervising others in the administration of nursing care, and teaching students, colleagues, and clients. They are primary care practitioners.

The community nurse's clients are the individual, the family, and the community. The term individual does not need to be defined, but there are so many definitions of the concept of the family and the community that for the purpose of this chapter they are defined as follows:

family A group of two or more people united by blood, marriage, adoption, or a commitment to exist as a family who reside together; a unit that maintains a common culture, derived from the general culture in which members learn and practice expected roles. A nuclear family generally consists of a mother, father, and children, although not all these members are necessary for the unit to qualify as a family. An extended family includes grandparents, aunts, uncles, and other relatives who reside with the nuclear family.
community A social group of any size whose members reside in a specific locality, share a government, and

have a common cultural and historical heritage; a social group sharing common characteristics and perceiving itself as distinct in some respect from the larger society within which it exists.[3] (The reader is referred to Chapter 7 for a detailed discussion on the nature of a community.)

For the most part, the community from which a nurse derives clients is either a small town (or even a group of small towns) or a section or a neighborhood of a larger municipality.

No one nurse can meet all the needs of a client. It is the purpose of this chapter to discuss *what* can be done by nurses and nursing, but it is up to individual practitioners and agencies to decide *how* and *by whom* various nursing functions will be carried out.

PURPOSES AND GOALS OF THE COMMUNITY NURSE
Improvement and maintenance of health

If we define health as the condition that enables an individual to function "normally," or if it is the active responses of physical and mental systems to their environment, or mental and social efficiency and well-being, then we need to define what we mean by improvement and maintenance. This is best done by describing four major concepts of nursing that enable the practitioner to function as a professional.[4]

conservation Maintenance of health status; a baseline from which to move; preservation of whatever functioning the client already has.
prevention Avoidance of changes in the health status that are harmful to the client.
restoration Helping the client return to an optimum state of health; recovering, to as great an extent as possible, whatever health functioning has been lost.
amelioration Improvement of the client's state of health; giving him what was never there in the first place.

Examples of the kinds of actions the nurse might perform to function within these four concepts are encouraging regular health examinations to *conserve* health functioning; making physical assessments in a well-baby clinic; participating in mobile chest x-ray or PAP test programs; counseling clients about the effects of smoking or overeating and the possible *prevention* of lung cancer or heart disease; engaging in the more traditional "laying-on-of-hands" role of the nurse to help *restore* the client's health; and giving a series of talks or classes to grammar school children on tooth decay to *ameliorate* their level of dental health.

In order to improve and maintain the health of individuals and the community, the nurse must be aware of the factors in the environment that contribute to poor health. Some of these factors include poor housing, employment hazards, street crime, and the great variety of environmental pollutants. Only by recognizing these factors can the nurse do anything to counteract them. The reader is referred to Chapter 11, which discusses several factors, both personal and environmental, that tend to make individuals and families high health risks. Chapter 8 deals with levels of wellness and factors that tend to push people to the illness end of the health-illness continuum. All the factors that tend to make us sick do not have to be what are traditionally thought of as negative. The coveted American affluence and leisurely life-style may also be killing us. According to the late John H. Knowles, who was president of the Rockefeller Foundation, "The next major advances in the health of the American people will come from the assumption of individual responsibility for one's own health and a necessary change in life-style for the majority of Americans."[5]

All these factors are obvious to community nurses. It is their responsibility as health educators and counselors and as client advocates to make the hazards obvious to the people in their care.

Helping people recognize and deal with health problems

It seems that many of the health problems in today's communities are either not recognized as such or are acknowledged but ignored for a variety of reasons. Health problems that are not recognized are perhaps the most tragic of all: a child who is a bright and active student in school suddenly be-

comes a behavior problem and begins to do poor academic work. An elderly man, living alone, develops headaches, blurred vision, and occasional slurring of his speech; he attributes these occurrences to advancing age and seeks no medical attention. An infant seems slow in its growth and development and is lethargic and not very responsive; the mother obtains her medical advice "over the back fence" and ends up with false reassurance from well-meaning but unqualified friends.

There are many reasons why people simply ignore health problems. As in the previous examples, if one does not know that a problem *is* a problem, it is easy to simply disregard it. The lack of money or the fear of lack of money is most likely one of the major reasons that health problems remain unattended. A little ache or pain may lead to fantasies of a major health problem and major bills. It is ironic that many Americans will bring their automobiles into a repair shop on hearing the slightest clunk or rattle, but they disregard the minor clunks and rattles in their own bodies. Health problems are also ignored because of a lack of medical facilities or other resources in an area. Even more disturbing, clients may not be aware of the resources and facilities that are available. This happens frequently in large metropolitan areas that are crowded with the most modern professional services and personnel, which may be underused by the people who need them the most. The availability and distribution of health care are discussed in Chapter 1, and various suggestions are offered. If one does not know that food stamps are available, starvation may be the result. If a client has no idea that amniocentesis can diagnose Down's syndrome in her unborn child, she will have no choice but to face and deal with the burdens and problems of mental retardation. The best facilities are useless if they are inaccessible to the client. A person who has to spend 2 hours on three or four buses to wait another few hours in a clinic might very well think it not worth the trip. A woman who has to decide between spending $10 for a baby-sitter while she visits the dentist and using the money for groceries will most likely make the latter choice. It is often the community nurse who has the best information about why people are not making use of available health services, and she can often best advise community planners or other health professionals on how to remedy the situation.

Another factor that prevents people from seeking medical attention is fear of the diagnosis. This characteristic crosses all socioeconomic boundaries; no matter how intelligent, well informed, and well educated a person is, there is the fear that something might really be wrong. If the fear is not discussed or even acknowledged to oneself, it is much easier to deny. It is not only the diagnosis that seems to alarm people but also the road to the diagnosis and the procedures that must be followed in the aftermath of the diagnosis. Diagnostic tests are becoming more time consuming, uncomfortable, and even painful, and they are expensive. Few people relish the thought of surgery, and almost no one reacts positively to various kinds of restrictive medical regimens. There is almost as great a variety of superstition and old wives' tales about health and the body as there is a variety of people. Helping clients to talk about and to work through their anxieties, fears, and false beliefs is one of the most important functions of the professional community nurse.

Contributing to improvement of nursing care

All professionals have the responsibility of continually improving and upgrading their profession. A career in professional nursing requires a lifetime of continuing education and reassessment of the profession of nursing, one's place in it, and reaction to it. The ways in which this task can be accomplished are discussed in the following section.

METHODS OF ACHIEVING THE PURPOSES AND GOALS
Increasing knowledge about health matters

This area has traditionally been known as the teaching function of the nurse and is more important today than ever before. The subjects about which the nurse most often teaches fall into two categories: health in general and specific health problems. These two categories are not discrete, and more often than not they should and do overlap.

If the nurse is the teacher, then the client—whether individual, family, or community—is the learner, and it would be beneficial to briefly discuss here some characteristics of the learning process. Sutterley and Donnelly[6] have defined five distinct characteristics:

1. Learning is a cognitive multisensory process. Human beings proceed through sensorimotor development, and the amount and kind of learning that takes place depends on the stage of development in which the learner is and on the kinds of experiences that have preceded each stage. Children learn in different ways from adults, but cognitive abilities do not decrease with advancing age; they merely become slower.

2. Learning is individual. Stereotypes about the learning abilities or disabilities of certain groups are almost always wrong. Studies have shown over and over that individuals vary as much in their ability to learn and in the speed at which they learn as they vary in other personality characteristics.

3. Learning occurs according to the readiness of the learner. There must be sufficient psychological and neurophysiological maturation for each new learning experience.

4. Learning requires feedback. Every learner needs to know whether he is meeting expected goals, assimilating the proffered information, winning approval of the teacher, and demonstrating what is considered appropriate behavior. There is positive and negative feedback, and, depending on what messages the teacher sends out and what the learner perceives, vastly different kinds of learning take place.

5. Learning requires an environment that provides stimulating and diverse experiences with regard to people, things, relationships, time, and space. We have all had the negative learning experience of the same person droning on and on for the same amount of time without varying teaching techniques and without using a variety of methods

to get the message across. Learning takes place more readily if the learner is stimulated by a variety of people from whom to learn and by a variety of experiences to assimilate.

The implications for nursing in these characteristics are enormous. No longer can the nurse be an authoritarian dispenser of knowledge. Consumers of health care are becoming less and less willing to accept a course of action merely because a health professional says it is a correct or good action. Consumers want to know why a particular course of action is being recommended. Nurses, in their role as client advocates, should encourage this realistic and healthy skepticism and should teach clients more about the health care system and how it can be made to function for the benefit of the client. Teaching today involves more than the mere imparting of information and the expectation that it will be unquestioningly received. It involves sharing thoughts, ideas, and feelings, experimenting with different ways of doing things, finding out what the learner wants and expects to learn, and searching for the kinds of motivation that exist for learning.

As a result of many years of teaching in a variety of settings, I have devised a set of flexible guidelines to be kept in mind when planning teaching of any kind. They are not applicable in every situation, but sooner or later they can all be put to use.

1. Find out what kinds of information are needed. Ask what the learner wants to learn. Investigate the purpose for which the information will be used. This is important in planning content and teaching techniques.

2. Find out who wants to know. The nurse will vary the teaching techniques depending on who are to be the recipients of the teaching, as well as their levels of ability.

3. Establish objectives. Without clearly defined objectives that are understood by both the teacher and the learner, teaching often becomes an aimlessly random hodgepodge of knowledge. Without objectives it is impossible to evaluate whether learning has taken place.

4. Determine the motivation of the learner. Find out the circumstances surrounding the request for information. The more important it is for the learner to learn, the more motivated he is likely to be.

5. Information has to be made useful to the learner. It cannot be too abstract, and it must be delivered in understandable terms. The use of jargon or unintelligible terminology is almost always inappropriate.

6. Begin at the learner's present level of knowledge, and do not be judgmental about information the client does not have. Clients are often embarrassed about their lack of knowledge or sophistication about health care. It is the nurse's responsibility to put the client at ease and to create an atmosphere of comfort in which learning can take place.

7. Be alert for teaching opportunities. They are everywhere: a group of clients sitting in a doctor's office or clinic waiting room, sports teams in school, or new mothers in a laundromat washing diapers.

8. Develop sensitivity to what the learners might be feeling or thinking. Many people are too shy to ask questions, and, if the teacher can anticipate what the learner might need to know, more learning could take place.

There are many situations in which the nurse is a teacher:

1. In a formal class setting: schools, clinics, consultation work, community center meetings

2. Structured but less formal situations: groups of parents at a well-child conference, sex education counseling at a high school, birth control discussion groups at Planned Parenthood offices

3. One-to-one planned teaching in clinics or on home visits

4. One-to-one impromptu teaching on a short informal basis in unplanned situations like going into a home and finding other than the expected situation

The various teaching techniques such as lectures, group discussions, and demonstrations are all appropriate in different situations. It is characteristic of a *professional* nurse to use judgment in selecting the technique that is best in each instance. It is also characteristic of the professional to be able to change and adapt the teaching method whenever the situation seems to warrant it. If a class of new mothers is falling asleep over a lecture on formula preparation, it might be well to begin a demonstration on a live, wiggly baby of how to change a diaper.

An important function of the nurse as a teacher is to raise the consciousness of clients. This is merely another way of saying that the nurse functions as a client advocate. Just as blacks in the fifties and sixties and women in the sixties and seventies were successfully motivated to begin constructive action by people who helped them to become more aware of their needs, so nurses can successfully motivate to constructive action the consumers of health care. The community must recognize and meet its own health needs, but it is the nurse who can lead the way. Following is an example of how she can do this. The community nurse hears from neighborhood mothers that children are not eating the hot lunches provided by the school. She and the school nurse discover the reason is that the children do not find the meals appetizing, so the two nurses, in consultation with the nutritionist, plan meals that children like. The result is better nutrition for the children who are not buying "junk food" at noontime, less waste of food in the school cafeteria, and the saving of family money because the lunches at school are free. This may be considered by some to be too abstract and impractical a concept of teaching, but it may very well be the best way a *professional* nurse can meet the needs of clients.

Client advocacy has become something of a cliché in the past several years—as if the client requires protection from other members of the health care team (for example, the physician as enemy is becoming a depressingly familiar theme in nursing). This is a rather paternalistic view of client advocacy, although in some situations it may be a necessary function of nursing. I prefer to think

of client advocacy as a partnership *with* a client, rather than the protection *of* a client. This partnership is goal-directed in that the nurse and client together, with the client's wishes always taking precedence of course, work out a plan of action to meet the client's health needs.

Provision of actual nursing services

The key concept here is meeting specific health needs. This can be done only through the use of the nursing process, which will be dealt with in greater detail in Chapter 13. The first two steps of the nursing process, collection of data and assessment of needs, are crucial to the determination of the kinds of services that will be required. This decision will be different for each situation encountered, but it is well within the scope of this chapter to discuss basic kinds of ways in which the community nurse can provide services to meet the health needs of clients.

THE HOME VISIT

The home visit is the classic and traditional preserve of the community nurse. It remains an excellent way (and is very often the only way) for the nurse to observe home situations, family interactions, and various positive and negative forces that operate on the client. People usually behave differently in their own homes than they do in public places. A sense of being "on one's own turf" can change modes of behavior and ways of relating to people and events. People behave more naturally in their own homes, and there is not the tension of having to display "party behavior." The nurse is a guest; she may be an uninvited one and be perceived as a threat, and whatever good intentions she brings along, she is still a stranger. This in itself places an entirely different character on the nurse-client relationship than that of a hospital, clinic, or office situation, where it is the client who is in strange territory and who is the "guest" of the agency.

The nurse in the home can fill a variety of roles and functions. She can provide direct nursing care that includes both physical and emotional aspects.

It may be on a short-term basis (a client recently discharged from the hospital who still needs dressing changes or injections) or on a long-term or permanent one, as in the case of the chronically ill or permanently disabled.

The home visit can serve as a teaching situation or as a review of teaching done in the hospital. A client may give every indication of having mastered the techniques involved in colostomy care, but in a different environment self-confidence can weaken or fall apart, and lessons can be forgotten. The nurse can assess what is needed and can reinforce teaching already done. When the nurse enters the home, there is an opportunity to determine in what areas of teaching she can be of help. She can also determine what other agencies or health professionals might be needed and can make the appropriate referrals.

The most important function of the community nurse in the home might very well not be the laying on of hands or "doing" something. The client's greatest need may be to talk. Problems arising from the home situation often recede when the client is out of the home, but they return with full intensity as soon as the client steps through the front door. It is only by making a home visit that the nurse can gain insight into the entire scope of the problem.[7] Sometimes during a home visit the nurse's most therapeutic act is simply listening. By making a home visit, she can often assess whether the client has the resources necessary (e.g., money, emotional stability, transportation, or living arrangements) to deal with the health problems at hand. Only by assessing the resources can the nurse assist the client to set up logical objectives to deal with whatever problems exist.

NURSE-CLIENT CONTRACTS

As contracts are made between teachers and students for grades in a course, so are contracts made between nurses and clients to meet health goals. It is essential, for the establishment of a workable contract, that both the client and the nurse have a clear idea of what the health problem is, the purpose of the nurse's visits, what the desired objectives are, and what means are to be used to reach the goal. The client and the nurse must have the same goals; unless there is agreement, there is no point to a contract. Contracts are extremely effective in some situations, but the nurse must carefully evaluate, each time she considers using the contract technique, whether it is appropriate.

Contracts are frequently used when clients must do something that is either difficult for them or that they do not want to do. It may be refraining from some kind of behavior such as smoking or eating forbidden foods, or it may be submitting to a test or procedure that is unpleasant or painful. A behavioral or contingency contract is a means of establishing consistently positive behavior by scheduling positive reinforcements. The contract can be written or verbal, although a written one lends an air of authenticity and importance. The contract states who is to do what and under what circumstances. The agreement is stated in behavioral terms with "rewards" clearly detailed. The time during which the terms of the contract will be fulfilled is also stated. Both parties in the contract are responsible for its fulfillment, and if either party fails to live up to the agreement, the other can request a reevaluation.

Following are some examples of the kinds of contracts that are made between community health nurses and their clients:

1. The nurse will make a home visit twice a week for four weeks to teach a mother about childhood diseases and the process of growth and development. By the end of that time all her children will have attended the well-baby clinic for examinations and will have begun their immunizations.

2. A bone marrow biopsy is necessary for a 23-year-old woman who is thought to have leukemia. She refused the test because she fears it and she is terrified of hospitals. The contract states that if the client agrees to the biopsy, the community nurse will arrange for it to be performed on an outpatient basis and will stay with the client during the entire procedure.

3. A 70-year-old widower who has had his leg amputated refuses to go out of the house because

he thinks people are laughing at the clumsy way he walks with his prosthesis. He is not getting enough exercise or practice with the prosthesis, and his socialization is declining. The contract states that if the man takes a half-hour walk every day for two weeks, the nurse will read aloud to him from his favorite books of poetry for a half hour each day for those two weeks.

At the end of the specified time period the terms of the contract are evaluated and examined. It may be necessary to make a new contract, or the client may have been sufficiently motivated to continue the behavior on his own without a contract.

THE CLINIC

The second traditional area in which community nurses function is the clinic, in either a hospital's outpatient department or ambulatory care unit or in a public health agency (Fig. 6-1). In the past clinic nurses have functioned, for the most part, as dispensers of directions and instructions, as assistants to the physicians, as interviewers to fill in the myriad forms, and as virtual clerical workers who make appointments and check health records.

The community nurse should function in the clinic in much the same way as in other settings: as a teacher, a provider of primary care, a health counselor, and as a client advocate. Primary care is usually considered preventive health care or health maintenance. Clients sometimes enter the health care system when they are in a relatively healthy state, and it is then that the community nurse as a primary care practitioner can be effective.

In the clinic nurses are in a uniquely advantageous position. They have a good overview of the kinds of health care needed by an entire community; they can gather statistics by observing and talking to groups of people; and there are large numbers of records available (more about the nursing audit in Chapter 14) to again assess health needs. By speaking with clients, nurses can often determine whether a home visit would be indicated, and they are privy in the clinic to a great deal

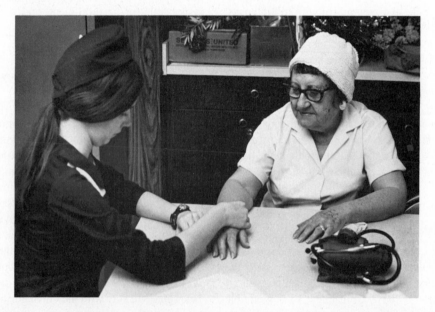

Fig. 6-1. Provision of nursing care by seeing clients in the clinic is a traditional and enduring function of the community health nurse. (Photograph by Ann Chwatsky; courtesy Editorial Photocolor Archives, Inc., New York.)

of neighborhood gossip. Listening to gossip, in our society, has been frowned on as a rather useless and negative pastime. Gossip, however, can be a positive and nondestructive source of information about what is happening in the neighborhood and in the community. The nurses can "recruit" clients; that is, nurses can hear about people whose health problems might have remained unknown and consequently unsolved. Present clients are often an excellent source of referral for other clients.

Community nurses are becoming more and more active in the provision of nursing services in indirect, innovative ways. With the exception of the discussion of physical assessment which follows, the remainder of this chapter will deal with the activities of the community nurse (Fig. 6-2) that involve other than the traditional concepts of nursing care. Nursing as a profession needs to recognize that nursing care is taking place even though the nurse does not appear to be "doing" something to or for the client.

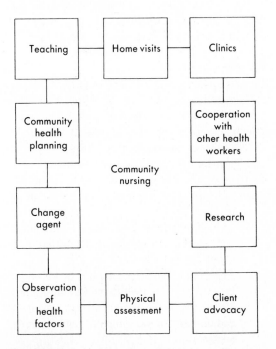

Fig. 6-2. Roles and functions of the community nurse.

Nursing care takes many forms. "The ability of nursing to place the needs of patients first and to respond directly to those needs, rather than the needs of medicine, government, or employing agencies, is the true test of maturity, that is, professionalism."[8,p.6] Nurses must consider clients' needs *as they are,* not as the nurse might like them to be. For example, in dealing with a family where there are multiple psychological and social problems, the nurse must find out what the *members of the family* want to do and then help them to do it. If a woman wants to find a job outside the home, the nurse could help meet her needs by suggesting child-care arrangements or perhaps even giving her ideas about the best way to look for a job. This may not be a traditional way of looking at nursing care, but it is truly nursing in its most professional sense. It is helping the woman to help herself, to become an independent human being, to meet her stated needs.

Another example is a family with a son in late adolescence. His parents have "caught" him frequenting homosexual bars, and he has admitted to them that he is indeed homosexual. The parents have implored the community nurse to find help for their son to "cure" him. But in speaking with the son, the nurse finds out that he does not consider himself sick and therefore feels no need to be cured. He sees the growing family conflict as his parents' problem for not being able to accept his life-style. In this instance the nurse should meet with the entire family to sort out what problems exist and what avenues there are for solving them.

Physical assessment

Two recent trends in professional nursing have resulted in more nurses doing formal physical assessment. Nurses have always assessed the physical conditions of their clients, but they have recently begun to perform entire physical examinations in a systematic way. This used to be the sole prerogative of the physician. The first trend is the great proliferation of nurse practitioner programs that lead to a master's degree or certification as a professional nurse practitioner in various fields.

The second is the increasing number of baccalaureate programs whose philosophy is to teach physical assessment so that their graduates will be prepared to function as primary care practitioners. It is not within the scope of this text to give detailed instructions on how to conduct a physical examination; there are many excellent guides for that purpose.

The reason the nurse does physical assessment is to detect and characterize abnormalities and to provide baseline data from which to make comparisons. An examination is done in three parts: a history, a physical examination, and ancillary procedures, usually called diagnostic tests. The three components are separate but very much related, and each serves no purpose without the other two. It is essential that the examiner establish rapport and trust with the client, which, of course, is much easier said than done. Clients often feel guilty or shameful about various physical symptoms and consequently may try to hide them. A nonjudgmental attitude is important. History taking, as well as the demeanor of the nurse during the procedure, is very important to the formulation of a nursing diagnosis, which is essential to the nursing process. (See Chapter 13 for details on how to take a health history.) Few people will admit to the possibility of venereal disease or to an alcohol problem if they think that the nurse is about to cast moral judgments on them. It is not enough for the nurse to simply state her nonjudgmental attitude; her behavior must corroborate it. Following is an example of a nonjudgmental way to handle an interview about a health problem that could be embarrassing for the client:

Nurse: Please describe what brings you to the clinic.
Client: Well, uh, I have, uh, well, you see, I have this problem . . .
Nurse (smiling): Can you tell me how you discovered the problem?
Client: Well, uh, a few days ago Mary and I were, uh . . . together. . . . I, uh, noticed the problem.
Nurse: You think the problem is connected with you and Mary being together?
Client: Yeah.

Nurse: I'd like very much to help you with your problem, but I can't unless I know what it is. You seem to want to tell me, but you're having difficulty putting it into words.
Client: Oh, yeah!
Nurse: I'm sorry you're feeling uncomfortable. Perhaps if you just take a deep breath and say it, we can talk about it and see how we can help solve it.
Client: Well, uh, you see I have this, uh, white stuff coming out of me, and every time I, uh, pee, it burns somethin' awful.
Nurse: This white stuff, a discharge, is coming out of your penis?
Client: Yeah, yeah, that's it. I'm scared half to death.
Nurse: There's no need to be that frightened, but I'm glad you came to see me about the problem.
Client: I feel like somethin' bad's happening to me.
Nurse: I understand how concerned you must be. I'm going to ask you some questions about your discharge and about how you think it might be related to being with Mary.

The nurse can then go on with the history. She has not given the client false reassurance that nothing is wrong, but neither has she reinforced his fear. She has not made fun of his embarrassment, but neither has she permitted him to become paralyzed by it so that she is unable to obtain a history. The nurse should remember that a nursing history is *not* the same as a medical history, and that the two are taken for different purposes. If the nurse will keep in mind that her aim is to provide nursing care for clients, not to cure disease, it is likely that she will obtain a better nursing history. A history consists of four major parts; interviewing techniques should be reviewed before embarking on any of them.

1. Statistical and informative data: the date and place of the examination, source of the information (it may not always be the client), and mental and physical condition of the client
2. The chief complaint: what it is that prompted the client to seek medical or nursing attention
3. The story of the present illness: the nature and duration of the symptoms and when they began
4. Background information: past history, family

history, review of systems, and personal and social history

During the physical examination four techniques are used:

1. Inspection: looking, both with the naked eye and with instruments
2. Palpation: pressing or kneading with the fingers or hands
3. Percussion: tapping with the fingers or with instruments
4. Auscultation: listening, either with or without a stethoscope

The sense of smell can also play an important role in physical assessment. Infections have a characteristic odor of putrefaction, and a client with a serious body odor may need teaching about hygiene.

As previously stated, this chapter will not contain a lesson on how to conduct a physical examination. The community nurse, however, should have a guideline to the assessment of all developmental and functional abilities, and it is up to the nurse to choose the ones that are applicable to the client as the physical assessment proceeds. Following are some of the items that are useful as a guideline:

1. General social background: ethnic group, religion, income, occupation, type of housing, contacts with social agencies, marital status, age
2. Family and peer group constellation: position in family, close friends, people with whom the client is living
3. Social development: gender, degree of independence, recreational interests, sexuality attitudes and practices, education
4. Mental and emotional status: level of consciousness and reactions to stimuli, intellectual development, mental skills, ability to think in the abstract, perception and understanding of health problem, beliefs and attitudes about health and disease, previous experience with and reaction to illness, patterns of relating to others, self-concept, drug and alcohol use
5. Environmental situation: mobility, permanent disability, exposure to infections or other hazardous conditions, safety of living and working environment
6. Sensory status: vision, ability to taste and smell, hearing, tactile senses, speech patterns
7. Motor status: mobility, artificial devices used for getting around, posture, range of motion, deformities, endurance
8. Nutrition: usual eating habits, appearance, economic status in relation to nutritional needs, appetite, cultural patterns, attitudes toward food, hindrances to eating, condition of teeth, digestion
9. Elimination: frequency, amount, color, consistency, drugs or devices used to aid in elimination, recent changes in bladder or bowel patterns, special problems
10. Fluid and electrolyte status: patterns of fluid intake and output, condition of skin, degree of thirst
11. Circulatory status: rate, quality, and rhythm of pulse; blood pressure and recent changes; skin color, chest or leg pains; fatigue after exertion; electrocardiogram
12. Respiratory status: rate, sound, and pattern of respirations; cough; smoking history; medications; devices used to aid breathing
13. Temperature status: stability
14. Skin: color, intactness, rashes, factors predisposing to breakdowns, appearance, condition of hair and nails, cleanliness of body exterior
15. Allergies: severity, duration of occurrence
16. Sleep and rest: usual patterns, mechanical aids to sleep, drugs
17. Female reproductive status: menarche and menopause, pattern of menstrual cycle, number of pregnancies and outcome, vaginal discharge, condition of breasts, regularity of PAP tests and breast self-examination

It must be noted that physical assessment is to be used only as a tool, one of many, to achieve better nursing care. It is not an end in itself, and the ability to carry out a physical examination is simply another technical skill the nurse learns, differing in degree only, not in kind, from such skills as measuring vital signs and giving various treatments. It is a skill that the nurse should indeed have, but it is not her primary goal.

Interaction with other health professionals

There are many ways in which the community nurse can interact and communicate with people to the ultimate benefit of the client. The client care conferences that take place at every well-run agency are an excellent way for the nurse to discuss the needs of the client with colleagues. It often happens that a nurse is so close to or so involved with a situation that she may be unable to see its components and consequently has difficulty making correct decisions. When the nurse discusses the case with colleagues, they frequently see a different picture of the situation and can offer suggestions or new approaches. Care conferences can also serve to reinforce decisions made by the nurse.

Frequently the community nurse deals with people from other professions or is at a meeting or conference attended by people not in the health field. This gives her an opportunity to act as an interpreter of the roles and functions of nursing in general and community nursing in particular. So often the general public has an erroneous concept of professional nursing, and the community nurse is in the unique and enviable position of being in constant contact with the public and can consequently do a great deal to correct wrong impressions.

The community nurse can serve as a coordinator of all health care the client receives so that the care is adequate but there is no overlapping of services. She can function as a "translator" when the client needs to deal with nonhealth agencies such as housing authorities or welfare boards. The client may need to have health problems interpreted to lay people. There is so much red tape and frustration in dealing with these kinds of agencies that in some instances the client truly needs the community nurse to function as an advocate.[9] The nurse usually has the closest and most frequent relationship with the client and is often best equipped to organize and preside over multidisciplinary conferences.

Another area of positive interaction for the community nurse is working with paraprofessionals: home health aides, licensed practical nurses, and physicians' assistants. It is often the case that the paraprofessional lives in the client's neighborhood and is a member of the same cultural group, whereas the professional nurse may be an ethnic stranger. If this is so, the paraprofessional can be a valuable ally in helping the nurse to recognize and understand some of the unique cultural needs of the client. Without this understanding, the nurse may not be able to communicate with the client as effectively.

Community health nurses also participate in consultation, either as the consultant or the consultee. No matter how experienced and how knowledgeable a person is, there are sometimes problems that cannot be worked through without help. A consultant is often able to shed new light on a situation or can put things into a different perspective. The consultee must be able to clearly define the needs and problems of the situation for the consultation process to work effectively.

Another way in which the nurse interacts with others for the benefit of the client is as a facilitator. By learning about the political structure of a community, the nurse can find out where the power lies and can use this knowledge to the client's advantage. This does not imply that the nurse should engage in unethical behavior, but knowing the intricacies of a system can often result in the cutting of a tremendous amount of red tape. If a nurse has participated in a health and welfare conference, a quick phone call on behalf of a client who needs emergency help to the administrator who also attended the meeting might save weeks of letter writing and frustration.

Participation in community health planning and facilitation of health care services

Planning consists of a logical sequence of events and is the third stage of the nursing process. As nursing care on an individual basis needs to be carefully planned, so does health care on a community basis (Fig. 6-3), perhaps even more carefully because the situations are so much more complex. Within the past decade health planning for existing and proposed communities has become such an important factor in society that it has developed into a large academic field with studies leading to a doctoral degree. The community nurse does not need a doctorate to make a meaningful contribution. Field experiences are valuable beyond measure. Tinkham and Voorhies[10] list guidelines for planning that are applicable in any situation but most particularly in community health planning:

1. Plans should be based on identified desires, needs, and interests of those for whom the plan is designed.
2. Those who will be involved in carrying out a plan should be involved in its inception.

3. Those who will have a major stake in the plan should be involved in the planning.
4. The plan should be realistic in terms of people, money, and resources available. Planners need to take into account the best way to do the job, the best people to do the job, and the best possible chance of success.

These are the essential elements involved in good planning, and it is a test of the creativity, judgment, and initiative of community nurses to adapt these guidelines to their particular situations.

There are several kinds of health planning in which the community nurse can be involved. Federal, state, and local agencies need consultation as they research and devise new health programs or change existing ones. Because the nurse is close to the client, she is in an extremely important and valuable position to advise on the kinds of programs and services needed. Many architects hire nurses as consultants as they design hospitals and ambulatory care facilities. Again, the nurse is in the best position to know what kinds of physical facilities are needed and how they can best be used. Private consulting firms also need nurses to plan

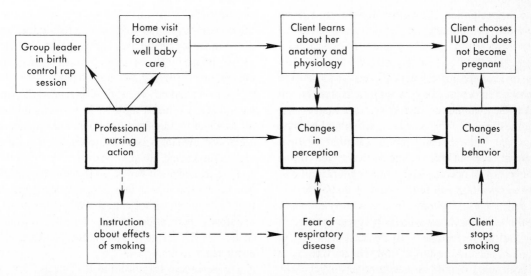

Fig. 6-3. Schematic representation of the ways in which nurses affect changes in perception with resulting changes in behavior.

health services and to evaluate the management of existing ones. On a community level there are all kinds of health planning committees and task forces, all the way from highly structured and well-funded conferences to neighborhood rap sessions at the laundromat. The nurse can and should become involved in health planning at all these levels.

There are many reasons why nurses should become involved. As a general rule they know more about the clients than do any other professional health workers; nurses are usually in more frequent and intimate contact with clients. Consequently they are best able to interpret the clients' needs to other health planners. Nurses, in the daily routine, have contact with the most people who can and do affect the lives of clients. This consequently gives nurses the greatest opportunity for interdisciplinary communication. They have the tools and skills (the nursing process) to assess the health problems they see, to draw inferences from them, and then to communicate these inferences to other health planners. Nurses deal with both clients and health professionals at the same time and can be in a position to interpret each group's needs and problems to the other. This sometimes puts the nurse into the position of a go-between, but there is often so much friction between the deliverers and consumers of health care that a cool professional head in the middle is often a necessity. Perhaps the best (or at least the most practical) reason to become involved in health planning is that the process will take place without us, and if we want what is best for the client and for ourselves, we should become involved in the system to try to get what we want from it. One can obtain more from a system if one knows how it operates and if one is an integral part of the operation and functioning of that system.

When nurses become involved in community health planning, they will soon become aware of the various forces that must be dealt with. There is often negative response from clients who seem to need help the most. As nurses review psychology and sociology, they will recall that people dislike and fear dependence on an impersonal system, es-

pecially a system that concerns itself with so crucial a matter as health. The paradoxical reaction to these feelings is often hostility toward the system and refusal to participate in it. For some reason nurses have traditionally believed that the political process has nothing to do with nursing directly. This is an incorrect assumption because *all* change comes about through the political process.

There are always political pressures of one kind or another to deal with. Nurses have in the past been naive about politics. They tended to think that the only people who "played politics" were elected officials in Washington or their state capital. Politics is the way in which social action and change takes place, and everyone is a politician in some sense of the word. It would seem practical that nurses become more aware of the political process so they can recognize it and deal with it in an effective and constructive way. A nurse need not run for public office to become involved in politics, but she does need to know the power structure of her community in order to bring about meaningful change in the health care system. The changing patterns of payment for health care are a strong force to be dealt with; high feelings always accompany the discussion of financial arrangements.

One of the most difficult and frustrating things the community nurse will have to face in the role of community health planner is resistance from health professionals who do not want or who fear change or progress. "We don't need this because we've never had it," or "This is the way it's always been done, so this is the way it will remain" are the kinds of feelings and behaviors one encounters when one evaluates health care services and tries to plan for change. People's tolerance of innovation and experimentation varies, and very often the crucial difference is how they perceive the presentation of the proposal for change. What can be done about these perceptions will be discussed in the last section of the chapter, which concerns the nurse as a change agent.

The roles and responsibilities of health professionals seem to change almost daily. It is difficult to keep up with who is supposed to be doing what, with whom, and how. The complexity of the health care system is increasing rapidly, and there does not seem to be any hope for simplification in the future. There is frustration concerning duplication of some services and total lack of other services. As many different priorities exist as there are health professionals—almost as many as there are kinds of people. The setting of priorities is a complex task and requires the cooperation of all health workers and the client. The nursing process is the ideal tool to be used. Consumers of health care can and should be vocal about plans that affect them. Any health planning conference, committee, or task force that does not include consumers and encourage their active participation will be ineffective.

How does one put nursing knowledge into action for community health planning? The answers are simple, even obvious, but they involve all the professional judgment the nurse has ever learned. The nurse must get to know the community: its resources, characteristics of the people and of the physical environment, influential people (everyone with influence does not necessarily have officially sanctioned power), what health services already exist and what is needed, what the future trends seem to be (is an area going to be razed for an expressway, thus wiping out homes and vital community services?), and what the people think about and care about.

Research to refine and improve nursing care

In addition to other characteristics, the hallmark of a profession is to engage in research for the benefit of clients and also to upgrade professional practice, which will ultimately benefit clients. Community nurses are in a unique position to do research because they have access to so much human data and because they are in a field that is constantly expanding and growing.

French has defined research as a "problem-solving process—a systematic, intensive study directed toward fuller scientific knowledge of the subject studied. In solving problems, research answers questions."[11,p.115] Basic research has as its goal knowledge for its own sake, and applied research tries to find ways to use the knowledge. It is with the latter that nursing is usually concerned. Research explores the different variables in a situation, how the variables relate to each other, and how they relate to the problem at hand.

Nurses traditionally have had a rather negative attitude toward research. It was usually thought of as something nasty to be gotten through to obtain a doctorate, and it involved the use of complicated and seemingly obscure statistical techniques. Students frequently balk at having to read research reports. There are, however, many imaginative research studies that make lively and interesting reading. These usually deal with small numbers of people with whom the researcher became actively involved. Nursing research in general involves human beings and their behavior and consequently has great potential for being interesting and important.

It is crucial that nurses engage in research. New and improved methods of nursing care need to be found and studied; these may or may not be based on current methods. Because it is obvious to everyone that the present system of delivering health care is ineffective, we must look for new techniques, and this can be done only through research. It is important also to evaluate results of existing techniques and methods of giving nursing care. We know very little about the consequences of our actions and need to do much more research on follow-up of client care. The nurse is also involved in epidemiological research; the reader is referred to Chapter 9 for a detailed discussion on epidemiology.

If research is a scientific process, then an orderly set of guidelines are followed. They consist of and are stated as follows:

1. The purpose of doing the research: what the researcher hopes to accomplish and why
2. A statement of the hypothesis[12]
3. Review of the literature: what others have done in the field and how this study will differ
4. Methodology: procedures used and the reasons for each; samples of tests, interviews,

questionnaires, and tests for statistical significance
5. Results: what was actually found out
6. Discussion of results obtained in view of the hypothesis and possible uses to which the results can be put
7. Recommendations for further study

It can be seen that these seven steps are very similar to, and follow the same order of, the nursing process. Solving clients' health problems, whether theoretically or actually, involves the same logical procedure of data gathering, assessment, implementation, and evaluation.

There are special considerations that are peculiar to nursing research. Nurses have always been action-oriented people who want to immediately remedy situations, to ''make things better.'' The urge to do something about a situation frequently supersedes the need to find out how things came to be the way they are. Nursing has not often taken the time to step back and analyze situations. Judgmental thinking and moralizing about clients' behavior has no place in research of any kind; it simply skews the results and gives an inaccurate picture of the problem.

Nurses attempting to do research sometimes have attended to too large an area of study, and when the task proved to be too monumental, the tendency was to drop the project instead of narrowing the area. Although professional nurse practitioners seem to be committed to doing research and are certainly to be commended, much of it seems to have a heavy emphasis on purely clinical practice and appears to be emulating medical research. What is needed is *nursing* research about how to personalize health care and how to avoid depersonalization and alienation in the health care system. The major thrust of nursing research should be finding better ways to solve health problems.

Sometimes nurses will engage in the kind of research that affects the subjects' basic physiological functioning; nurses must be aware of certain ethical considerations, which were explored and discussed in Chapter 5.

SUMMARY: THE NURSE AS A CHANGE AGENT

Speaking of the nurse's role as a change agent as if it were a separate nursing function is redundant. Almost every nursing action taken results in change. Some are for the better, and some actions would have been better not taken.

Raising the consciousness of clients about health hazards and other influences in their environment leads to a change in their perceptions about the world in which they live and may or may not result in a change in behavior.

Bringing to light situations that the nurse sees as a health problem but that the client does not can lead to a change in the way in which the client perceives the situation and may result in his obtaining professional health care.

Telling clients about health services and resources (or directly providing these services) can lead to a change in the way the client deals with the health problem (Fig. 6-3). This can bring professional health care to the client where none was previously available.

Teaching about health can change the amount and kind of information clients have about their bodies and should result in better care of those bodies. Teaching works two ways. The nurse as a teacher learns about what the clients had previously believed, which leads to a change in the nurse's perception of the clients. This in turn changes the way the nurse relates to the clients and what and how she teaches.

Client advocacy can result in clients getting the health services they need and can also result in their learning how to be more adept in the various social and political maneuverings that everyone must employ to get what he wants and deserves. The change seen is usually better health care.

A home visit can lead to a change in the nurse's perception of the client's health problems and perhaps will result in a change in the client's perception of the nurse. If the client behaves differently at home, so does the nurse. The relative informality of the situation can lead to a change in the relationship between the client and the nurse and possibly to a change in the way in which the health problem is solved.

The nursing contract can lead to changes in the way nursing care is given and health services provided.

Making a physical assessment almost always results in changes in information the nurse has about a client. In the past nurses had to request and wait for the results of a physical examination from the physician. Now nurses can do their own examinations and can discuss their findings with the physician. There is also a change in the kinds of actions nurses can take on an independent basis, as well as a change in the rapidity with which the action can be taken. The information that nurses seek is immediately available when they obtain it themselves.

Communicating with other health professionals often leads to changes in the way the professionals relate to each other. There is usually a change in the perception of roles, functions, and expected abilities.

Consultation leads to changes in the ways and the speed in which health problems can be solved.

Participation in community health planning usually results in changes in the kinds of services offered to clients and often in changes in the nurses' perception of themselves.

Political action can change the health system, or it can change nurses' knowledge of how the system works so they can learn to function more effectively within the system.

NOTES

1. Rines, Alice R., and Montag, Mildred L.: Nursing concepts and nursing care, New York, 1976, John Wiley & Sons, Inc.
2. Henderson, Virginia: The nature of nursing, The American Journal of Nursing **64:**64-68, August, 1964.
3. Random House dictionary of the English language, New York, 1966, Random House, Inc.
4. These concepts were developed and refined by the faculty of the Department of Nursing at Rutgers University Camden College of Arts and Sciences.
5. Kotulak, Ronald: The good life: biggest killer of Americans, Philadelphia Inquirer, June 20, 1976.
6. Sutterley, Doris, and Donnelly, Gloria: Perspectives in human development, Philadelphia, 1973, J.B. Lippincott Co.
7. See Chapter 12 for techniques of crisis intervention.
8. Marram, Gwen D., Barrett, Margaret W., and Bevis, Em O.: Primary nursing, ed. 2, St. Louis, 1979, The C.V. Mosby Co.
9. The term *advocate* is used so frequently in this book, and the concept of client advocacy is so integral a part of the book's philosophy, that the term should be defined: "One who defends, vindicates, or espouses a cause by argument; upholder; defender; one who pleads for or on behalf of another." (From Random House dictionary of the English language, New York, 1966, Random House, Inc.)
10. Tinkham, Catherine, and Voorhies, Eleanor: Community health nursing: evolution and process, ed. 2, New York, 1978, Appleton-Century-Crofts.
11. French, Ruth M.: The dynamics of health care, New York, 1974, McGraw-Hill Book Co.
12. A hypothesis is an assertion subject to verification or proof; a proposition stated as a basis for argument or reasoning; a premise from which a conclusion is drawn; conjecture. (From Random House dictionary of the English language, New York, 1966, Random House, Inc.)

BIBLIOGRAPHY

Archer, Sarah, and Fleshman, Ruth: Community health nursing: patterns and practice, ed. 2, N. Scituate, Mass., 1979, Duxbury Press.

Bates, Barbara: A guide to physical examination, ed. 2, Philadelphia, 1979, J.B. Lippincott Co.

Benson, Evelyn, and McDevitt, Joan: Community health and nursing practice, ed. 2, Englewood Cliffs, N.J., 1980, Prentice-Hall, Inc.

Collins, Mattie: Communication in health care: understanding and implementing effective human relations, ed. 2, St. Louis, 1981, The C.V. Mosby Co.

Epstein, Charlotte: Effective interaction in contemporary nursing, Englewood Cliffs, N.J., 1974, Prentice-Hall, Inc.

Fielo, Sandra: A summary of integrated nursing theory, New York, 1975, McGraw-Hill Book Co.

Freeman, Ruth B.: Community health nursing practice, Philadelphia, 1970, W.B. Saunders Co.

French, Ruth M.: The dynamics of health care, New York, 1974, McGraw-Hill Book Co.

Gentry, W. Doyle: Applied behavior modification, St. Louis, 1975, The C.V. Mosby Co.

Hobson, Lawrence B.: Examination of the patient, New York, 1975, McGraw-Hill Book Co.

Kotulak, Ronald: The good life: biggest killer of Americans, Philadelphia Inquirer, June 20, 1976.

Leahy, Kathleen M., et al.: Community health nursing, New York, 1977, McGraw-Hill Book Co.

Malasanos, Lois, Barkauskas, Violet, Moss, Muriel, and Stoltenburg-Allen, Kathryn: Health assessment, ed. 2, St. Louis, 1981, The C.V. Mosby Co.

Marram, Gwen D., Barrett, Margaret W., and Bevis, Em O.: Primary nursing, ed. 2, St. Louis, 1979, The C.V. Mosby Co.

Milio, Nancy: The care of health in communities, New York, 1975, The Macmillan Co.

Murray, Ruth, and Zentner, Judith: Nursing concepts for health promotion, Englewood Cliffs, N.J., 1975, Prentice-Hall, Inc.

Rines, Alice, and Montag, Mildred: Nursing concepts and nursing care, New York, 1976, John Wiley & Sons, Inc.

Shontz, Franklin C.: The psychological aspects of physical illness and disability, New York, 1975, The Macmillan Co.

Sutterley, Dorris C., and Donnelly, Gloria F.: Perspectives in human development: nursing throughout the life cycle, Philadelphia, 1973, J.B. Lippincott Co.

Tinkham, Catherine, and Voorhies, Eleanor: Community health nursing: evolution and process, ed. 2, New York, 1978, Appleton-Century-Crofts.

7

THE NATURE OF A COMMUNITY

WILLIAM HARRIS TUCKER

HEALTH CARE AND THE COMMUNITY

Humor frequently results from differing interpretations of the same word. A New Yorker visiting the Midwest is hit by a car at an intersection. As he lies injured in the street waiting for an ambulance, a local policeman bends over, covers him with a blanket, and inquires solicitously, "Are you comfortable?" "Well . . . I make a nice living," is the Easterner's reply. To New Yorkers, *comfortable* is a commonly used synonym for *affluence,* but clearly the victim's financial status was not the subject of the officer's query. Nevertheless, both usages of the term share an underlying connotation of ease: in the one case physical; in the other financial.

Some words touch so many diverse phenomena that they are both practical and impractical at the same time. *Community* is such a word, applicable in a wide variety of situations and so quite versatile but prone to multiple connotations and, therefore, easily misunderstood. The term is frequently used both in speech and writing with just a vague assumption that everyone has approximately the same idea of what community means or what the community is. It is such assumptions that lead to the much-lamented breakdowns in communication. In contrast to the situation in which the disparate intentions of policeman and pedestrian become immediately apparent through the rather comical in-

congruity of the latter's response, extended discussions concerning the community often take place in which, unknown to each other, the participants lack agreement on who or what is meant by *community.*

USES OF "COMMUNITY"

This is hardly a surprising state of affairs in view of the many different entities designated by the single generic term community. Nomadic tribes, isolated rural hamlets, affluent suburbs, gigantic industrial and commercial centers, ethnic groups, professional groups: all are lumped together in the same category. Thus it is common to speak about the black community, the academic community, the Washington, D.C., community, the South Bronx community, the rural community, the urban center community, the business community, and the medical community all as meaningful kinds of communities. These many uses result from three distinctly different approaches to the concept of community: as a spatial unit, as an ethnic group with a common culture, and as an aggregate of people with shared values, interests, and goals.

Professional community

Considering these approaches in inverse order, the last named refers to a community whose organizing factor is neither a geographical nor an

173

emotional tie but rather some common intellectual or professional bond. It is in this sense that Goodman speaks of the community of scholars,[1] Kuhn discusses the community of scientists,[2] or economic analysts speculate on the reaction of the business community to some new government policy. Studying the sociology of such communities is often the key to understanding change in the substantive areas (science or business) with which they are concerned. A careful analysis of the interests, values, and sociologic dynamics of the medical community would certainly provide some insights into the nature of health care in the United States.

Ethnic community

The use of the term community to refer to an ethnic group has led to some confusing and controversial situations. Sometimes, bordering on an abstraction, it is meant to refer to the group in its totality, as in "The black community in this country has been oppressed for centuries." At other times, while retaining the characteristic of membership in an ethnic group, it stresses a specific locality as being the black community: the section of town where the majority of the area's black population resides. Thus, much to the consternation of government planners and agency administrators who attempt to structure minority group participation onto health planning boards, one of the most common complaints is that appointees to such boards do not really represent their ethnic community. "Oh, sure, so-and-so is a Puerto Rican," goes the refrain, "but he does not live in the Puerto Rican community." The person is a member of the minority community (i.e., group) but does not live in the minority community (i.e., place). Frequently implicit, though not usually stated as a part of this dualistic use of the concept of an ethnic community, is the issue of socioeconomic class. Since most minorities tend to be poor—indeed, phrases like the "urban poor," "the ghetto," or "the welfare mess" are often just euphemisms for blacks, Chicanos, and Puerto Ricans—vertical mobility, especially if it results in an upper—middle class

life-style, is often seen as a cultural defection from as well as a physical desertion of the community.

Community as locale

Finally, there is the community as a geographical unit: a locale (Fig. 7-1). This approach is no doubt the closest to the common-sense concept of community held by that mythical average person in the street. It involves a specifically designated area that contains residential structures, probably shops of various kinds, perhaps buildings for work, and, of course, the inhabitants: "community people." This definition of community is dependent on street names and map coordinates. Because such an approach is particularly advantageous in a public health context, where one can define the community served by a given hospital, health planning agency, or neighborhood health facility by precise boundary lines, it is the view of the community that this discussion will use. Many sociologists do not feel that such a simple approach is sufficient to define community, even in the geographical sense. One frequently quoted definition is that "the community consists of persons in social interaction within a geographic area and having one or more additional common ties."[3] This insistence on "additional common ties" presents problems. It suggests that a monolingual Spanish Puerto Rican welfare mother and a middle-class WASP college professor who live on the same block but have no other cultural/demographical characteristic in common are not part of the same community. Moreover, such a definition may foster the temptation to assume that residents of a specific area are ipso facto like one another in the sense that they share common beliefs, values, and aspirations. Although this may be the case when a particular geographical community is composed predominantly of members of the same culture, often the social reality is quite different.

To many people this view of community is probably unsatisfying. It suggests that by placing pins on a map, one can artificially create a community that may not coincide with the boundaries of the "real" community known to those who live there.

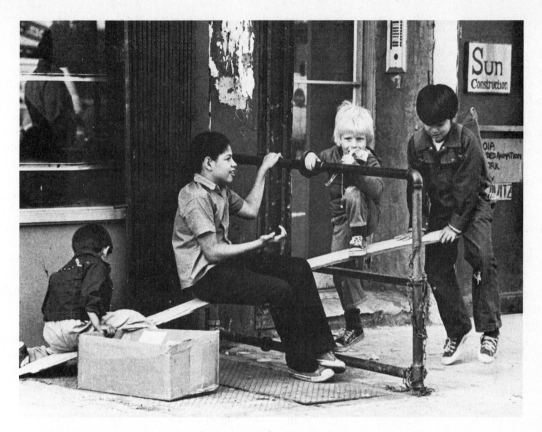

Fig. 7-1. Community can mean social and cultural values as well as locale; the two concepts coexist (Photograph by Laima Druskis; courtesy Editorial Photocolor Archives, Inc., New York.)

Only by talking to the residents, according to the objection, can one find whether the real boundaries grow out of a politically defined area, ethnic groupings, or natural geographical bounds. However, the political reality is that numerous government groups (e.g., sanitation departments, post offices, and health agencies) carve up an area in order to best fit their own projects. Although such gerrymandering is done to serve the interests of those making the delineation with little regard for the possible fragmentation of the "natural" communities, ironically, a greater cohesiveness often grows out of the interaction (conflict or cooperation) with the agency or institution itself. Especially in the field of health, some geographical area

is often labeled a community on the basis of its proximity to a medical center. Perhaps it is not a community in the social or psychological sense of having "additional common ties," However, in time, "by shared experiences and a common enemy (usually some arm of the medical establishment) the target area might become a cohesive unit . . . much to the chagrin of the medical establishment."[4,p.213]

How large an area constitutes a community is also unclear. One sociological text informs the reader that a community is larger than a neighborhood but smaller than a society.[5] Another suggests that a larger social unit, an urban center together with its satellite suburbs, for example, might be designated a community complex,[6] but does not offer any guidelines for deciding whether a particular social unit is sufficiently large and complex to be categorized as a community complex rather than a community. There is no compelling necessity for delimiting a community to a given size as long as the exact dimensions of the community being discussed are made clear. Thus, if one is advising a health systems agency, it would be quite appropriate to consider, for example, the southern New Jersey community, even though it consists of seven counties, at least as many fair-sized cities, and 1.5 million people. At the other extreme, a neighborhood health center might be organized to serve a community of only a few square miles.

Finally, one further qualification is necessary in the specific context of public health. When health care groups or agencies use the term community, they typically intend to exclude those associated with the health profession itself. As one physician clearly states in the *American Journal of Public Health*, "By the community we mean the consumers of health as distinct from the professional providers."[7] Thus for the remainder of this chapter community members will refer only to persons who live in the designated locale and are not health professionals. Although this may seem in some ways arbitrary—after all, if a physician lives in the defined area, by what capricious fiat should he be exluded from membership in the community?—there is a defensible rationale. Contemporary health projects of various kinds usually seek some degree of community involvement: *input* seems to be the currently popular, though vague, term. Health care professionals by their very position already have the opportunity to make some kind of impact on these projects, and consequently, further input, as a community member, is seen as unnecessary or even undesirable.

Within the context of the local community, that is, people living within a geographically defined area, there may be one or more separate and well-defined communities. This is especially evident in cities where neighborhoods are changing. For example, in many large American cities such as Washington, D.C., San Francisco, Cleveland, St. Louis, and others there exists a movement known as "gentrification," "neighborhood rehabilitation," or some other regional phrase. Gentrification is the process by which affluent people (usually young professionals and sometimes but not necessarily white) buy dilapidated and seedy houses in run-down neighborhoods for a very low price. Then they repair the house to its original (or better) condition and either live in it themselves or sell it for a tidy profit. Other people follow suit, and in a decade the character of a neighborhood has changed completely. The people who had been living in the houses (always poor, usually older, and many times black) are forced to move to even worse neighborhoods. However, while the area is in a state of transition, there are many types of people living there, frequently in disharmony, and they represent many different communities even though their geographical locale is the same.

In addition, for some people there is an emotional dimension to the phrase "the community" that transcends any denotative meaning, both a glorification and a romanticization of a sense of closeness perhaps associated with some idealistic concept of community, what is referred to by the German word *Gemeinschaftsgefühl*. Thus an inherent sense of goodness is sometimes attached to the concept of community. To be pro-community is to be on the side of the angels; opposition to the community is viewed as similar to opposition to motherhood. Such a view is in reality part of a political ideology which posits that many contemporary social problems result from the overinstitutionalization of our society and that the solution to these problems lies in the community movement: the active reclamation by the nonprofessional individuals in the community of control over institutional processes that affect their lives. Some take this position because they believe that it is the only way to make even well-intentioned professional people, responsive to the needs of the community in which they work; others more cynical agree with George Bernard Shaw that "All professions are conspiracies against the laity."[8,p.16]

Community as client

"Community as client" has become somewhat of a catch phrase in the jargon of community health professionals, almost as if the community itself (that amorphous combination of bricks, mortar, institutions, and people) had a health problem that required assessment, intervention, and evaluation on the part of a nurse or other health professional. In a metaphorical sense, this is true, and we see continuing evidence that many communities have many serious problems that are having a devastating impact on the lives of people. However, the problems that affect communities as wholes, rather than the individuals, families, and institutions that comprise the community, are so complex that they are not within the scope of this text. What is essential for the nurse to learn, however, is how to distinguish the problems of the community itself from those of its composite parts.

COMMUNITY INVOLVEMENT IN HEALTH CARE

In medicine, as well as in such other diverse areas as education, day care, and even law enforcement, there is heard the cry for some kind of community participation. Although some who raise this concern have been dismissed by those in control of institutions as extremists or agitators, others have such unimpeachable establishment credentials that such a characterization cannot possibly be taken seriously. Shirley Chisholm, for example, the congresswoman from Brooklyn, New York, speaking at the Health Conference of the New York Academy of Medicine,[9] pointed out:

It is no longer an issue whether the community can or cannot, or should not, or even will or will not participate in the planning and implementation of the delivery services to itself. The issue now before us is: How can the community best participate in the planning and implementation of those services that most crucially and directly affect its life and well-being.

Civil rights movment

The current trend toward the establishment of community health centers had many of its roots in the social upheavals of the 1960s. The civil rights movement pressed for, among other demands, better health care. As millions of black Americans vigorously asserted their refusal to stand for second-class services, community health centers seemed to be one route to redressing grievances against hospitals and other standard providers of health services. Such centers were envisaged not only to focus on the health needs of the poor, but also to include intensive participation by and involvement of the population to be served, both in policy making and as employees. The legislative vehicle that initially provided the resources for such centers was the Economic Opportunity Act of 1964, Lyndon Johnson's most highly touted weapon in the war on poverty. The purpose of this legislation was to provide the federal government with an opportunity to support the development of new ways for dealing with traditional problems. While not originally intended as one of OEO's major efforts, proponents of the poverty syndrome point of view succeeded in adding health to the other program emphases on employment training and education, and in 1967 Senator Edward Kennedy sponsored an amendment to the original act allocating funds to support the

development and implementation of comprehensive health services programs focused upon the needs of persons residing in urban or rural areas having high concentrations of poverty and a marked inadequacy of health services.[10]

Consumer movement

Some further impetus for community involvement in the health care system also came from the consumer movement led by Ralph Nader. Some health organizations (e.g., health maintenance organizations) are beginning to substitute the term *consumer* or sometimes *client* for the traditional *patient*. This change in terminology reflects a relatively new underlying orientation toward obtaining a service while maintaining the nonsubordinate relationship to the provider of that service, as described in Chapter 1. But, although Nader and company have made the consumers of health services money and quality conscious, there are definite limitations to the consumerist mentality applied to health care. As Illich[11] points out, consumers of medical services often cannot learn from experience. They cannot return the service to the seller or have it repaired. Health services are not advertised, and comparison shopping is discouraged. Also, once having decided on purchase, consumers cannot have a change of mind in the midst of treatment. In most cases they even have to rely on the evaluation of the supplier to inform them if they have been well served. Whereas consumers who feel quite competent to look under the hood of a car and make judgments about the performance of General Motors may band together to demand changes in engine structure and a cleaner exhaust system, they feel much less qualified, even as an organized group, to decide what ought to be done to their stomachs or kidneys.

One of the chief sources of dissatisfaction with health care is its impersonality. Clients want time, sympathetic attention, and concern for themselves as individuals from health professionals. When mothers were interviewed at a Los Angeles pediatric clinic, they reported lack of warmth or friendliness, failure to understand their worries, inadequate explanations of illness, and confusing medical terms as principal causes of their dissatisfaction.[12] Evidently it is the lack of family physicians that disturbs people most. Consumerism has not always been the best antidote for this complaint because of its previous emphasis on the sale of a product or impersonal service (automobiles and their repair are the classic examples), and it is precisely the commodification of medical care that is the major source of the complaints. According to Illich,[11,p.166] before such commodification, the sick person

could still find in the eyes of the doctor a reflection of his own anguish and some recognition of the uniqueness of his suffering. Now, what he meets is the gaze of a biological accountant engaged in input/output calculations.

Thus to some degree a consumer approach, conceived originally in the struggle to make producers and servicers of objects responsible, acquiesces to the view of client as object, a defective commodity to be repaired. Illich goes so far as to suggest that dying can be considered the ultimate form of consumer protest,[11] since it is only at this point that the consumer must be finally written off as a total loss to the medical business.

These limitations prevent the consumer movement from dealing with a medical corporation in the same way that was so effective with General Motors: no hospital will recall its appendectomies, regardless of the number of complaints. However, it has organized significant activity directed toward community participation in health care delivery, especially in the planning and financing stages. Rather than pursuing the civil rights strategy of organizing new quasialternative institutions, consumer groups have opted for efforts at local representation on the boards of already powerful institutions like Blue Cross. Such efforts were formed as much by the desire to hold down the skyrocketing cost of health care as by the interest in influencing other aspects of its delivery.

Federal government

One final factor had been especially influential in the mid-1970s in involving the community in health care: the federal government. Civil rights activists and, to a lesser extent, consumerists have been social reformers who advocated varying degrees of community participation both because they believed that it was the community's right to have some kind of input into local health care institutions and because they believed that these institutions would be considerably more effective with such input. In contrast, the government's motivation has been predominantly one of cost cutting during a period of unprecedented increase in health care expenditures.

However, during the 1960s and 1970s government did not succeed in its cost-cutting goals; in fact, the result was the opposite of that intended. Following the enactment of Medicare and Medicaid in 1966, vast sums of money poured virtually without control into hospitals and other health care institutions. *The American Health Empire*,[14] a report from the Health Policy Advisory Center, presents a detailed description of how hospitals grew by leaps and bounds, building new facilities, enlarging old ones, adding new beds, exotic equipment, and increased staff, hiring public relations firms, and virtually anything else they wanted, almost all at the taxpayer's expense. This was hardly surprising, since the legislation was shaped by the hospital people—the American Hospital Association and its financing arm, Blue Cross—precisely to relieve the hospitals' financial difficulties. Medicare and Medicaid accomplish this purpose by reimbursing health institutions on the basis of their cost of operation without stringently specifying what makes up that cost.

Thus, Medicare/Medicaid provided an attractive bonanza not only for hospitals but also for drug companies, vendors of surgical equipment, electronic data processors, and all the other interests which comprise the medical-industrial complex. Two Tufts Medical School professors[13,p.311] were prompted to comment that "Medicare has proved a better mechanism for insuring the provider than the patients." The spending became so free and easy that in Virginia Medicare was billed for at least part of the cost of entertainment for Blue Cross executives (alcoholic beverages, theater and sports tickets), the Blue Cross company picnic, and even Blue Cross/Blue Shield monogrammed golf balls.[13]

In response to such an unbridled outpouring, the federal government had no choice but to step in, tentatively at first and then more assertively, to stem the tide. Attempts to contain and rationalize this system have led to planning agencies and councils that feature community representation. Knowing that it can rely on public support in the effort to contain increasing costs, the federal government has fostered a planning structure through which such agencies can decide where facilities will be located and who will do what in health care. There can be little doubt as to the government's primary motivation for encouraging such planning. The

chapter on "Planning for Community Health" in the public health service book, *Community Health Services*, begins with the obligatory statement about the necessity for planning to enhance the well-being of people in an industrial society characterized by rapid growth and increasing complexity, but it quickly gets to the meat of the issue on the next page:

> Planning helps to ensure proper return for expenditure. . . . Although many health professionals are reluctant to evaluate their activities in economic terms, all health agencies are obliged to keep expenditures within the limits of their budgets. There is also growing recognition that the size of expenditures made in the nation for health purposes necessitates assurance that they are economically sound. No community has enough resources to be able to spend them without considering cost. . . .*

MODES OF INVOLVEMENT

Although these separate forces have each proposed some kind of community involvement in health care, naturally there have been major differences in the form and character of the involvement. Basically three different types of participation have been advocated: the civil rights activists and the social reformers who followed in their tradition have pressured for some kind of community participation in the policy and administration of local health facilities; the consumer movement has lobbied for representation on the directing boards of hospitals and major financing agencies like Blue Cross; and the federal government's desire to cut costs has led to community participation on health planning councils.

Neighborhood health centers

The OEO legislation cited earlier enabled the creation of some sixty neighborhood health centers, although funding and operational control for them

---

*From Herman, H., and McKay, M.E.: Community health services, Washington, D.C., 1968, p. 209. Copyright 1968 by the International City Manager's Association. Reprinted by permission.

was later transferred to the Department of Health, Education, and Welfare. These projects ranged in size from storefront operations to multimillion-dollar complexes, the largest of which (Dr. Martin Luther King Health Center in the Bronx, New York, and the South Central Multipurpose Health Services Center in Watts, Los Angeles) even featured extensive training and research components.[15] The centers were intended to be a radical departure from the condescendingly traditional approach of ministering to the needs of the poor, substituting in its place the concept of "maximum feasible participation" in the program by the community.[15] The differing interpretations of this phrase, from token representation on an advisory board to complete community control, produced controversy and confrontation at most of the neighborhood centers at one time or another.

The mechanism for getting a neighborhood health center funded involved a grantee agency (e.g., medical center or hospital), which submitted a proposal to OEO. The requirements for OEO support included not only a focus on the needs of the poor but also their involvement. The administrative guidelines for the Comprehensive Neighborhood Health Services Programs stated, "Programs must be developed, conducted, and administered with the full and active participation of the persons served, to the end that the program becomes truly responsive to the needs and wishes of those it is designed to serve."[16,p.4] Although there were a few exceptions, more typically the community was not consulted in any way during the development stage; preliminary feasibility studies and the initiation of the proposal was the work of the sponsoring agency. However, the guidelines made clear that in the administration of the project the community had to be involved in one of two ways: either

the governing board of the administering agency is structured so that at least one third of its members are persons eligible to receive services from the project and at least one half of its members are either persons eligible to receive services or are representative of community

groups, such as social service organizations and labor or business organizations . . .

or

a Neighborhood Health Council, which acts as a policy advisory board to the administrative agency, is structured so that at least one half of its members are persons eligible to receive services from the project.[16,p.6]

Implementing these guidelines invariably resulted in some degree of conflict between the health professionals and the community. H. Jack Geiger, one of the original OEO consultants on health and general director of two community health centers, points out that most professionals have the attitude that they run the services while clients provide the illnesses.[17] Even those who believe in local residents' participation have one view of the community's role (the health workers will set the goals, and the community can participate in the means), whereas some community activists may be thinking about setting their own goals and meeting needs as *they* see them. Geiger suggests that the conflict goes through specific stages.[17] In the first stage the professional organization, perhaps believing in the principle of community involvement but more often under pressure from OEO, seeks instant community participation. In doing so, the first group it meets is inevitably that sector of the community including activists, teachers, ministers, and antipoverty workers who have some organizational sophistication and experience in dealing with institutions and agencies. They usually are the more articulate of the community residents and may or may not have a constituency of any size, but, more significant than either of these considerations, their selection as community representatives hardly ever involves a majority of the community's population in any systematic way. (Much of that population, at least in the communities in which the projects were placed, characteristically showed little interest in who ran the project at the outset; the provision of the services was initially more important than their organizational control.) For the first period of operation (Geiger estimates it may last from six weeks to six months) these two groups function in a symbiotic calm because each has met its immediate aim. The professionals are rubbing elbows with the folk and can point pridefully to their advisory group of community representatives, while those representatives have preserved their relative status as leaders of the community.

This state of calm shows its first signs of disintegration as the local representatives begin to realize that, in truth, they have little, if any, control over policy-making decisions and have far less power than might be considered desirable. In addition, more of the previously uninvolved people in the community typically begin to express dissatisfaction with the performance of their self-appointed representatives in getting them jobs, increasing services at the center, and handling their complaints. When the community representatives begin to voice their own discontent to the health professionals over their lack of any real control, a new stage in the relationship between the two groups begins, often marked by severe animosity and the "you-people" syndrome on both sides.

Although some concessions are usually made by the professional group, this period of conflict generally goes on for quite some time. Community representatives continue to demand real power over budgets, hiring, and firing, while the medical personnel respond that there are some decisions that cannot be intelligently made by lay people. According to Robb Burlage, former director of the Health Policy Advisory Center, if OEO intervenes in the conflict, it is always on the side of the professionals.[18] Although the government bureaucrats are very displeased and will probably lecture the center sternly on its lack of good community relations, nevertheless, when the chips are down, they characteristically back off on letting the ordinary people gain control over hiring, firing, and budget.

The conflict may be terminated in various ways. Occasionally the community may develop sufficient political clout to actually take control of the center after it has become operational. In Los Angeles the South Central Multipurpose Health Services Center was established in the Watts community through an OEO grant to the University of Southern California. This action by the university, which had shown no previous interest in the community's problems, was not greeted favorably. On the contrary, it was met with resistance and actually served to unify the community around a common enemy.[19] After a protracted struggle around a number of issues, a community corporation was formed to directly receive and control funds for the health center. At this point an interesting thing occurred: with real control of the center finally in their possession, the community opted to allow the university personnel to continue in their administrative functions rather than attempting to immediately take over themselves.[19]

More often some compromise is reached as to how power will be shared by the two groups. This usually requires that the community group receive some kind of technical training, whereas the professional group must relinquish some of the privileges of rank. In the Columbia Point section of Boston, such a resolution was formalized in a contractual agreement between the professionals, Tufts University School of Medicine, and the Columbia Point Health Association, a group composed of elected community representatives.[17]

Two major exceptions to this sequence have occurred when the plan for the center was actually initiated in the community and the center consequently remained under community control. The Hunt's Point Multi-Service Center, Inc., in the southeast Bronx was the first community-controlled health delivery system in the United States.[19] The original proposal developed through a series of confrontations between groups from the community and city health officials. It created a community corporation whose policy is set by a board of directors elected by and accountable to the community. Since the health clinic is only one of a number of components of the corporation, the board chooses from its members a health committee. The medical director of the health clinic answers directly to this committee, and all personnel must be approved by it.[19]

The other exception is truly remarkable for the tactical sophistication shown by the local group.

An east Baltimore community organization wanted to exert pressure on Johns Hopkins Hospital to use some of its vast resources to meet the health needs of those who lived in the hospital's immediate vicinity. The first problem this group faced was to acquire recognition from Johns Hopkins as *the* community group; others were also approaching the hospital claiming to represent the local interests. In order to accomplish this, the east Baltimore group, marshaling its base in the community, attended a meeting with Johns Hopkins officials that had been called by the strongest competitor. At a given signal all those aligned with the former group departed, leaving the Johns Hopkins people with only a handful of remaining local residents but with a clear picture of who had the community's support.[23] Next the group needed to gain the support of the thirteen general practitioners in the local area. These physicians viewed the developing health center as a threat to their own practices, especially since the center staff would have admitting privileges at Johns Hopkins, whereas they did not. Rather than just ignoring these local physicians, the community won their support by informing the hospital that there would be no program unless the hospital granted them such privileges. Although at the time such a request was unprecedented—general practitioners simply were not given admitting privileges at Johns Hopkins— and the hospital's initial response was an adamant refusal, seventeen meetings later the medical people acquiesced.[20] Further lengthy negotiations over administrative responsibility and funding finally culminated in a health center completely owned and operated by the East Baltimore Community Corporation, which controls the money and the personnel decisions.[20]

In a few instances controversy has caused a neighborhood health center to be terminated. Most frequently this happened because no agreement or compromise could be reached between the community and the professionals, but on occasion more powerful political forces intervened to protect what they perceived as their own interests. In Mississippi the Delta Health Center (actually developed by

Tufts University School of Medicine in Boston) merged with a local hospital to form the Delta County Hospital and Health Center governed by a board of local residents. State officials intervened in an attempt to revoke the group's charter and organize a new board operating under state control.[15] Here the local conflicts were resolved, but state government felt that there was too much or, more likely, the wrong kind of community control (most of the board members were militant civil rights activists) and sought to cut off OEO funds, preferring to shut down the health facility rather than see it continue under its community board.[15]

Since almost all of these neighborhood health centers were started as demonstration projects, they tended to form a rather uncoordinated patchwork, their locations dependent on wherever some local organization (medical school or hospital) took the initiative to put together a proposal. Although the many reports and evaluations of these projects concurred that the quality of care provided was from good to excellent,[21] their cost ruled out any serious consideration of systematic replication across the country.

By 1977 no new centers were being funded by the government. However, on May 4, 1977, a bill was introduced in Congress that if approved would recreate the neighborhood health center cencept in a more highly systematized fashion. The Health Service Act sponsored by Representative Ronald V. Dellums (HR 6894) provides for community-based health care with national financing. It would establish a United States Health Service Organization as a nonprofit corporation mandated to provide comprehensive health services, including occupational health advocacy services, without charge to everyone in the country. The organization would be governed from below through a process referred to as *community federalism* that would parallel the health care delivery structure. The basic governing bodies would be elected community health boards, communities being defined in this act as geographical areas containing 25,000 people (a smaller number would be used for isolated rural areas). These local boards would oversee the provision of primary outpatient health care as well as nursing homes and other multiservice community facilities. In addition, district hospitals would be supervised by district health boards also elected from the population served.[22] More than any other piece of health care legislation, the Dellums bill would allow community participation in the determination of health care needs. The American Public Health Association, which is a 50,000-member organization of public health workers, the United Electrical Workers, and the Gray Panthers, a senior citizens organization, have all gone on record in favor of the principle embodied in the bill.[22] Between the introduction of the bill and adjournment of the 95th Congress, it was referred to eight congressional committees and subsequently died. On March 14, 1979, Representative Dellums introduced it again (renumbered HR 2969), and it has again been referred to eight committees, although there were two days of hearings in the subcommittee on Health of the Ways and Means Committee. It seems unlikely, given this history, that the Health Service Act will become law.

Consumer activity

The consumer movement has made strenuous efforts to gain local representation on the boards of hospitals and health insurers. Although the insurers serve only their subscribers rather than all residents of an area, their policy decisions often have such a far-reaching impact that everyone is affected. Blue Cross, the nation's largest single health insurer, covers 80 million persons, almost 40% of all Americans, and through Medicare and Medicaid programs it administers benefits for another 32 million.[23] Moreover, Blue Cross also plays an important role in determining health policy through its representatives on governmental advisory and congressional committees.

Almost half the members of the boards of directors of the seventy-four local Blue Cross plans are representatives of hospitals.[23] No doubt this is one of the reasons that these boards have such a poor record of support for consumer concerns such as cost and quality control. Some health care an-

alysts like Sylvia Law in *Blue Cross: What Went Wrong?* have argued convincingly that hospital representatives have no proper role on Blue Cross boards.[24] Such representatives have a primary responsibility to their own hospital, not to the subscribers or the general public, and thus it is unrealistic to expect that, as Blue Cross members, they will challenge their own policies on cost control or planning.

Furthermore, the so-called public representatives on Blue Cross boards constitute an elite group, in most cases appointed by the hospitals' representatives or the incumbent board. Of 824 such members in 1971, 806, or about 98%, were men, and 585, or about 64%, came from the ranks of business executives, bankers, investment advisers, real estate brokers, physicians, and lawyers.[24]

Attempts to change the composition of such boards in order to make them more representative of the subscribers and sensitive to the needs of the community have been met with resistance. The consumer movement's struggle with the Philadelphia Blue Cross board is a typical example. In 1970 this thirty-four-member board included six physicians, one hospital administrator, fifteen hospital trustees, and three former hospital trustees, for a total of twenty-five people who were then or had been active in the health care business.[25] Although the board's bylaws provided that a majority of its members come from the public, that is, persons not affiliated with hospitals who represent the interests of subscribers, incredibly the public members included the hospital trustees on the grounds that there is not a direct affiliation with the hospital and thus implies no conflict of interest for them. Even the commissioner of the Pennsylvania Insurance Department, as part of a ruling on a Blue Cross rate increase request, recommended that the "board of directors more truly reflect the broad spectrum of the community. . . ."[26]

Many of the Philadelphia Blue Cross board members had other interests that could be said to conflict with their Blue Cross board responsibilities. One member was chairman of the board of directors of a large Philadelphia pharmaceutical company,[25] and there were several others who were major stockholders in companies that did business with hospitals.[27] The consumer advocates took the position that it was not possible for these board members to make decisions in the interest of the public when they had direct affiliations with profit-making organizations dependent on Blue Cross financing for much of their income. Furthermore, eight members of the Philadelphia board also served on the board of trustees of major Philadelphia banks, and two of these bank trustees had extensive involvement in real estate corporations. Banks and real estate developers both profit from hospital construction. Indeed, overconstruction of hospitals and related facilities is the greatest single factor contributing to national hospital cost inflation.[31] In many hospitals as much as $3 a day of a client's bill does not pay for any direct services; it goes directly to the bank for interest payments.[23]

Perhaps prompted by this board's request for a large rate increase, a number of consumer actions ensued. A suit was filed against Blue Cross of Philadelphia requesting release of information on board members and their voting records, especially on the rate increase resolution, an opportunity to examine the corporation's books and minutes, and a change in the bylaws dealing with the selection of public members.[29] A letter was sent to each provider (i.e., hospital-associated) nominee for the new board explaining that the selection process was being challenged in court and asking whether the nominee felt that he could honestly fulfill an obligation to the subscriber by acting in a decision-making position with Blue Cross, "a public serving community trust," while at the same time representing the institution that stands to profit financially by every Blue Cross decision to increase subscriber rates. The letter closed with the request that each nominee give serious personal consideration to a refusal to accept membership on the board.[33] A different letter was sent to each nominee for public representative, detailing a number of the consumer grievances concerning the lack of dis-

closure of the board's affairs to the public, its generally unrepresentative composition and undemocratic selection procedures, and its tendency to rubber stamp whatever the hospitals and the paid staff presented. This letter concluded with the plea that the nominee accept membership on the board only if he were willing to accept the responsibility of serving the subscriber.[31]

On February 16, 1971, about three weeks after these letters were sent out, a number of community groups recommended the following in a formal statement to Blue Cross:

1. Blue Cross of Philadelphia should create immediately subscribers' councils as a regular decision-making element of the corporation.

2. Such councils should establish a relationship with the areawide council hubs, with the neighborhood council hubs, with the community action councils, with the district health and welfare offices, and with the consumer policy groups of the district offices of the Philadelphia Department of Health.[32]

This flurry of activity produced only one concession from Blue Cross: in 1971 the procedure for selection of new board members was changed to an election by the subscriber population.[24]

It is unclear why hospitals and financing institutions are so adamantly opposed to broadening representation on their policy-making boards. The most frequently repeated explanation emphasizes that nonprofessional community residents lack administrative skills and technical know-how. They cannot effectively participate in such organizations without the necessary attributes, and being a union member, poor person, minority, or representative of a community group does not constitute adequate credentials for making health care policy. Although this seems to be the "good" reason, the real reason more likely concerns the unfortunate stereotype of the activist who seeks to be a community member of such boards. An article printed in the American College of Hospital Administrator's journal, *Hospital Administration*, entitled "Giving the Consumer a Voice in the Hospital

Business"[33] states that a common occurrence these days is the meeting where the successful executive

finds himself on the same board as a man dressed in work clothes, necklace, turtleneck topped off with sunglasses and beard, who talks and curses without restraint, and continually projects the image of being ready to throw a Molotov cocktail.

More balanced board representation will certainly not begin to materialize until such stereotypes are overcome.

ASSESSING THE HEALTH OF A COMMUNITY

Assessing the health of a community is a concept and phrase that is in vogue; however, not only is its precise meaning unclear, but also the process of the actual assessment is hotly debated. Some even doubt that it is possible to assess a community's health, and given the complexity of the concept of community that we have just discussed, they may be correct. If, however, the health of a community can be assessed, it is a tremendously complicated task involving professional groups other than those concerned with health. It is not ordinarily a function of professional nursing, but nurses should be aware of the concept and the criteria that can and should be taken into consideration.

Because the nature of a community changes so frequently, any health assessment must first contain an account of *who* the community members are; that is, certain demographic information must be obtained, such as the distribution of age, race, occupation, income and educational levels, type of housing, marital status, and the like. In addition to the demographic data, one would want to know the health history of the members of the community including contagious diseases and certain endemic ones such as cancer, heart disease, sexually transmitted diseases, and others. It is necessary to survey the health *habits* of members of the community in order to determine vulnerability to various diseases, and one must also know the kinds of environmental hazards that exist that might ultimately affect the health of a community. For example, are there large numbers of chemical manufacturing plants in the area; do large numbers of people work in situations where they must stare at cathode ray tubes all day; is the community an urban, suburban, or rural one?

Is the community aware of its own health problems or potential for problems? This depends to a great extent on the educational and occupational level of the people who live in the community. For example, a community of middle and upper level professionals, executives, and business people will tend to do more to keep themselves healthy and will be more aware of factors causing decreased health than will a community of less knowledgeable people.

Those assessing the health of a community must also know the extent to which the people who live there are willing to take *action* to do what must be done to improve their own chances for good health. For example, are they willing to assess and perhaps change personal health habits, and are they willing to take community action, for instance, to institute health-related programs in the schools, to try to convince the local government to change traffic patterns so heavy industrial traffic will not be routed down residential streets, or to insist that factories use air pollution control devices?

It is obvious that to assess accurately the health of an entire community takes the combined efforts of the whole community health team, and the process may take several years. Community nurses, in the course of their daily work, may have general impressions about a particular community's health, but they should understand that until these impressions are substantiated by empirical data, they cannot be used for community-wide health programs.

Health planning

During the same congressional session in which Medicare and Medicaid were enacted, Congress also passed the Partnership for Health Act, formally titled the Comprehensive Health Planning and Public Health Services Amendments of 1966

(Public Law 89-749). Although the federal government's interest in health planning dates as far back as the Hill-Burton Act of 1946, the 1966 act was the first law to mandate consumer participation in the planning process. Accompanied by some inspiring rhetoric on the necessity to ensure the highest level of health attainable for every person, the legislation allowed the creation in each state of a hierarchical network of CHPs, comprehensive health planning agencies. The state-level CHP was to be advised by a health planning council, a majority of whose members had to be consumers of health services. Funds were also made available for regional, county, metropolitan, or other local area CHPs, again with the stipulation that each such agency have an advisory council with a consumer majority selected from the designated community. According to DHEW guidelines, these local councils were to be broadly representative of the community or area's population and had to provide "balanced representation of the traditionally influential and the previously unheard."[15,p.28] Each CHP was to develop a health plan for its area stating area-wide health goals and policies, specific recommendations based on these goals and policies, and the activities required to implement these recommendations. The plan was also to describe and analyze the area's current and projected health needs and health system components, recommend necessary changes in the health system, and delineate specific actions to meet area health needs.[34] The associated advisory councils were to have the right to review and comment on all program activities of the planning agency.

The results of this legislation were largely symbolic. For the first time hospital representatives, physicians, and members of the community sat down at the same table and addressed local health problems together. However, although the participation of the community was a major feature of the health planning structure on paper, the reality of power in these councils was quite different. An investigation by the government's General Accounting Office found that retired physicians, members of hospital boards, administrators of homes for the aged, and others with ties to the health services industry were often listed as the consumer members,[35] and, consequently, the health care professionals on the council tended to dominate local decision making either by numerical superiority or by virtue of their expertise. Even on occasions when the nonprofessionals took issue and were able to muster a majority of votes on the council, it turned out that the council had no power to really control or veto the use of funds; they were purely advisory.

This lack of power meant that when there was a conflict between the interests of health care institutions and the local communities they served, the resolution was typically in favor of the former. In 1973 the local planning council in Durham, North Carolina, documented the major needs as, first *accessible* primary care, followed by emergency services and preventive health programs, and it pointed out a clear lack of need for increase in the number of hospital beds.[36] Nevertheless, the next major expenditures in the area were earmarked for a medical research center, more specialists, and a new hospital miles away from the center of the city but conveniently located in an area owned by a leading real estate broker and the city's biggest banker, who, together, are promoting suburban residential development there.[36] In Oklahoma City even the local CHP staff, normally no enemy of hospital interests, advised the planning council that further hospital expansion was not in the community's interest. An independent consultant was called in. His report concluded that expansion was unnecessary, would waste $35 to $50 million on capital expenses, would limit the hospitals' ability to explore new forms of health care because of the size of the debt incurred for unused beds, and would exert pressure on the hospitals to make use of the beds, resulting in unnecessary hospitalization.[28] Again, the council, composed of physicians, hospital trustees and administrators, and consumers, some of whom were clearly involved in conflict of interest (one such member was also on the board of directors of a local hospital[35]), decided to move ahead with additional construction.

The ineffectiveness of the CHP network in regulating or systematizing the health industry set the stage for the passage of the National Health Planning and Resources Development Act of 1974 (Public Law 93-641), the major health planning legislation in effect as of 1977 and the strongest statement yet from the federal government concerning the role of the nonprofessional in health care decisions. This act creates a network of HSAs (health systems agencies) across the country on over 200 regional and local levels. The governing body for each HSA is a board that, again, must have a majority of consumers who must be broadly representative of the social, economic, linguistic, and racial populations, geographical areas of the health service area, and major purchasers of health care.[37] Since the HSA serves a large region—each area with an HSA has a population between 500,000 and 3 million—consumer representatives are often selected from local councils that are based on much smaller communities.

Each HSA is to gather and analyze data and prepare a health system plan, a detailed statement of goals for improving the health of its residents and increasing the accessibility and quality of health services while restraining costs. In addition the HSA must develop an annual implementation plan setting forth its objectives for attaining these goals and the priorities among the objectives.[38] In preparing these plans, the HSA must review the appropriateness of services provided by health institutions in the area and make findings as to the need for new institutional services and the unnecessary duplication of existing ones. Most important, the new planning legislation gives HSA governing boards some real clout. Although the old CHPs sometimes became HSAs merely through a change in their letterhead, the new boards are no longer just advisory; they can grant or withhold the all-important certificate of need for any large capital expenditure and can approve or disapprove expenditures of federal funds in the region,[39] which means that the boards are not just rubber stamps. They can play a major role in deciding where and how money on health care is spent.

It is too early to make any substantial judgment about the performance of the HSA structure: many of them are still in the starting-up phase. Preliminary indications are that they are not going to be the handmaidens of the hospitals that the CHPs were. Drafts of hard criteria for judging the appropriateness of expansion requests have been distributed to some local boards, and already a number of such requests have been refused. However, some of the old problems remain. The professionals still tend to dominate the discussion if not the decisions, especially at regional-level HSAs in which the social planning and medical jargon tend to confuse the nonprofessional; even if this obstacle were overcome, it is doubtful that in the larger and more formally conducted HSA meetings the dialogue will ever become more informal. Also, the regional HSAs sometimes become a battleground for local or institutional interests. If only one piece of major equipment (e.g., a CAT scanner) or only one specialty facility (like a perinatal center) can sensibly be placed in a region, the representatives from local areas and hospitals struggle over its location.

Because of the philosophy of the Reagan administration we are beginning to see not only cutbacks in the amount of federal money available for such community-based health groups but also the way in which available funds are administered. The goal is to decentralize government, to let states and municipalities do as they please with funds allocated (this phenomenon is known as "block grants," that is, blocks of money granted to states with few or no restrictions on how it is to be spent), and to remove federal control and render many current regulations more or less impotent. This appears to be a political rather than a social maneuver, and it is too early to tell if it is a change for the better in the provision of health services.

COMMUNITY HEALTH SERVICES AND MINORITY ETHNIC GROUPS

The practice of medicine is to a large degree a social relationship conditioned by the backgrounds and attitudes of the different parties to the relationship. When the client comes from a different sociocultural milieu than the health worker, there is a great likelihood that the two will begin their relationship with quite different views about the behavior appropriate to each role and even about illness and its treatment. For this reason operating an effective health program requires an intimate knowledge of the social systems of the community and an ability to communicate effectively with local residents (Fig. 7-2). It was the recognition of this requirement that motivated many of the neighborhood health center activists to demand community control over hiring and firing. Such local control was to ensure the selection of health personnel who would have an understanding of and a sensitivity to the cultural backgrounds of community members.

Culture and mental illness
MENTAL RETARDATION

Although a lack of such understanding and sensitivity has often been a serious obstacle to the delivery of quality health services, in the case of mental illness it has sometimes been the cause of oppression and suffering. Physical sickness is confined to the body and can be characterized in an anatomical, physiological, and genetic context

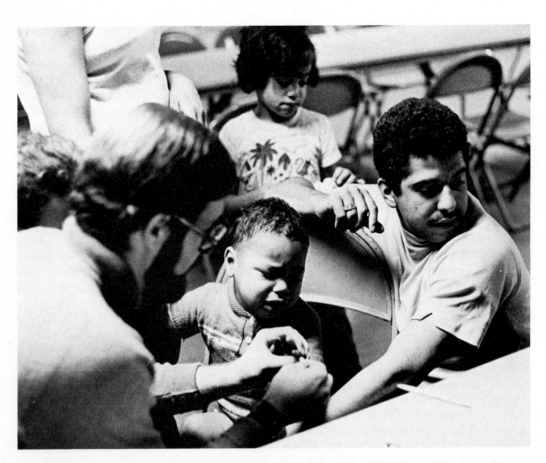

Fig. 7-2. Community nurses must understand the cultural values of the individuals and the community they serve. (Photograph by Bruce Anspach; courtesy EPA Newsphoto, Division of Editorial Photocolor Archives, Inc., New York.)

without any reference to a value system. (Some theorists, notably Illich,[11] feel that no diagnostic procedure is value free and complain that those who raise the question of the culture-bound nature of mental illness as a disease have rendered it more difficult to raise the same question about disease in general.) In contrast the status of mental illness as a sickness depends almost entirely on the judgment of a health professional. Thus the diagnosis of "mental illness" is not necessarily universal, objective, or reliable. (Studies of the reliability of diagnosis of mental illness have shown remarkably little agreement when different mental health professionals diagnose the same patient[40] and, furthermore, that such judgments can be easily influenced by the opinion of others.[41]) Quite the contrary, diagnoses are value and culture bound, often ethnocentric or perhaps even Anglocentric, and reflect the preconceptions and social biases of the diagnosers as much as they are valid categorizations of the characteristics of clients.[42]

Consider the diagnostic category "mentally retarded." Actually, two different models are used for making such a diagnosis. In the pathological model a pattern of biological symptoms interfering in some physically measurable way with the health or preservation of the organism is recognized and organized into a syndrome with a specific label, Down's syndrome or Klinefelter's syndrome, for example.[43] Although identification of the syndrome is made by the observation of patient symptoms, the pathological condition exists regardless of whether it has been diagnosed and labeled by anyone.

In the statistical model diagnosis proceeds entirely from the concept of normal, which is derived from frequency distribution in a large population. Norms are always culturally and socially defined and actually represent *average* behavior or activities. Retardation in this model thus becomes an artifact of the statistical properties of the normal curve. Even if no one were "really" retarded, a certain percentage of the population would nevertheless be so labeled solely because they scored below the large majority on whom the test was standardized. Such a norm-referenced test procedure arbitrarily categorizes the bottom 2% of the population as retarded whether or not they conform to any other criteria of mental retardation, which were arbitrarily established in the first place. If an analogous process were applied to a physical attribute like height, it would suggest that every adult whose height is below some point (probably approximately 5 feet 6 inches) would be two standard deviations below the mean, cutting off the bottom 2% of the United States adult population and would be labeled "height retarded" or "abnormally small" or the victim of a "height disease" even if there were no evidence of some genetic or biological condition responsible for the lack of growth.

Being labeled mentally retarded can have serious consequences for the stigmatized individual: twenty-seven states have sterilization laws applicable to the mentally retarded; thirty-seven states prohibit marriage of some persons so classified; eight states permit the annulment of the adoption of a child found to be retarded; and in many states mentally retarded individuals cannot be issued a driver's license and are not allowed to vote, hold public office, or serve on juries.[43]

COMMITMENT

Many other behaviors that are easily understandable viewed from the ethnic or class culture prevalent in the community may be labeled "abnormal" or "sick" by the health professional acting, despite the best of intentions, as an agent of his own sociocultural milieu. Such labeling is far more serious than that of a diabetic or a coronary case. The diagnosis of mental illness can result in loss of liberty: involuntary commitment to a mental hospital deprives an individual of many of the constitutional protections and the rights to due process that are normally associated with incarceration in our society. Although the United States Supreme Court has recently ruled in *Donaldson v. O'Connor*[46] that only the likelihood of danger to oneself or others constitutes justification for such commitment, nevertheless, many health professionals continue to consign members of ethnic cultures to hospitals against their will because they are too loud, too quiet, too confused, too emotional, or too angry by the norms of the dominant culture.

Following is a description of the judicial review of the involuntary commitment of Larry, a 19-year-old black youth from an almost entirely black section of a small Eastern city.[47]

Before Larry entered the room, the hospital's chief psychiatrist and the treating psychiatrist discussed his case with the others present—legal personnel, hospital employees, and observers. Larry's behavior was characterized as "sullen, hostile, uncooperative, suspicious, and angry," and he was diagnosed a paranoid schizophrenic. Then Larry walked in and was seated. He glared defiantly at the staff members and brusquely inquired, "Am I getting out today?" At this "confirmation" of his diagnosis the chief psychiatrist looked knowingly at the others, raised his hands in a gesture of long-suffering resignation, and commented, "See?" Seemingly benign questions like "How are you?" produced a surly "I'll be just fine when I get out of here!" Attempts at discussing Larry's "problems" with him received a similar response: "There's nothing wrong with me that getting out of here won't cure." The chief psychiatrist began to explain the commitment to Larry: "You see, you've been diagnosed as a case of nervous . . ." "Ain't nothin' wrong with my nerves 'cept bein' in this place," cut in Larry. "Now am I getting outta here or not?" "Not today," was the reply. "You're not ready yet." Larry got up and stalked angrily out of the room, slamming the door behind him. A lawyer now turned to the treating psychiatrist and inquired, "Do you think that this boy's obvious hatred for you would be an obstacle to successful therapy?" "Oh, no," was the doctor's incredible response. "I'm confident that on a conscientious regimen of medication, we will soon see progress."

That Larry was angry is undeniable. He had good reason to be, a black ghetto youth surrounded by a group of middle-class professionals who were deciding whether he should be forced to remain incarcerated in the hospital or be allowed to return home.

However, it was also obvious that Larry was not being kept in the hospital because he was mentally ill. The real reason for continuing his commitment was his belligerent manner and lack of respect for the authority of the staff physicians. If Larry could only have been present for the previous case hearing on the same day, he would have seen the culturally approved behavior for successfully interacting with psychiatrists. Patients who were judged ready to be released were extremely deferent to the staff, admitted the existence of serious problems, and promised to adhere faithfully to their prescribed medication and return regularly for outpatient services.

Imposition of majority norms on the members of minority cultures has led to numerous similar cases. Some social scientists have suggested that rather than being the result of mere insensitivity, such an "imperialist" imposition may have a deliberate and sinister purpose:

Casting persons in the sick role is regarded as a powerful, latent way for the society to exact conformity and maintain the status quo. For it allows a semi-approved form of deviance to occur which siphons off potential for insurgent protest and which can be controlled through the supervision or, in some cases, the "enforced therapy" of the medical profession.[42, p. 18]

Community mental health centers

Because mental health professionals have sometimes been unprepared to serve communities with sizeable concentrations of ethnic minorities, considerable support has mounted for the community mental health center (CMHC). (Certainly a person prepared for a career in health care should have a marked sensitivity to cultural differences. It is true that he might not have specific knowledge, but this can be obtained in the orientation and in-service education program.) Such centers have been established in local areas and often employ members of the surrounding community in paraprofessional roles. The concept of the CMHC was not only to bring quality mental health services closer to community residents, but also to confront oppressive institutions within the community. That is, the approach was to include both a social action and a mental health component.[48]

Evaluative reports on the CMHCs are predominantly favorable, although dissenting voices can be found. The use of paraprofessionals who reside in the community ensures greater sensitivity to the language, values, culture, and needs of community members. The paraprofessionals are given some training in basic mental health skills (counseling or even testing[49]) and then may assist the health professionals or sometimes function independently. One mental health worker complains that, although the paraprofessionals were more successful in establishing a close initial relationship with clients as a result of familiarity with the language and culture, these paraprofessionals were often "upwardly mobile individuals . . ." and, as a result, "were often unsympathetic towards their lower-class clients whom they considered to be unambitious."[50] Another psychologist[51] claims that the concept of paraprofessionals is a type of co-optation which selects neighborhood leaders who may be activists for social change and defuses their potential by incorporating them into the structure of a system they would otherwise oppose.

Influence of culture on health care

Although the mental health area is a striking example, familiarity with the ethnic cultures present in the community is essential for the effective provision of all health services. To illustrate this contention, the values and beliefs of one minority group, Puerto Ricans, will be discussed in a little more detail.

Between 2 and 3 million Puerto Ricans now live on the mainland, concentrated generally in urban areas. Although many speak English fluently, there are still large numbers who are monolingual Spanish, especially those who were born in Puerto Rico and now live in a predominantly Spanish-speaking community. Thus overcoming the linguistic barrier should be a major consideration for health workers. Unfortunately, health personnel do not always realize the importance of this communication problem. Survey research commissioned by Paul Kimball Hospital, a medical complex that serves a northern New Jersey community with a large Puer-

to Rican population, found that the staff did not regard language barriers as a serious concern. However, 71.4% of the Puerto Ricans interviewed stated that they did not understand physicians and nurses, while 75.8% felt that "doctors and nurses think they understand me but they really do not."[52] Overcoming the language difference is not easy. The optimal solution is to have bilingual health personnel, but people with such qualifications are often scarce. Other possibilities are the training of local residents to be paraprofessionals as in the community mental health center or the employment of interpreters in critical positions such as emergency medical service units. Of course, any printed material on public health, such as pamphlets, posters, and handouts, should be stated in both languages. All health workers should also have some kind of brief bilingual reference of medical terms for emergency use on occasions when there are no bilingual personnel available. Such lists, no more than twelve pages long (six English-Spanish and six Spanish-English), are already in use in the emergency rooms of some large hospitals. Finally, all public health staff who serve Spanish-speaking community residents should receive some type of in-service orientation so that they can at least pronounce the names of clients correctly and address them appropriately (Señor José Rivera Colón, for example, may be addressed as Mr. Rivera Colón or Mr. Rivera, but not as Mr. Colón, his mother's maiden name).

As with other ethnic groups, Puerto Rican culture has a set of core values. However, these traditional values are gradually changing under the effects of urbanization, industrialization, and increased intercultural relations with the larger society. Consequently, many younger, more assimilated Puerto Ricans do not adhere to them as much as do the older, more traditional folk. The family is one of the institutions most resistant to change and is the keystone of Puerto Rican culture. Typically, the man is the undisputed head of the house; he is concerned with the family's "external" relations, setting schedules of work and play for his children outside the home.[53] Institutional personnel who do not realize or respect this custom quickly lose the opportunity to establish any rapport with the family. A fluently bilingual school social worker in an Eastern city visited a traditional Puerto Rican home to talk about the oldest child's problems in school. She was met at the door by the father and explained the purpose of her visit in impeccable Spanish. When the father invited her in and sent his wife to the kitchen to make coffee for the visitor, the social worker intervened to countermand the father's directive: "Oh, no, Senõra. Please stay and listen. It's important that you hear this also." End of communication with that family.[54] Many public health workers will no doubt find such male domination difficult to tolerate and perhaps even offensive, but it is essential for them to show respect for a particular family's choice of values if any productive interaction is to take place.

Unlike the typical American nuclear family of parents and offspring, the traditional Puerto Rican extended family may also include aunts, uncles, cousins, and grandparents. This extended family has been referred to as the Puerto Rican social security plan.[55] It is a source of great strength and support for a people in the process of migration, transplanted to a different culture in a sometimes hostile environment. However, for medical personnel who do not understand the support rendered by the extended family, it can be an exasperating experience when fifteen distraught people arrive at a clinic or emergency room, even though only one of them is sick or injured. Health professionals who serve communities with many Puerto Rican families must not only expect and be able to cope with such a situation, they must understand the therapeutic benefits for the client.

Puerto Rican culture places great emphasis on the inner worth of every individual. This intrinsic value, or *dignidad* (dignity), is complemented by *respeto* (respect), a pattern of almost ritualistic politeness observed by all but exceptionally close friends. *Respeto* is shown to others just as it is expected from them, and a deviation from it, as in the example of the school social worker, is considered unacceptable and possibly even insulting.

For this reason, out of *respeto* a Puerto Rican may express verbal agreement with the opinion or directive of an authority figure even in the absence of any intention to comply with it.[56] Thus when a client deferentially agrees to adhere to a particular treatment regimen prescribed by a physician but then ignores it at home (some reasons for this will be discussed later), this may be characterized as deceit by some, but from the Puerto Rican point of view it is not considered to be at all dishonest. The emphasis on individual value is also expressed in the importance placed on personal contact, *personalismo,* in any relationship. A Puerto Rican is much more likely to respond to a referral if it directs him to a named person rather than an institute or agency.[56]

The socialization of the Puerto Rican woman stresses modesty. Consequently, she may be reluctant to undergo a physical examination and especially a breast or pelvic examination even if conducted by another female.[57] Family planning agencies and advisers in particular must be sensitive to this characteristic because it can create a communication barrier between husband and wife on the topic of sex and birth control. One study of Puerto Rican families found that almost half the wives never discussed birth control with their husbands.[53]

When a highly stressful situation occurs, one involving extreme tension and anxiety or intense grief, a common cultural reaction among Puerto Ricans is the *ataque de nervios* (attack of nerves), a sudden episode of hysteria possibly characterized by hyperkinetic seizure, temporary loss of consciousness, paresthesia, mutism, or even aggressive behavior.[56] The *ataque* is often misdiagnosed by physicians unfamiliar with the language and culture as a serious personality disorder or even a psychotic episode.[57] This latter diagnosis is frequently made when the seizure is accompanied by uncomprehensible or bizarre (to the health professional) statements about spirits and spells, both of which are also a common part of Puerto Rican culture.

Espiritismo, or spiritism, is actually a part of Puerto Rican folk medicine in which the medium plays a role similar to psychotherapist in the larger society. Mediums perform a diagnosis by describing and interpreting the problems of cult participants and then heal by invoking the protection of some spirits or exorcising the *malas influencias* (the evil influences) of others.[58] Sometimes these problems are bodily aches and pains, possibly psychosomatic in origin, for which a physician has not been able to provide relief. More typically they are difficulties in personal relationships with family members, other community residents, or fellow workers, and, like psychotherapy, the medium-patient process can be viewed as "a means through which a distressed individual can achieve changes in the way he relates to other individuals."[59] Recognizing the therapeutic benefits, the reduction of anxiety and frustration achieved by the medium, some health professionals regularly refer Puerto Rican clients to these folk psychotherapists.[60] One medical writer suggests that spiritists may constitute an untapped resource and even proposes that some training in psychotherapy to supplement their own skills would result in better mental health services for the community.[58]

In addition to these general cultural traits, many Puerto Ricans, again depending on how traditional their view, adhere to a special set of medical beliefs and practices, the hot-cold theory of disease, in which illnesses are classified as hot or cold, while food and medications are grouped into categories of hot, cold, and intermediate or cool. In this system an illness of one type should be treated by prescribing substances from the opposite classification. A diet and/or medication that does not agree with this approach may represent a violation of the client's concept of appropriate treatment and thus be disregarded. In the *Journal of the American Medical Association*[61] Harwood has presented a detailed discussion of the hot-cold theory and the implications of the theory for understanding and treating patients who subscribe to it. He suggests that rather than attempt to educate patients to abandon their old beliefs, a more effective approach would be to work within the hot-cold system to achieve the desired behavior. For example, penicillin is classified with hot substances because it can cause "hot" symptoms (a rash or diarrhea), and thus a Puerto Rican client may not readily accept it as a treatment for an illness in the same category. Encouraging the client to take the medication with cold fruit juice would be perceived as appropriate in the hot-cold system, since the cold liquid would "neutralize" the hot medication. Harwood describes a number of other situations in which a treatment regimen might possibly conflict with the folk system and suggests ways of working out a resolution within the system. Health professionals who work in communities with many Puerto Rican residents obviously must be aware of the hot-cold theory and, when working with a particular client, should allude to it in a nonjudgmental way to determine whether that client adheres to it and whether it will pose problems in treatment.

Even this brief discussion of the culture of one ethnic group makes it clear that the delivery of effective health services requires a thoughtful understanding of cultural differences. However, unfortunately, much of the contact between health professionals and minorities in the community occurs under stress-oriented conditions that are not conducive to the development of sensitivity. Hence in-service cultural awareness programs for health personnel are an essential need in communities with ethnic minorities.

FINAL COMMENT: ADVOCATING FOR THE COMMUNITY

Psychologist William F. Ryan[62] has proposed two contrasting approaches to the analysis and solution of social problems: one focusing on the idiosyncratic characteristics of individuals who "have" the problem, the other viewing the problem as the result of an imperfect social arrangement. The former view, which Ryan terms *exceptionalist*, implies solutions designed to change the individuals in some way: to remove or remedy the unique personal defect that involves them in the difficulty. The latter, labeled *universalist*, suggests that, rather than modify the affected individuals, public action should be taken to restructure the social arrangement so that the problem will be eliminated.

Most health care is exceptionalist in nature. It is designed to provide remedial treatment for the unique group of persons who fall prey to a particular illness or, through some kind of screening and detection process, to ferret out special individuals who show preliminary signs of such vulnerability. Universalist health measures, designed to change the environment that creates the difficulty, have often become incorporated into the culture so that they are a result of legislative action or can be applied independently of health professionals. Among such measures are water purification and fluoridation.

Community health nurses often employ only exceptionalist activities in dealing with current community health problems. Consider the example of lead paint poisoning, a condition that has been termed epidemic in a number of poor urban communities.[63] The exceptionalist approach stresses education, early detection, and treatment; pamphlets are distributed throughout the community warning of the dangers of ingesting lead paint chips and urging parents to be extremely watchful over children who play near flaking walls and windowsills. Now danger of lead poisoning is the lead from gasoline, so homes near freeways and heavily traveled streets have lead deposits on the grass and roadway. Children playing here and putting objects in their mouths after they have dropped to the ground may also be exposed to a great quantity of lead. This may be a hazard in small communities of the Midwest and West with heavily traveled highways. Television commercials may carry a similar message; mass testing is done throughout the community to find undetected cases, asymptomatic cases, or subclinical cases of increased blood lead level; appropriate treatment is rendered for cases identified through the screening, even though lead in paint has been outlawed for several decades, and it is houses that were built before 1940 that are the hazard. Essential though these measures may be, a universalist approach, the rigid enforcement of housing codes mandating the removal of lead-based paint from residential structures, would eventually prevent the great majority of such cases.

Universalist approaches are effective but difficult to follow. Rather than conferring on their advocates the plaudits and awards that accompany the discovery of a cure for a major disease, such measures often evoke opposition and outrage. (Sometimes the innovator of a universalist solution may even be ostracized by medical colleagues. Semmelweis, the first gynecologist to use antiseptic procedures, was dismissed by other physicians who were offended at the thought that they could be carriers of infection.[11]) Typically the opposition comes from vested interests who foresee that universalist measures would lead to personal or political loss. Thus a clique of slum landlords, real estate speculators, and local political officials often obstruct vigorous enforcement of the prohibitive statutes on appropriate housing and clean environment.

Not all health personnel see universalist measures as appropriate to their role primarily because there are government agencies and offices (e.g., the Occupational Safety and Health Administration [OSHA]) whose designated mission is to determine the necessity of such measures and arrange for their implementation, and there are health professionals employed by OSHA and other agencies. Yet, despite the existence of governmental regulations for health and safety, one continues to hear and read of a new menace to some community's health resulting from the unwillingness of vested interests to take appropriate preventive action.

There are many hazardous occupations because of the explosion of chemical technology. Kepone, phosvel, Nemagon, asbestos, BCME, and polyvinyl chloride are examples of chemicals that in the past few years have caused serious disability such as cancer, nervous system deterioration, sterility, and lung disease, not only to the plant workers in daily contact with them, but also to many others in the surrounding community.[64-68] Medical researchers and investigative reporters have documented in detail both the suppression of undeniable evidence concerning the danger of these industrial substances and the ineffectiveness of government agencies, either from complicity or understaffing, in establishing appropriate safeguards and demanding compliance with the standards that are established.[64,66,67] In his discussion of the contemporary cancer "epidemic," Glasser concludes that 75% to 85% of the cases of this dreaded disease result "solely from exposure to environmental causes and industrial pollutants"[65,p.viii] and that today "the enemy is no longer bacteria or viruses but man."[65,p.176] The same observation could be accurately made about many other currently widespread illnesses.

The implication for community health workers is inescapable; the most meaningful preventive actions, those most effective in producing a safe and healthy existence for the community, are universalist, that is, political. Exerting pressure on companies, government agencies, and politicians to take measures restraining the cause of disease at its source will have much greater impact than only tending to the casualties. In addition to their traditional duties, community health nurses must be prepared to provide technical advice and assistance to the worker and community groups taking such paths. Participation in these activities will involve some risk, but use of the nursing process in working with these interested individuals and groups will contribute significantly to an improvement in community health.

NOTES

1. Goodman, Paul: The community of scholars, New York, 1962, Random House, Inc.
2. Kuhn, Thomas S.: The structure of scientific revolutions, Chicago, 1962, University of Chicago Press.
3. Hillery, G.A.: Definitions of community: areas of agreement, Rural Sociology **20:**111-123, 1955.
4. Conflict and roles. In Curriculum on community control sourcebook, vol. II, Washington, D.C., The Institute for the Study of Health and Society (undated).
5. Nelson, L., Ramsey, C.E., and Verner, C.: Community structure and change, New York, 1960, The Macmillan Co.
6. Clark, T.N.: Community structure and decision making: comparative analyses, San Francisco, 1968, Chandler Publishing Co.
7. Haynes, M.A.: Professionals and the community confront change, American Journal of Public Health **60:**519-523, 1970.
8. Shaw, George Bernard: Preface to The doctor's dilemma, Baltimore, 1965, Penguin Books.
9. Chisholm, Shirley: Community health and community participation, Bulletin of the New York Academy of Medicine **46:**1144-1148, 1970.
10. Schorr, L.B., and English, J.T.: Background, context and significant issues in neighborhood health center programs, Milbank Memorial Fund Quarterly **46**(3):289-296, 1968.
11. Illich, Ivan: Medical nemesis, New York, 1976, Bantam Books, Inc.
12. Korsch, B., Gozzi, E., and Francis, U.: Gaps in doctor-patient communication: doctor-patient interaction and patient satisfaction, Pediatrics **42:**855-871, 1968.
13. Hodgson, G.: The politics of health care: what is it costing you? In Kotelchuck, David, editor: Prognosis negative: crisis in the health care system, New York, 1976, Vintage Books.
14. Ehrenreich, B., and Ehrenreich, J.: The American health empire: power profits and politics, New York, 1971, Vintage Books.
15. Borsody: Legislative methods of community participation in control of health facilities, Philadelphia, 1973, unpublished paper on file at the Health Law Project.
16. OEO Guidelines No. 6128-1, Washington, D.C., March, 1970, U.S. Government Printing Office.
17. Geiger, H. Jack: Community control or community conflict? American Lung Association Bulletin, pp. 4-10, November, 1969.
18. Burlage, Robb K.: Participant in Community Control of Health Services, panel discussion at the Orientation of the Cleveland Student Health Project. In Curriculum on community control sourcebook, vol. II, Washington, D.C., The Institute for the Study of Health and Society.
19. Community response: examples of community efforts to provide health care. In Curriculum on community control sourcebook, vol. II, Washington, D.C., The Institute for the Study of Health and Society.
20. The OEO neighborhood health center: two examples. In Curriculum on community control sourcebook, vol. II, Washington, D.C., The Institute for the Study of Health and Society.
21. Sparer, G., and Johnson, J.: Evaluation of OEO neighborhood health centers. American Journal of Public Health **61:**931-942, 1971; Morehead, M.A., Donaldson, R.S., and Seravalli, M.R.: Comparisons between OEO neighborhood health centers and other health care providers of ratings of the quality of health care, American Journal of Public Health **61:**1294-1306, 1971.
22. In These Times, p. 15, August 17-23, 1977.

23. Kotelchuck, David. The structure of American health care. In Kotelchuck, David, editor: Prognosis negative: crisis in the health care system, New York, 1976, Vintage Books.

24. Law, Sylvia: Blue Cross: what went wrong? In Kotelchuck, David, editor: Prognosis negative: crisis in the health care system, New York, 1976, Vintage Books.

25. Conflicts of interest on the 1970 Blue Cross board, Philadelphia, unpublished paper on file at the Health Law Project.

26. Some legal and policy problems of the recent Blue Cross board of director's election and annual meeting, Philadelphia, unpublished paper on file at the Health Law Project.

27. Barnhart, R.: Getting a fix: the U.S. drug monopoly. In Kotelchuck, David, editor: Prognosis negative: crisis in the health care system, New York, 1976, Vintage Books.

28. Nichols, B.: Oklahoma crude: everything's gushing up hospitals. In Kotelchuck, David, editor: Prognosis negative: crisis in the health care system, New York, 1976, Vintage Books.

29. Barnet Lieberman v. Blue Cross of Greater Philadelphia, Philadelphia County, 1970, Court of Common Pleas.

30. Lieberman, Barnet, and over 200 other subscriber members: Letter to nominees for provider directors, Philadelphia Blue Cross, Philadelphia, February 3, 1971, on file at the Health Law Project.

31. Lieberman, Barnet, and over 200 other subscriber members: Letter to nominees for public directors, Philadelphia Blue Cross, Philadelphia, January 29, 1971, on file at the Health Law Project.

32. Humphrey, M.: Statement to the Blue Cross board meeting, Philadelphia, February 16, 1971, unpublished mimeographed statement.

33. Johnson, E.A.: Giving the consumer a voice in the hospital business, Hospital Administrator **15**(2):15-26, 1970

34. Comprehensive health plan for southern New Jersey, part I, 1974. Excerpts from the Federal Requirements for Areawide Comprehensive Health Plans.

35. Ensminger, B.: The $8-billion hospital bed overrun: a consumer's guide to stopping wasteful construction. In Kotelchuck, David, editor: Prognosis negative: crisis in the health care system, New York, 1976, Vintage Books.

36. Bermanzohn, P., and McGloin, T.: Southern empire: cool handed duke. In Kotelchuck, David, editor: Prognosis negative: crisis in the health care system, New York, 1976, Vintage Books.

37. PL93-641: implications and strategies for health services management and board members, a self-instructional guide, Bellmawr, N.J., October, 1976, Southern New Jersey Health Systems Agency, Inc.

38. Department of Health, Education, and Welfare: The consumer and health planning, DHEW Publication No. (HRA) 76-14020, Washington, D.C., 1976, U.S. Government Printing Office.

39. Duval, M.K.: The provider, the government, and the consumer. In Knowles, John H., editor: Doing better and feeling worse, New York, 1977, W.W. Norton & Co., Inc.

40. Ash, P.: The reliability of psychiatric diagnoses, Journal of Abnormal and Social Psychology **44**:272-276, 1949.

41. Temerlin, M.K., and Trousdale, W.W.: The social psychology of clinical diagnosis, Psychotherapy: Theory, Research and Practice **6**(1):24-29, 1969.

42. Fox, Renée C.: The medicalization and demedicalization of American society. In Knowles, John H., editor: Doing better and feeling worse, New York, 1977, W.W. Norton & Co., Inc.

43. Mercer, J.: Labeling the mentally retarded, Berkeley, 1973, University of California Press.

44. Wechsler, D.: Wechsler Intelligence Scale for Children (manual), New York, 1949, Psychological Corp.

45. Donaldson, K.: Insanity inside out, New York, 1976, Crown Publishers, Inc.

46. Personal observation at Lakeland County Hospital, Blackwood, N.J., May, 1976.

47. Peck, H.B., Kaplan, S.R., and Roman, M.: Prevention, treatment and social action: a strategy of intervention in a disadvantaged urban area, American Journal of Orthopsychiatry **36**:57-69, 1966.

48. Allerhand, M.E., and Lake, G.: New careerists in community psychology and mental health. In Golann, S.E., and Eisdorfer, C., editors: Handbook of community mental health, New York, 1972, Appleton-Century-Crofts.

49. McSweeny, A.J.: Including psychotherapy in national health insurance: subsidy to the rich? IV. Insurance guidelines and other proposed solutions, presented at the American Psychological Association, Washington, D.C., September, 1976.

50. Statman, J.: Community mental health as a pacification program. In Agel, J., producer: The radical therapist, New York, 1971, Ballantine Books, Inc.

51. Health care consumer survey of the Paul Kimball Hospital, Lakewood, New Jersey, Camden, N.J., 1975, Rodriguez Associates.

52. Brameld, T.: The remaking of a culture, New York, 1959, Harper & Brothers.

53. This incident was personally related to me by José Jimenez, coordinator of ESEA (Title VII) Bilingual Program, Camden, N.J.

54. Thomas Marie, Sister: Puerto Rican culture, Philadelphia, 1975, unpublished paper.

55. Thillet, I.C.: Some culture related characteristics and "syndromes" of the Puerto Rican, presented at the Forum on Community Health and Cultural Awareness, Camden, N.J., February 19, 1976, Rutgers University.

56. Leavitt, Ruby Rohrlich: The Puerto Ricans: culture change and language deviance, Tucson, 1974, University of Arizona Press.

57. Fisch, S.: Botanicas and spiritualism in a metropolis, Milbank Memorial Fund Quarterly **46**:377-388, 1968.

58. Koss, J.D.: Therapeutic aspects of Puerto Rican cult practices, Psychiatry **38:**160-171, 1975.
59. Borrello, M.A., and Mathis, E.: Botanicas: Puerto Rican folk pharmacies, Natural History **86**(7):64-73, 1977.
60. Harwood, Alan: The hot-cold theory of disease, Journal of the American Medical Association **216:**1153-1158, 1971.
61. Ryan, William F.: Blaming the victim, New York, 1971, Vintage Books.
62. Rothschild, E.O.: Lead poisoning: the silent epidemic, New England Journal of Medicine **283:**704-705, 1970.
63. Agran, L.: The cancer connection, Boston, 1977, Houghton Mifflin Co.
64. Glasser, Ronald J.: The greatest battle, New York, 1976, Random House, Inc.
65. Brodeur, Paul: Expendable Americans, New York, 1974, The Viking Press.
66. Randall, W.S., and Solomon, S.D.: Building 6, Boston, 1977, Little, Brown & Co.
67. In These Times, p. 6, August 31-September 6, 1977.

BIBLIOGRAPHY

Agran, L.: The cancer connection, Boston, 1977, Houghton Mifflin Co.

Allerland, M.E., and Lake, G.: New careerists in community psychology and mental health. In Golann, S.E., and Eisdorfer, C., editors: Handbook of community mental health, New York, 1972, Appleton-Century-Crofts.

Ash, P.: The reliability of psychiatric diagnoses, Journal of Abnormal and Social Psychology **44:**262-276, 1949.

Barnet Lieberman v. Blue Cross of Greater Philadelphia, Philadelphia County, 1970, Court of Common Pleas.

Barnhart, R.: Getting a fix: the U.S. drug monopoly. In Kotelchuck, David, editor: Prognosis negative: crisis in the health care system, New York, 1976, Vintage Books.

Borello, M.A., and Mathis, E.: Botanicas: Puerto Rican folk pharmacies, Natural History **86**(7):64-73, 1977.

Borsody: Legislative methods of community participation in control of health facilites, Philadelphia, 1973, unpublished paper on file at the Health Law Project.

Brameld, T.: The remaking of a culture, New York, 1959, Harper & Brothers.

Brodeur, Paul: Expendable Americans, New York, 1974, The Viking Press.

Burlage, Robb K.: Participant in Community Control of Health Services, panel discussion at the Orientation of the Cleveland Student Health Project. In Curriculum on community control sourcebook, vol. II, Washington, D.C., The Institute for the Study of Health and Society (undated).

Chisholm, Shirley: Community health and community participation, Bulletin of the New York Academy of Medicine **46:**1144-1148, 1970.

Clark, T.N.: Community structure and decision making: comparative analysis, San Francisco, 1968, Chandler Publishing Co.

Community response: examples of community efforts to provide health care. In Curriculum on community control sourcebook, vol. II, Washington, D.C., The Institute for the Study of Health and Society (undated).

Comprehensive health plan for southern New Jersey, part I, 1974. Excerpts from the Federal Requirements for Areawide Comprehensive Health Plans.

Conflicts of interest on the 1970 Blue Cross board, Philadelphia, unpublished paper on file at the Health Law Project.

Conflict and roles. In Curriculum on community control sourcebook, vol. II, Washington, D.C., The Institute for the Study of Health and Society (undated).

Department of Health, Education, and Welfare: The consumer and health planning, DHEW Publication No. (HRA) 76-14020, Washington, D.C., 1976, U.S. Government Printing Office.

Donaldson, K.: Insanity inside out, New York, 1976, Crown Publishers, Inc.

Duval, M.K.: The provider, the government and the consumer. In Knowles, John H., editor: Doing better and feeling worse, New York, 1977, W.W. Norton & Co., Inc.

Ehrenreich, B., and Ehrenreich, J.: The American health empire: power profits and politics, New York, 1971, Vintage Books.

Ensminger, B.: The $8-billion hospital bed overrun: a consumer's guide to stopping wasteful construction. In Kotelchuck, D., editor: Prognosis negative: crisis in the health care system, New York, 1976, Vintage Books.

Fisch, S.: Botanicas and spiritualism in a metropolis, Milbank Memorial Fund Quarterly **46:**377-388, 1968.

Florio, J.J.: Accent on health: state of our nation's health, Congressman's Special Report, August, 1977.

Fox, Renée C.: The medicalization and demedicalization of American society. In Knowles, John H., editor: Doing better and feeling worse, New York, 1977, W.W. Norton & Co., Inc.

Geiger, H. Jack: Community control or community conflict? American Lung Association Bulletin, pp. 4-10, November, 1969.

Glasser, Ronald J.: The greatest battle, New York, 1976, Random House, Inc.

Goodman, Paul: The community of scholars, New York, 1962, Random House, Inc.

Harwood, Alan: The hot-cold theory of disease, Journal of the American Medical Association **216:**1153-1158, 1971.

Haynes, M.A.: Professionals and the community confront change, American Journal of Public Health **60:**519-523, 1970.

Health care consumer survey of Paul Kimball Hospital, Lakewood, New Jersey, Camden, N.J., 1975, Rodriguez Associates.

Herman, H., and McKay, M.E.: Community health services, Washington, D.C., 1968, International City Manager's Association.

Hillery, G.A.: Definitions of community: areas of agreement, Rural Sociology **20:**111-123, 1955.

Hodgson, G.: The politics of health care: what is it costing you? In Kotelchuck, David, editor: Prognosis negative: crisis in the health care system, New York, 1976, Vintage Books.

Humphrey, M.: Statement to the Blue Cross board meeting, Philadelphia, February 16, 1971, unpublished mimeographed statement.

Illich, Ivan: Medical nemesis, New York, 1976, Bantam Books, Inc.

In These Times, p. 15, August 17-23, 1977.

In These Times, p. 6, August 31-September 6, 1977.

Johnson, E.A.: Giving the consumer a voice in the hospital business, Hospital Administrator **15**(2):15-26, 1970.

Kamin, Leon J.: Heredity, intelligence, politics and psychology, presented at the Eastern Psychological Association, Washington, D.C., 1973.

Knowles, John H. Introduction. In Knowles, John H., editor: Doing better and feeling worse, New York, 1977, W.W. Norton & Co., Inc.

Korsch, B., Gozzi, E., and Francis, U.: Gaps in doctor-patient communication: doctor-patient interaction and patient satisfaction, Pediatrics **42:**855-871, 1968.

Koss, J.D.: Therapeutic aspects of Puerto Rican cult practices, Psychiatry **38:**160-171, 1975.

Kotelchuck, David: The structure of American health care. In Kotelchuck, David, editor: Prognosis negative: crisis in the health care system, New York, 1976, Vintage Books.

Kuhn, Thomas S.: The structure of scientific revolutions, Chicago, 1962, University of Chicago Press.

Law, Sylvia: Blue Cross: what went wrong? In Kotelchuck, D., editor: Prognosis negative: crisis in the health care system, New York, 1976, Vintage Books.

Leavitt, Ruby Rohrlich: The Puerto Ricans: culture change and language deviance, Tucson, 1974, University of Arizona Press.

Lieberman, Barnet, and over 200 other subscriber members: Letter to nominees for provider directors, Philadelphia Blue Cross, Philadelphia, February 3, 1971, on file at the Health Law Project.

Lieberman, Barnet, and over 200 other subscriber members: Letter to nominees for public directors, Philadelphia Blue Cross, Philadelphia, January 29, 1971, on file at the Health Law Project.

McSweeny, A.J.: Including psychotherapy in national health insurance: subsidy to the rich? IV. Insurance guidelines and other proposed solutions, presented at the American Psychological Association, Washington, D.C., September, 1976.

Mercer, J.: Labeling the mentally retarded, Berkeley, 1973, University of California Press.

Morehead, M.A., Donaldson, R.S., and Seravalli, M.R.: Comparisons between OEO neighborhood health centers and other health care providers of ratings of the quality of health care, American Journal of Public Health **61:**1294-1306, 1971.

Nelson, L., Ramsey, C.E., and Verner, C.: Community structure and change, New York, 1960, The Macmillan Co.

Nichols, B.: Oklahoma crude: everything's gushing up hospitals. In Kotelchuck, David, editor: Prognosis negative: crisis in the health care system, New York, 1976, Vintage Books.

OEO Guidelines No. 6128-1, Washington, D.C., March, 1970, U.S. Government Printing Office.

The OEO neighborhood health center: two examples. In Curriculum on community control sourcebook, vol. II, Washington, D.C., The Institute for the Study of Health and Society (undated).

Peck, H.B., Kaplan, S.R., and Roman, M.: Prevention, treatment and social action: a strategy of intervention in a disadvantaged urban area, American Journal of Orthopsychiatry **36:**57-69, 1966.

PL 93-641: Implications and strategies for health services management and board members, a self-instructional guide, October, 1976, Southern New Jersey Health Systems Agency, Inc.

Randall, W.S., and Solomon, S.D.: Building 6, Boston, 1977, Little, Brown & Co.

Rothschild, E.O.: Lead poisoning: the silent epidemic, New England Journal of Medicine **283:**704-705, 1970.

Ryan, William F.: Blaming the victim, New York, 1971, Vintage Books.

Schorr, L.B., and English, J.T.: Background, context and significant issues in neighborhood health center programs, Milbank Memorial Fund Quarterly **46**(3):289-296, 1968.

Shaw, George Bernard: Preface to the doctor's dilemma, Baltimore, 1965, Penguin Books.

Some legal and policy problems of the recent Blue Cross board of director's election and annual meeting, Philadelphia, unpublished paper on file at the Health Law Projects.

Sparer, G., and Johnson, J.: Evaluation of OEO neighborhood health centers, American Journal of Public Health **61:**931-942, 1971.

Statman, J.: Community mental health as a pacification program. In Agel, J., producer: The radical therapist, New York, 1971, Ballantine Books, Inc.

Temerlin, M.K., and Trousdale, W.W.: The social psychology of clinical diagnosis, Psychotherapy: Theory, Research and Practice **6**(1):24-29, 1969.

Thillet, I.C.: Some culture related characteristics and "syndromes" of the Puerto Rican, presented at Forum on Community Health and Cultural Awareness, Camden, N.J., Rutgers University, February 19, 1976.

Thomas Marie, Sister: Puerto Rican culture, Philadelphia, 1975, unpublished paper.

Wechsler, D.: Wechsler Intelligence Scale for Children (manual), New York, 1949, Psychological Corp.

Who will pay your bills? A health/PAC special report on national health insurance. In Kotelchuck, David, editor: Prognosis negative: crisis in the health care system, New York, 1976, Vintage Books.

8

LEVELS OF WELLNESS AND THE HEALTH-ILLNESS CONTINUUM

HEALTH, WELLNESS, AND ILLNESS

Although people have been feeling well or not so well since the beginning of time, the concept of levels of wellness is fairly new. In the past, people were either sick or well, and before the advent of modern medicine, sick often meant shortly dead. There was no acknowledgment of any stage between sick and well. There was the concept of being "sickly" or "doing poorly," but these phrases usually applied to women who were not of great consequence (except in their role of bearers of children) in the business or economic sphere of life, and therefore their state of health "didn't count." If one was well, one was expected to be fully functional, and if one was sick, one was looked on as a liability. The sick individual was regarded as a financial and social burden.

As social systems became more sophisticated and as health and social welfare programs developed with increasing complexity, health educators and planners, policymakers, and theoreticians saw that health is not merely an absence of illness, that one could be not healthy while still not being acutely ill. Various professions such as nursing, medicine, and social work devised definitions of health as did government and international agencies. The definitions were similar to each other while not being precisely the same. This was confusing but

surely in accord with a pluralistic society. However, social policy, because it reflects social and cultural mores, tends to change constantly, and health professionals now tend to speak of "wellness" instead of "health." The terms may be equally confusing to some, and this chapter will attempt to dispel some of that confusion by discussing the concept of wellness as it relates to the way people function.

We recognize almost an infinite number of levels of wellness, and health professionals think of their clients as being at a particular place on the health-illness continuum at any given time. This continuum is an abstract horizontal line along which an individual's health moves during his lifetime; one end of the continuum is optimum health functioning, and the other end is death or total disability. Fig. 8-1 illustrates the continuum.

A totally objective discussion of wellness and illness is impossible because the topic itself is so subjective, and even a conjectural analysis is difficult. A person may be perfectly healthy, pass all the diagnostic tests with flying colors, be told by his physician that there is absolutely nothing wrong, and at the same time feel dreadful. Conversely, it is possible, perhaps even likely, for an individual to feel in perfect health, even feel capable of running the 4-minute mile, and be very close to death. The way we *feel* is not always

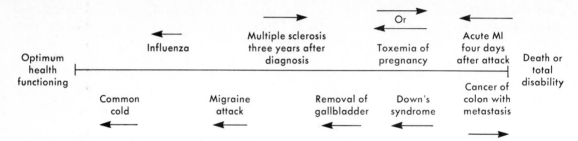

Fig. 8-1. Conception of the health-illness continuum with the location of the continuum of various deviations from optimum health. The arrows indicate the *probable* direction the course of events will follow; for example, people almost always recover from a cold and return to their optimum health functioning.

indicative of the way we *are,* but at the same time our feelings are accurate enough that we should give them credence. If a client says he does not feel well, he likely is not well. I can well remember a grim experience in a newborn nursery. A nursing colleague with a great deal of neonatal experience mentioned to a physician that a certain baby "just didn't look right." The physician examined the baby but ordered no laboratory tests because he found the baby not to be ill. The nurse protested and argued (hospital policy did not, and still does not, give a nurse authority to order laboratory tests), but no blood was drawn. The baby was dead 12 hours later of severe hyperbilirubinemia. The nurse said she "just knew" there was something dreadfully wrong with that baby. In some hospitals nurses can order laboratory tests, or there is a mechanism by which the tests will be ordered. However, in most instances, nurses' hands are still tied, and they are dependent on physicians' judgments. Fortunately, this is far less true of the community health nurse's mode of functioning.

Garfield,[1] in an article on clients' entry into the health care system, uses the terms *well, worried well, early sick,* and *very sick.* These terms, however, are difficult, if not impossible, to define. If well is optimum health functioning, how optimum is it? The answer seems to be that it varies from individual to individual. It is too facile an answer to explain that for a person with multiple sclerosis, optimum health functioning might be simply climbing a flight of stairs; for a college student it might

be running five miles every day; for a person with acute psychotic depression, it might be simply getting out of bed and dressed in the morning.

When we think about it further, the concept of optimum health functioning becomes more complex. For each individual it is not always the same. We have all experienced changes, day by day or even hour by hour, in what we feel able to do. If a person with multiple sclerosis does not feel capable of climbing the stairs on a particular day, is he still not functioning at optimum capacity for that particular day? How does one measure capacity for optimum health functioning, and thus measure a level of wellness, at any given time? Fluctuations in levels of wellness or in feelings of wellness, which may or may not be the same at any given time, are attributed to a variety of factors, some physical and some psychologic. Among these is the concept of the circadian rhythm which is abstract and complex.

Although we do not know what organization integrates the body's many rhythmic changes into the harmony that we experience as a steady sense of well-being, we know that it is the maintenance of this delicate balance that we call normal health or sanity. Deviations from normal rhythmicity may serve as clues to illness and dysfunction, since many diseases are now known to follow specific individual rhythms.[2,p.206]

If a person is well, what turns him into a person who is worried well? A little ache, a little pain, a vague symptom, the neurotic enjoyment of worrying about one's health? And when does an individual perceive himself to be early sick (the point at which, according to Garfield, he usually enters the health care system) instead of worried well? And how sick does one have to be to cross the line from early sick to very sick? Again, the answers are subjective, individual, and dynamic.

Levels of functioning

One way to look at health, wellness, and illness is to equate an individual's level of wellness with his level of functioning within a given set of circumstances and in relation to a variety of factors (Fig. 8-2). Many factors affect one's level of wellness. The presence of physical or mental disabilities[3] is perhaps the most obvious one. There are few people who do not have a disability of one kind or another. The need for eyeglasses is a visual disability. About 25% of all Americans function every day with the disability of being more than 10% overweight. It is the level of functioning within that disability that is an indicator of the level of wellness.

One's living habits and general life-style can affect and influence one's level of wellness. It stands to reason that if we stopped smoking and decreased our intake of cholesterol, our level of wellness would improve. The kind of work one

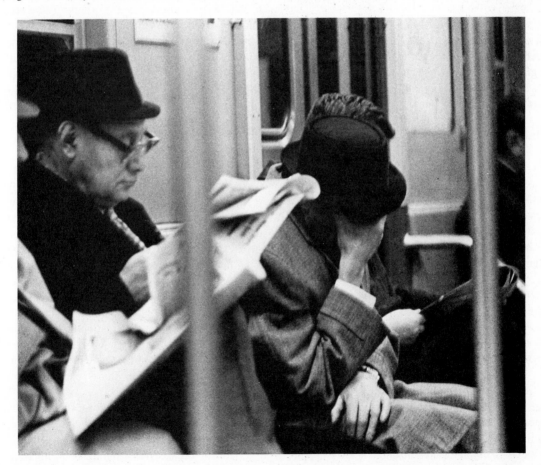

Fig. 8-2. People function at varying levels of wellness. How they feel and their general level of wellness affect their everyday functioning. (Photograph by Michelle Stone; courtesy Editorial Photocolor Archives, Inc., New York.)

does (inhaling particles in an asbestos factory all day cannot contribute in a positive way to the level of wellness) and the amount of exercise one gets contribute in large measure to the level of wellness.

Health functioning is, to a great degree, dependent on heredity. In addition to the obvious fact that congenital anomalies or hereditary disabilities change an individual's optimum level of functioning, other hereditary factors exist. Degrees of stamina, basal metabolism, and inherited diseases or traits all contribute positive and negative factors toward one's level of wellness.

The health care system that is available and the way in which it is used also affects the level of wellness, although some would argue that it has more to do with sickness than with wellness. Sickness, however, can be interpreted as an absence of wellness, and we are right back to where we started. It does stand to reason that if a health care system does not encourage maintenance of health and wellness, the population it serves is likely to have a lower level of wellness than one in which health maintenance is encouraged.

The environment in which we live has a tremendous influence on our level of wellness. City dwellers in particular are fighting a losing battle with pollution of every kind. Statistics on the increase in respiratory disease and certain kinds of cancer in highly industrialized areas should speak volumes about our levels of wellness. Socioeconomic conditions play a large part in one's level of wellness. Living in a crowded dirty ghetto most certainly does not contribute to one's mental, physical, or emotional health.

Wellness can also be interpreted as a result or a function of homeostasis. Homeostasis, a characteristic of all living beings, is the ability to maintain the constancy of one's internal milieu, despite changes in the external milieu. It usually refers to the physical and chemical properties of body tissues and fluids, but emotional homeostasis is a definite and palpable entity. Organisms must interact with but be discrete from their environment. If the self-regulatory mechanism is working, wellness exists. If it goes out of control, sickness (or nonwellness) exists. Although homeostasis is usu-

ally defined in physical terms, a kind of mental or emotional homeostasis exists; psychologists call it adjusted or adaptive behavior. Psychological processes can and do lead to changes in psychological homeostasis. Physical illness, on the other hand, has an attendant decrease in homeostasis that can cause psychological disturbances. The Latin adage *mens sana in corpore sano*[4] is still very much operative.

The fear of illness or the fear of exacerbation or worsening of an illness often results in a self-fulfilling prophesy. A person who is paralyzed with fear or self-pity as a result of disease sometimes is simply unable to recover. It is not unusual to die of fear, to be literally scared to death. There are a number of documented cases of people who expressed extreme terror of surgery and who said they feared dying on the operating table who actually did die. It is now standard procedure to cancel surgery if the client seems unduly frightened or truly convinced that he is going to die.

Stages of wellness and illness

Suchman lists characteristics and behavior patterns in various stages of wellness and illness[5]:

1. Symptom experience. The stage in which the individual perceives that something is wrong; he evaluates the degree of severity and responds emotionally.
2. Assumption of the sick role. The individual decides to adopt the sick role and seeks confirmation from others that he is sick; validation of the role leads to health care contact.
3. Health care contact. The individual seeks both treatment and validation of his assumption of the sick role.
4. Dependent patient role. The decision to undergo treatment for illness makes the sick person a patient.
5. Recovery and rehabilitation. The individual must renounce any pleasure he received from being dependent on others and leave the sick role or be classed as a malingerer; with a cure, the patient regains health and adulthood.[6]

These characteristics can be conceived of as a type of health-illness continuum on a circular rather than a linear basis. Although there is no concept of optimum health functioning and no designated place for death or total disability, all individuals move round and round the circle, in and out of various stages and severity of illnesses, throughout their lifetimes. The stop at various places can be for shorter or longer periods of time, and the direction around the circle can be reversed at any time and for any duration. Fig. 8-3 illustrates the circular continuum.

Biofeedback is a new technique in the perception and awareness of wellness and illness. According to Brown:

Only now are we learning that if we provide man with accurate and recognizable information about the dynamics of his functioning being as part of his external environment, he can experience himself. That is, he can verify certain relationships between himself and the internal, nonexternal world, and then interact with himself. The biological phenomenon which underlies this

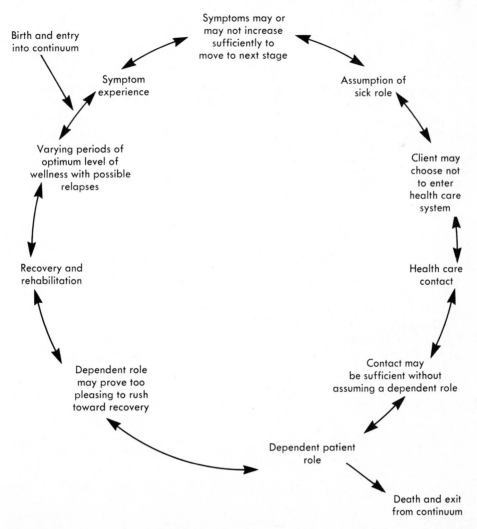

Fig. 8-3. Schematic representation of one conception and analysis of Suchman's behavior patterns in various stages of wellness and illness.

confrontation is the revelation by biofeedback of the ability of individuals to regulate and control a wide variety of their own physiologic functioning once information of such functioning is presented in a form that can be perceived by that same individual.*

By the use of biofeedback, internal signals can be translated into external signals that can be sensed, perceived, recognized, and acted on. Individuals can become acquainted with what is going on inside their own bodies; thus they can become more aware of their level of wellness. If this level appears to be in jeopardy, it may be that something can be done about it. One interprets one's own biofeedback in relation to the way one feels, not in relation to the way a physician interprets assessment data, thus letting us know how he thinks we *should* feel.

One of the great potentials of biofeedback techniques is to prevent some illnesses and to detect some other illnesses while they are in an early stage. These techniques are highly complex, involving sophisticated electronics, and will not be dealt with in this book. (Readers who are interested in further information about biofeedback are referred to Brown's book in the Bibliography.) As effective communication with others leads to good mental health, so effective communication with our own bodies can lead to good physiological (*and* mental) health.

We have all been ill; we have all seen people who are ill, and as nurses we have been rather intimately concerned with illness. But how do we define it? Wu, in her study of behavior and illness, defines illness as ''an event or happening that offers content for scientific observation and study, i.e. an experience that evokes a certain class of behavior.''[7, p.6] This is an abstract definition and could apply to almost any phenomenon that might possibly lead to scientific investigation. Wu stated that the definition is purposefully abstract so it can be studied from a variety of perspectives.

To further define illness, Allport[8] has developed

*From New body, new mind: bio-feedback: new directions for the mind, p. 3, by Barbara Brown, Ph.D.; copyright © 1974 by Barbara B. Brown. By permission of Bantam Books, Inc.

a set of descriptive criteria having to do with an individual's perception of illness, that is, how an individual knows he is ill and by what processes the conclusion was reached.

1. A change in sensory quality. The individual's ability to hear, see, and feel is somehow altered. There might be such perceptions as pain, nausea, or dizziness, and these subjective feelings can be referred to in terms of site, intensity, duration, and clarity. Generally the individual experiences feelings that have come to be known as symptoms.

2. A comparison of perceived feelings with some objective standards. This is a subjective and difficult comparison to make and to describe, and often the individual needs prompting by a skilled interviewer. The individual must be able to compare how he feels with how he *should* feel.

3. A decision of whether the perceived feelings fit the individual's concept of illness. The individual must ask himself, ''Is this feeling a sickness?'' How does one know what a heart attack feels like if one has never experienced one or has never done any reading on what the symptoms may be like?

4. An interrelatedness and configuration of all the perceived dimensions to a sequence of events and feelings. This is an extremely abstract concept, and the individual goes through this stage on a purely subconscious level.

5. The identification of feelings with past experiences or abstract knowledge. This is similar to, but more positive than, the perceptions described in stage 3.

The behavior of sick individuals has been well described in many different places, and the reader should be acquainted with many of these behaviors. What about the behavior, however, of a well or healthy person? What does he *do* to remain healthy? Taking care of one's body is the most obvious behavior. Healthy individuals will ensure their own adequate nutrition, will get enough rest, sleep, and exercise, and will avail themselves of preventive health measures such as dental prophylaxis, PAP tests, and annual physical examinations. They also engage in activities that minimize exposure to illness, such as avoiding contact with contagious diseases and receiving appropriate immunizations. Healthy people try to strike a balance in their activities among work, pleasure, and rest. They also follow recommended health advice, including taking prescribed medication and returning to the physician for checkups. Healthy individuals also accept their vulnerability to illness but do not dwell on it, and these same individuals teach health maintenance to their children, mainly by setting a good example.

FACTORS, VARIABLES, AND OCCURRENCES THAT CAUSE FLUCTUATIONS ALONG THE HEALTH-ILLNESS CONTINUUM

There is almost nothing that happens to human beings which will not affect their level of wellness or their place on the health-illness continuum. Every time we get out of bed in the morning, we subject ourselves to experiences that can affect our health in a variety of ways. In the following discussion some factors, variables, and occurrences are examined. The order in which they are discussed is not indicative of their relative importance.

Anxiety

Anxiety can be a positive and creative force in an individual's day-to-day experiences, or it can be a crippling and destructive force (Fig. 8-4). Anxiety is a feeling tone of anticipation, generally unpleasant, that is physiologically manifested by the "fight or flight" mechanism of the autonomic nervous system. Without a certain level of anxiety, much of our work would not be accomplished. Students studying for an examination or athletes preparing for competiton are spurred on by anxiety that is the result of a need to succeed. On the other hand, free-floating anxiety, which is not derived from reality, can become such an obsession that all creative and productive effort is blocked. School phobia in children is an excellent example of this. Something at school or in the thought of going to school so frightens the child that he is unable to attend. Vomiting, hysterics, and feigned illness in the morning are common symptoms of a school phobia. Adults are often consumed by anxiety

about their physical well-being, and this anxiety can frequently turn into hypochondria.

Aging

Aging most certainly is a factor that affects one's place on the health-illness continuum. Although aging does not necessarily imply the presence of illness, it is more likely for an elderly person to become ill than it is for a younger person. Chronic illness tends to push the elderly toward the illness end of the continuum. Diabetes, arteriosclerotic cardiovascular disease, stroke, and degenerative musculoskeletal diseases all tend to be depressing, debilitating, and sources of concern. At the same time there may be sensory deterioration, the psychic stress of growing older, loneliness from the loss of one's family and friends, and depression. It is not uncommon for elderly people, especially those who live alone and have few friends, acquaintances, and activities, to lose the will to live. To have given up life and to merely wait for death is to be almost at the end of the continuum. Problems related to aging are discussed in detail in Chapter 17.

Stress

Stress can be defined as any stimulus that upsets either the body's or the mind's homeostasis; it, almost more than anything else, can affect wellness. Each individual has his own methods of coping with and adapting to stress. The methods may succeed or not depending on a number of variables: the state of the person's physical and mental health, the amount and kind of stress, the life situation at the time of the stress, past experiences with the same kind of stress, what kind of support is received and from whom, and an almost unlimited range of other variables. Most people most of the time react to stress in a healthy and adaptive way. The failure to adapt to stress will be discussed in succeeding paragraphs (Fig. 8-5).

PHYSIOLOGICAL STRESSORS

There are various kinds of physiological stressors: allergy, infection, disruption or failure of any of the body's organs or systems, trauma, prolonged

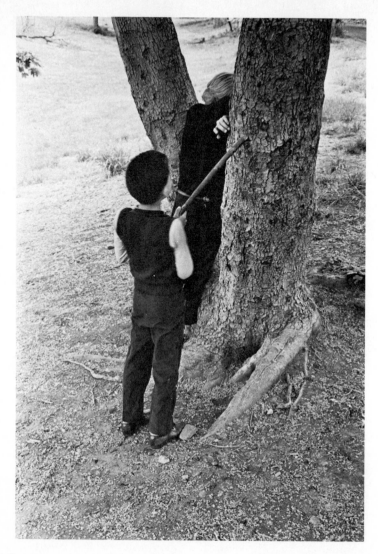

Fig. 8-4. Tension, anxiety, and stress are the greatest psychological factors affecting people's wellness. (Photograph by James Carroll; courtesy Editorial Photocolor Archives, Inc., New York.)

hunger or malnutrition, prolonged lack of sleep, surgery, pregnancy, climacteric, fluid and electrolyte imbalances, abortion, or any other major or minor event that befalls the body.

PSYCHOLOGICAL STRESSORS

Psychological stressors are more varied and much less easy to describe and define. All physi- ological stress causes psychological stress, so the mere fact of being ill is a psychological stressor. Hospitalization compounds the stress and adds some that is unique to itself. Loss of independence, the sense of vulnerability and helplessness, and the need to comfort to behaviors that are neither un- derstood nor explained all create an extremely stressful situation with which even the most

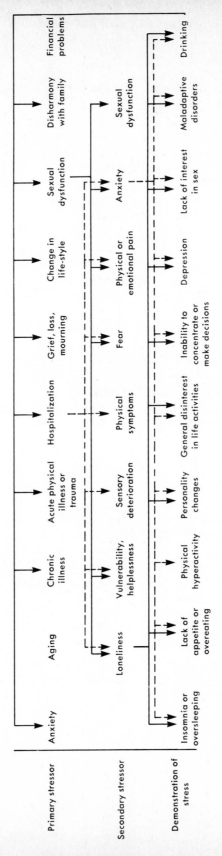

Fig. 8-5. Schematic representation of causes, effects, demonstrations, and results of stress. Note that some primary and secondary stressors are identical. Demonstrations of stress often themselves become primary stressors. The cause and effect of stress then becomes a circular pattern. Only portions of each interconnecting web are shown in order to avoid making the chart unreadable. A few samples are sufficient to demonstrate the process.

adaptive people have difficulty coping.

Grief, loss, and mourning are all strong psychological stressors, and often individuals are temporarily unable to function at all. A definite series and sequence of events surrounds grief and mourning[9] that may even involve physical symptoms. The adaptation to loss takes a varying length of time, but there is almost always full recovery.

A change in one's life-style or life situation produces a tremendous amount of stress. Marriage, divorce, pregnancy, a new job, being fired from a job, moving out of the nuclear family onto one's own: these are all major changes that are accompanied by a great deal of stress.

Sexual dysfunction (impotence or the inability to achieve orgasm) is a psychological stressor, as is infertility. Another major source of stress is a change in one's sexual identification, that is, changing from heterosexual to homosexual or vice versa or functioning as a bisexual. Sex is such an important part of our lives, and we spend so much time thinking about it, that any alterations in our patterns of sexual behavior, even positive and desired ones, produce stress.

Disharmony with one's family and friends is a great negative stressor and can consume enormous amounts of energy that could have been used to more productive and positive ends.

Financial problems cause psychological stress, and with the exception of sex, more marital fights and problems are concerned with money than with any other matter. The necessity of making an important decision is a source of stress. The larger the consequences of the decision, the more stress there is likely to be.

People demonstrate in many different ways that they are undergoing stress. Some of the more common clues are insomnia or sleeping for excessively long periods; lack of appetite or overeating, fidgeting, handwringing, and other forms of physical hyperactivity; changes in personality such as irritability; lack of enthusiasm for activities formerly of interest; inability to concentrate; depression; lack of interest in sex; and excessive drinking.

PSYCHOSOMATIC ILLNESS

The study of psychosomatic illness concerns itself with the relationship between physical illness and the emotions and how individuals react to and adapt to stress, both biologically and psychologically. Many investigators feel that there is no fundamental difference between physical and mental illness, that all diseases have components of both, with either the physical or the mental aspect predominating at various times. Psychosomatic diseases are often called *maladaptive disorders,* and there are no special treatments for them. A prolonged stress response places increased strain on some organs or systems, which can result in disease. This is particularly true if the organ or system has been previously diseased or injured.

It had been believed that particular diseases or syndromes were caused in whole or in part by psychologic stress. Notable among these are cardiovascular disease, asthma, certain gastrointestinal disorders, and even cancer. However, recent literature[13] indicates that most of the evidence for a causal relationship between stress and physical illness is based on retrospective or uncontrolled studies. Prospective studies, which would be more appropriate and accurate, have tentatively indicated that no direct causal relationship can be assigned to psychologic stress and physical illness. Rather, the relationship is based on complex and interlocking factors. However, once the course of a physical illness is underway, stress and other psychologic factors *do* play a role in the duration and severity of the illness. In general, the higher the degree of stress the more severe the illness.

THE ENVIRONMENT

There is a wide variety of socioenvironmental factors and variables that affects health. We are living in a much freer and more permissive society than ever existed before in the United States. Modes of behavior and thinking are permitted now that in the past were not only frowned on but illegal. In this area we have a long way to go. Many forms of behavior, mainly sexual acts, are illegal, even among consenting adults, in many states. And there are many behaviors that are permitted by law but are not yet condoned by most people. More people are having sexual contact with more people, thus leading to a tremendous increase, of epidemic proportions, in the number of cases of venereal disease (sometimes referred to as sexually transmitted disease). The increased tolerance for "deviant" behavior can create an atmosphere of comfort for drug addicts. This atmosphere, combined with better methods of growing, refining, and transporting opium-derivative drugs, has led to the increase in the number of drug addicts in the United States.

Our polluted environment—air, water, and food —gives us cancer, mercury poisoning, respiratory diseases, and all manner of unhealthy living conditions, thus pushing us all a bit further down the continuum toward illness (Fig. 8-6). Not only does the pollution cause disease in and of itself, but it also lowers resistance to other forms of illness. More and more cars are on the road, and we spend more time in them; naturally there are more accidents.

The growing tension under which we live causes us to take record numbers of tranquilizers, smoke greater numbers of cigarettes, and to lose our tempers with increasing frequency, often with disastrous results. Most of the murders committed today are "crimes of passion" where the murderer and victim are known to each other. Child abuse is increasing with frightening speed. The Child Abuse Prevention Effort (CAPE) in Philadelphia states that there are over 2 million *reported* cases of child abuse each year. Deaths from cardiovascular disease are multiplying, and there is mounting evidence that some forms of cancer may be related to stress.

The climate and weather affect our level of wellness a great deal, to which anyone with arthritis or bursitis can attest. People's moods and tension levels are often dependent on the weather. Large-city police departments will verify that when the weather is bad and people are cooped up with each other indoors, more physical violence occurs. Our health and wellness are, of course, definitely functions of our income, living conditions, and lifestyle.

Food habits play an important role in health. In several surveys of Japanese people, it was found that when the people lived in Japan and ate diets that were relatively low in animal fats, incidence of cardiovascular disease was low. When the people moved to the United States and began consuming cholesterol in greater quantities (and at the same time began living at a faster, more hectic, and tension-filled pace), the incidence of cardiovascular disease increased proportionately. Cultural and religious responses to health and illness also affect the level of wellness, as do race and physical growth and development. Body stature affects personality, which in turn affects the level of wellness.

Body repair mechanisms determine in large measure how fast we move back and forth along the health-illness continuum. If every time an individual becomes ill, it takes two or three times longer than average to regain his health, he will spend less time in a state of health. The mere fact of a long recovery is a psychological stressor that in itself can delay recovery.

Human behavior is an enormous factor in health, wellness, and illness. It is not within the scope of this chapter to discuss behavior and personality disorders or psychological maladaptation. Suffice it to say that an individual's temperament, personality, methods of relating to others, mood swings, feelings, and outlook on life are very much a part of his mental and physical health.

Although situational and maturational crises will be discussed in detail in Chapter 12, it must be stated here that these crises affect one's level of wellness a great deal. A crisis is a turning point, a problem that cannot be readily solved by an individual's usual coping mechanisms. Stress, tension, and anxiety continue to increase until a solution to the problem is found. Every human being experiences crises and stress; it is the way in which

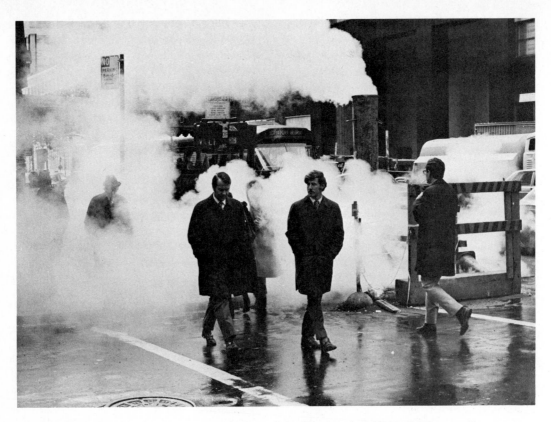

Fig. 8-6. Noise and air pollution push us toward the illness end of the health-illness continuum. (Photograph by Michos Tzovaras; courtesy Editorial Photocolor Archives, Inc., New York.)

they are dealt with that affects the individual's place on the health-illness continuum.

GENERAL ADAPTATION SYNDROME
Description

The following discussion is based on work done by Hans Selye and on his description of the syndrome of reactions and responses to physical and psychic stress.[10] Much of Selye's work was done on individual cells and on certain biological systems, although he goes into a rather extensive application of the General Adaptation Syndrome (GAS) theory for psychosomatic medicine. Following a general review of Selye's work will be a discussion of how the community nurse can apply the GAS theory to working with clients.

In order to define the GAS, one must first define stress; it is interesting that Selye[10] found it necessary to define what stress is *not* before he tried to define what it is. Stress is not any of the following:

1. Nervous tension. Stress reactions occur in lower animals that have no nervous systems.
2. An emergency discharge of hormones from the adrenal medulla.
3. Anything that causes a secretion of corticoids from the adrenal cortex. ACTH can produce a discharge of corticoids without any evidence of stress.
4. The nonspecific result of damage. Normal activities can produce stress without causing damage to the organism.
5. Any deviation from homeostasis. Any bio-

logical function causes marked deviation from the normal resting state in active organs.[11]

6. Anything that causes an alarm reaction. It is the stressor that does this, not the stress itself.

7. Identical with the alarm reaction or with the GAS as a whole. These reactions are characterized by stress and therefore would not themselves be stress.

8. A nonspecific reaction. The pattern of stress reaction is specific and predictable.

9. A specific reaction, since it can be produced by almost any agent.

Now that everything stress is not has been eliminated, it would seem that the definition would be too abstract and vague to be of much practical use. Selye defines it as essentially the rate of all wear and tear on an organism caused by life, or "stress is the state manifested by a specific syndrome which consists of all the nonspecifically induced changes within a biologic system."[10,p.54] It is a state manifested by a syndrome, so, although stress cannot actually be seen or felt, the effects and patterns of the syndrome are such that it becomes evident that the organism is undergoing stress. Stress has its own form and composition, and the elements of this form are the visible changes that occur in the organism as a result of stress.

The General Adaptation Syndrome of reactions and responses to stress consists of three stages:

1. Alarm reaction. This is a bodily expression of a generalized call to arms of the organism's defensive forces; no living organism can maintain itself continuously in alarm reaction. Either death occurs, or, more likely, the organism enters the second stage of the GAS.

2. Stage of resistance. This stage is physiologically opposite to the stage of alarm reaction. The adrenal cortex accumulates an adequate reserve of corticoids instead of (during the alarm reaction) discharging corticoids to the point of depletion.

3. State of exhaustion. In many organisms this is the stage of premature aging caused by the wear and tear of the stress; physiologically it resembles the alarm reaction and may possibly result in the death of the organism.

With the exception of extreme physical exercise, most people go through only the first two stages of the GAS the majority of time when subjected to stress. We have all, however, had the experience of feeling totally exhausted and depleted as a result of a stressful experience that was not a result of physical exercise. The GAS encompasses all specific and nonspecific changes as they develop throughout the continued exposure to stress: a kind of kaleidoscope of actions and reactions.

It is not within the scope of this book to detail all the physiological and biochemical phenomena that take place during the GAS. It is, however, interesting that Selye distinguished between the fundamentally different kinds of biological adaptations to stress:

1. Developmental adaptation (also called homotrophic adaptation). A simple, progressive adaptive reaction accomplished by the enlargement and multiplication of preexisting cell elements without a qualitative change, this is the response that occurs whenever a tissue is called on to increase the activity for which it is already adapted, for example, a muscle that is required to perform more work.

2. Redevelopmental adaptation (also called heterotrophic adaptation). This occurs when a tissue is forced to readjust itself to perform an entirely different kind of activity such as phagocytosis, which is the ingestion and digestion of bacteria and particles by phagocytes.

Application

Selye sees three distinct kinds of application of the GAS theory. The somatic applications are perhaps the most obvious. If the body can meet various kinds of aggression and stress with the same adaptive-defensive mechanism, then it should be possible to dissect the reaction and learn how to combat disease by strengthening the body's defense against stress. To some extent this has already been accomplished by the process of immunization against certain diseases. However, if one assumes (and there is a large school of thought which does) that all disease is the body's reaction to stress of one kind or another, then it becomes necessary to link the kind of stress with the reaction produced, and theoretically a prevention for the particular disease under observation should emerge.

In the psychosomatic implications of the GAS theory, investigators look at emotional stress. If one could distinguish between the part played by the stressor and the part played by our own adaptive reactions, tremendous insight could be gained about the *way* in which people react to the kinds of stress to which they are subjected. Then by the use of various psychoanalytic or behavior modifications techniques, people's reactions to stress could be altered.

The philosophical implications of the GAS theory are extremely important and far-reaching. Our responses and reactions to stress are very much a function of our personality development and our individuality. The more one knows and understands about these aspects of the self, the more one can control the reactions to stress.

THE NURSE'S USE OF GAS PRINCIPLES

In order to best demonstrate how the community nurse can use knowledge of the health-illness continuum, levels of wellness, and the factors that influence health, wellness, and illness, case histories will be presented. The cases involve families, all of whose members are at varying levels of wellness, all of whom are subjected to various kinds of stress, and all of whom experience different reactions to stress. After the description of each family situation will be a short discussion of how the community nurse might begin to analyze the family situation and what could be done to alleviate some of the problems. This is not meant to be an exhaustive analysis, and it is greatly hoped that the readers' own ideas, creativity, ingenuity, and professional judgment will be applied toward solving some of the families' problems.

SITUATION ONE: THE COHENS

The Cohen family is composed of Arthur, a 31-year-old middle management executive with a pa-

per company; his wife, Susan, 29, who teaches high school English; Larry, a first grader; and Sarah, a 3-year-old with Down's syndrome. They also have two cats, a collie (Samson), and an ever-proliferating family of gerbils.

Sarah can do very little for herself. She is not toilet trained, cannot even help with putting on her clothes, and her efforts to feed herself are disastrous. She is, however, a most happy and loving child. She has a smile and a hug for everyone, almost never cries, and is greatly loved by her family. Her favorite family member is the dog, and the only task she has been able to master is filling his water bowl and putting it on the floor. Samson, in turn, is totally devoted to Sarah.

The Cohens have always been a rather close family unit, but in the past several months definite signs of tension have begun to appear. Arthur, who almost never drinks, has taken to stopping in a tavern for a beer on his way home from work. Susan has less and less patience with her students and is not receiving the job satisfaction she once did. Larry's friends sometimes poke fun at Sarah, so he does not bring them home as often.

Sarah's maternal grandmother stays with her during the day until Susan comes home from work, and a cleaning woman is present three times a week. Even though Sarah is fed separately, the dinner hour is chaotic, and there is no peace in the house until both Sarah and Larry have fallen asleep. By that time Arthur and Susan are exhausted, and even if finding a babysitter were not such a problem, they would be too tired to go out. They rarely can relax enough to make love in a satisfying manner, so television has become their major source of entertainment.

The status quo cannot continue for much longer. Sarah's grandmother is aging rapidly, Sarah is physically growing and becoming more active, Larry is demanding more attention, and the marital relationship cannot stand much more strain.

Discussion

It seems that until the past few months, the Cohen family's level of wellness was good (even with the presence of Down's syndrome), but it is now deteriorating rapidly. The major cause is most likely the stress resulting from the burgeoning peripheral problems of a mentally retarded child. The problems are compounded and enlarged by the passage of time. Sarah will keep growing, the grandmother will keep aging, Larry will keep maturing and developing more sophisticated needs, and the marriage will become more and more stressful. Either something must be done to remove or lessen the source of stress, or the family and some of its members will collapse.

In addition to the family's level of wellness, the community nurse must assess and deal with each individual's level of wellness. Sarah is most likely not functioning at her optimum level even though she is happy, physically healthy, and is the recipient of loving care and affection. Most people with Down's syndrome can be trained and even educated to function at a much higher level than would be thought possible. Larry seems well, but already his socialization (an important developmental task for a 6-year-old) is suffering. This could easily lead to emotional problems and difficulty functioning in school. He is evidently not receiving the attention he requires at home, which can also lead to emotional problems. We know little about Arthur's level of wellness except for one important clue: his drinking, specifically public drinking, which he never did before. The need to drink before facing a stressful situation is one of the first indicators of potential alcoholism. Most likely few of his emotional, spiritual, and other human needs are being met. It is quite possible that he is having difficulty concentrating on his work, which could lead to severe employment problems. He and Susan must both be worried about Sarah, about how she will spend the rest of her life, about who will care for her, and about how this care will be paid for. Susan's level of wellness seems to be just about what Arthur's is: deteriorating. Her reactions to stress are manifested by her increasingly poor performance at school. So it becomes obvious that not only does the nurse need to attend to the family's problems, but to those of each individual member as well.

In order to relieve the stress, some specific decisions need to be made by the Cohen family. Specific actions will then be taken as a result of these decisions. There are ways in which the community

nurse can be of help. The major problem to be confronted is what to do about Sarah, how to give her the best possible life, which her family so obviously wants for her. Should she or should she not be institutionalized? In this kind of situation the community nurse can serve her most important function. She can sit down with the family members and help them to look at their situation and come to grips with the direction in which they are headed. There are alternative courses of action to be considered, and the nurse should be able to help the family think through the alternatives and their various ramifications, although the nurse must never make a decision for the family. The community nurse might arrange for the Cohens to look at institutions in which Sarah might live and might arrange for them to speak with other families of children with Down's syndrome in order to share feelings and experiences. The Association of Parents of Retarded Children is an excellent support group, but there are also others in most communities. Sometimes people with similar problems can help each other make appropriate decisions for care. It might well be the nurse who is astute enough to convince an institution's administrator that Samson should move in with Sarah.

Whatever decision the family makes, a great deal of stress will be involved, and it is the nurse's function to somehow lessen the stress and to help the family deal with it in a way that will result in an improved level of wellness.[12] She must provide emotional support (or, if the nurse cannot provide it herself, then arrange for another source of support) for the family during its period of crisis. The crisis is the consideration of the alternatives, the making of the decision, and the action taken as a result of the decision. The family must have a guide while they work through their feelings; for some members the exploration of these feelings may be uncharted emotional territory.

Although the decision about Sarah is the most pressing one and some of the other problems may take care of themselves as a result of the decision, there are other factors to be considered. Larry's needs must be attended to before he develops serious emotional problems, and the nurse, with her knowledge of other members of the health team, should be able to arrange for some kind of child guidance. The school nurse could possibly be of help here. She might be one person to whom Larry can relate, and she could consult with the community nurse and with Larry's parents. Susan and Arthur need desperately to have some stress-free time together, to share their feelings, to make love, to have fun, to relax, and to attend to the growth and development of their marriage. Marriage counseling is indicated in this situation, and if the nurse is not equipped to handle the counseling, then the couple should be referred to a marriage counselor.

The Cohen family has many of the resources necessary to maintain a high level of wellness, and with professional nursing intervention, there is no reason why the family cannot establish and achieve goals that will lead to wellness.

SITUATION TWO: GWEN AND GEORGE

Gwen is 37; her husband George is 41. They have been married for fifteen years and have three children. George is a sales representative for a large steel company and spends almost half his time traveling. Sometimes he takes Gwen, but mostly he does not. His salary and other benefits are about $40,000 a year, so even the partial support of his mistress is a bit of a squeeze. George also indulges in other sexual liaisons on his travels but tries to be discreet.

Gwen used to have an interesting and well-paid job as the assistant editor of a literary journal; it kept her busy and gave her much satisfaction. Shortly after their first child was born, George insisted that she quit her job and devote full time to the household and to him. Gwen resisted, and several weeks of bitter fighting ensued. George had his way, however, and Gwen is now on all kinds of charity committees and does volunteer hospital work one afternoon a week. Gwen and George are both attractive people and are considered by their friends to be an "ideal couple."

The reality of their marriage, however, is less than ideal. When they do see each other, there is almost no conversation, and the aura of hostility is palpable. The terrible screaming fights that were

common a few years ago have almost totally stopped; they have been replaced by indifference.

Their two growing children are in school or at camp, and about a year ago the loneliness began to press in on Gwen, so she became pregnant. George was not part of her decision; she simply stopped taking her contraceptive pills. Several weeks ago Gwen had a daughter who was so beautiful at birth that she was named Beau.

The community nurse was referred to this family as part of a routine neonatal visit. As she walked into the house, she had the distinct feeling that it was only Gwen's innate good manners that prevented her from slamming the door in the nurse's face. Their home was beautiful, and Gwen was impeccably dressed. Beau, who was in a playpen in the living room, was a beautiful child who gave the nurse a tremendous smile. During the visit Gwen cuddled Beau in her lap; she was such a happy baby that it was obvious that she is very much loved. The way Gwen related to her daughter confirms the observation.

The visit lasted for more than two hours, and Gwen gradually relaxed and began to talk. Beau is being adequately cared for by a pediatrician, and the nurse soon saw that it is Gwen who needs the professional help. She is quite guarded and protective of her feelings, but she did tell the nurse that she knows of her husband's affairs and that they no longer love each other. Divorce was not mentioned. She has not sought professional marriage counseling because she thinks "they're all a bunch of charlatans," but she did admit that the strain of the marriage is becoming unbearable.

The nurse introduced several alternative areas of help, which Gwen rejected. The nurse sensed a flicker of interest, however, and the rejection seemed less than total. When the nurse asked if she might return in a few days, she was glad to see Gwen agree, though reluctantly. As the nurse left, she saw that Gwen was making an effort to fight back tears.

Discussion

Although this family's physical health is perfectly fine, their level of wellness is not fine at all. There are a multitude of problems, but the outstanding one is a lack of communication, both between the husband and wife and, because the children are away so much, between the parents and the children. The only people who seem to communicate well are Gwen and Beau. Lack of trust is a serious problem in a marriage and in a family, and George's infidelity compounds this missing ingredient. Childbearing should most assuredly be a mutual decision, and we might assume that Beau is a child unwanted by one of her parents. The child was born out of her mother's loneliness and frustration, not a healthy reason for having a child. One of the major reasons for becoming and remaining a family is that the people involved wish to live and to grow together; there seems to be none of that feeling here, and the lack of it is a good reason to assume a poor level of wellness. The *character* of the marital unhappiness has changed. Fighting, if it is not overly destructive, can be a healthy outlet for releasing anger, hostility, and aggression. Indifference in a marriage is never a healthy situation.

In looking at the individuals' wellness, Gwen's appears to be poor. Again, she is perfectly physically healthy, but the stress under which she is living pushes her further and further toward the illness end of the health-illness continuum. She is experiencing the extreme stress of boredom, the need to accede to George's demands, inability to assert herself enough to meet her own needs, loneliness, a feeling of uselessness, and perhaps resentment of George's life: his business, his busyness, his lovers, and his indifference. Gwen may also be feeling the stress of sexual frustration if George's lovers are sufficiently meeting *his* needs.

George's level of wellness is more difficult to assess. A moralist might point out that his attitude toward his marriage in general and toward his wife in particular is unhealthy, even sick. Another person may point out that George seems to be meeting his own needs and is therefore extremely healthy, but the only accurate way to assess George's level of wellness is to find out how he feels about his activities and his life-style. If he is unhappy in his marriage and his current life situation, then it would

seem to be unhealthy to sustain the status quo. His life-style may very well meet his needs; it is a moral judgment to say that the kind of dishonesty that George is exhibiting is in itself unhealthy. If the behavior produces guilt, which in turn is a stressor, then it is indeed unhealthy. His behavior may not be considered to be worthy, but it is not necessarily unhealthy.

George faces additional stress: the need to succeed in business, to earn money, to make sexual conquests, and apparently to live up to his image of masculinity, regardless of whether that image is an accurate one. Perhaps this is not what George wants, and he is suffering from the additional stress of forcing himself to do something he doesn't want to do. His indifference toward Gwen may be the result of his anger and resentment and his inability to verbalize it. All this, however, is conjecture until we find out what George is feeling.

The community nurse is faced with a difficult situation. It seems that a priority is to find out why Gwen and George are still married, and to do this, George's presence is required. How indifferent is he really? He has to come home sometime, and it would seem a good idea for the nurse to spend some time with the two of them in the evening. It is essential for them to confront the problem, to get the hostilities, resentments, and anger, as well as the good feelings, out into the open. This, of course, cannot be accomplished in one evening, but what *can* be done fairly quickly is to determine whether they want to go on with help to see if their marriage can be salvaged. If they want marriage counseling, then the community nurse can make the appropriate referrals or can begin crisis intervention therapy herself. If Gwen and George do not want further help, and this is their choice to make, the nurse can do little except to leave the door open for future changes of mind. The other alternative is to see if either Gwen or George would consider beginning individual therapy. The nurse might also take some action to help Gwen explore her own feelings of worth as a person and as a mother. The nurse can do this therapy herself or refer her to a community mental health center or to a variety of religious and secular parent support groups. If Gwen and George do decide to separate, Parents without Partners can provide emotional support, practical help, and new acquaintances.

SITUATION THREE: MARY AND HER FAMILY

Mary is 23 years old, black, and pregnant for the fourth time. She is in the hospital in her seventh month because of occasional vaginal bleeding. The community nurse has been asked to see her in the hospital because of her history and many home problems.

She is married but is not living with her husband. He has just been released from prison, where he served two years for manslaughter for the death of two of their children. Mary is living with her parents, and she must sleep in the living room on a club chair because there are not enough beds. She tells the nurse that she is happy to be in the hospital where there is a bed, clean sheets, and enough food to eat. Both her parents are alcoholics; Mary does not drink at all. As a child she was severely beaten by her parents, and her father still hits her when he is drunk.

Two of Mary's children are dead by her husband's hand, and Mary watched the deaths of both of them. One was beaten, and one was forced to drink a lethal dose of kerosene. The third child was beaten so badly that both his legs were broken, and he sustained a skull fracture. He is in a foster home.

As the nurse sat by the bed and this story unfolded, she noticed several scars on the parts of Mary's body not covered by the nightgown. They were of various shapes and sizes and in varying stages of healing. Mary related (with almost no emotion in her voice) that her husband beat her regularly when he came to see her at her parents' home. She refuses to divorce her husband because "I need the sex." When it was pointed out that other men could provide sex, she said that sex with a man other than one's husband was against her religion (Jehovah's Witness). She also stated that it would be wrong to divorce and remarry. She seems fatalistic about the trap she is in; she does not enjoy being beaten but seems powerless to do anything to stop or prevent it.

She seems to sincerely want the child she is carrying, and when the nurse mentioned that the child might likely suffer the same fate as the other three,

Mary merely shrugged and said something about "God's will." She was converted to her religion several years ago but seems to know nothing about it aside from the fact that she may not receive blood. Since her medical problem is recurrent vaginal bleeding, it is quite possible that she will need a transfusion.

Later in the day her husband came to visit. He looked about 40 and frequently fell asleep abruptly, sometimes in midsentence. When the nurse tried to engage him in conversation, he was monosyllabic, noncommunicative, and seemed totally uninterested in the nurse, in Mary, and in his surroundings. Mary seemed to be trying to please and placate him.

Mary impressed the nurse as a woman who is desperately unhappy, trapped in a situation she is unwilling or unable to control, and extremely fatalistic about her future. The nurse had the distinct feeling that *she* had stronger feelings about Mary's life than Mary did. She was open about her story, appeared to experience no shame and no guilt about what happened to her children, and was an extremely pleasant person.

Discussion

This story is quite horrifying in its implications of what human beings are capable of doing to themselves and to each other. It is a true story (I personally interviewed the client, whose name was not Mary), and it is the kind of situation that is not uncommon. Child abuse and wife beating are quite common, not just among the lower classes or among certain ethnic groups; they are increasing at an alarming rate.

Nurses in general are one of the groups of people who see other people at their lowest ebb, at their meanest, at their saddest, at their most vulnerable, and every now and then they see people at their best. Community nurses in particular, because they have a broader and more comprehensive view of their clients, see horror, pain, and the results of "man's inhumanity to man." How one can grow accustomed to seeing and dealing with all the horror without becoming indifferent to or calloused by it is a problem each individual nurse must solve. If we are sensitive and empathetic people, we find ways to help people help themselves. We might let a family know we know that they have a big problem and that they are strong people simply to survive for another day in their situation. A nurse can do this only if she has an effective support system. Either her supervisor or fellow staff members help her to beleive she is doing all she can and that perhaps in some situations just standing by is all that can be expected. Perhaps we expect change in things for which we do not have responsibility. The nurse is only one member of the community health team and therefore may mistakenly believe she can do more than is indeed possible.

Mary's family's level of wellness is obviously poor, and they are living close to the sickness end of the health-illness continuum. In fact they are barely functioning. Mary is living with her extended family, which used to be her nuclear family, and this in itself is a source of stress. The fact that her parents do not provide her with even the bare rudiments of living, such as a bed to sleep on, indicates that she is not wanted in their home. Her husband, in his own way, is telling her that he wants neither her nor their children. Mary's parents are alcoholics, which surely lowers their level of wellness and contributes to an extremely unhealthy atmosphere in the home. The one surviving child seems doomed to a perpetually low level of wellness. If he remains in the foster home, he will face a myriad of social, emotional, and legal problems. If he returns to his mother and father, his life is in jeopardy. The same kind of situation is facing the unborn child. At best he could anticipate an atmosphere of physical and emotional violence and abuse. Even though Mary's husband did the actual beating of the children, Mary, for whatever reason, apparently made no effort to stop it, so the mother will not be a haven of safety for the child.

This family's low level of wellness is also most graphically demonstrated by the generational aspects of the child abuse. It is likely that Mary will herself eventually abuse her children. Verbal communication in this family is practically nonexistent, but the nonverbal communication is demonstrative. The level of wellness here will most likely never improve until the family members begin talking to each other. The interlocking sadomasochistic re-lationships between parent and child and between husband and wife are complex and contribute to the family's unhealthy level of functioning.

It is difficult to conceive of an individual's level of wellness that is worse than Mary's. Although her physical health is not generally poor and her present condition is only potentially serious (if she is steadfast in her refusal to receive blood, she could possibly hemorrhage to death, although the presence of the fetus could pose a medical, ethical, and legal dilemma), Mary does face the possibility of a premature or stillborn infant. This would be just one more stressor in her life. As it is now, she is facing about as much stress as one human being can be expected to bear and more than many people could actually deal with. The feelings she must have experienced over the death of her children, particularly the way in which they died, could be an overwhelming stressor. Although she is able to express little emotion, watching one's husband murder one's children is bound to lead to feelings of extreme guilt, sadness, remorse, and shame. The stress of feeling an obligation to remain married to a man like her husband must be another incredible burden. Perhaps the intensity of the stress is having an almost paralyzing effect; hence her inability to break away from him. She is a convert to a religion that she neither knows nor understands and which could possibly cost her her life. The subhuman conditions under which she is living are another monumental stressor that in itself could be conceived of as unbearable. Mary is subjected to constant and unremitting physical and mental abuse. I remember distinctly being amazed that Mary was able to function at all, let alone carry on a conversation in a pleasant and lucid manner.

The husband's level of wellness is so poor, and he is so far down the health-illness continuum, that it would take the highly specialized skills of many people to work with him. The therapy, help, and rehabilitation that he needs are far outside the sphere of expertise of most community nurses, or for that matter, of most individuals. The community nurse's most appropriate action would be to refer him to a local mental health center *if* the nurse could establish any kind of communicative contact with him at all. The nurse must consider the possibility that Mary's husband is beyond help, beyond being reached by another human being, and that she should concentrate her therapeutic efforts on Mary. Each nurse has only a given amount of energy, and it must be used where it will do the most good.

The health problems in this family are so many, so varied, and so severe that it is difficult to establish priorities. Without the establishment of communication and a trusting relationship with a therapist over a long period of time, it would be impossible to find out how Mary perceives all of the stressors and what she wants to do about them. The therapist can only shed some light on the situation, help Mary see her life through someone else's eyes and perception, offer alternatives for living, give emotional and practical support, and demonstrate that she cares. But the therapist *cannot* provide motivation for Mary to alter her life. Mary has to want and to need to improve her level of wellness, and it may well be that she will not want to.

In this eventuality, the nurse will have to cope with her own feelings of rejection and helplessness and perhaps even anger and resentment. The nurse then needs someone with whom she can share her thoughts and feelings; in a well-run community health or nursing agency, the client care conference, or even simply informal talks with colleagues, can serve this purpose.

In this situation, as well as in many others, the nurse is dealing with a set of values and standards of behavior that are most likely different from her own. The vast majority of people consider murder, child abuse, wife beating, and other forms of physical violence to be highly immoral and wrong, and of course they are illegal. When confronted with direct evidence of this behavior, how does the nurse react? What does she say and do? Professional nurses have always been taught not to impose their own standards and values on other people, and by and large this is an excellent rule. However, it sometimes needs to be circumvented. Each nurse would have to relate to Mary in her own way,

depending on the beliefs and past experiences she brought to the situation. It will not be of any therapeutic value to castigate Mary for what happened to her children, but neither can it be construed as acceptable human behavior. Obviously, the nurse or other therapist will need a great deal of support and counseling while she works with this family.

SUMMARY

The concept of health, wellness, and illness is best illustrated by the health-illness continuum, which is an abstract horizontal line along which an individual's health moves during his lifetime. One end of the continuum is optimum health functioning, and the other end is death or total disability. The continuum can also be circular; individuals move around the circle in different directions and stop at different points for varying lengths of time.

The topic of wellness and illness is subjective; it is impossible to establish definite criteria or behaviors for a well or an ill person. One may *feel* well but not *be* well, and a well person may feel sick. The level of functioning within a given set of circumstances is a more accurate way to measure wellness than the establishment of specific parameters. Levels of functioning, however, change frequently, whereas the level of wellness may remain the same.

Many factors and variables affect levels of wellness, including the presence of physical or mental disabilities, heredity, the kind of health care available and the way in which it is used, environment, weather, socioeconomic conditions, anxiety, aging, stress and tension (physiological and psychological), financial problems, sexual dysfunction, and all manifestations of psychosomatic disease.

Individuals exhibit various behavior patterns as they travel along the continuum. Each set of behaviors is characteristic of various stages of wellness and illness; a perceptive health worker might be able to partly assess a client's level of wellness by the way he is behaving. Biofeedback is a new technique by which some areas of the level of wellness can be assessed. Human beings also have a series of inner perceptions that give them clues about how they are feeling; if the person pays attention to these clues (some are more subtle than others: a raging headache is more quickly discerned than a gradual loss of stamina), he will know when he is becoming ill.

Selye's General Adaptation Syndrome (GAS) is a description of the syndrome of reactions and responses to physical and psychic stress. Most of his work was done on individual cells and on isolated biological systems, but the GAS can be applied to the total human organism as it reacts to the various stresses of life.

The community nurse can use knowledge of the characteristics of health, wellness, and illness as well as the application of the GAS to analyze and solve clients' health problems, many of which are the result of some kind of stress.

NOTES

1. Garfield, S.R.: The delivery of medical care, Scientific American **222:**15-23, 1970.
2. Sutterley, Doris C., and Donnelly, Gloria F.: Perspectives in human development: nursing throughout the life cycle, Philadelphia, 1973, J.B. Lippincott Co.
3. The much used term *handicap* is to be avoided because it imparts an extremely negative connotation.
4. *Translation:* A healthy mind in a healthy body.
5. Suchman, E.A.: Stages of illness and medical care, Journal of Health and Human Behavior **6:**114-128, 1965.
6. The term patient instead of client is used here to denote a certain dependent sick role. It implies passivity, not the active participation in health care of a client.
7. Wu, Ruth: Behavior and illness, Englewood Cliffs, N.J., 1973, Prentice-Hall, Inc.
8. Allport, Floyd H.: Theories of perception and the concept of structure, New York, 1955, John Wiley & Sons, Inc.
9. Refer to *On Death and Dying,* by Elisabeth Kübler-Ross.
10. Selye, Hans: The stress of life, New York, 1956, McGraw-Hill Book Co.
11. This is slightly contradictory to other authors' concepts of homeostasis, which has been previously described as a state of balance (which could be disturbed by stress) rather than simply a resting state. An organism at rest is not necessarily in a state of homeostasis, and homeostasis is not necessarily disturbed by the organism not being at rest.
12. See Chapter 12 for techniques of crisis intervention therapy.
13. Hurst, Michael W.: The relation of psychological stress to onset of medical illness. In Garfield, Charles A.: Stress and survival: the emotional realities of life-threatening illness, St. Louis, 1979, The C.V. Mosby Co.

BIBLIOGRAPHY

Aguilera, Donna C., and Messick, Janice M.: Crisis intervention: theory and methodology, ed. 3, St. Louis, 1978, The C.V. Mosby Co.

Allport, Floyd H.: Theories of perception and the concept of structure, New York, 1955, John Wiley & Sons, Inc.

Archer, Sarah, and Fleshman, Ruth: Community health nursing: patterns and practice, N. Scituate, Mass., 1975, Duxbury Press.

Brown, Barbara B.: New body, new mind: bio-feedback: new directions for the mind, New York, 1974, Bantam Books, Inc.

Dunn, Halbert L.: High level wellness, Arlington, Va., 1961, R.W. Beatty.

Fielo, Sandra B.: A summary of integrated nursing theory, New York, 1975, McGraw-Hill Book Co.

Garfield, Charles A.: Stress and survival: The emotional realities of life-threatening illness, St. Louis, 1979, The C.V. Mosby Co.

Garfield, S.R.: The delivery of medical care, Scientific American **222:**15-23, 1970.

Hymovich, Debra, and Barnard, Martha: Family health care, New York, 1973, McGraw-Hill Book Co.

Murray, Ruth, and Zentner, Judith: Nursing assessment and health promotion through the life span, Englewood Cliffs, N.J., 1975, Prentice-Hall, Inc.

Murray, Ruth, and Zentner, Judith: Nursing concepts for health promotion, Englewood Cliffs, N.J., 1975, Prentice-Hall, Inc.

Schwartz, Lawrence H., and Schwartz, Jane L.: The psychodynamics of patient care, Englewood Cliffs, N.J., 1972, Prentice-Hall, Inc.

Selye, Hans: The stress of life, New York, 1956, McGraw-Hill Book Co.

Suchman, E.A.: Stages of illness and medical care, Journal of Health and Human Behavior **6:**114-128, 1965.

Sutterley, Doris C., and Donnelly, Gloria F.: Perspectives in human development: nursing throughout the life cycle, Philadelphia, 1973, J.B. Lippincott Co.

Wu, Ruth: Behavior and illness, Englewood Cliffs, N.J., 1973, Prentice-Hall, Inc.

9

EPIDEMIOLOGY

GRACE WYSHAK

COMMUNITY MEDICINE AND EPIDEMIOLOGY

Community medicine is the field concerned with the study of health and disease in human populations. In some settings it is referred to as population medicine, preventive medicine, or social medicine. Its goal is to identify the totality of health problems and needs of defined populations and to consider mechanisms by which these needs are or should be met. In contrast to clinical medicine, which focuses largely on the care of individuals, community medicine focuses primarily on groups of individuals or the community and is concerned with evaluating the health of all members in a defined community, including those who do not seek health care.

Just as the clinician needs knowledge about the disease in relation to the individual client in order to make a correct diagnosis, information about the illnesses prevalent in groups is needed to answer important questions relating to the etiology and prevention of disease in the community. Epidemiologists need to collect data about the allocation of health resources and personnel in order to evaluate the effectiveness of health care. Community medicine is a systematic way of studying the diseases present in a community and the patterns of delivery of care, both of which influence the amount and nature of disease. Epidemiology is the discipline that provides this systematic approach.

Epidemiology is defined as the study of the distribution and determinants of disease frequency in humans. Historically, epidemiology was concerned with studying infectious diseases such as cholera, plague, smallpox, yellow fever, and typhus, which until the twentieth century were the most important threats to human life and health. In the past the term epidemic was used to describe an acute outbreak of infectious disease. However, epidemiology has expanded greatly in scope, and the definition of epidemic now stresses the concept of excessive prevalence of disease as its basic implication. Epidemiologists are now concerned not only with infectious diseases but also with those presumed to be noninfectious, among which are coronary heart disease, diabetes, accidents and injuries, cancer, and mental illness. The shift in epidemiological effort has occurred in part because in most developed countries acute infectious diseases have been largely controlled, whereas other diseases, chiefly chronic in nature, have increased in both relative and absolute importance. For example, in the United States two seemingly noninfectious diseases, coronary heart disease and lung cancer, are of epidemic proportions, since they satisfy the criterion of excessive frequency. Lung cancer is thirty times more common in the United States today than it was fifty years ago; coronary heart disease accounts for nearly one third of all deaths in the United States, although there are areas in the world in which it is relatively infrequent.[1]

In addition to their traditional concern with the elucidation and containment of disease, epidemiologists are now studying health care systems in order to prevent and anticipate health problems and to learn new approaches to health care.

In brief, epidemiology is said to be now concerned with all health and illness in population groups and with the factors, including health services, that affect them.[2] The aims of epidemiology include knowledge of the distribution of disease in order to elucidate causal mechanisms, explain local disease occurrence, describe the natural history of a disease, and provide guidance in the administration of health services.

Following are human characteristics that are of concern to epidemiologists:

1. Biological characteristics such as biochemical levels of the blood, including antibodies and enzymes; cellular constituents of the blood; and measurements of physiological function of different organ systems of the body
2. Demographic characteristics such as age, sex, race, and ethnic group
3. Social and socioeconomic characteristics such as socioeconomic status, education, occupation, and nativity
4. Personal living habits such as tobacco use, diet, and exercise

Factors other than personal characteristics useful in epidemiology for administrative purposes and for the study of the etiology of disease include place or geography of the existence of an illness and its time or secularity. The interaction between person, place, and time are also important in studying the causes of disease.

According to Morris,[3] uses of epidemiology include the following:

1. To study the history of the health of populations and the rise and fall of diseases and changes in their character.
2. To diagnose the health of the community and the condition of people; to measure the distribution and dimension of illness in terms of incidence, prevalence, disability, and mortality; to set health problems in perspective and to define their relative importance; and to identify groups needing special attention. New methods of monitoring must be constantly sought.
3. To study the working of health services with a view to their improvement. Operational research shows how community expectations can result in the actual provision of service. The success with which the services achieve their stated goals and the effects on community health have to be appraised in relation to resources. Action research can lead to future plans for better services.
4. To estimate the risks of disease, accident, and defect, and the chances of avoiding them.
5. To identify syndromes by describing the distribution and association of clinical phenomena in the population.
6. To complete the clinical picture of chronic diseases and describe their natural history.
7. To search for causes of health and disease by comparing the experience of groups that are clearly defined by their composition, inheritance, experience, behavior, and environments.

One of the most significant purposes of epidemiology is to acquire knowledge of causation of disease. Consideration of a disease, tuberculosis, for example, illustrates that causation is rarely simple or based on a single factor. Tuberculosis is not merely caused by the tubercle bacillus; not everyone exposed to the tubercle bacillus becomes ill with tuberculosis. Other factors that have been identified as clearly contributing to the occurrence of the disease are poverty, overcrowding, malnutrition, alcoholism, and genetic factors.

. . . the tubercle bacillus as a species; its strain-determined pathogenicity, the genetic character of the host, his age, sex, and state of nutrition, the operation of various stress phenomena; the extent of human contact in homes and places of work; the inadequacy of ventilation and sunlight; the lack of medical care and proper nutrition are just a few of the determinants of tuberculosis.[4,pp.33-34]

Every disease has multifactorial causes, and it is up to the epidemiologist to sort out these causes so the etiology of the disease can be systematically studied. One way to view causation of some diseases, particularly infectious ones, is in terms of an ecological system. Ecology is defined as the study of the relationship or organisms to each other as well as to all other aspects of the environment. A model used for describing the ecological system is the epidemiological triangle: host, agent, and environment (Fig. 9-1). The model implies that each component must be analyzed for comprehension and predictions of patterns of disease. When the focus of epidemiological studies was limited to infectious diseases, the infecting organisms were

separate from environmental factors and identified as agents of disease. With the current epidemiological emphasis on conditions, such as mental illness, coronary heart disease, and rheumatoid arthritis, that have not been linked with specific agents, the agent is considered an integral part of the total environment, and new models stress the multiplicity of interactions between host and environment.

Another epidemiological view of disease etiology is as a "web of causation" (Fig. 9-2). This concept considers that effects never depend on single isolated causes, but rather develop as the result of chains of causation in which each link itself is the result of a complex genealogy of antecedents. These chains of causation represent only a fraction of the reality, and the whole complex may be thought of as a web that in its complexity and origins lies quite beyond our understanding. Fortunately, it is not necessary to understand causal mechanisms completely to effect preventive measures. An example is the prevention of scurvy by a ration of limes. The occurrence of scurvy in epidemic proportions on board British ships during long sea voyages was correctly traced to a nutritional deficiency in 1753. Effective prevention did not depend on a full understanding of the dietary lack; vitamin C was not isolated until 1928.[5]

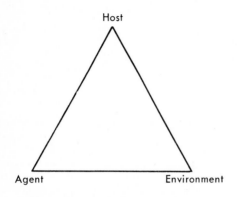

Fig. 9-1. The epidemiological triangle.

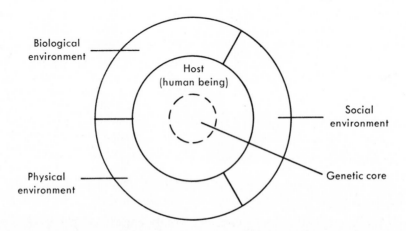

Fig. 9-2. Wheel model of man-environment interactions. (Modified from Mausner, Judith S., and Bahn, A.K.: Epidemiology: an introductory text, Philadelphia, 1974, W.B. Saunders Co.)

BASIC METHODS OF EPIDEMIOLOGICAL STUDY

The uses of epidemiology encompass two main components:

1. The systematic collection of health data (including the utilization of data collected for other purposes)
   a. Identification of health problems and assessment of priorities in allocation of resources, including surveillance
   b. Detection of new problems or changes in frequency of existing problems
   c. Identification of risk factors enabling efficient distribution of resources assigned to a particular problem
   d. Evaluation of effectiveness of control programs
   e. Formulation of hypotheses regarding the reasons for nonrandom disease distribution (disease etiology)
2. The search for causes of ill health
   a. Identification of alterable causes
   b. Identification of susceptible groups for special surveillance
   c. Identification of disease entities
   d. Identification of early manifestations of disease or disease syndromes

The collection of health data and the search for causes of ill health can be considered in terms of a basic model of health: exposure $\rightarrow$ disease $\rightarrow$ treatment $\rightarrow$ cure. Causes can be an etiological agent, a preventive agent, or a therapeutic agent. The effects of the model are disease, nondisease, or cured disease.

The nature of data can be shown so that cause is related to effect, and collection of data can be made in terms of a clinical approach, an epidemiological approach, or an experimental approach. The clinical is concerned with assessment of cause and effect in sick persons. Epidemiology is concerned with assessment of cause and effect in persons with and without cause, or in assessment of cause and effect in persons with and without effect. The experimental approach is interested in the assessment of cause and effect in persons with and without cause.

The effort of epidemiologists and medical scientists to understand the etiology of disease and develop appropriate therapy involves a study of relationships of one type of event or characteristic or "variable" to another; here the relationship is between cause and effect. In a two-variable relationship one is usually considered the independent variable, which affects the other (dependent) variable. Relationships that are studied need not only be between one variable and a second. Often the investigator must be concerned with the interrelationship of three or more variables.

Observational and experimental studies

Epidemiological approaches to relationship studies fall into two broad categories: observational and experimental studies. In observational studies the amount and distribution of disease within a population by person, place, and time are noted. In experimental studies the investigator intervenes and actually changes one variable and observes what happens to the other: the investigator controls the condition. Epidemiology includes both observational and experimental studies, examples of which follow.

DESCRIPTIVE AND ANALYTICAL OBSERVATIONAL STUDIES

Observational studies fall into two main classifications: descriptive and analytical. Descriptive studies usually involve the determination of the incidence, prevalence, and mortality rates for diseases in large population groups, according to characteristics such as age, sex, race, and geographical area. For descriptive studies data on both cause and effect in an individual are often *not* known.

Analytical studies attempt to explain disease, for example, determining the reasons for relatively high or low frequency of disease in specific groups. The starting point for any analytical study is often a descriptive finding that raises certain questions or suggests certain hypotheses that require further investigation. With analytical studies the investigator has a specific question or group of questions that he sets about to answer. For an analytical study, data on both cause and effect in an individual are known.

However, the distinction between descriptive and analytical studies is not clear-cut. A large-scale descriptive study may provide abundant and impressive data that give a clear answer to specific questions. Data collected incidentally may be of great descriptive interest and raise further questions for investigation. Although the distinction between descriptive and analytical studies is not clear-cut, the classification is useful. In other words, the two broad categories of epidemiological studies are (1) descriptive, which study the *amount* and *distribution* of disease within a population by person, place, and time, and (2) analytical, which focus on the *determinants* of or *reasons* for the relatively high or low frequency of disease in specific groups. Descriptive studies usually involve a more diffuse, superficial, or general view of a disease problem; for this reason it was said before that data on both cause and effect in an individual are not known. Analytical studies on a specific question may require a more rigorous study design and data analysis. Thus, we say that data on both cause and effect in an individual are known. The study design and the data analysis provide the answer to the specific questions of interest.

Types of analytical studies. Nonexperimental analytical studies are those in which nature determines the exposure; the investigator does not intervene or control the conditions. Cross-sectional or prevalence and longitudinal studies comprise the main classification of nonexperimental studies. Prevalence or cross-sectional studies examine the relationships between diseases and other characteristics or variables of interest as they exist in a defined population at one particular time. The presence or absence of disease and the presence or absence of the other variables are determined in each member of the study population or in a representative sample at one particular time. The relationship between a variable and the disease can be examined in two ways, either in terms of the prevalence of disease in different population subgroups, or in terms of presence or absence of the variable in the diseased versus the nondiseased. A critical feature of cross-sectional or prevalence

studies is that the time sequence between cause and effect is not known, and measurement of cause and effect is made at the same time. In contrast, for longitudinal studies the time sequence is known; cause and effect relate to two different points in time, even if both items of information are collected simultaneously.

Case-control studies, a type of analytical study, are similar to cross-sectional studies in that they assess the relationship of existing disease to other variables or attributes. Selection is on disease, that is, cases. After the initial identification of cases (persons with the disease), a suitable control group or comparison group of persons without the disease is identified. The relationship of an attribute to the disease is examined by comparing the diseased and nondiseased with regard to how frequently the attribute is present or what the levels of the attribute are in the two groups.

The case-control study is often called a retrospective study because it compares cases and controls with regard to the presence of some element in their past experiences. The purpose is to determine if the two groups differ in proportions of persons who had been exposed to a specific factor or factors. The term case-control method indicates the way in which the study group is assembled.

The case-control study first starts with people (cases) with a given disease and compares them with appropriate controls, usually people without the disease that is being studied for history of the suspected cause. For example, one suspected cause of lung cancer is smoking. The method is called retrospective because the investigator looks backward at the history of smoking in both groups. The larger the series of cases the better, and they should be as typical of the disease as can be defined and found. The assumption is that the controls belong to the same population as the cases, differing only in terms of the disease in question, so they too must be drawn carefully.[1] Sources of bias are endless; the safest course may be to study as large a group of people as possible and to make the cases and controls as random as possible, matching only for sex and age and any other attributes not being studied. This way there will be less chance of biasing the controls with people suffering from diseases having their own systematic connections with the suspected cause.

Cohort studies

A second major method of testing a hypothesis on causation of disease starts by defining a population free of the disease, each individual of which is characterized by the cause or causes, smoking, for example. The whole cohort, as it is called (a cohort is simply a group of people, therefore the term *cohort analysis),* is then followed to see who developed the disease as defined and how this is associated with smoking habits; the incidence of disease is observed and compared in smokers and nonsmokers. This approach is sometimes called "prospective," looking ahead.

The essential difference between case-control and cohort studies lies not in the time sequence but rather in the way the study groups are assembled. In case-control studies (often called retrospective studies) diseased and nondiseased groups (cases and controls) are selected and compared for presence or absence of an antecedent factor. In cohort studies (often called prospective studies) we begin with individuals who are free of the disease being studied. They are classified by exposure or nonexposure to a factor and followed for the development of disease. With either method of study, if there is a positive association between the factor and the disease, those exposed will tend to develop the disease, whereas those not exposed will not.

Historical retrospective studies are also cohort studies. Such studies consist of the identification of a group at some point in the past and analysis of their subsequent disease experience. To conduct such a study, it must be possible to identify from records the membership of some previously existing group, such as employees of a given industry who were exposed to a suspected cause at a time in the past. Second, it is necessary that the factors of interest had been recorded adequately at that time or can be reconstructed. Third, it must be possible to obtain the needed information about outcome (disease or death) for the cohort. This method employs previously assembled data, but it is essentially longitudinal; the longitudinal information covers a time interval extending from past to present rather than present to future as in the conventionally termed prospective study or cohort study. It is likely that an increasing number of studies will be based on already existing cohorts as large numbers of people come under medical care in health maintenance organizations.

Analysis of results from case-control and from cohort studies

Analytical studies are designed to determine if an association exists between a factor and a disease and what the strength of the association is. A difference between case-control studies and cohort studies is that incidence rates of the disease can be determined only if there is a denominator (population at risk), and there frequently is not an identifiable denominator in a case-control study. Because of the way the study group is assembled, the groups in such studies do not represent the total populations exposed and not exposed to the factor. The ratio of the rates can often be determined and is known as the relative risk.

Under the following assumptions, (1) the controls are representative of the general population, (2) the cases are representative of all cases, and (3) the frequency of the disease in the population is small, it can be shown that the ratio yields reasonable approximation of the relative risk.[6]

In cohort studies a study population consisting of persons exposed or not exposed to a factor is selected. For example, in a study of malformations in infants, the study population is pregnant women who took a particular drug and some who did not. The groups are observed to determine how many exposed and how many nonexposed infants (when they were fetuses) developed malformation. The comparison made is between the proportion of malformed infants in the nonexposed group with the proportion in the exposed group. This method permits the determination of the magnitude of risk for the populations exposed and not exposed. The excess risk resulting from exposure to a given factor can be calculated directly. The two major ways are relative risk and attributable risk. Cohort studies also permit calculation of incidence rates among those exposed and those not exposed.

CHOICE OF STUDY METHODS

Each of the types of study in the preceding discussion can make a distinctive contribution to finding causes of disease. The most appropriate strategy depends on such factors as the state of existing knowledge about a disease, its incidence, the interval between exposure and development of the disease, and the nature of the factors to be studied from possible etiological significance. The advantages and disadvantages of case-control and cohort studies are given in Table 9-1.

Survivorship in chronic disease

Prognosis or outcome is an important aspect of any disease. Different criteria may be used, such as survival versus death or survival with or without recurrence. Most often only two outcomes are considered: survival or death. For chronic diseases where the course of the disease is characteristically long and variable, a cohort life table method of analysis is used to determine the probability of surviving or dying within specified time periods after diagnosis. This method takes into account follow-up of people for unequal periods of time because of loss to follow-up, migration, or late

entry into the study. Five-year survival is commonly used as an end point, particularly for evaluating survival after treatment for cancer, but other end points, for example, one, two, or ten years, can be used (Fig. 9-3).

EXPERIMENTAL STUDIES

The essential feature of an experiment is that the conditions are under the control of the investigator. A system is subjected to manipulation; this creates an independent variable whose effect is then determined through measurement of a subsequent event in the system. The subsequent event is the dependent variable. In epidemiology there are two types of experiments: prophylactic trials designed to prevent disease and therapeutic trials to treat established disease processes.

The first step in any experimental trial is the development of a standard study protocol. The protocol defines the question or questions to be answered and specifies all details of the selection of subjects and of procedures. It should include an explicit statement of the characteristics of the subjects to be recorded.

Studies are usually carried out only if the results can be applied to a larger group than the one included in the study. The group of interest is the reference population; the group actually studied is the experimental population that is chosen from among the reference population. There may be some difficulty in deciding the extent to which re-

Table 9-1. Advantages and disadvantages of case-control and cohort studies

STUDY	ADVANTAGES	DISADVANTAGES
Case-control	Relatively inexpensive Smaller number of subjects Relatively quick results Suitable for rare diseases	Incomplete information Biased recall Problems of selecting control group and matching variables Yields only relative risk
Cohort	Lack of bias in factor Yields both relative risk and incidence Can yield associations with additional disease as by-product	Possible bias in ascertainment of disease Requires large numbers of subjects Long follow-up period Problem of attrition Changes over time in criteria and methods Very costly

sults from a study may be generalized. It is also necessary to ensure that an adequate sample is correctly determined.

Some of the principles of experimental studies in epidemiology are basic to all experiments, whether conducted in the laboratory on rats or with humans. A basic principle is the random allocation of subjects to the appropriate subgroup. In the simplest model, two groups are formed; the experimental or study group receives a drug or other procedure; the other group, often referred to as a control group, receives no treatment or sometimes a placebo. Random allocation is used so the groups can be expected to be generally alike at the beginning of the experiment. A control, or nontreated, group is necessary in order to know what the results would be if there were no treatment. It is desirable that the investigator not know which group is treated and which is not so that he will not consciously or unconsciously favor one group or another. If the experimental treatment is surgery, this is difficult, but if one group is being given a

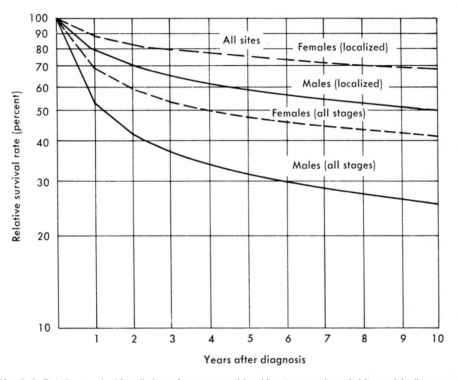

Fig. 9-3. Relative survival for all sites of cancer combined by stage and sex (whites only), diagnosed 1955 to 1964. In order to portray survival patterns for a period of years after diagnosis, survival curves are used. The table above presents relative survival curves for all sites combined and sites with the highest incidence, by stage and sex, plotted on a logarithmic scale. The slope of the relative survival curve reflects changes in the force of cancer mortality. A steep slope indicates that cancer mortality is high; a shallow slope indicates that cancer mortality is moderate. A horizontal curve segment would indicate that excess mortality resulting from cancer is no longer operative. Examination of the relative survival curves reveals the same relationships as previously observed; that is, females have a higher survival rate than males, and patients with localized tumors have a more favorable survival rate than patients whose cancers are no longer confined to the site of origin. (From Department of Health, Education, and Welfare: Cancer rates and risks, ed. 2, DHEW Publication No. (NIH) 76-691, Washington, D.C., 1976, U.S. Government Printing Office.)

drug, the control group can be given a placebo. An experiment is the model or ideal on which observational studies must be based; however, even if well done, experiments may not yield conclusive results.

In experiments with humans several other principles are basic:

1. Ethics (see Chapter 5).

2. Ability to generalize. If the experiment is conducted on a representative sample of the total population, it is possible to make generalizations. If only a small sampling of persons participate, the results will not be widely applicable.

3. Double blindness. In a double-blind study, neither the investigator nor the subjects know who receives the study treatment and who receives the control treatment. In addition, the outcome is measured in such a way that the type of treatment is not known. Thus no bias is introduced by the investigator or subject. Although double blindness is desirable in experiments with human subjects, it is not always possible.

EXAMPLES OF STUDIES
Case-control study

A recent study[7] employing the case-control method relates to carcinoma of the vagina, a rare disease in young women, but one which is more likely to occur in women past 50 years of age. Between 1966 and 1969 seven cases of adenocarcinoma of the vagina were seen in women ages 15 to 22 years. Because this was most unexpected, a case-control study was designed to investigate the factors related to the disease occurrence. Subjects were compared with controls matched by sex, date of birth, hospital of birth, and type of hospital service (private versus ward). In this example four controls were matched with each of the cases. These subjects (those with adenocarcinoma of the vagina) were found to differ from the controls with respect to their past history. All except one of the subjects and none of the controls had been exposed in fetal life to DES (diethylstilbestrol), a drug that had been administered to their mothers because of bleeding, prior pregnancy loss, or both. This is an example of a case-control study for a rare disease

that was based on a small number of cases and was relatively inexpensive to carry out.

An example in which either the case-control method or the cohort method might be used is a study to answer the question of whether the proportion of malformed infants is higher in the offspring of mothers who took a particular drug than in the offspring of those who did not. In a case-control study, a study population consisting of some infants who are malformed (cases) and some who are not (controls) is selected. The investigator then determines the frequency with which the mothers of the two groups took the drug. The alternative approach would be the cohort study in which the investigator may select a study population consisting of some pregnant women who took the drug and some who did not. The groups are observed over time to determine how many exposed and nonexposed infants develop malformations. We can then compare the proportion of malformed infants in the nonexposed group with the proportion in the exposed group.

Cohort study

Doll and Hill (1956)[8] studied the mortality experience of British doctors by comparing smokers and nonsmokers. Smoking histories were obtained by mail questionnaires; the response rate was 68%. A ten-year follow-up to determine mortality has been carried out.[9] Cohort studies such as this permit observations on many outcomes. Cohort studies of smokers and nonsmokers were originally designed to detect association of smoking with lung cancer; however, they also showed that smoking is associated with the development of other diseases: coronary heart disease, peptic ulcer, emphysema, and cancers of the larynx, oral cavity, esophagus, and urinary bladder.

Therapeutic study

A recent and still controversial experiment (clinical trial) was designed to compare the experience of diabetics treated with insulin (a generally accepted form of treatment for diabetes since the 1920s) with oral hypoglycemic agents and with a placebo.[10]

The study was a collaborative trial known as the University Group Diabetes Program. This was a multicenter trial with twelve collaborating centers. Persons with diabetes were told about the study and the reasons for it. If they agreed to participate, they would be randomly assigned to one of four treatment groups involving two types of insulin, an oral agent, and a placebo. When insulin was the assigned treatment, it was not possible for the diabetic or the doctor to be blinded because injections were given; however, neither client nor doctor knew who was given the oral agent and who the placebo. After about five years, it became apparent that the clients treated with the oral agent were dying at a higher rate than clients treated otherwise; the major cause of death was cardiovascular disease. This difference continued to increase for about eight years, and it was decided to stop the study.

Interpretation of the data from this study has been extremely controversial. Tolbutamide, the oral agent, is widely used, and clinicians have become convinced of its value. The study also suggested that diet may be sufficient treatment for diabetes because there was no difference in mortality rates of those treated with insulin and those treated with the placebo. This study illustrates the problems one may encounter in experimental epidemiology. The study was well designed and executed. The results were not likely to be biased because the investigators, if anything, expected that the oral agent was of value in preventing cardiovascular complications of diabetes. A major argument against the study was that it did not mimic clinical practice; once a patient had been assigned to a treatment group, he remained there. In practice a physician has the option of switching therapies.

PREVENTIVE EPIDEMIOLOGY: SCREENING

Screening programs to detect persons with early, mild, and asymptomatic disease have been established. "The basic purpose of screening for disease protection is to separate from a large group of apparently well persons those who have a high probability of having the disease under study, so that they may be given a diagnostic work-up and if diseased brought to treatment."[11] Screening tests are designed to be applicable to large population groups; thus they must be simple, rapid, and inexpensive. Screening is carried out in the belief that detection in an early or asymptomatic stage will lead to appropriate treatment and therefore less disability and mortality. The main role of the epidemiologist is to evaluate the results of screening.

There is considerable skepticism about the benefits of screening. Critics point out that many persons discovered by screening did not receive adequate or appropriate treatment afterward. Also, persons correctly or incorrectly labeled as having a disease would be caused worry and anxiety, often to no purpose. There is also the possible risk of harm to the client from the procedure. A technique known as mammography to detect breast cancer at an early stage was started in 1963.[12,13] It is now considered by some to be of questionable value as a screening technique because of the harm of low doses of x rays.

A generally accepted principle is that screening should be done only if it can be integrated with the health care program where it is carried out. The characteristics of screening tests that relate to accuracy are important to note. The two measures of accuracy that are commonly used are sensitivity and specificity. Practicing physicians are in the habit of dividing distributions of findings from laboratory tests and other quantitative measurements into two parts, "normal" and "abnormal." Normal has more than one meaning: one is good, desirable, or healthy; another is usual or frequent; and still another has to do with a curve used in the study of human populations, the normal or Gaussian distribution. A method used to define "normal-healthy" is to determine the "normal-usual." A better way is to determine test values in two groups, one that is healthy and one which has the disease of interest. The result is two overlapping distributions. If a client's value falls in the overlap area, he has a possibility of falling into either the normal or abnormal group. Any cutoff will result in errors, and one hopes to choose a cutoff point that will minimize the errors of classification. The two types of errors are termed sensitivity and specificity of a test. Sensitivity is the proportion of truly diseased people who are called diseased by the test. Specificity is the proportion of truly nondiseased who are classified as nondiseased by the test. Related to sensitivity and specificity are the concepts of false positive, persons who do not have the disease but are classified as having the disease by the test, and false negative, those with the disease for whom the test was negative. False negatives, persons with undetected disease, may be deprived of therapy; false positives may be subject to needless worry.

Another important concept is the predictive value. The predictive value of a positive test is the likelihood that a person with a positive test has the disease. The predictive value of a negative test is the likelihood that a person with a negative value on the test is nondiseased. It has been shown that when prevalence in the population is low, even a highly specific test will give a relatively large number of false positives because of the many nondiseased persons tested. Therefore, screening is generally directed toward high-prevalence groups; for example, diabetes screening programs are often limited to high-prevalence groups such as persons over 40, the obese, or those with a family history of diabetes.

QUANTITATIVE METHODS IN EPIDEMIOLOGY

Epidemiology is an applied discipline and is concerned with the solution of practical problems. Since it is defined as the study of the distribution and determination of disease and injuries in humans, it needs the contribution of other disciplines (clinical medicine, pathology, and behavioral sciences), as well as basic sciences such as biochemistry, physiology, and the quantitative sciences such as biostatistics.

Rates

As a quantitative science, epidemiology requires methods of measurement to assess the amount of disease in a population and to describe groups of persons. Epidemiological statements often consist of fractions or rates. By expressing measurements in terms of rates, the amount of disease is related to some population base. The numerator of the fraction is the number of persons with the particular disease, and the denominator is the population base at the same time. The numerator is derived from the denominator.

Rates or proportions are useful for comparing and describing groups (Table 9-2). They are also useful in studying the determinants of disease and for studying the etiology of disease. For example, the virtual absence of carcinoma of the cervix among nuns in contrast to the high rate among prostitutes suggested that sexual activity was probably an important etiological factor. A rate is defined by the following relationship:

$$\text{Rate} = \frac{\text{number of cases or deaths}}{\text{population in same area}} \text{ in a time period}$$

Note that in the preceding formula some time relationship is involved.

Two frequently used rates in epidemiology are the prevalence rate and the incidence rate.

$$\text{Prevalence rate} = \frac{\substack{\text{existing cases of a number} \\ \text{of persons with disease}}}{\text{total number in group}} \text{ at a point in time}$$

Prevalence describes the number of people in a population who have the disease at a given time. It is like a snapshot of an existing situation.

$$\text{Incidence rate} = \frac{\substack{\text{number of persons} \\ \text{developing disease}}}{\text{total number at risk}} \text{ per unit of time}$$

The incidence describes the number of new illnesses that occur in a group over a period of time. In contrast to prevalence at a point in time, incidence describes a continuing process over a given time period. Not everyone in a study population may be at risk for developing a disease. Some diseases are lifelong in duration, so that once an individual has the disease, he cannot develop it again.

Table 9-2. Major public health rates*

RATES	USUAL FACTOR	RATE FOR UNITED STATES 1975
Rates whose denominators are total population		
Crude birth rate = $\dfrac{\text{number of live births during year}}{\text{average (midyear) population}}$	Per 1,000 population	14.8
Crude death rate = $\dfrac{\text{number of deaths during year}}{\text{average (midyear) population}}$	Per 1,000 population	9.0
Age-specific death rate = $\dfrac{\text{number of deaths among persons of given age group in a year}}{\text{average (midyear) population in specified age group}}$	Per 1,000 population	5-9 years, 0.4 65-69 years, 29.7
Cause-specific death rate = $\dfrac{\text{number of deaths from stated cause in a year}}{\text{average (midyear) population}}$	Per 100,000 population	Diseases of the heart, 339.0 Malignant neoplasms, including neoplasm of lymphatic and hematopoietic tissues, 174.4
Rates and ratios whose denominators are live births		
Infant mortality rate = $\dfrac{\text{number of deaths in year of children less than 1 year of age}}{\text{number of live births in same year}}$	Per 1,000 live births	16.1 (estimated)
Neonatal mortality rate = $\dfrac{\text{number of deaths in year of children less than 28 days of age}}{\text{number of live births in same year}}$	Per 1,000 live births	11.7
Fetal death ratio = $\dfrac{\text{number of fetal deaths† during year}}{\text{number of live births in same year}}$	Per 1,000 live births	14.2 (1970)‡
Maternal (puerperal) mortality rate = $\dfrac{\text{number of deaths from puerperal causes in year}}{\text{number of live births in same year}}$	Per 100,000 (or 10,000) live births	10.8 (estimated per 100,000)
Rates whose denominators are live births and fetal deaths		
Fetal death rate = $\dfrac{\text{number of fetal deaths during year}}{\text{number of live births and fetal deaths during same year}}$	Per 1,000 live births and fetal deaths	13.3 (1971)§
Perinatal mortality rate = $\dfrac{\text{number of fetal deaths 28 weeks or more and infant deaths under 7 days of age}}{\text{number of live births and fetal deaths 28 weeks or more during the same year}}$	Per 1,000 live births and fetal deaths	27.6 (1971)§

*From Department of Health, Education, and Welfare: Monthly vital statistics report, provisional statistics annual summary for the U.S., 1975, Publication No. (HRA) 76-1120, **24**(13), Washington, D.C., June 30, 1976, National Center for Health Statistics, U.S. Government Printing Office.

†Includes only fetal deaths where the period of gestation was twenty weeks or more or was not stated.

‡From Department of Health, Education, and Welfare: Facts of life and death, Publication No. (HRA) 74-1222, Washington, D.C., 1974, U.S. Government Printing Office.

§From Mausner, Judith S., and Bahn, A.K.: Epidemiology: an introductory text, Philadelphia, 1974, W.B. Saunders Co.

Persons with such a disease are usually removed from the denominator, or population at risk. Persons who are not susceptible by virtue of immunization, for example, are also excluded from the denominator, which consists of persons who are at risk of developing the disease under consideration.

One of the central concerns of epidemiology is to find and enumerate appropriate denominators in order to describe and to compare groups in a meaningful and useful way.

Thus incidence measures occurrence of new disease; prevalence measures the "residual" of such disease: the amount existing at a given time. Prevalence depends on two factors: the number of people who have developed the disease in the past and the duration of the illness or disease. If only a few people develop the disease and the disease is chronic, the number of diseased persons will mount. In contrast, if the disease is of short duration (acute) either because of recovery, death, or migration from the area, the prevalence will be relatively low.

The utility of one rate over another is dependent on the problem under study. Prevalence is important in administrative situations and for the planning of facilities and manpower needs. For example, an administrator may need to know how many people with a given disease exist in the community. For purposes of elucidating the causal factors, the incidence rate is fundamental because incidence rates provide a direct measure of the rate at which disease occurs and because causal factors necessarily operate prior to the onset of disease. Thus the closer in time that the stage of disease at which incidence is measured comes to the time of actual onset, the more directly will the measure be influenced by the operation of causal factors. By comparing incidence rates of a disease among population groups varying in one or more identified factors, one can get some notion about whether a factor affects the risk of acquiring a disease and, if so, about the magnitude of the effect. This is not so for prevalence data.

Prevalence is affected by factors that influence the duration of a disease as well as its development.

Incidence reflects only the factors that affect its development. Thus the introduction of a treatment that prolongs life (e.g., insulin for treatment of diabetes) might lead to an increase in prevalence. Since incidence reflects only the development of disease, it would remain unchanged by the new treatment.

Other rates often used in epidemiology are considered next. Period prevalence is constructed from prevalence at a point in time plus new cases (incidence) and recurrences during a succeeding time period (e.g., a year).

$$\text{Period prevalence} = \frac{\text{number of persons with disease during a period of time}}{\text{total number in group}}$$

In other words, period prevalence of a disease in a given year is the prevalence at the beginning of the year plus the annual incidence during the year. Period prevalence is frequently preferred to point prevalence or incidence for analyzing data on mental illness because of certain problems in the measurement of mental diseases. Exact data needed for onset are difficult to determine, and it may not be possible to state whether mental illness was present on a given day (point prevalence). Period prevalence may also be useful for purposes of planning hospital beds for cancer patients, both old and new, that may be anticipated during a given year.

In constructing incidence rates, a number of other considerations are important. Time of onset as indicated is necessary for studies of incidence (new occurrences of disease). This may be relatively simple for influenza or myocardial infarction. But for some conditions, such as cancer, determination of onset is not. For such conditions date of onset is defined by the date of definitive diagnosis, not date of first symptoms or date when a physician may have become suspicious.

Incidence rates are stated in terms of a definite period of time, usually a year. Under certain circumstances a population may be at risk of a disease for a limited period of time only. The limitation may result from the duration of an epidemic, such as an outbreak of food-borne disease. When this occurs, the incidence rate is called the *attack rate*.

Studies that require the observation of persons over long periods of time may have problems of attrition: people die, move away, become lost to follow-up, or they may be enrolled at different times during the course of the study. Because persons may be observed for varying lengths of time and therefore may not contribute equally to the population at risk, the period of observation for each individual is weighted according to the person's contribution to the study; a person-time unit or person-year unit is constructed for the denominator of rates calculated. In a ten-year study of the incidence of a disease, if three people were observed for three, eight, and ten years, respectively, they would contribute a total of twenty-one person-years to the denominator of the incidence rate. The assumption involved in adding all subjects' person-years into one denominator is that the disease risk remains relatively constant over time.

The size of the numerator and denominator affects the incidence rate.

1. Denominator. If the denominator population is growing or shrinking during the time period for which the rates are to be computed, it is usual to use the population size at the midpoint of the time interval as an estimate of the average population at risk. If an incidence rate is to be computed for the year 1977, then the population at risk as of July 1, 1977, is used for the denominator.

2. Numerator. In some instances more than one event can occur to the same person within the time period. For example, one person can develop two colds during a year. Two incidence rates can be constructed:

$$\frac{\text{Number of people who developed a cold}}{\text{People at risk}} \text{ in a one-year period}$$

Each tells something different. The first gives the probability that a person will develop a cold in a year; the second is the number of colds

to be expected among the group of people in that year.

Other rates

The most commonly used rate is the mortality or death rate.

$$\text{Mortality or death rate} = \frac{\text{number of persons dying due to particular cause or due to all causes}}{\text{total number in group}} \text{ per unit of time}$$

When the rate applies to the total population, it is known as the total death rate or crude death rate. It is crude because it is a summary rate based on the actual number of events in a total population over a given time period. Rates may apply to any subgroup of the population, for example, a particular age group, in which case it is termed an age-specific mortality rate:

$$\text{Age-specific mortality rate} = \frac{\text{number of persons dying in particular age group}}{\text{total number in same age group}} \text{ per unit of time}$$

Related to the mortality rate is the case fatality rate:

$$\text{Case fatality rate} = \frac{\text{number of persons dying due to particular cause}}{\text{total number with disease}} \text{ per unit of time}$$

The case fatality rate refers to the proportion of persons with a particular disease who die of that disease.

In most rates the numerator must include only persons who are derived from the denominator population. The denominator is the total population at risk of being or becoming one of the numerator. Rates such as these can be seen as a statement of the probability that a condition exists (prevalence) or will develop (incidence) in the population at risk. Some rates, for convenience or because of the data available, depart from having the numerator derived from the denominator. An example is the maternal mortality rate:

Maternal mortality rate =

$$\frac{\text{number of deaths from puerperal causes during a year}}{\text{number of live births during same year}}$$

Crude, specific, and adjusted rates are frequently used by epidemiologists. Crude rates, as noted before, are summary rates based on the actual number of events in a total population over a given time period. Specific rates are the rates for a subgroup of the population; for example, age-specific rates for ages 25 to 34 or sex-specific rates for female and male subgroups of the total population. Adjusted rates, also called standardized rates, are fictitious summary rates constructed to permit fair comparison between groups differing in some important characteristic.

COMPARISON

In comparing rates, one may simply note which rate is larger than the other; by subtracting one from the other, one may obtain the magnitude of the difference. The method of measuring the difference between two rates is termed attributable risk or risk difference. In a study of coronary heart disease among heavy smokers and nonsmokers, the annual death rates per 100,000 persons were 599 and 422, respectively; the attributable risk, 599 minus 422, is 177. This is the coronary heart disease risk attributable to heavy smoking, if heavy smoking were the only important difference between the groups in factors affecting the development of coronary heart disease. Only the excess rate in heavy smokers should be attributed to smoking, not the entire death rate, since nonsmokers also develop coronary heart disease.

A second method of comparing rates is to divide one rate by another, that is, to form the ratio of the two rates. The ratio of two rates is called the relative risk, risk ratio, mortality ratio (if the rates are mortality rates), or morbidity ratio (if the rates are morbidity rates). In the example cited previously, the rates were 599 and 422, respectively; the relative risk is 599/422, or 1.4.

Risk ratios and risk differences are different measures of the risk of disease and are used in different ways. If one wishes to assess the role of a suspect agent in the causality of a disease, the risk ratio is useful. The relatively low risk ratio of 1.4 suggests that prevention of coronary heart disease would require alteration of other factors in addition to smoking. In contrast, the relative risk for lung cancer is 23.7, evidence of a strong association between smoking and lung cancer. The risk difference or attributable risk is used to measure the cost to society of a disease. Although the risk ratio is relatively low, nevertheless, because death from coronary heart disease is so common among nonsmokers (annual death rate of 422/100,000 persons), even a fairly small relative increase in this rate attributable to smoking can create an absolute increase in the death rate that is as large as that for lung cancer. If the observed association is a causal one, the attributable risk gives a better idea than does the relative risk of the impact that a successful preventive program might have. If the associations of smoking with lung cancer and with coronary heart disease are both causal in nature, then elimination of smoking would prevent even more deaths from cardiovascular disease than from lung cancer.

Risk ratios and risk differences should not be compared with each other. The first is a relative measure, the second an absolute measure. The concepts should be kept distinct.

QUANTITATIVE ATTRIBUTES

Counts that we have been considering are discrete, qualitative measurements such as presence or absence of disease or possession of one attribute versus another. Other measurements that can be used to characterize groups are quantitative measures such as height, weight, and blood pressure. Quantitative measurements are best summarized by a distribution that tells how many persons in the group observed were found to have each one of the possible values. The descriptive statistics that are most useful are mean (the average), median (the middle value in a set of values ordered according to magnitude), mode (the value occurring with the greatest frequency), and standard deviation (measure of variability or spread). Other descriptive measures include range, quartiles, and percentiles.

SOURCES OF DATA ON COMMUNITY HEALTH

Epidemiology encompasses all aspects of illness and health and is useful to administrators and health planners for identifying health problems and needs, allocating resources, and measuring the effectiveness of new procedures. For these purposes data are required in three areas: (1) the population and its demographic components; (2) health status, illness, and deaths; and (3) health resources, manpower, and facilities. In this section the concern will be with the first two areas.

The census

The importance of accurate information on population is recognized by governments everywhere. In the United States a decennial census has been taken since 1790. The original purpose was to count heads in order to apportion the number of legislators each state would send to the House of Representatives. The census now has dozens of purposes, one of which is the allocation of federal funds as a result of health and welfare legislation. Since its beginning, the census has been gradually expanded to encompass data on many characteristics of the population. Census information is analyzed and presented for the country as a whole and for progressively smaller subdivisions. In addition to decennial censuses, monthly sample surveys of approximately 50,000 households known as the Current Population Survey are undertaken. There is interest in reducing the interval between total population censuses to five years. Valuable compilations of world census and vital data for many countries are published in the United Nations Demographic Yearbooks.

Vital statistics

Probably the major source of information about the health of a population is its vital statistics. Vital statistics, or vital records, are the certificates of birth, death, marriage, and divorce required for legal and demographic purposes in most industrialized countries. In the United States the content of these records is determined by the individual states and certain independent registration cities, but most areas follow the standard certificates developed by the National Center for Health Statistics (NCHS) of the United States Public Health Service (USPHS) after consultation with registration authorities. The standard certificates were last revised in 1968.

DEATH CERTIFICATES

The introduction of death registration was the foundation of modern epidemiology. Even today changes in the death rate may give the first indication of epidemic conditions, and cause-specific rates are the single most useful source of information on the distribution of many diseases.

Recording of the fact of death is virtually complete in North American and European countries. But this is not the case in most areas of the world, and differences in completeness of registration must be considered when evaluating statistics based on death certificates. Even in countries where levels of registration are generally high, it may be deficient in small ethnically or culturally isolated groups.

Historically, registration of vital events goes back a variable length of time for the different states. In Virginia and Massachusetts registration of births, marriages, and deaths had been instituted by the middle of the seventeenth century. The federal government began to compile national statistics on deaths in 1880 and on births in 1915 on the basis of copies of certificates submitted by the states. By 1933 the quality of reporting of births and deaths had improved to the extent that all states were included in the birth and death registration area. Sincedeath rates vary by state as well as by time, changes in the registration area must be considered in the interpretation of time trends. Trends for the years between 1900 and 1933 are most accurately determined for the ten states that provided acceptable data throughout the period. Beginning with 1933, all data cover events occurring within the forty-eight contiguous states. In 1959 the figures included Alaska, and the next year Hawaii.[14]

Cause of death. Unlike the fact of death, cause of death as recorded on death certificates cannot be accepted without question. Ascertainment of cause of death is complex and depends on concepts of what constitutes a cause, adequacy of diagnostic acumen, classification of disease, and other questions that have much broader implications than the interpretation of death certificates. In addition, there is the question of how much of what the certifying physician knows is recorded on the certificate. Autopsy findings, for example, usually do not enter into cause as recorded on the certificate, at least in the United States, since the certificate is usually completed prior to autopsy. The physician's major contribution to the death certificate is certification of cause of death. For each death one condition must be assigned as the underlying cause. There is also provision for reporting immediate cause of death as well as other significant conditions that contributed to the death. The diagnostic terms used on the certificate must follow an internationally accepted classification, the International Statistical Classification of Diseases, Injuries, and Causes of Death (ICD). This is revised every ten years.

The successive revisions of the ICD may profoundly influence the apparent trends of mortality of certain diseases as reported in published material. This is particularly true with respect to the sixth revision in 1948. Before 1949 if more than one cause of death was recorded on a death certificate, the cause was assigned according to a system of fixed priorities. Since 1949 the cause of death, which is incorporated into all statistics, is the one recorded on the death certificate by the physician as underlying cause. The effect on some diseases was profound. For example, there was an apparent sudden drop in mortality from diabetes; deaths attributed to this cause were reduced by almost 50%. About half of the deficit was accounted for by assignment to arteriosclerotic heart disease, the other half to several other conditions. In contrast, rates for malignant neoplasms showed an abrupt upward shift.[6] Changes attributable to such revisions are usually identifiable by the abruptness of the changes and their coincidence with the institution of revisions.

BIRTH CERTIFICATES

The registration of births is one of the major components of the system of vital statistics. Not only does it provide identification essential to individuals as citizens (proof of birth is required for obtaining a passport and for school entrance), but also for epidemiological and demographic purposes. Until recently a major epidemiological purpose was to provide denominators (number of live births) for the comparison of rates of diseases of infancy. The variation that may occur from year to year in the number of births points to the importance of such denominator information for comparison with diseases of infancy and for predicting changes in the size of various age groups in the population.

The standard certificate of live birth contains two parts: the first is an open public record and primarily identifies the child and the parents. A second section, marked confidential for medical and health use only, contains information useful for epidemiological study. This has information on race and education of the parents, previous pregnancies, amount of prenatal care, birth weight, complications of pregnancy and delivery, and congenital abnormalities. Most of this information was added to the standard certificate only recently, although it was previously gathered by some states.

Many studies of the distribution of congenital malformations have used information from birth certificates. Information on severe malformation of unequivocal diagnosis are relatively good, but birth certificates are inadequate for surveillance of congenital malformations as a whole, even those obvious at birth.[15] Maternal complications of pregnancy are even less well reported. On the other hand, population variations on the distribution of birth weight and multiple births are problems in which a great deal of knowledge has been gained from studies using birth certificate information.

CERTIFICATE OF FETAL DEATH

In most countries with well-developed registration procedures, fetal deaths are legally required to be certified. Statistics on fetal deaths provide some information on fetal wastages. However, these data are inferior to those on births and deaths in completeness and in comparability of different areas. In the United States certificates are required in most jurisdictions for deaths after the twentieth week and in some areas for all fetal deaths, regardless of the length of gestation. The definition of fetal death adopted by the World Health Assembly includes all fetal deaths regardless of age of gestation. The National Center for Health Statistics excludes fetal deaths from birth and death certificates. Fetal death figures include only fetal deaths for which the period of gestation was given as twenty weeks or more or was not stated.[14]

Morbidity surveys

The U.S. National Health Survey was established in 1956 and has provided data on the health of the American population continuously from 1957. It is conducted by the National Center for Health Statistics and includes several major survey programs.

Health Interview Survey. This is a continuous survey in which individuals in some 40,000 different households (about 120,000 individuals) are interviewed each year. Each week, interviews are conducted with approximately 800 households throughout the country. The methods of sampling are such that short-term trends can be followed closely, and data can be accumulated by month or year. The interview is based on a questionnaire containing a core of questions relating to current or recent acute illness and injury and information on chronic illness and disability. A major limitation of the HIS is that the diagnostic information is given by the respondent, and there is no attempt to obtain confirmation from medical sources.

Health Examination Survey. The Health Examination Survey is designed to augment the information from the HIS. Additional population samples are studied through physical examinations supplemented by laboratory tests and include physical examination and measurements such as blood pressure, electrocardiogram, hearing and visual activity, and blood chemistry. The examinations are carried out in specially designed mobile units. They have been done in cycles, each requiring approximately two years to complete. The first cycle, completed in 1962, covered adults ages 18 to 79; the second, 1963 to 1965, covered children 6 to 11; the third, 1966 to 1970, youths 12 to 17. In 1971 a new cycle, the Health and Nutrition Examination Survey (HANES), was begun; in this survey persons 1 to 74 years of age will be examined with particular attention to the detection of nutritional deficiency. Limitations on epidemiological usefulness arise from the fact that prevalence rather than incidence is measured and that the sample sizes are such as to allow analyses for only the most frequent diseases and abnormalities.

Health Records Survey. This was designed to supplement the findings of the HIS and HES, primarily by sampling records of institutions such as hospitals, nursing homes, and homes for the institutionalized elderly. The purpose of these surveys is to construct a record of health services provided by the various facilities themselves and to delineate the characteristics of people being served, discharge diagnoses, and surgical procedures.

National Family Growth Survey. This is a biennial household survey of fertility patterns and trends and family planning practices.

Surveys linked to vital records. These are follow-back surveys in which information supplementary to birth or death certificates is obtained from the family, physician, or hospital.

Ambulatory Medical Care Survey. This is a sample survey of office-based physicians. Participating physicians will be asked to report on demographic characteristics and medical problems of clients seen in office visits during one week of practice.

Analysis of data. Analyses of data from the National Health Survey are published periodically. Despite limitations, the NHS is the only source of nationwide data on minor illnesses, disabilities, functional deficits, physiological measurements, and patterns of utilization of health care. To provide data of greater value to the states and local areas, cooperative arrangements among the various levels of government are being developed: the Cooperative Health Statistics System.

Routine statistics on morbidity. Information for a number of sources is available, including hospital records, records of private physicians, data from insurance programs, health plans, school records, and federal agencies such as the armed forces or the Veterans Administration. Disease registers or rosters have been established for diseases of public health concern, including tuberculosis, cancer, mental illness, and rheumatic fever.

Disease notification and registration

Certain diseases have been considered of sufficient importance to the public health to require that their occurrence be reported to health authorities. This procedure was initiated for the control of infectious disease. The selection of infectious diseases to be reported is mostly a local matter except for six diseases, the reporting of which is required by international sanitary regulation: cholera, plague, louse-borne relapsing fever, smallpox, louse-borne typhus fever, and yellow fever. In the United States about forty infectious diseases are reportable; reports are generally made by practicing physicians to local health authorities and are transmitted to the Centers for Disease Control of the U.S. Public Health Service in Atlanta. Weekly summaries are prepared for about twenty-five diseases and published in the Morbidity and Mortality Weekly Report. On a worldwide basis information on infectious disease is published by the World Health Organization. Generally the number of cases of notifiable diseases reported is far lower than the number occurring, the proportion varying with the time and place, as well as with the disease. This deficiency may not seriously impair the value of the system, since the beginnings of an epidemic may be apparent in a trend even if only a small proportion of the cases is reported, and such data can lead to hypotheses about the etiology and mode of transmission of disease, for instance, viral hepatitis.

Linked health records

The various sources of data cited so far lead to fragmented records for many individuals. A person's birth certificate may be on file in one jurisdiction, his marriage certificate in another, his children's birth certificates in a third, and so on. The possibility of integrating all this information into one record system is termed *record linkage*. The term was first used by the chief of the National Vital Statistics Office of the United States[16] in discussing a comprehensive approach to linking events of significance for health. "Each person in the world creates a Book of Life. This book starts with birth and ends with death. Its pages are made up of the principal events in life. Record linkage is the name given to the process of assembling the pages of the book into a volume." With the advent of computer technology, it becomes reasonable to consider the feasibility of linking records on vital statistics and health events of the entire population. The term record linkage implies an ongoing procedure in which records from two or more sources are routinely searched for linkage, usually by computer. Programs of this kind are common in business and government; probably the largest such effort is that of the Internal Revenue Service. In health fields efforts are still small and experimental. Data banks of computer-linked vital statistics and health records theoretically have great potential for studies in epidemiology, demography, and health services. However, the costs are high, and there are ethical problems revolving around the need to protect the individual from breach of confidentiality or misuses of information.

INFECTIOUS DISEASES

The early efforts of epidemiology were related to study of infectious diseases; recently in developed countries infectious diseases have been brought under reasonably good control, and epidemiologists have turned their attention to chronic diseases, which are now the leading causes of death and disability.

Nevertheless, infectious diseases are still important problems in developing parts of the world, and dangerous infectious disease outbreaks continue to occur in industrialized nations like the United States. Epidemiologists, community health nurses, and others are still called on to investigate specific disease outbreaks to determine the conditions or factors that may be responsible. The control of communicable disease has long been accepted as a critically important health department function. Related to the investigation and control of infectious disease is the study of the occurrence of diseases according to their distribution by time and place.[17]

ENVIRONMENTAL HAZARDS

In addition to the time-honored study of infectious diseases, more recently the epidemiological investigation of environmental hazards has assumed an important role in community health. In recent years there has been considerable concern that technology has contributed to the pollution of air, water, and land. Pollutants include such substances as industrial wastes, exhaust products from burning fuels, trace metals, chemical pesticides, and radioactive materials. It is also known that a variety of chemicals in such forms as preservatives and medicinal drugs are ingested by the population. Epidemiological studies are playing a role in the quantitative determination of the effects of these substances on human health and the assessment of the risks involved. Examples of projects that were designed to study the relationship between specific substances and a particular disease include the prevalence study of thromboembolic disease in relation to oral contraceptives and a cohort study of the occupational hazard of x-ray exposure. These are examples of studies where the environmental hazard is already under suspicion.

The proliferation of new chemicals has led to concern about hazards of which we are currently unaware. As a result, epidemiologists have begun work in the new area of research called "monitoring," the purpose of which is to detect adverse effects as soon as they appear, thus providing an early warning system. The federal government through the Food and Drug Administration, the Environmental Protection Agency (EPA), the National Institute for Occupational Safety and Health (NIOSH), and the Consumer Safety Products Commission is concerned with environmental and occupational hazards.

SUMMARY

As Morris[3, p. 264] has said:

Epidemiology is the basic science of *Community Medicine*. Using epidemiological methods greater understanding will be sought of population health and necessary information provided for plans to improve it, to prevent disease and deliver medical care. The success of services in reaching stated standards will be assessed, and what in fact are the benefits to health and the relief of suffering in relation to resources consumed. Such a contribution to rationality (and fairness) is an urgent requirement in the management of health services and for ordering their priorities. Epidemiology thus is basic to the training of community medicine specialists.

Epidemiology is also basic to preparation of community health nurses and all other members of the health team. Community nurses play an important role in epidemiological studies. They often may be the ones to initiate a study and more frequently assist in the data collection. The community nurse often is cast in the role of interpreting study findings to families, schools, industry, and others. In actual practice the community nurse is considered the "foot soldier" in the army of epidemiology. The epidemiologist in the state health department is dependent on the local community health nurses for follow-up on various conditions.

NOTES

1. MacMahon, B., and Pugh, T.F.: Epidemiology principles and methods, Boston, 1970, Little, Brown & Co. Includes full discussion of the selection of controls for case-control studies.
2. Acheson, R.M.: The need for comparability in international epidemiology, Milbank Memorial Fund Quarterly **43:**11-17, 1965; American Journal of Public Health **66:**1201, 1976.
3. Morris, J.N.: Uses of epidemiology, ed. 3, Edinburgh, 1975, Churchill Livingstone.
4. Fox, J.P., et al.: Epidemiology: man and disease, London, 1970, Collier-Macmillan Ltd.
5. This is how British sailors earned the nickname "limeys."
6. Mausner, Judith S., and Bahn, A.K.: Epidemiology: an introductory text, Philadelphia, 1974, W.B. Saunders Co.
7. Herbst, A.L., et al.: Association of maternal stilbestrol therapy with tumor appearance in young women, New England Journal of Medicine **284:**878-881, 1971.
8. Doll, R., and Hill, A.B.: Lung cancer and other causes of death in relation to smoking; second report on mortality of British doctors, British Medical Journal **2:**1071-1081, 1956.
9. Doll, R., and Hill, A.B.: Mortality in relation to smoking: ten years' observation of British doctors, British Medical Journal **1:**1399-1410, 1964.
10. Cornfield, J.: The University Group Diabetes Program. A further statistical analysis of the mortality findings, Journal of the American Medical Association **217:**1676-1687, 1971.
11. Thorner, R.M., and Remein, Q.R.: Principles and procedures in the evaluation of screening for disease, U.S. Department of Health, Education, and Welfare Public Health Monograph No. 67, Washington, D.C., 1961, U.S. Government Printing Office.
12. Shapiro, S., and Shrax Pand Venet, L.: Periodic breast cancer screening in reducing mortality for breast cancer, Journal of the American Medical Association **215:**1777-1785, 1971.
13. Breslow, L., et al.: The final reports of the National Cancer Institute Ad Hoc Working Group on Mammography in Screening for Breast Cancer, Journal of the National Cancer Institute **59:**467-541, 1977.
14. Department of Health, Education, and Welfare: Facts of life and death, DHEW Publication No. (HRA) 74-1222, Washington, D.C., 1974, U.S. Government Printing Office. Provides a useful summary of vital statistics data through 1972.
15. Milham, S., Jr.: Underreporting of incidence of cleft lip and palate, American Journal of Diseases of Children **106:**185-188, 1963.
16. Dunn, H.L.: Record linkage, American Journal of Public Health **36:**1412-1416, 1946.
17. Benenson, A.S.: Control of communicable diseases in man, ed. 12, Washington, D.C., 1975, American Public Health Association.

BIBLIOGRAPHY

Daniel, Wayne W.: Biostatistics: a foundation for analysis in the health sciences, New York, 1974, John Wiley & Sons, Inc.

Fox, John Perrigo, et al.: Epidemiology: man and disease, New York, 1970, The Macmillan Co.

Friedman, G.D.: Primer of epidemiology, New York, 1974, McGraw-Hill Book Co.

Lilienfeld, Abraham M.: Foundations of epidemiology, New York, 1976, Oxford University Press.

MacMahon, B., and Pugh, T.F.: Epidemiology principles and methods, Boston, 1970, Little, Brown & Co.

Mausner, Judith S., and Bahn, A.K.: Epidemiology: an introductory text, Philadelphia, 1974, W.B. Saunders Co.

Morris, J.N.: Uses of epidemiology, ed. 3, Edinburgh, 1975, Churchill Livingstone.

10

THE FAMILY AND THE NURSE

FAMILY STRUCTURE AND ORGANIZATION

The family is the basic unit of society in almost all cultures of the world, and it is the central and most important social and psychological factor in community health nursing. For this reason it is important that the nurse understand the structure and function of the American family, that is, who the members of the family are and how they relate to each other. To what internal and external forces are they subject, and how are the structure and function of the family shaped by these forces?

There are many ways to define "family" as well as many different groups of persons who think of themselves as a family, but we will be concerned here with the nuclear family in the United States. A nuclear family is described in the abstract as a group of people who come together to share each other's lives and who are bound to each other by a series of emotions such as love, duty, loyalty, obligation, caring, and the like. A more traditional and pragmatic definition of "family" is a group of people consisting of a man and a woman, who are married to each other, and their children. There are also several variations on this basic unit such as the existence of stepparents and children, half-relatives, and parents who are not married to each other. For the present, however, we will define "nuclear family" in the traditional way described above.

One of the most significant occurrences in the development of a family is the change in role that takes place when a child of one family becomes a marriage partner and eventual parent of a different family. This change typically occurs between the ages of 18 and 25 when, in the United States, one is expected to become a full member of the adult community by the acts of marriage and childbearing. Many cultures have specific and formal rites of passage, usually accompanied by religious rituals, but in Western culture the transition is more ambiguous. Two of the specific behaviors that signify entrance into adulthood are marriage and parenthood, although the absence of one or both of these does not negate adulthood. They are, however, considered the norms in Western culture, and those who choose not to participate in one or both of these institutions are frequently looked at askance.

The transition from being single to being one of a couple involves several distinct stages, as well as a host of thoughts, feelings, and behaviors. The first stage is dating or courting, in which two people find themselves physically, emotionally, and intellectually attracted to each other and thus decide to spend time together. Dating is, or should be, a kind of "experiment in intimacy" in which the two people spend increasing amounts of time together in a variety of settings and share a variety of experiences. Of course, not all dating ends in marriage;

that is why the phrase "experiment" is used. If the two people find they are not compatible and do not wish to share each other's future, the relationship as such is terminated, and the experiment begins again with someone else.

Should the two people decide they are "meant for each other," a period of increasing intimacy ensues. This intimacy occurs in three general spheres: sexual, social, and emotional. The most important aspect of developing sexual intimacy is self-knowledge. Understanding one's own sexual values, needs, and desires will generally contribute to a more effective meshing of one's own sexuality with that of another person, resulting in increased likelihood of greater overall happiness. With the advent of the "sexual revolution" of the late 1960s and 1970s, sanctions against premarital sexual intimacy have been greatly decreased. It is not the purpose of this chapter to maintain what a person *should* do in regard to developing sexual intimacy, and it is obvious to observers of the American social scene that the sexual revolution has been a double-edged sword. However, many persons have taken advantage of the greater opportunities to "practice" sexual intimacy before making the serious decision to commit themselves permanently to another person. Increased opportunity for choice is almost always good; exercise of that choice depends on values and other factors. Conflicts, however, do exist in regard to decisions about sexual intimacy.

On the one hand, American society values individualism, and changes do take place regarding sex roles, yet an opposing force—that of conformity to group pressures and adherence to certain kinds of sex-role behaviors—coexists and is still rewarded. The individual seeking intimacy is faced with a dilemma: to live up to the stereotyped and often times rewarded norms and conceptions of one's gender versus behaving according to one's own conceptions, that is, breaking the norms and risking isolation. Any anxiety or conflict regarding one's gender is apt to affect the development of sexual intimacies. Anxiety inhibits behavior, and conflict leads to vacillation, which, in some cases, can paralyze.[1]

Sexual attitudes play a large role in future sexual, emotional, and social relationships. Malewska,[2] in a study of cultural and psychological determinants of sexual behaviors, found that the impact of the first sexual experience may be even more significant than later sexual experiences even if that first experience was "casual." The data suggested that the more pleasurable the perception of the first erotic petting experiences and the first intercourse, the more satisfying are later sexual experiences. The reason posited for this correlation is that the pleasure of the first experience encouraged the women studied to go on to learn and experience an increased range of responses. The study also reported that those women who were in loving relationships with their first sex partner generally experienced a higher degree of sexual satisfaction with subsequent partners. These findings are easily understood in a culture that places a high value on romantic love.

Social intimacy is another sphere in which the couple operates. Although it has unique aspects, it is also inextricably intertwined with both sexual and emotional intimacy. Social intimacy can be characterized as getting to know the other person: how he behaves in a variety of situations, what he likes to do with his time, what his life goals are and how he proposes to achieve them, the people with whom he associates, his relationships with friends and family, how much of a sense of adventure he has, where he likes to vacation, what his taste in the arts is, and an almost infinite variety of other social phenomena. Complete social intimacy can come only through living with someone. Whether living together begins before or after marriage is a personal choice, but it does have definite pragmatic overtones. It is easier to dissolve a "live-in" love relationship, if the increasing social intimacy reveals characteristics that point to a desire not to continue the relationship, than it is to obtain a divorce. This observation should not, however, be construed as an endorsement of people living together before marriage. Social intimacy is the next step when dating has continued for a period of time and there is an indication that the relationship may become permanent. This is the time to begin to scrutinize the nature of the relationship and the place that sexuality will occupy in it. The couple needs to discuss what the sexual encounter means to each partner and how it is used. Is sex seen as a means to communicate feeling and to increase trust, or is it viewed as an obligation or an activity engaged in because it is "the thing to do" in view of the circumstances? The answers to these questions will have a profound effect on the quality of the relationship.

Emotional intimacy in a relationship can be best characterized by a developing trust: the willingness to reveal vulnerability, to share those parts of oneself to which no one else is privy and to care intensely about the welfare of another human being without permitting one's own ego to be completely subsumed in that of another. Emotional intimacy is the most perilous of the three and usually develops last. It should be noted that some couples achieve it only partially and some not at all. Although emotional intimacy can be frightening because it reveals a person's innermost core, it is also the source of the greatest human satisfaction.

Somewhere along the continuum of developing intimacy the two persons choose to make a commitment to each other. This usually involves an announcement of an engagement and subsequent marriage, although commitment does not necessitate a legally sanctioned marriage, as when the relationship is a homosexual one, if a man or woman see no personal value in marriage, or if one of the partners is already married (the reader is not to assume that adultery is advocated [just as homosexuality is not advocated], but it *does* exist and cannot be ignored because it is distasteful to some). However, as marriage is the norm in American society, we shall proceed with the assumption, for the purpose here, that marriage follows commitment. Because marriage is so crucial a decision and is one of the major milestones in one's life, several issues must be seriously considered:

1. Are *both* partners ready to take this step, which involves both a drastic change in life-style and the foreswearing of other sexual partners? Although the divorce rate is rising rapidly in the United States (approaching 50%), one hopes that the intent of marriage is permanence.

2. Is the commitment freely chosen, or is there an element of pressure from society, parents, or oneself (for example, "I'd better marry Jack because he seems okay, and maybe no one better will come along"). Does the couple really want to be married, or does it seem the appropriate thing to do at the time?

3. There is in today's society a conflict about commitment. On one hand, there is an increasing fascination with independence and emotional remoteness and a simultaneous desire for closeness without commitment and permanence. On the other hand, there is the universal need for love, fidelity, and bonds of security. These needs and desires are often incompatible with each other, and the couple should recognize that conflict exists and resolve it before marriage.

For the young adult, the dilemma and challenge seems to center around finding a personally appropriate balance. To feel and express genuine love, care, and concern for another and to have the other's interests in mind does not preclude the possibility or the inevitability of changing feelings and readjustments to those changes. It implies taking responsibility for one's own behavior along with keeping the best interests of the other in mind. But we must also remember that it implies that we love ourselves and have our own interests in mind, as well. If one's behavior or needs stunt another's growth, neither is doing a service to the other by staying in the relationship. In such a case, separation is the sane choice.[1,p.240]

IMPLICATIONS AND RESPONSIBILITIES OF MARRIAGE

Marriage is a drastic change of social, emotional, and legal status and brings with it, in addition to pleasure, conflict and a paradoxical sense of insecurity (Fig. 10-1). Being a marriage partner is a societal role, but as personal freedom in the United States increases, the behaviors and expectations involved in that role change and loosen. This phenomenon of social change sometimes makes

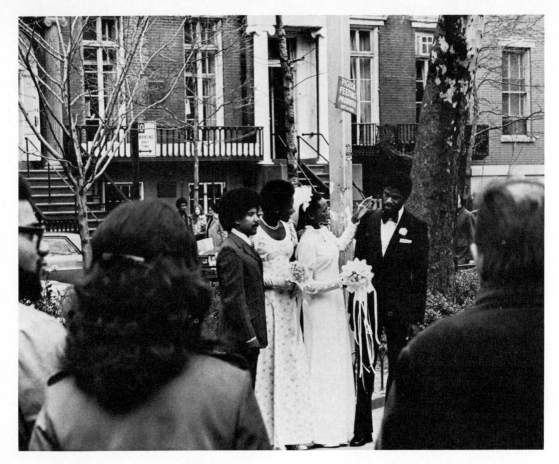

Fig. 10-1. A wedding ceremony is not a Hollywood movie ending. It is the beginning of new developmental tasks. (Photograph by Dan O'Neill; courtesy Editorial Photocolor Archives, Inc., New York.)

adaptation difficult. As an analogy, imagine an actor playing Hamlet if suddenly the ghost of Shakespeare appeared on stage and whispered, "No need to worry about my exact words; just use your judgment and wing it!" The actor would likely stand there with his mouth agape, not knowing what to say. So too with marital roles. Until the mid-1960s roles were well defined, and each partner knew what behaviors were expected. (In some cultures these role expectations have not yet changed, but the participants must surely be aware of the enormous social upheaval taking place around them.) True, life was somewhat restrictive and stultifying,

and today's freedom is much more exciting and challenging. But it can also be frightening not to know what is expected and to know that societal roles and customs are changing rapidly. This can lead to a sense of being cast off from one's social moorings.

Marriage itself, regardless of role expectations, changes thoughts and behaviors. Individual preferences now must sometimes be subordinated to those of a partner, and compromises need to be worked out. The extent to which this is necessary or desirable also produces conflict. For example, if a husband likes noisy, crowded parties and his wife abhors them, they have a social conflict. If they always go to these parties together, the husband may enjoy himself while the wife resents being "dragged along." If they refuse all invitations to such parties, he may resent being deprived of a social activity he likes, and if he goes to the party and she stays home or does something else, they sacrifice an activity as a couple. Whatever compromise is reached should have come about as a result of a free and open discussion of feelings and a decision that is as mutually agreeable as possible.

The first year of marriage is critical for establishing behaviors and modes of communication on which to base future intimacy. Rapoport and Rapoport[3] have delineated critical transition phases for the establishment of a family. The first two phases are the engagement and honeymoon. The third phase, early marriage, involves establishing a home while at the same time engaging in day-to-day living, that is, learning about each other while working or continuing an education. The stress of this "breaking-in" period can be enormous, compounded by the fact that it is totally unexpected. The American myth surrounding the first year of marriage involves unmitigated bliss. The myth, however, is tarnished by the reality of stress and conflict. The first year may be a time when decisions about childbearing are made, that is, to have or not to have children, how many, and what the spacing will be. A sexually satisfying relationship also should be developing. The *form* that the marital relationship is to take will be established early; therefore this phase is crucially important. This is not to say that the form of the marriage cannot be changed in later years, but it is more difficult to change roles and modes of functioning after they have become firmly established.

The traditional role expectations of a husband and wife will not be discussed here; it is assumed that the reader is well aware of them from the study of psychology and sociology. What is important here, particularly for the community nurse to understand, is how people interpret and react to role expectations. Roles are interpreted and acted out in an almost infinite variety of ways and are affected by such factors as age, culture, socioeconomic background, education, and satisfaction with the *perception* of a traditional role. Troll[4] found that men with only an elementary school education do not become as emotionally involved with their marriages as do men with a college education. The former view their role as husband only as it pertains to financial support, whereas the latter provide emotional and social support as well. Women with an elementary school education are more satisfied with the traditional role of wife than are women with a college education.

Since both the traditional male and female roles have both positive and negative elements, it would seem that a societal move toward androgyny, that is, the blurring of sharply drawn lines between the sexes, would be a move toward increased mental and social health. Men need to learn how to be soft, tender, and emotionally vulnerable, while women need to learn to be assertive, independent, and emotionally self-reliant. Not only are these developmental characteristics essential for the husband and wife as they relate to each other, they are necessary for the ability to teach children to reach their full potential as human beings. It is not enough for the wife to have a job outside the home or for the husband to be also responsible for child-rearing, these androgynous values should also be communicated and taught to children.

There are, however, families that would be made uncomfortable by rethinking or changing traditional societal roles. The way in which one lives is essentially a matter of personal preference or choice as long as no one is being harmed.

Developmental aspects of marriage

After the initial form of the marriage has been established, the function of the marriage requires constant nurture and development.

If the nurturance is not there, the system becomes deficient and may ultimately collapse and fail. In opposition to the settled-for relationship of the settled-in couple is the couple who continually attempts to make changes and shifts that will improve the partners' relationship. Desiring to be a better mate is no different from desiring to be a better worker, teacher, or doctor. Keeping up with or expanding one's role as wife or husband is as necessary as keeping up with the changes in one's environment or in one's working situation.[1,pp.247-248]

The marriage will change as the partners grow and develop and as the characteristics of the family change, most notably by the addition of children. Marriage is one of the most difficult states of human affairs to maintain successfully, and although this discussion is not intended to be exhaustive in terms of the components of a happy marriage, there are some generalizations of which the community nurse should be aware. First, and most important, is the desire by *both* partners to achieve a successful marriage. Both husband and wife must be willing to devote the time and energy required; both must be willing to share roles, functions, and responsibilities; both must compromise; and both must commit themselves to honesty, even though the resultant vulnerability can bring transient unhappiness and pain.

Second, both partners must be able to see the marriage through each other's eyes and must try to visualize what the other is thinking and feeling. Although one's ego should not become hopelessly blurred as a result of marriage, one cannot be so self-involved that no attention is paid to the partner's needs.

Third, there must be excitement in the marriage. This is not meant to imply that there has to be a constant change of scenery or companions or that the couple embark on a high adventure every year. What is meant is that there is change, variety, and growth. This can be accomplished in a number of ways: taking advantage of educational and cultural opportunities in the community, opening oneself to new people and experiences, eating new foods, and choosing a vacation locale at random. There must also be excitement and variety in the sexual relationship. This does not refer to the frequency of sexual activity but to the degree of satisfaction experienced by both persons. Sexual inadequacy and dissatisfaction usually has little, if

anything, to do with physical prowess but almost everything to do with modes of communication and love. Sex is something partners must teach each other and want to learn from each other. A good sexual relationship will not in itself be the cause of the success or failure of a marriage, but it can add immeasurably or detract from overall happiness.

Fourth, the existence of growing and deepening love is a necessary ingredient for marital success. There are, of course, marriages that are arranged for political or economic reasons which do not depend on the existence of love, but these are not the usual and will not concern us here. The community nurse will work with couples who married because they loved each other, and the existence of love will play a key role in the continuation of their marriage. Fromm, in the *Art of Loving*,[5] states that love requires knowledge, care, respect, responsibility, discipline, charity, faith, hope, and patience on the part of the people involved. Love can be frightening because rejection is always a possibility. Knowing that one has close to a 50% chance of being divorced adds to the fear and perhaps to a false security of not permitting oneself to love for fear of rejection. There is sacrifice involved in a deepening love as well as ongoing loyalty to a commitment. As the marriage develops, relationships are formed outside the marriage and must somehow be brought within the circle of the marital bond. This can be another source of conflict. For example, both husband and wife will have business associates and friends of their own with whom the partner is expected to socialize. A woman may be asked to have dinner with her husband's business partners whom she dislikes and finds boring. This calls for both sacrifice and compromise. If the socialization is important to the husband's career and if the wife wants her husband to be successful, she may have to sacrifice her needs and endure an occasional evening of boredom. By the same token, however, the husband must compromise by not asking her to do this too frequently. And he must give up an occasional evening of tennis to help his wife entertain her business associates.

PARENTHOOD

Assuming the role of parent is a monumental decision and one which should be considered long and carefully if the couple are to be responsible, loving, and caring parents. Almost all life decisions can be reversed or terminated; parenthood cannot, and it is for this reason that the decision-making process is so important. Parenthood is a culturally and socially accepted norm and is in fact necessary for the perpetuation of the species. But it is *not* necessary that everyone become parents, and those persons who do not wish to have children, for whatever reason, should not. It is admittedly difficult to "buck" society's pressure to become a parent once the marriage is established, but to have children when the desire to do so is absent is unfair to both the parent and the child.

Motivations for parenthood are many and complex: the desire to care for and nurture another human being; the need to leave a legacy in the form of a person; the belief that a child will provide security in one's old age; societal pressure or the need to please one's spouse; the need to see a "little me" as an extension of one's ego; or a belief in the media fantasy of what childrearing is like. It is much too facile to say that some of these motivations are healthy and some are not; there are elements of neurosis and "normalcy" in all of them. It is most essential that the parent(s) understand the motivations for childbearing and how the relationship to the child is viewed.

The role of parent is as complex as are the motivations to become one. It is a reciprocal role; that is, parent and child take from and give to each other in a variety of ways and degrees (Fig. 10-2). It is a mistake to try to balance the amount of pleasure and displeasure derived from parenthood because this balance constantly shifts and frequently seems one-sided for long periods of time. There is great pleasure in holding a warm and cuddly infant who nestles its head under its parent's chin and sighs with contented ecstasy. There is displeasure in trying to comfort this same infant when he is bright red and screaming for no apparent reason at 3:30 AM, and the parent has a crucial business meeting in a few hours. The goal of parenthood, of course, is to have more pleasure than displeasure, but children do not always turn out the way their parents hope and expect, and this is one of the gambles that must be considered when the decision for parenthood is made.

One of the most important requirements for parenthood, and perhaps the hardest to adjust to, is the switch from self-centered concerns (some of which, of course, concern the spouse) to child-centered concerns. Children's needs *must* be attended to, some of them instantly and without question. They are completely dependent on their parents for safety and physical and emotional development, which makes parenting a 24-hour responsibility even though one may not necessarily be with the child for that amount of time. Parents must adjust their entire lives to the presence of this third person in the home.

Tolerance levels for and the handling of all types of stressors need to be appropriate if the parent-child relationship is going to be relatively sane and succesful. Furthermore, the new stressors presented to the new parents also affect the husband-wife relationship. Therefore, parents must be able to adjust to innumerable interruptions in work, play, and time spent with the mate. In addition, the adult parent is expected to exhibit a fair amount of control over certain feelings and behaviors, such as anger or aggression, despite the innumerable sources of frustration contributing to these feelings.[1,pp.252-253]

In addition to the demands made by this new person in the household, the relationship between husband and wife is irrevocably changed. These changes can be both positive and negative, and the responsibility of parenthood can draw the couple closer together or drive a wedge between them. Although changing societal values no longer make it a foregone conclusion, the mother still has primary responsibility for the care of the child(ren) in most instances. This is in itself an unjust situation and can lead to sources of friction between husband and wife. The injustice of the situation comes in assuming that a woman will have primary *childrearing* responsibility simply because she has

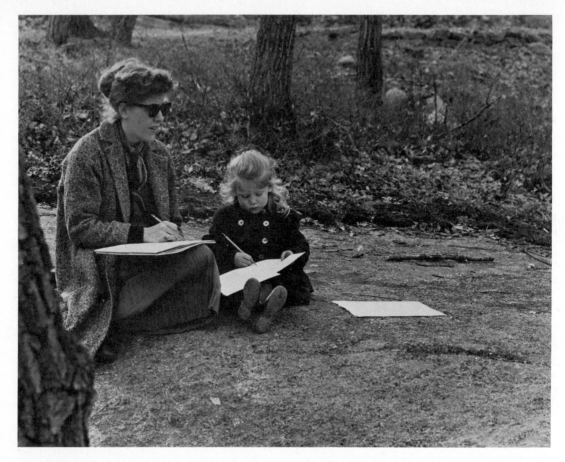

Fig. 10-2. Parents serve as role models for children, who should be encouraged to be everything they can be. (Photograph by Raimondo Borea; courtesy Editorial Photocolor Archives, Inc., New York.)

childbearing capability. This assumption is illogical in that the considerable talent and skill needed to raise a child is not necessarily strictly a feminine characteristic and has little to do with biological structure and function. Many marriages cannot survive the strain placed on them by the presence of children, and even though divorce may not occur, the marriage as a viable partnership is ended.

FAMILY DEVELOPMENT

The family is the single most important influence on the socialization of human beings. Outside sources such as school, peer relationships, the media, and the world at large can also influence a child's development, but it is the family from which the person derives social class, human values, and his initial and continuing ideas of himself as a human being.

The first significant social relationship in a person's life is that of parent-child, and it continues to be the most enduring, although of course others intervene and surpass it in social and emotional importance. The feeding experience is the one from which the infant first develops a sense of trust and security *if* his needs are met. It is socially irrelevant whether the infant is breast or bottle fed; what is important, however, is that the feeding situation is as relaxed and loving as possible and that the parent is responsive to the needs of the child. During feeding the infant learns how it feels to be held and stroked by another person and thus develops a sense of physical affection. He responds to the parents' facial expression and tone of voice, both during feeding and at other times, and thus senses approval or disapproval. In this way he begins a rudimentary experience with his effectiveness as a person; that is, if his cries of hunger are ignored he may be left with a negative impression of his effectiveness which, if parents ignore other needs, can be reinforced as he matures. If, however, his cries of hunger are attended to, he sees that he can affect his limited environment and will be encouraged to continue experimenting with this power to affect others.

The person(s) who nurtures and feeds the child is the one with whom he makes his first strong attachment, but soon the child's horizons expand to other family members and to persons in his "community." The child's learning experiences in the early years are the most important because it is then that he learns *how* to learn; that is, the more stimulating and enriching the environment, the more indications there are that the world is a stimulating place to be and the more excited the child will be to learn about that world. It is not appropriate in this text to delineate all the developmental stages of childhood, but it is important to understand here that each family participates in developmental tasks and that parental obligations are owed to children. There is a good deal of controversy about what kinds of obligations parents owe children (and even greater controversy about what, if anything, children owe parents in return), but parental obligations *do* exist and appear to fall into several categories:

1. Parents must give their children the opportunity to develop into their full selves, not into carbon copies of their parents or the persons their parents want them to be. The chance for self-determination is essential for a successful parent-child relationship.

2. Parents must give their children survival skills so they can make their own way in the world.

These survival skills will depend on values and social class, and it is not so much the nature of the skills that matters but rather that the child learn how to earn a living and deal with the exigencies of everyday life.

3. Parents must provide the child with social skills. This does not necessarily mean which fork to use for the fish course at dinner (although etiquette is an important social skill) but rather how to relate to other human beings as persons, to have respect for others' personal privacy and rights, and how to live successfully in the human community.

4. Parents must instill a sense of morality or conscience in their children. This cannot be left to religious organizations and schools or ignored in the hope that the child will "pick it up along the way." The child must be taught that certain actions are permissible and certain others are not and that both self-discipline and social controls are mandatory (Fig. 10-3). Children must be disciplined and have limits set for them.

5. Parents are not obligated to love their children, but they are obligated to respect them *as persons* no matter how old they are. Children must be given autonomy, always of course within the bounds of safety and good judgment. Children must be permitted to exercise choice whenever it is appropriate, and the more choices the child is permitted to make, the more control he is able to exercise over his own life and thus the more likely he is to develop into a responsible adult.

6. Parents must serve as positive role models for children. Children imitate actions more often than they do stated values. Therefore, if a parent tells his child that stealing is wrong and then boasts to his friends how much he cheated on his income tax, the child has an inadequate and confusing role model. Children who grow up in homes where stated values are not practiced are likely to experience serious social and moral conflict when they become adults.

7. Parents must learn to let go, and this task starts far earlier than one might expect. It begins when the child first squirms out of his parent's lap and sets off to explore his world. The wise parent

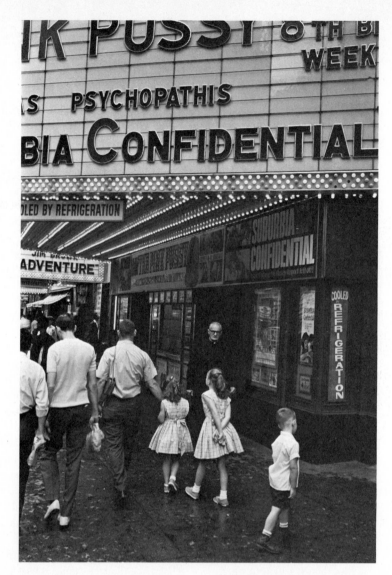

Fig. 10-3. Children are subjected to many influences outside the home that can be a source of frustration to parents. (Photograph by James Carroll; courtesy Editorial Photocolor Archives, Inc., New York.)

will keep a loving watch over the child while encouraging the exploration. There are many major and minor milestones along the path to the final leave-taking, for example the first day of school, the first summer at overnight camp, the first date, the driver's license, and the first major life decision made alone. It is difficult to allow children increasing independence and can make the parents feel old and useless or even rejected. But parents owe children this developing ability to live their own lives.

The challenge of living successfully in a family is one of the most complex that any of us faces. The family can be a source of security, nurtur-

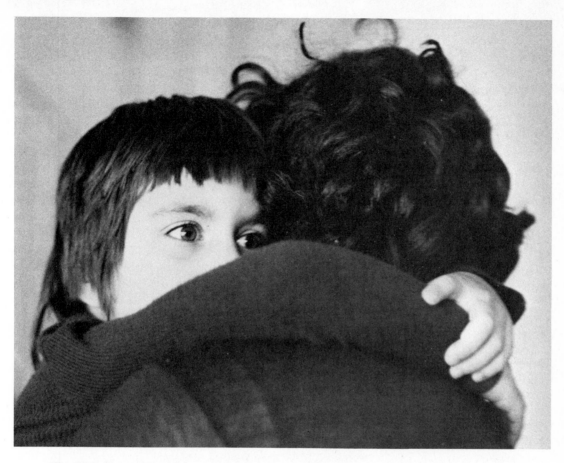

Fig. 10-4. The warmth of an enveloping hug and the feeling of security that accompanies it creates a positive self-image and is essential to the psychoemotional development of the child. (Photograph by Peggy Bliss; courtesy Editorial Photocolor Archives, Inc., New York.)

ance, and love, or it can be a trap of fear, abuse, and tragedy. For every happy child playing with trucks and dolls on the living room floor, there is another one huddled in a corner after having been savagely beaten by a parent. For every family enjoying a peaceful dinner eagerly sharing the news of the day, there is another eating grimly and silently, not speaking with each other and not caring about each other. For every child tucked cozily into bed with a teddy bear, there is another who dares not close his eyes because he fears an incestuous sexual attack that he has experienced before. For every child who is hugged and kissed and swung up to his daddy's shoulders so he can see the pa-

rade better, there is another who has been told he was unwanted and whose parents barely acknowledge his existence. All these children, the happy and the sad, will be irrevocably affected by the families in which they grew and were nourished. The kind of person they become depends, in large measure, on the family that nurtured them (Fig. 10-4).

ALTERNATIVES TO THE TRADITIONAL NUCLEAR FAMILY

The trend toward alternatives to the traditional nuclear family is increasing for two major reasons: (1) the traditional mode of family living fails in many instances and for a wide variety of reasons, and (2) the greater degree of societal and cultural freedom makes experimentation with other modes of living more acceptable. Several nontraditional life styles are common in the United States today.

Remaining single

More people are staying single longer and more women are living alone. About 25% of all unmarried women between the ages of 25 and 29 live alone.[6] This represents a considerable change from life-styles in the past decade, due partly to the freedom of choice encouraged by the women's movement and partly to the increased economic independence of women. Women are increasingly likely to remain single or to delay marriage when there is an attractive alternative.[7]

There are, however, consequences of being a "norm-breaker." Radloff[8] found that single men who had been previously married and were now separated or divorced were more depressed than married men. Single women heads of households were less depressed than men, but single women who were not heads of households were more depressed than men. This depression in single women could be accounted for by the fact that they had problems relating societal expectations to their own personal goals. Single people who live alone must contend with a set of problems that is as unique as are married persons' problems to them. Because single people may not have a consistent "live-in" love relationship, they must face all or most of life's problems and exigencies on their own. Although family and friends can sometimes be counted on to help, for the most part they must depend on their own strength and do not have the luxury of falling apart in a crisis, knowing that someone else will always be there to carry on.

One woman fell and broke her wrist on a Sunday morning. She was taken to the emergency room by the friend at whose home she had the accident, but after that she was on her own. She had to find an orthopedist, make arrangements to have her car driven back to her house, find someone to take her to another hospital for surgery, arrange to have her cat fed during her hospitalization, and pack a suitcase, all while she was in a temporary cast from fingertips to axilla. This took an entire day and evening, during which she could not permit herself to cry or reflect on how much pain she was experiencing. She had refused pain medication in the emergency room because she needed a clear head to make all these arrangements. By the time she had collapsed into a hospital bed at 11:00 that evening, she was far too tense and anxious to relax and cry. She said, "I felt cheated out of being able to sob into my pillow, which I felt I truly deserved by then."

Single persons must maintain their own emotional balance by dealing with the issues of love, companionship, and life as effectively as they are able. People must learn how to be alone and how to function when alone. This means being alone with the self. We must learn that we belong to ourselves; we have ourselves, existentially speaking. What we need to accept is that it is "okay" to be alone. In fact, in certain cases it is the only rational way to be, depending on the situation and the time.[1,p.263]

There are, of course, distinct advantages to being single and living alone. There is complete freedom of life-style and opportunities for movement and change without having to consider another's needs. Independence and autonomy provide a chance for personal growth and development, and one can enjoy as many or as few sexual experiences as one wishes. And the addition of a child to one's life is not an impossibility.

Single parenthood

One of every six children lives in a single parent family, and in 95% of the cases that parent is the mother.[9] Although there is an increasing number of children and fathers living together, that trend still is not statistically significant. The major reason for this large proportion of single parent families is a combination of the rising divorce rate and a social climate that makes divorce permissible. Many couples now no longer feel compelled to stay together "for the sake of the children." Heatherington, Cox, and Cox,[9] in a study of women as single parents, found that even when the father shared the financial burden of raising children, most or all of the stresses of parenthood shifted onto the mother after divorce, and some women stated that being a single parent restricted social, recreational, and career opportunities. In comparison, divorced men who won child custody felt restricted for the first few months and then experienced a surge of activity. By two years after the divorce their activity level was about the same as that of women. Both men and women reported intense loneliness as a result of the single parent experience.

Divorce and the subsequent single parent family obviously also affects the parent-child relationship. The younger the child, the more potential there is for serious deleterious effects. In the study of single parents cited previously[9], it was found that communication and affection are reduced, and discipline tended to be more inconsistent when the child had only one parent. This study showed that sex role development is also affected. The effect on boys of the absence of a father seems to be a "feminization"; that is, boys engage in less aggressive activity than they do when the father is present in the home.[10] Girls tend to become extremely shy and anxious around men when they grow up in a home without a father. It was also found that instead of reacting to men with shyness, girls could also become "inappropriately" assertive. These sequelae of divorce, however, are by no means universal phenomena and should not be interpreted as such. Divorce is no doubt a source of disequilibrium for the parent-child relationship, and it should also be noted that widowhood creates the same sorts of problems in addition to the ones created by loss and grief.

In some cases single parenthood is the deliberate choice of a person who has never been married (the choice is then the result of one of two decisions: either consciously deciding to become pregnant or, having become pregnant by accident, deciding not to abort the fetus). A woman who finds herself pregnant and who does not have an abortion for a variety of psychological or ethical reasons, will find single parenthood a more stressful situation than will the woman who plans her pregnancy but does not wish to be married for one or several reasons. The reason for this is that the woman who plans a pregnancy can be assumed to have a greater motivation for parenthood than the woman who becomes pregnant by accident. Motivations for single parenthood (this discussion necessarily implies only motherhood) are wide-ranging: indecision about abortion thus resulting in "motherhood by default"; the idea that motherhood is a personally creative accomplishment or that it is a socially desirable or productive act; a bid for attention or a failed attempt to induce a reluctant man into marriage; an altruistic response to a need to give affection to a child; or a desire to express feelings of nurturance. For some, children are seen as fun and a challenge to raise well, as well as a source of emotional satisfaction. No matter what the motivation, the actual fact of single motherhood is frequently difficult and lonely. Society, with all its new liberalism in some quarters, is not generally ready to accept the single mother who deliberately chooses this way of life. The conventional view of marriage as the appropriate milieu for childbearing is strongly ingrained.

Childless marriage

Other couples believe that the world is already overpopulated and that it is irresponsible to bear more children. And there are vast numbers of people (probably far more than are willing to admit it) who simply do not like children. There are those who do not dislike children but who are not willing to give up the social, emotional, and financial freedom and independence of a childless marriage. In American society those couples who choose to remain childless and who verbalize this choice are, to a great degree, scorned (the expression of scorn varies in kind and degree with socioeconomic status and culture). However

People have a choice, and this freedom of choice can and should be exercised. Why should someone feel guilty about *not* wanting to do something that might be painful, harmful, or destructive to themselves and/or to the child?

Not having children and craving to do so or having children and regretting it is senseless in times when we can get to know our minds and feelings and then make a reasonable choice. Parenthood is not the issue; the issue, the task, is *responsible* parenthood.[1,p.265]

NURSING CARE AND THE FAMILY
Assessment of family problems

There is no family that does not have problems interacting with and relating to each other; family dissention seems to be an American way of life. Most family problems are like individual neuroses: they are simply assimilated into everyday functioning and are either ignored or accommodated. However, some family problems, like some neuroses, grow severe enough to interfere with effective functioning and create general unhappiness for family members. The crucial element in nursing assessment is to recognize when this dividing line has been crossed and when the family needs professional help. Sometimes the nurse knows the family well and can see problems brewing; sometimes the problems are glaringly obvious, even on first contact with the family; sometimes they are difficult or impossible to recognize. Recognition of problems also depends in large measure on the astuteness of the nurse. There are, however, some clues that should alert the nurse that all is not well within the family:

1. Signs of obvious ongoing tension within the family, attested to by strained or nonexistent communication
2. Indications that family members do not trust or support each other
3. An obvious physical problem of one family member that has a continuing effect on all other members
4. Severe economic problems
5. Signs that the power and control mechanism of the family is not working to the satisfaction of all members
6. Conditions in the home that are clearly substandard, such as inadequate plumbing or a dangerous physical structure
7. One or more members involved in illegal, antisocial, or personally counterproductive

activities (for example, dropping out of school, "petty" juvenile crime, and the like)
8. Evidence of child abuse or neglect
9. Significant social isolation

These clues may exist with varying degrees of overtness or covertness; they may be obvious to the nurse on her first home visit or they may not become apparent for weeks or months. Sooner or later, however, the astute nurse will notice something amiss, and what she does about her observations and intuitions can significantly affect the success of the intervention. An example should be illustrative.

The community health nurse makes an initial visit to the Solis family because Maggie Solis has just given birth to her second child. The other child is 18 months old. She arrives in midafternoon just as Maggie's husband Lucky is going off to his job as a spot welder on an automobile assembly line (Lucky's real name is Alphonso, but no one ever calls him that; he got his nickname when he was a child and fell off the garage roof and walked away literally without a scratch.) The older child was napping, and Maggie and Lucky were just finishing a late lunch in the kitchen, where the baby slept in its basket next to the kitchen table. Lucky kissed Maggie very affectionately, left for work, and Maggie and the nurse sat in the kitchen drinking coffee. Everything seemed to be going well for the Solis family, although they did not expect this new baby quite so soon. Maggie rather sheepishly admitted to a haphazard use of her diaphragm but seemed open to a discussion of other contraceptive methods. The visit went smoothly and pleasantly with routine child care discussions and talk of supplementary formulae and immunizations. Then the baby woke up hungry and when Maggie opened her blouse in preparation for nursing, the nurse noticed a large sore-looking contusion on Maggie's breast. When the nurse asked about it, Maggie blushed, averted her eyes, and mumbled, "Oh, it's nothing." The nurse was struck by a note of discord but chose to say nothing because Maggie was so obviously embarrassed. The nurse said she would stop by in a few weeks to see how everything was and to see if Maggie had made a decision about contraception.

On the next visit when Maggie opened the door,

the nurse immediately noticed that she had a black eye and several serious bruises on her cheek. When she asked what happened, Maggie said she had fallen down the stairs, but her eyes filled with tears and her chin trembled when she spoke. The nurse said, "That must have been very frightening for you." Whereupon Maggie began to cry and immediately excused herself and left the room. When she returned a few minutes later, she was smiling and said she was "touchy" because the baby kept her up at night and she was beginning to feel the effects of a lack of sleep. During the rest of the interview Maggie made it verbally and nonverbally clear that she did not wish to discuss the bruises on her face. When the nurse left, she made certain that Maggie knew where to reach her and that she was available for discussions about *any* kind of problem. When they said good-bye at the door, Maggie kept her eyes downcast.

The next week the nurse was driving past the Solis' house on her way to another family when she saw that the Solis' front door was open and Maggie and Lucky were standing in the doorway arguing loudly. Lucky raised his arm as if to strike Maggie, while at the same time slamming the door closed. The nurse drove on but was not certain she should have done so.

The nurse's suspicions are now pretty well confirmed, and she is able to make a fairly accurate diagnosis of wife abuse. There are now several choices of action available, each of which results in consequences. The nurse can:

1. Do nothing and base this decision on the fact that the altercation did not take place while she was making a home visit. Or she can convince herself that it is none of her business.
2. Immediately go back to the Solis home, tell them what she saw in the doorway, and ask them if they want to discuss the problem.
3. Do nothing now, but when she is next alone with Maggie, she can relate her observations and perceptions and ask Maggie what she wants to do.
4. Call the police and let them handle it.

Wife abuse is, of course, a crime as well as a serious family health problem. For this reason the nurse is obligated to do something; thus the first option is an untenable one. The action she takes, however, will depend on her relationship with this family (which is friendly but still somewhat superficial), the resources available in the community, and how Maggie and Lucky view the problem and what they choose to do about it.

If the nurse goes back to the Solis' home right then and confronts them with what she saw, she runs the risk of exacerbating an already highly emotionally charged situation. On the other hand, she might be protecting Maggie and prevent even further physical harm. The nurse must also realize that Lucky is not in a rational state and might also turn on her. If she chooses the third option, she is most likely to be able to broach the subject during a time of relative calm. But the urgency of the need to do something has abated considerably, and there is a tendency to minimize the seriousness of the problem. The fourth option poses a dilemma. Since wife abuse (assault and battery) is a crime, the nurse should report it. However, since it is also a human relations problem, there are community agencies far better equipped to deal with it than the police. However, Maggie should be made fully aware of her right to press criminal and civil charges against Lucky if she chooses.

Although professional judgment and experience are the community nurse's most effective assessment "tools," there are observations to be made and guidelines to follow when assessing family health. A few of those observations and guidelines follow:

1. Notation should be made of who the family members are, where they live (the fact that some family members do not live at home may or may not be significant), and how they are related to each other. There also may be nonfamily members living in the home, and the nurse needs to know their relationship to the family.

2. The nurse should know the educational level of the family members, as well as their occupations and general income levels. Contrary to what we might prefer to believe, these factors *do* have a bearing on how the family perceives health problems and the way in which they go about solving

them. These three factors—education, occupation, and income—are the primary determinants of social class, which in turn provides the major backdrop for one's world view and resultant mode of functioning in the world.

3. Modes of communication can be an important indicator of present or potential problems. Family members who stop sharing thoughts and feelings with one another are almost invariably headed for trouble.

4. The nurse should know how the family spends its time together (and indeed whether it *does* spend leisure time together doing things as a family group) and what kinds of activities are preferred.

5. The nurse will want to know how important ethnic and religious experiences are to the family (see Chapter 18 for a further discussion of cultural diversity). What the family's religious and cultural beliefs and practices are is not as important as how they feel about them and what they do to perpetuate the uniqueness of the culture. Identification with a religious or cultural group can be an important source of support when a problem or crisis exists.

6. Of particular importance is the way children are treated as persons and as family members. Much can be learned about a family's values by observing how they treat children. Disrespect for children signals the existence of serious problems.

7. Patterns of coping with crisis should be observed and discussed with the family. Past coping mechanisms can be used to help solve current problems.

General concepts of family nursing

Family nursing falls almost entirely within the province of community health nursing. It began to develop as a serious object of study after World War II when psychological and sociological research provided much empirical evidence regarding the importance of the family as a social and developmental unit. Both the National Organization for Public Health Nursing and the National League for Nursing influenced nursing educators to increase the role of family nursing in the curriculum, especially in baccalaureate programs.[11] The

American Nurses Association, through its emphasis on the advancement of nursing through research, also encouraged the study of family nursing.

The growth of family nursing as a field of study and practice in large measure is dependent upon powerful, dynamic, social forces. The expanding knowledge base about man and technology, the evolving philosophies of equality and humanism, the changing value system, the concern for population growth and the environment all have their impact. One of the most remarkable influences today is the demand to activate the long-enunciated democratic philosophical concept of equality for all—including health care. The implications of this are not only for the development of quality health services, but also for health care to be comprehensive and primarily oriented toward the promotion of health and the prevention of disease.[11,p.95]

Efforts to provide the kind of health care described above must center around the family, both in terms of nursing *in* the community and in more formalized community institutions such as neighborhood health centers and the like. The provision of health care can be seen, in some views, as a metaphor for the attempted democratization of society. Although individual nurses have and do recognize the family as the essential social unit, many people believe that the attempt for the most part has failed and that the delivery of health care is more expensive, elusive, and elitist than ever. There are, however, islands of success in this sea of failure, and it is family nursing that has been responsible for most of them. Because family nursing is based on a foundation of family organization and function, that is, dealing with families as they really are, it can employ some fairly sophisticated nursing techniques, such as contractual arrangements, complex sets of assessments and interventions, use of a wide variety of therapeutic techniques, and predictions of future development and function. The current shift in thinking to the delivery of primary health care should create an even greater role for the family nurse practitioner. She has the opportunity to be a leader in this new trend because primary care always has been the traditional goal of community health nursing.

Ford[11,pp.100-102] has made some predictions about what the next decade will hold for the future of family nursing. She believes that the increasing number of health maintenance organizations will create an atmosphere in which "families are partners with the health professionals." That is, families and providers of health care will be equally anxious to preserve and maintain health because illness is costly in economic, physical, and emotional terms. Moreover, health benefits (beyond the illness-oriented benefits commonly seen today) will be negotiated into labor contracts. In addition, management will be interested in providing healthier working conditions for employees because refusing to do so will result in decreased worker health and increased cost to industry. It should be noted, however, that industry is not likely to provide employee health benefits unless it has empirical evidence to prove that the benefits will be financially advantageous to industry.

Although the philosophies of baccalaureate nursing programs have for many years stated a commitment to the family as a basic unit of care, there has been little opportunity to put that commitment into practice because of the heavy emphasis on hospital-based nursing activities. However, now with the ascendance of primary care in the curriculum, a commitment to the family should have a chance to be realized. Society is slowly changing to permit individuals to exercise more control over their lives in regard to health care. This means that the individual is morally and legally responsible for making health care decisions; thus he will look to his family for support and guidance. The family in turn will need to be informed about the issues, and it is the family nurse who can and should provide much of this information.

The family in the decade ahead and those professionals who attempt to serve it will need to adopt a philosophy of becoming to accommodate the inevitable changes. The professional nurses who serve best will be those who research well the problem of daily living and dying that families face and can help families find innovative and creative ways to deal with the internal and external stresses and strains of complex, multidimensional relationships of the difficult to define family within contemporary society.[11,p.102]

It may be advantageous at this point to explain some terms of the many used in regard to family nursing. Bowns[12] defines (her definition is based on that of the American Nurses Association) the nurse practitioner (NP) as an independent health care professional, certified as such by the ANA, and prepared at the baccalaureate, masters, or doctoral level. The NP is in active practice and engages in continuing education to keep abreast of current knowledge and technology.

The *nurse practitioner in primary care* is formally prepared to give comprehensive, continuous, personalized care to consumers at the point of entry to the health care system. As independent functionaries they are accountable within solo, group, or agency practice to make sound judgments while providing care to the consumer in ambulatory settings (ANA, A-FNP, Scope of Practice, 1976).[12,p.254]

Bowns goes on to define primary care as that care the consumer receives at the entry to the health care system and the continued ambulatory care of the individual. Primary care can also be distinguished from secondary or tertiary care in that the former is the provision of accessible and equitable health services for the purpose of health maintenance and promotion while the latter generally are concerned with cure and rehabilitation. The family health clinical specialist, according to the ANA's "Scope of Practice," is a licensed family health nurse practitioner who has been prepared in a formal NLN accredited graduate program to provide primary care within the discipline of community health nursing.

If this wide variety of nurse practitioners engaged in family nursing seems confusing, it is. More and more nurses have independent practice as a goal, and some are achieving that goal. Most, however, work within established community health agencies and practice nursing with renewed emphasis on the family as a client. It matters less what a nurse's title is than the fact that she perceives the family as the essential focus of her practice.

Some readers will want to know, since the concept of wellness is becoming so prominent in baccalaureate curricula, what the role of the nurse is with the well family. Most often the nurse does not come in contact with the family that has no physical problems and only rarely does she see families with nonphysical problems that might be considered well by less trained observers. Most well families continue merrily on their way without ever perceiving a need for nursing intervention. And most of the time, aside from health maintenance services and health education, there is no need for the nurse to intervene. In those instances where there are observable potential problems, although the family would still be considered well, the nurse's role is anticipatory guidance and counseling. These well but potentially problematic families usually come to nurses' attention through health maintenance organizations and clinics of various kinds and through informal referrals by other members of the community health team who are astute enough to recognize well families that might not remain so.

SUMMARY

The family is the basic social unit in almost all the world's cultures, and it is the central focus of community health nursing. Family structure and organization follow a variety of patterns depending on geography, culture, religion, race, social class, and other variables, but there are certain commonalities, almost all relating to personal and interpersonal development. The social and psychological changes that one experiences in the process of moving from being a child of one family to single adult to marriage partner and then to parent are profound and are the cause of much anxiety and frequently many health problems.

Marriage carries with it several implications and responsibilities, not all of them resulting in or from unbridled happiness. The decision to bear children is a serious one, and increasing numbers of couples are deciding to remain childless or to have only one child. With or without the presence of children the marriage will undergo many changes and will be subjected to many stresses. The divorce rate in the United States is approaching 50%; for this reason and others many people are deciding to experience life-styles that are alternative to the traditional nuclear family.

The community health nurse's responsibility toward the family lies mainly in recognizing and assessing problems and then in implementing appropriate nursing interventions. There are many effective ways to accomplish this, and of course much of the success depends on the nurse's professionalism and creativity.

NOTES

1. Mazurkewicz, Dolores T.: The family. In Fromer, Margot J.: Community health care and the nursing process, St. Louis, 1979, The C.V. Mosby Co., p. 236.
2. Malewska, Hanna: Cultural and psychological determinants of sexual behavior, Social Science and Medicine **2:**319-335, 1968.
3. Rapoport, R., and Rapoport, R.: Work and family in contemporary society, The American Sociological Review **30:**381-394, 1965.
4. Troll, Lillian: Early and middle adulthood, Monterey, Calif., 1975, Brooks/Cole Publishing Co.
5. Fromm, Erich: The art of loving, New York, 1956, Bantam Books, Inc.
6. Bernard, J.: Note on changing lifestyles, Journal of Marriage and the Family **37:**591, 1975.
7. Bernard, J.: Women and the public interest: an essay on policy and protest, New York, 1971, Aldine-Atherton, Inc.
8. Radloff, Lenore: Sex differences in mental health: the effects of marital and occupational status. Presented at the American Public Health Association, New York, October, 1974.
9. Hetherington, E., Cox, Martha, and Cox, R.: Beyond father absence: conceptualization of effects of divorce. In Hetherington, E., and Parke, Ross, editors: Contemporary readings in child psychology, New York, 1977, McGraw-Hill Book Co.
10. Many people view this decrease in boys' aggression as a positive result of divorce.
11. Ford, Loretta C.: The development of family nursing. In Hymovich, Debra P., and Barnard, Martha U., editors: Family health care, vol. 1, General perspectives, ed. 2, New York, 1979, McGraw-Hill Book Co., p. 92.
12. Bowns, Beverly H.: Community health family nursing. In Hymovich, Debra P., and Barnard, Martha U., editors: Family health care, vol. 1, General perspectives, ed. 2, New York, 1979, McGraw-Hill Book Co., pp. 254-256.

BIBLIOGRAPHY

Anderson, W.: Comments on developments in the teaching of human sexuality, Teaching of Psychology 2(1):22-24, 1975.

Bach, G., and Wyden, P.: The intimate enemy: how to fight fair in love and marriage, New York, 1969, William Morrow & Co., Inc.

Bandura, A., and Mischel, W.: Modification of self-imposed delay of reward through exposure to live and symbolic models, Journal of Personality and Social Psychology 2:698-705, 1965.

Bandura, A., and Walters, R.: Social learning and personality development, New York, 1963, Holt, Rinehart & Winston.

Baumrind, Diana: Child care practices anteceding three patterns of preschool behavior, Genetic Psychology Monographs 75:43-88, 1967.

Becker, W.C.: Consequences of different kinds of parental discipline. In Hoffmann, M.L., and Hoffmann, Lois W., editors: Review of child development research, New York, 1964, Russell Sage Foundation.

Bee, Helen: Social issues in developmental psychology, New York, 1975, Harper & Row, Publishers.

Benedek, Therese: Psychosexual functions in women, New York, 1952, The Ronald Press Co.

Berger, P., and Kellner, H.: Marriage and the construction of reality, Diogenes 46:pp. 1-25, 1964.

Bernard, J.: Women and the public interest: an essay on policy and protest, New York, 1971, Aldine-Atherton, Inc.

Bernard, J.: Note on changing lifestyles, Journal of Marriage and the Family 37:591, 1975.

Bieliauskas, V.J.: Recent advances in the psychology of masculinity and femininity, Journal of Psychology 60:255-263, 1965.

Blauner, R.: Alienation and freedom: the factory worker and his industry, Chicago, 1964, University of Chicago Press.

Bowns, Beverly H.: Community health family nursing. In Hymovich, Debra P., and Barnard, Martha U.: Family health care, vol. 1, General perspectives, ed. 2, New York, 1979, McGraw-Hill Book Co.

Bronfenbrenner, U.: Freudian theories of identification and their derivatives, Child Development 31:15-40, 1960.

Bronfenbrenner, U.: The changing American family, presented at the meeting of The Society for Research in Child Development, Denver, 1975. In Hetherington, E., and Parke, Ross, editors: Contemporary readings in child psychology, New York, 1977, McGraw-Hill Book Co.

Brown, D.: Sex-role development in a changing culture, Psychological Bulletin 55:232-242, 1958.

Brunswick, Ann: Adolescent health, sex and fertility, American Journal of Public Health 61:711-729, 1971.

Butler, E., McAllister, R., and Kaiser, E.: The effects of voluntary and involuntary residential mobility in females and males, Journal of Marriage and the Family 35:219-227, 1973.

Byrne, D.: The attraction paradigm, New York, 1971, Academic Press, Inc.

Carlsmith, Lyn: Effect of early father absence on scholastic aptitude, Harvard Educational Review 34:3-21, 1964.

Christiansen, Kathryn E.: Family epidemiology: an approach to assessment and intervention. In Hymovich, Debra P., and Barnard, Martha U.: Family health care, vol. 1, General perspectives, ed. 2, New York, 1979, McGraw-Hill Book Co.

Clausen, J.A.: Family structure, socialization and personality. In Hoffmann, M.L., and Hoffmann, Lois W., editors: Review of child development and research, vol. 2, New York, 1966, Russell Sage Foundation.

Clausen, John: Perspectives on childhood socialization. In Clausen, John, editor: Socialization and society, Boston, 1968, Little, Brown & Co.

Coffin, P.: The young unmarrieds. In DeLora, J.S., and DeLora, J.R., editors: Intimate lifestyles: marriage and its alternatives, Pacific Palisades, Calif., 1972, Goodyear Publishing Co., Inc.

Constantine, L.L., and Constantine, J.M.: Multilateral marriage: alternate family structure in practice. Unpublished paper cited in Bernard, J.: The future of marriage, New York, 1973, Bantam Books, Inc.

Coopersmith, S.: Antecedents of self-esteem, San Francisco, 1967, W.H. Freeman & Co., Publishers.

Coopersmith, S.: Studies in self-esteem, Scientific American 218:96-106, 1968.

Edison, Carolyn E.: Family assessment guidelines. In Hymovich, Debra P., and Barnard, Martha U.: Family health care, vol. 1, General perspectives, ed. 2, New York, 1979, McGraw-Hill Book Co.

Ehrmann, W.: Premarital dating behavior, New York, 1959, Holt, Rinehart & Winston.

Erikson, E.H.: Childhood and society, New York, 1950, W.W. Norton & Co., Inc.

Erikson, E.H.: Eight ages of man. In Levitas, G.B., editor: The world of psychoanalysis, vol. 1, New York, 1965, W.W. Norton & Co., Inc.

Ford, Loretta C.: The development of family nursing. In Hymovich, Debra P., and Barnard, Martha U.: Family health care, vol. 1, General perspectives, ed. 2, New York, 1979, McGraw-Hill Book Co.

Friedman, D.: Parent development, California Medicine, 86(1):25-28, 1957.

Fromm, Erich: The art of loving, New York, 1956, Bantam Books, Inc.

Furstenberg, F.: Birth control experience among pregnant adolescents: the process of unplanned parenthood, Social Problems, pp. 192-203, April, 1971.

Gillespie, D.: Who has the power: the marital struggle, Journal of Marriage and the Family, pp. 445-458, August, 1971.

Glueck, S., and Glueck, Eleanor: Unravelling juvenile delinquency, New York, 1950, Commonwealth Fund.

Goethals, G., and Klos, D.: Experiencing youth, Boston, 1976, Little, Brown & Co.

Goffman, E.: The presentation of self in everyday life, New York, 1959, Doubleday & Co., Inc.

Goode, W.: Family disorganization. In Festinger, Leon, Back, K., and Schacter, S.: Social pressures in informal groups: a study of human factors in housing, New York, 1950, Harper & Brothers.

Goode, W.: The contemporary American family, New York, 1971, Franklin Watts, Inc.

Hetherington, E., Cox, Martha, and Cox, R.: Beyond father absence: conceptualization of effects of divorce. In Hetherington, E., and Parke, Ross, editors: Contemporary readings in child psychology, New York, 1977, McGraw-Hill Book Co.

Hicks, M.W., and Platt, M.: Marital happiness and stability: a review of the research in the sixties. In Broderick, C.B., editor: A decade of family research and action, Washington, D.C., 1971, National Council on Family Relations.

Hoffmann, Lois W., and Wyatt, F.: Social change and motivations for having larger families: some theoretical considerations, Merrill-Palmer Quarterly 6:235-244, 1960.

Hoffmann, M.L.: Parent practices and moral development: generalizations from empirical research, Child Development 34:295-318, 1963.

Homans, G.C.: Social behavior: its elementary forms, New York, 1961, Harcourt, Brace & World, Inc.

Hymovich, Debra P., and Barnard, Martha U.: Family health care, vol. 1, General perspectives, ed. 2, New York, 1979, McGraw-Hill Book Co.

Kantner, J., and Zelnik, M.: Sex and reproduction among U.S. women, Draper World Population Fund Report, No. 1, pp. 13-15, 1975.

Kaplan, Alexandra, and Bean, Joan: Beyond sex-role stereotypes: readings toward a psychology of androgyny, Boston, 1976, Little, Brown & Co.

Kerchoff, A., and Davis, E.: Value consensus and need complementarity in mate selection, American Sociological Review 27:295-304, 1962.

Kogan, B.: Human sexual expression, New York, 1973, Harcourt Brace Jovanovich, Inc.

Kohlberg, L.: Development of moral character and moral ideology. In Hoffmann, M.L., and Hoffmann, Lois W., editors: Review of child development research, vol. 1, New York, 1964, Russell Sage Foundation.

Kramer, Rita: The no-child family, New York Times Magazine, pp. 28-31, December 24, 1972.

Lerner, B.R., Raskin, D., and Davis, E.: On the need to be pregnant, International Journal of Psychoanalysis 48:288-297, 1967.

Levinger, G.: A social psychological perspective on marital dissolution, Journal of Social Issues 32(1):21-47, 1976.

Lott, Bernice: Who wants the children? Some relationships among attitudes toward children, parents and the liberation of women, American Psychologist, pp. 573-582, July, 1973.

Lynn, D.B.: Divergent feedback and sex-role identification in boys and men, Merrill-Palmer Quarterly 10:17-23, 1964.

Mackinnon, D.W.: Violation and prohibitions. In Murray, H.A.: Exploration in personality, New York, 1938, Oxford University Press.

Malewska, Hanna: Cultural and psychological determinants of sexual behavior, Social Science and Medicine 2:319-335, 1968.

Matteson, D.: Adolescence today. Sex roles and the search for identity, Homewood, Ill., 1975, Dorsey Press.

Mazurkewicz, Dolores T.: The family. In Fromer, Margot J.: Community health care and the nursing process, St. Louis, 1979, The C.V. Mosby Co.

McKeighen, Rosemary J.: Principles of family counseling. In Hymovich, Debra P., and Barnard, Martha U.: Family health care, vol. 1, General perspectives, ed. 2, New York, 1979, McGraw-Hill Book Co.

Mischel, W.: A social learning view of sex differences in behavior. In Maccoby, E., editor: The development of sex differences, Stanford, Calif., 1966, Stanford University Press.

Moran, R.: The singles in the seventies. In DeLora, J.S., and DeLora, J.R., editors: Intimate lifestyles: marriage and its alternatives, Pacific Palisades, Calif., 1972, Goodyear Publishing Co., Inc.

Mussen, P.H.: Early socialization: learning and identification. In New directions in psychology, vol. 3, New York, 1967, Holt, Rinehart & Winston.

Navran, L.: Communication and adjustment in marriage, Family Process 6:173-184, 1967.

Newton, N., and Newton, M.: Psychologic aspects of lactation. In Gordon, I.J., editor: Readings in research in developmental psychology, Glenview, Ill., 1971, Scott, Foresman & Co.

Nutt, R.L., and Sedlacek, W.E.: Freshman sexual attitudes and behaviors, Journal of College Student Personnel 15:346-351, 1974.

O'Neill, G., and O'Neill, N.: Open marriage, New York, 1972, Avon Books.

Otto, H.: Communes—the alternative lifestyle, Saturday Review, April 24, 1971.

Palme, O.: The emancipation of man, Journal of Social Issues 28:237-246, 1972.

Parsons, Talcott: Family structure and the socialization of the child. In Parsons, Talcott, and Bales, R.F.: Family socialization and interaction process, Chicago, 1955, Free Press.

Piaget, Jean, et al.: Moral judgment of the child, transl. by Gabain, Marjorie, Chicago, 1948, Free Press.

Pineo, P.C.: Disenchantment in the later years of marriage, Marriage and Family Living 23:3-11, 1961.

Pleck, Joseph, and Sawyer, Jack, editors: Men and masculinity, Englewood Cliffs, N.J., 1974, Prentice-Hall, Inc.

Poland, Ronal G.: Human experience: a psychology of growth, St. Louis, 1974, The C.V. Mosby Co.

Rabin, A.I.: Motivation for parenthood, Journal of Projective Techniques and Personality Assessment 29:405-411, 1965.

Rabin, A.I., and Greene, R.J.: Assessing motivation for parenthood, Journal of Psychology 69:39-46, 1968.

Radloff, Lenore: Sex differences in mental health: the effects of marital and occupational status, presented at the American Public Health Association, New York, October, 1974.

Rains, Prudence: Becoming an unwed mother, Chicago, 1971, Aldine-Altherton, Inc.

Rapoport, R., and Rapoport, R.: Work and family in contemporary society, American Sociological Review **30:**381-394, 1965.

Rogers, Carl: Becoming partners, New York, 1972, Dell Books.

Rosenkrantz, P., Bee, Helen, Vogel, Susan, and Broverman, D.: Sex role stereotypes and self concepts in college students, Journal of Counseling and Clinical Psychology **32:**287-295, 1968.

Rossi, Alice: Equality between the sexes: an immodest proposal, Daedalus **93:**607-652, 1964.

Rossi, Alice: Transition to parenthood, Journal of Marriage and the Family **30:**26-39, 1968.

Rossi, Alice: Family development in a changing world, American Journal of Psychiatry **128:**1057-1066, 1972.

Rubin, Isadore: Implications for the education of adolescents, Journal of Marriage and the Family **27:**185-189, 1965.

Rubin, Zick: Measurement of romantic love, Journal of Personality and Social Psychology **16:**265-273, 1970.

Rubin, Zick: Liking and loving: an invitation to social psychology, New York, 1973, Holt, Rinehart & Winston.

Sears, Robert R.: Identification as a form of behavioral development. In Harris, D., editor: The concept of development, Minneapolis, 1957, University of Minnesota Press.

Sears, Robert R.: Relation of early socialization experiences to self-concept and gender role in middle childhood, Child Development **41:**267-289, 1970.

Sears, Robert R., Maccoby, Eleanore, and Levin, H.: Patterns of child rearing, Evanston, Ill., 1957, Row, Peterson & Co.

Smart, Mollie, and Smart, R.: Children: development and relationships, New York, 1977, Macmillan, Inc.

Swiger, Mary, Quinlas, D., and Wexler, Sherry: Abortion applicants: characteristics distinguishing dropouts remaining pregnant and those having abortions, American Journal of Public Health **67:**142-146, 1977.

Troll, Lillian: Early and middle adulthood, Monterey, Calif., 1975, Brooks/Cole Publishing Co.

Veroff, J., and Feld, S.: Marriage and work in America: a study of motives and roles, New York, 1970, Van Nostrand Reinhold Co.

Walters, J., and Stennett, N.: Parent-child relationships: a decade review of research. In Brodereck, C., editor: A decade of family research and action, Minneapolis, 1971, National Council of Family Relations.

Whitley, Marilyn, and Poulsen, Susan: Assertiveness and sexual satisfaction in employed professional women, Journal of Marriage and the Family, pp. 573-581, August, 1975.

Winch, R.F.: Mate selection: a study of complementary needs, New York, 1958, Harper & Brothers.

Wyatt, F.: Clinical notes on the motives of reproduction, Journal of Social Issues **23:**29-56, 1967.

11

HIGH-RISK FAMILIES AND SITUATIONS

"High-risk" is a phrase that is commonly used in the delivery of health care today. It should be self-explanatory; that is, an individual or family can be considered high-risk if, because of certain intrinsic or extrinsic factors, they have a greater than average chance of falling ill. But what are these factors, and in what ways do they create the propensity for illness? It is obvious that all factors that might cause increased chances of illness can be resisted with various degrees of success, and everyone is not affected to the same degree by the same factors. For example, if three people are in a room and one has a bad cold, the other two people do not run exactly the same risk of catching that cold. Their resistance to the cold depends on many variables, among them nutritional status, when they last had a cold, sleep patterns, general health, and current emotional stresses.

Resistance to all major or minor illness is highly individual and frequently highly unpredictable, but there are general factors that usually will create an increased risk of poor health; poverty, unemployment, lack of education, existing physical illness, the inability to be a productive part of the community, maternal and child health problems, inability to control reproduction, and mental illness.

POVERTY

In this country of extreme wealth and abundance, there are millions of poor people. Who are

they? How are they recognized, and how is their poverty defined? Is there a definition of the word *poverty* that will include all people who are poor and that will exclude all those who are not poor? What is the difference between feeling poor and actually being poor? Perhaps it is the difference between buying clothes on sale to save money and not sending a child to school because his shoes do not fit and there is no money to buy another pair.

There is no objective definition of poverty. It could be said that the condition of being poor is not having the financial resources necessary to provide for basic needs. But this is so subjective. What are financial resources? An actual job or the prospect of getting one? A salary that may be cut off at any time, or an unending income from inheritance capital? Which needs are basic, and which are not? The answer, of course, differs with every person. One family may be satisfied with simply having food on the table, whereas another family may consider it absolutely necessary to eat at a restaurant once or twice a week. What one person considers a basic need may be a luxury to another.

The Social Security Administration and several other government agencies every year compile and publish statistics about exactly how much money is needed to raise a family above an arbitrary poverty level. The statistics tell how many families are poor, to what ethnic and racial groups they belong, and in what sections of the country they live (Table

11-1). But numbers do not tell the whole story. It is true that the amount of income must be the major criterion for the measurement of poverty, but what happens to the income is equally important. For example, there are two families of four, each with an income of $20,000 a year: not much in today's economy. One family lives on a stringent budget; there is always more rice and pasta on the table than meat; the only entertainment is that which is practically free: television, sports in the public park, and, infrequently a trip to a dollar movie. If a meal is eaten out, it is at McDonald's, not at a downtown French restaurant. Clothes are bought in budget departments on sale and are worn until they no longer can be mended. The other family has the same income, but the father is out almost every night in a bar drinking with his buddies, buying them rounds, and flirting with the women who are attracted to his apparently free style of spending. These nightly adventures are expensive, his wife and children often literally go to bed hungry, there is frequently not enough money to pay the electric and phone bills, and the children never have new clothes. Which family is poor and which is not? It depends on who is making the judgment. A stranger seeing a man in a bar every night may assume he has plenty of money for such frivolity and not know that his family is literally starving. A black woman on welfare with six children might look at a family eating hamburgers in a restaurant and be envious. A physician's wife living in the affluent suburbs might think that a family that cannot afford to send its children to college is living in abject poverty. Poverty is relative, and there is no way that the question "How much is enough?" can be answered. It is in the nature of the vast majority of people always to want more than they have. There are always greener economic pastures, and most people, when asked if they can afford everything they want, will say no.

Who are the poor in the United States? The elderly are poorer than younger people. Women are poorer than men. Nonwhites are poorer than whites. Statistics from 1976 indicate that the median income of an elderly family is about half that of a nonelderly family. Of people over age 65, 15% are below the poverty level (more than three times as many blacks as whites fall into this category). More than half of all families headed by a person over age 65 had an annual income below $8,311.[1] (The double-digit inflation of recent years affects the elderly's expenditures but not income.) People who are born poor generally remain poor. The poor are most often the socially and culturally disadvantaged: the ones who, no matter how hard they try, have less of a chance to rise out of poverty than do others. There are many complex social, cultural, and psychological factors operating to make this so, but it seems that it all boils down to the fact that some groups of people hold opinions about other groups of people. If some groups of people hold negative opinions about other groups, social and economic discrimination is bound to occur, forcing the disliked group into an economic position that is worse than the group doing the disliking. And if a population imbalance exists, that is, if the disliked group is a minority, the economic distinctions will be heightened.

The young do not like elderly people very much. There are many reasons—not wanting to be reminded of the future, the nearness of death that is inherent in the elderly, and the fear of physical

Table 11-1. Distribution of income in the United States (1976)*

TOTAL MONEY INCOME	PERCENTAGE OF FAMILIES
Under $3,000	3.9
$ 3,000-4,999	6.5
5,000-6,999	7.8
7,000-8,999	8.0
9,000-11,999	11.9
12,000-14,999	12.1
15,000-19,999	19.1
20,000-24,999	12.9
25,000 and over	17.8

*From Bureau of the Census statistical abstract of the United States, ed. 98, Washington, D.C., 1977, U.S. Government Printing Office.

frailty. Partly because of this essential dislike, elderly people are forced out of their jobs at a certain age, removed from the nuclear family, given a fixed amount of money on which to live, and are generally ignored. And the people we do not like, we do not want to see. So we establish old-age homes in high-rise buildings, which are remote and impersonal, and "leisure villages" way out in the country where we never go. We do not like elderly people, so we hide them away, do not permit them to earn a living, and then we dislike them even more when their poverty reaches a point at which they can no longer survive on their own and are forced to come back to young people for help. (See Chapter 17 for a more complete discussion of the problems of aging.)

During the course of American history, women have been placed by men in socially and economically subservient positions. They have been kept dependent by men and also perhaps by their own inertia and timidity. The fact remains that, for whatever reason, they have been more dependent than independent; it could be interpreted that men do not like women very much, and, as dependent people, women become even more unlikable. Consequently they are kept poor.

White people do not like nonwhite people. This is evident from the course of our history, but it is a defeatist kind of philosophy. Because white people dislike blacks and other nonwhite people, the cycle of events described in regard to the elderly is the same. Consequently nonwhites are objects of derision and contempt. So it could be argued that blame for the existence of poverty should be placed on the nonpoor, *not* because they are not poor, but because they need, for a variety of reasons, to keep other people poor.

Causes

People who are born poor tend to remain poor, and the cycle is perpetuated, for several reasons. There is ignorance about the opportunities (which may be few and far between, but they *do* exist) to break out of poverty. Those who have no experience with the way in which business and industry operate do not know how to benefit from the system. For children growing up in a ghetto, there is barely a knowledge that an outside world exists. Even if there is awareness of another way of living, the skills to live another kind of life are absent, and so one must remain where one is.

People ignorant of the choices today work in jobs where their productivity is so restricted as to leave them below the poverty line. If they were aware of other opportunities, many could move to jobs where their productivity and income would rise above the poverty line. People ignorant of impending change in their present jobs are not currently training in the skills that would maximize their productivity in the future. Unprepared for the change, some of these people will drop below the poverty line when change comes. If they know of prospective changes, they could begin to train now for the future.[2,p.90]

Something else that tends to keep people poor is the absence of achievement motivation. Sheer laziness, although it certainly exists in all of us at one time or another, is not all there is to the lack of motivation. The fear of inevitable doom or failure is a strong reason not to make an effort. It is easy to say, "I'm black and a woman, so no one will hire me anyway." Since black women have had a notoriously hard time climbing out of poverty, this is not an unrealistic and unreasonable attitude. It is simply not a very productive one. Achievement motivation is a behavior learned at home during childhood, so if a father is content to collect unemployment or welfare and chooses not to work, there is small likelihood that his son or daughter will be motivated to do much else. Or if the child is somehow motivated, there may not be much encouragement from the parent, and motivation can die. Someone who comes from poverty may be aware of the goal of nonpoverty and may even have the desire to develop the skills to achieve this goal. But the journey to the goal may be so lond and so arduous that the sustained motivation is lacking. If there is no experience with the establishment of subgoals and no tools to achieve them, motivation may die.

Family obligations also can keep people poor. This is especially true of women who are made to feel obligated by society to stay home and care for children. The feminist slogan, "Every married woman is only one man away from welfare," may seem overly dramatic, but it is true. A woman who is totally dependent on her husband for money is poor. While he is working *and* while he is married to her, she may not feel poor. But if he dies, leaves her, or loses his job, she *will* be impoverished (Table 11-2). Few life insurance policies provide enough money for a widow to support herself and her children without having to look for a job outside the home. If she has never held a job and has no marketable skills, she is not much better off than the ghetto woman who has always struggled for survival. The "affluent" widow does not even have the survival skills that the ghetto woman has learned over the years.

In most states alimony has been abolished or severely altered.[3] Women are being awarded alimony for only fixed, short periods of time, and they are expected to use the time and money to get a job or to train for one to prepare for the day when alimony stops permanently. Women who have been married for twenty to forty years suddenly find themselves competing on the job market with much younger people who have commercially valuable skills. When the older woman's alimony stops and she still has not found a job, her only alternative is welfare.

Table 11-2. Median income by race and sex, 1970*

	TOTAL	WHITE	BLACK
United States	$ 9,870	$10,200	$6,300
Men (full-time)	8,965	9,375	6,600
Women (full-time)	5,325	5,490	4,675
Families (1972) with women heads	5,115	5,840	3,645
Men heads (wife not working)	10,930	9,976	6,500

*Reprinted with permission of Macmillan Publishing Co., Inc., from The care of health in communities, by Nancy Milio. Copyright © 1975 by Nancy Milio.

Income (percent of distribution)

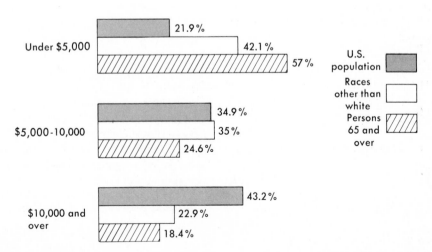

Fig. 11-1. Annual income by minorities and aged, 1970. (Reprinted with permission of Macmillan Publishing Co., Inc., from The care of health in communities, by Nancy Milio. Copyright © 1975 by Nancy Milio.)

The idea of punitive alimony . . . is almost extinct in fault and no-fault states. The guiding principle now is neither passion nor punishment, but economics, defined in the divorce courts as who needs how much, and who has it to give?[4]

It is usually the woman who needs money and the man who has it to give, and no matter how much alimony she receives or for how long, the woman's earning power will almost always be less than her husband's. With the divorce rate climbing steadily, a whole new category of poor people is emerging: formerly married women. And what of the woman who is still married and whose husband loses his job? She, too, becomes instantly poor, and if he cannot find work soon, she remains poor. If he no longer provides income for her, the married woman with the jobless husband is infinitely worse off than a widowed or divorced woman, who at least has alimony or insurance benefits, no matter how small.

Some circumstances utterly beyond people's control perpetuate poverty (Fig. 11-1). An unhealthy economy leads to high unemployment, and it is, of course, the people who are least employable who remain unemployed and continue to be poor. Personal disasters contribute to poverty. Poor people cannot afford fire and theft insurance, and they live in neighborhoods where the rates of robbery and arson are high. So when they are robbed or when their houses burn down, their poverty is exacerbated. Poor people also do not have health insurance, and if they have no jobs, they have no paid sick time, so not only must they pay for their own medical treatment (even in clinics there is a charge, and many people have never applied for Medicaid benefits), but they are also losing money by not being able to work. And people with chronic diseases are chronically unable to work. So the poverty cycle goes on.

Helping the poor to become nonpoor

How can a poor person become nonpoor? According to the medieval scholar Moses Maimonides (1135-1204)[5,p.369]:

There are eight degrees in the giving of charity. . . . The highest degree . . . is to take hold of a man who has been crushed . . . enter into partnership with him, or to find work for him, and thus to put him on his feet so that he will not be dependent on his fellow men.

It is as true today as it was in the twelfth century that the endless giving to and supporting of poor people will never help them to become nonpoor. Dependence never leads to independence.

The social welfare programs in this country (e.g., disability benefits from Social Security, various kinds of welfare, unemployment insurance, and workman's compensation) were all designed to help tide people over until they could again earn their own income. They were to prevent poverty for short periods of time, to put food in people's mouths while they looked for work. That original purpose has somehow become lost; now there does not seem to be any way to lessen the large numbers of people who are surviving solely on welfare, unemployment insurance, and the like. Welfare has, in many cases, become a trap. An unskilled laborer earns a salary so low, and taxes and other deductions are so high, that in many cases he can make more money from welfare than he can from a job. A woman with small children, no one to support her, and no way of leaving her children to look for work has no choice but to remain on welfare. A person with a physical disability of some kind has difficulty finding work, so he must remain on Social Security payments and live at a poverty level. The cycle is endless: poverty causes lack of education and poor preparation for jobs, so the person is forced onto welfare, which permits a standard of living that is well below the poverty level and fosters an attitude of dependence that keeps people mired in poverty.

PUBLIC AND PRIVATE TRANSFERS

The term transfer payments is used by economists to describe payments for which no work, goods, or services are received in exchange: charity. Short-run transfer payments *can* be used to give people the boost they need to rise out of poverty.

There are several different kinds of transfer payments. Private transfers within families extend all the way from the support of nonproductive children (college and professional students are included) to elderly relatives who can no longer work to other nonproductive family members: those with physical disabilities or those who simply choose leisure instead of work. Private nonfamily transfer payments are from charitable organizations, mostly springing from religions (e.g., National Jewish Welfare Board and National Conference of Catholic Charities) and from disease-oriented organizations such as the American Cancer Society or the Kidney Foundation. There are also miscellaneous charities such as the Salvation Army, which has a variety of services, including soup kitchens for down-and-out alcoholics and family-centered maternity hospitals; Goodwill Industries; and the Red Cross. They are all organized to give short-term financial help to people who are temporarily "crushed," in Maimonides' words. None are designed to support people forever, but it has come to be that without the continuing partial help of these agencies, many poor people would not be able to survive.

Although millions of dollars pass from the nonpoor to the poor every year through private transfers, the sum is but a drop in the bucket compared with the billions involved in government transfers.

These government transfer programs originally were designed to provide income to persons who might otherwise be made poor by the operation of the market system. However, the following is true:

1. A large portion of transfer funds (about 40%) go to people who would *not* be poor in the absence of these programs.
2. A large number of people are poor but are not helped by these programs. . . .
3. Many poor people remain poor after receiving government transfers[2,p. 145]

In addition to the government transfers mentioned previously, including Medicare and Medicaid discussed in another chapter, there are veterans' benefits, food stamps, distribution of surplus food, hot lunch programs for schoolchildren, various kinds of public housing assistance, and all kinds of counseling and social services. It is entirely possible for an individual to be born into a family that is supported by government transfers, grow up in this family learning the system, and then spend the rest of his life being supported by government money. Even if he works long enough to contribute to Social Security and to be eligible for unemployment benefits, he is not essentially an independent human being, and he still needs the government transfers to survive. This is not a value judgment; it is merely a demonstration of how the original philosophy of government transfers has changed and become distorted. Most of the programs were developed in the 1930s during the Depression when there was widespread unemployment and impending starvation. The programs were thought to be stopgap measures until the economy improved. The system, however, snowballed partly because many of those made poor by the Depression never recovered and partly because of the liberalization of the general social and cultural climate. Bureaucracy tends to perpetuate itself, and as the system grew, the need and demand grew. Only about one third of the poor are lifted out of poverty by government transfers, one third are helped but remain poor, and one third are not helped at all.[2] And because the poor still pay taxes on income that is not from government transfers, they are actually contributing to the support of other poor and even of nonpoor people. As a result they have an even greater need for government and private transfers. The cycle of poverty goes on.

EMPLOYMENT

The most obvious way for a poor person to become nonpoor, now that we have seen that transfers are not the answer, is to put him to work so that he will become independent. This is easier said than done, but there are some human and economic measures that could help. Increasing the demand for employment by increasing the productivity of goods and services is one way. As unemployment drops, consumer spending increases, and production demands increase. Job opportunities *do* exist, but if people are not aware of them, the jobs go begging. There must be improved methods of publicizing jobs and training people to do them. It is a simple matter of arithmetic to see that it is cheaper for the government to train a person for a job than it is to feed, house, and clothe him for the rest of his life. There also needs to be increased mobility to where the jobs are. It does no good to be stuck in a city ghetto when there is work available building interstate highways in the country. It would behoove the government to provide subsidies to help people to move to areas of the country where there is employment. The obstacles to participating in the labor force should be reduced. More quality day care is needed so women with young children can work. The subject of racial and ethnic discrimination in employment can and does fill volumes and need not be discussed here. Suffice it to say that discrimination is a tremendous obstacle to work and should not be tolerated for economic if for no other reasons.

PERSONAL ATTITUDES

The development of human potential is another, even less tangible, way for the poor to become nonpoor. Education, values, ethics, and attitudes in the home passed from parent to child are perhaps the greatest influence on either keeping people poor or motivating them to become nonpoor. The government, of course, has no right to step into the privacy of one's home to try to change attitudes, and great controversy exists about whether any person has the right to try to change any other person, or even if essential personality change is possible after a certain age. As nurses we should be concerned with improving people's lot in life, but it is impossible to break the bonds of poverty without changing attitudes. As community nurses we are among the few professional health workers who can go into people's homes in a nonpunitive manner. Welfare workers go into homes to "check up" on welfare recipients and to see how many people are actually living there and what the relationships are. Credit companies go into repossess furniture and appliances. Building inspectors and sanitation

workers are looking for reasons to condemn buildings. Only community nurses have no "ax to grind." We can establish long-term relationships with poor families, and, although in the vast majority of instances we can make no permanent impact, there *are* those shining moments when our intervention has caused someone to make a decision that will permanently improve the course of his life. Many studies in social psychology have shown that attitudinal changes are extremely difficult to accomplish; there is no doubt that attitudes learned at home are the single most powerful influence on how a person lives.

Poverty and health

How does poverty increase the health risk of individuals and families? The obvious superficial answer is that poor people get sick more frequently because they have inadequate, if any, health maintenance (Fig. 11-2). They stay ill longer because they have limited access to health care facilities, and the facilities to which they have access are generally of lower quality than those which are available to nonpoor people.[6] The United States National Health Survey (NHS) reports higher morbidity and mortality among poor people than among the nonpoor. Chronic illness sufficient to cause a limitation of function is four times higher among the poor, and the number of days lost from work because of illness is almost twice as high.[7] "As measured by periods of disability spent in bed, the upper income person has a rate of 5.2 days per year, compared with 12.0 in the poor person. In terms of types of 'restricted activity,' the higher income person loses 13.1 days per year, compared with 29.1 days for the poor person."[7,p.238] According to the NHS the six leading types of chronic illness in the United States are heart disease, arthritis and rheumatism, mental and nervous conditions, high blood pressure, visual impairments, and orthopedic impairments. For all six of these conditions, the heaviest burden is on the poor.

The reasons for the higher incidence of illness and death among the poor are many and complex: the handicaps of inadequate housing; not enough

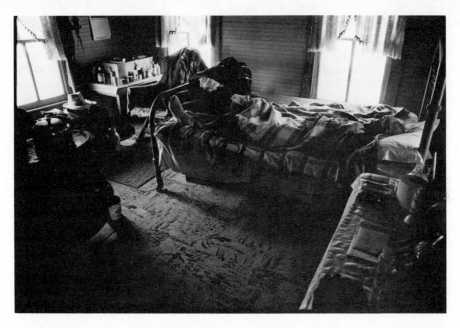

Fig. 11-2. Poverty and loneliness increase the incidence and severity of all health problems. (Photograph by Michael D. Smith; courtesy Editorial Photocolor Archives, Inc., New York.)

heat in winter; insufficient clothing; poor nutrition; being forced to work in unhealthy occupations (few professional and white-collar workers contract silicosis, or "black lung" disease); lack of health education and inadequate knowledge about how to prevent disease; the refusal, for a variety of reasons, to seek medical attention while an illness is in the beginning stages; and a generally unhealthy life-style.

Health services available to the poor and the comparison of these services with those of the non-poor have been discussed in various places in this text, but it should be emphasized that even though services are available, the poor do not take advantage of them at the rate one would expect and hope. Health care today is so technologically sophisticated that even a routine physical examination, with its attendant thumping, prodding, poking, and blood taking must be tremendously frightening to someone who has no idea of what is going to happen. And all the reassurance in the world may have no effect. Consider this analogy: I know intellectually that a roller coaster ride is not fatal. It is, in

fact, extremely safe, and passengers always come back no worse for their experience. There is, however, not a ghost of a chance that I will *ever* willingly go on a roller coaster: I simply have too much "gut fear." This fear may well be akin to people's beliefs about a trip to the doctor. Poor people who do not have the education and experience may not know that they should see a physician when something is wrong. If one does not know that chest pains are a symptom of heart disease, no action is taken until it may be too late. Prescribed drugs are taken at a lower rate by poor people partly because a trip to the corner druggist for a patent medicine is quicker and cheaper than a trip to the doctor and partly because people distrust ingesting strange substances as a result of lack of knowledge about what the drug will and will not do.

An interesting fact about the health care of the poor is that two thirds of health expenditures for poor people go to hospital care and one third for outpatient care. Among nonpoor people the ratio is exactly the opposite.[7] In addition, once admitted to the hospital, the poor person stays longer. There are several reasons for this: his illness is usually at a more advanced state by the time he is admitted, so recovery takes longer; the poor person is likely to be "teaching material" for the interns and residents, so he is kept longer to be more thoroughly studied; and his home conditions are apt to be so unhealthy that a relapse would be likely, so he is kept in the hospital until his recovery is more complete. All these factors tend to make a rather traumatic hospital stay, and the poor client is often discharged after an intensely negative experience, vowing never to go near the medical establishment again.

The poor, because of their lack of health knowledge and sophistication, tend to be easily bamboozled by quacks, chiropractors, herbalists, and other cultist practitioners, who promise quick cures from potions that are useless at best and downright dangerous at worst for what seems like very little money. These charlatans abound in poor neighborhoods, bilking the gullible and ignorant out of their money *and* thus preventing them from seeking legitimate medical care.

There is no doubt that poverty itself is one of the main causes of the high incidence of morbidity and mortality among the poor. Some of the causes of illness could be eliminated with the eradication of poverty, but, since this is not likely to happen in our lifetime, there must be some special effort made to provide quality health care for the poor. There are two competing philosophies about how to do this: the "separatists" and those who prefer the "mainstream" approach.

Separate health facilities for the poor have existed for many years, first in the form of municipal hospitals with their outpatient departments (or special clinics in voluntary hospitals) and then later in the form of neighborhood health centers like those funded through the OEO. There are great financial disadvantages to the separate facilities approach. This was well demonstrated in June, 1977, when the Philadelphia General Hospital closed its doors after almost a hundred years of continuous operation. The city could no longer afford to maintain the hospital, and the decision was made after years of fighting in city council. Neighborhood health centers almost always operate in the red and are constantly plagued by crime and vandalism. I visited one not long ago, and there were two attack-trained guard dogs in the waiting room. The atmosphere was far less than neighborly. As was mentioned in Chapter 1, there is a problem finding quality medical and nursing personnel to staff the separate facilities.

But problems also exist when poor people are treated in mainstream health facilities. They tend to be segregated within an institution and receive less than optimum care. Clients who would formerly have been admitted to Philadelphia General Hospital are now distributed among several area voluntary hospitals, where they are put into separate units and are resented by hospital administrators because they are an added strain on the already overburdened financial resources. If outpatient clients are to receive the highest quality health care, they need to come to the great medical centers where the facilities and personnel are located, but then they face all the logistical problems that have already been discussed. The only possible solution to the problem is a drastic alteration in the nature of health care delivery.

UNEMPLOYMENT
Causes

If one is unemployed, one is poor, and we have seen how poverty adversely affects health. The obvious answer is to reduce unemployment; if everyone had a job (everyone, that is, who is mentally and physically capable of holding one), everyone's mental and physical health would improve. The economy would improve; billions of tax dollars would be saved because people would not require so many government transfer payments, and the general self-esteem of the country would be better.

Increased productivity leads to increased employment, which leads to increased consumer spending and therefore even greater productivity. It all seems so simple and straightforward. Why, then, is the rate of unemployment so high? What causes a capitalist economy to slow down, close its factories, and leave millions out of work? According to John Maynard Keynes (1883-1946), the brilliant British economist, an advanced capitalist society like the United States has a tendency to reach equilibrium with high unemployment. There is no built-in mechanism in the capitalist system to bring about full employment, so the government must intervene to compensate for inadequate private demand. With enough government spending, full employment, in principle, could be achieved. The government could spend money on housing, military buildup, or devising new ways to play baseball. It would not matter what the government spent money on, as long as jobs were provided. The economic impact would be the same, whatever the job; only the social and psychological influences would vary. The Keynesian philosophy is firmly implanted in the economic policies of the United States and most capitalist countries. The use of government expenditures (money received from the taxes of citizens) controls the level of employment and unemployment, and in this way the economy is controlled. Capitalist governments now have a goal of stabilizing unemployment at levels they see as politically acceptable, and the question of inequality of income has become unimportant.

The alternative to this system is, of course, Marxist socialism, and even the most casual observer of the Russian economic system since the revolution in 1902 will see the slow but steady trend toward the increase of capitalist practice in a supposedly socialist economy. So we are left with an imperfect economic system; the challenge is to reduce unemployment to the lowest possible level without causing the system to collapse. Keynes did much of his conceptualizing about his economic theories during the period between the stock market crash in 1929 and the outbreak of World war II. We are heir to his concept of what the capitalist system should be.

For my own part, I believe that there is social and psychological justification for significant inequalities of incomes and wealth, but not for such large disparities as exist today. There are valuable human activities which require the motive of money-making and the environment of private wealth-ownership for their full fruition. Moreover, dangerous human proclivities can be canalised into comparatively harmless channels by the existence of opportunities for money-making and private wealth, which, if they cannot be satisfied in this way, may find their outlet in cruelty, the reckless pursuit of personal power and authority, and other forms of self-aggrandisement. It is better that a man should tyrannise over his bank balance than over his fellow-citizens; and whilst the former is sometimes denounced as being but a means to the latter, sometimes at least it is an alternative.[8,p.120]

Keynes had some notions about human nature, greed, and personal power that seem fairly naive when viewed with today's knowledge of organized crime and its encroachment on legitimate business, the dangerous by-products of the drive to ever increase profits—pollution in our atmosphere, dangerous chemicals in food, automobiles that fall apart under stress—and the evident need of big business to control our lives, all in the name of "money-making and private wealth."

As President Herbert Hoover said, "Business is the business of America," and if we must continue to live with the Keynesian philosophy and a capitalist economy, then there should be a way to provide jobs for those who want them. It is, however, in the nature of capitalism to generate wealth and poverty and employment and unemployment at opposite ends of poles.

This law of capitalist development, which is equally applicable to the most advanced metropolis and the most backward colony, has of course never been recognized by bourgeois economists. They have rather propagated the apologetic notion that a levelling-up tendency is inherent in capitalism. . . . This is where the second part of the explanation becomes relevant. At the root of capitalist poverty one always finds unemployment and underemployment—what Marx called the industrial reserve army—which directly deprive their victims of income and undermine the security and bargaining powers of those with whom the unemployed compete for scarce jobs.[9,p.165]

This is obviously a Marxist view of economic philosophy, but it actually bears out what Keynes was espousing as a desirable state of affairs. So it seems that both the capitalists and Marxists agree that unemployment will always be with us, and the problem still remains of what to do about it. Economists generally agree that an unemployment rate of 4% is ideal for a stable economy, and greater employment would lead to wage increases and inflation. However, during the 1970s, inflation increased drastically while the unemployment rate also increased, although at a slower rate. It seems that inflation will always be with us whether we have "full" employment (4% unemployed) or the 8% to 9% unemployment that was common in the last decade and that threatens to rise higher in this decade. Those who want to see the eradication of unemployment argue that prices should be permitted to rise in the social interest of full employment; those who fear rampant inflation want to halt rising production with its consequent high employment. The economic issue is whether we are willing to risk higher prices in order to achieve full employment.

Possible cures

If the Keynesian philosophy is to be carried to its practical conclusion, the government would intervene and provide jobs by inventing avenues of production. The government money that would ordinarily be spent on transfer payments for the poor and unemployed could be used to provide jobs. Would it not be better, economically, socially, and culturally, to use tax revenues to help people become independent by providing them with jobs than to use the same money to encourage people to remain dependent by reinforcing existing patterns of behavior? This may seem like a simplistic view and is an obvious anathema to big business, but general tax revenues *do* come out of the pockets of citizens who should have a voice in how their money is to be spent.

One of the ways to counteract the effects of unemployment is the negative income tax devised by the University of Chicago economist Milton Friedman. The approach is simple, although there are many drawbacks. He recommends setting an arbitrary annual income on which a family could live and paying the difference between what is actually earned below that level and the determined income. Because everyone would have at least the minimum income, Friedman would abolish all existing government transfer payments and legislative reforms like welfare, Social Security, minimum wage laws, public housing assistance, Medicare, and all other government programs. In theory the need for these programs would be eliminated because everyone would be able to pay for everything out of their minimum income. But in practice, poor people might remain poor, or their situations could become even worse. A family with several dependent children, an unemployed mother, and a disabled father might receive a higher income from the combined benefits of Aid to Dependent Children, unemployment insurance, and Social Security disability payments than they would from whatever arbitrary minimum income was established. Friedman thinks the negative income tax is advantageous because it gives help in its most useful form, cash, and, although he admits that it reduces the incentive of people to help themselves, it does not entirely eliminate the incentive. The negative income tax would indeed be less costly to the taxpayer, but if the people who are theoretically to be helped are worse off than they were before, there is no point in saving money. According to Friedman[10.p.295]:

The major disadvantage of the proposed negative income tax is its political implications. It establishes a system under which taxes are imposed on some to pay subsidies to others. And presumably, these others have a vote. There is always the danger that instead of being an arrangement under which the great majority tax themselves willingly to help an unfortunate minority, it will be converted into one under which a majority imposes taxes for its own benefit on an unwilling minority.

The race riots of the 1960s gave way to civil rights marches and rallies in which blacks, women, and other disadvantaged people demanded jobs and other forms of equality. Since the people who were demonstrating were the ones who were out of work, the eventual response of government and big business made a temporary difference in the numbers of people unemployed. Boycotts of products manufactured by companies who discriminated against minorities eventually had an effect. It is now difficult to find a large company that does not have its "do-good" activities. Part of this new attitude is dictated by the federal government's affirmative action program, and part is dictated by good business sense: if a group of people is threatening to burn down your factory, it seems a good idea to hire some of them. The National Association of Manufacturers instituted a program to teach school dropouts in Harlem how to read, write, type, and then apply for jobs in civil service, banks, and other businesses. Many large companies hire unemployable adults, train them in a skill, and also pay for completion of a high school education. In this way the company assuages the ranks of the unemployed by demonstrating a sincere attempt to help people become employable; it also assures itself a steady stream of trained employees. Continuing pressure from militants and activists ensures that these programs are not simply pilot projects that never take off.

In 1968 a group of United States senators proposed legislation that would create, in areas of the country where unemployment is high, corporations for the poor in which the community would own and operate essential services such as day-care centers, job counseling and placement, and banks. Federal "seed money" would be provided, and the stock would be owned by community members who ran the businesses. There would also be provisions for tax advantages for companies that set up plants in areas designated as having high unemployment. The companies would then sell the plant to the community development corporation, which would, in turn, be lightly taxed. The New York Urban Coalition is an excellent example of about 150 business, labor, and civil rights leaders who provide assistance for community development corporations in the ghettos. They raise millions of dollars of private money to provide jobs and training for the hard-core unemployed.

There are 8,500 building-trade unions in this country (this is building trade only and does not include the thousands of other trade unions, such as teamsters, garment workers, and steel and auto workers) that have systematically discriminated against blacks and have contributed to the unemployment problem. So many discrimination suits were being filed against the unions that the AFL-CIO decided to take some positive action to recruit blacks.

During the mid-1960s the Ford Motor Co. in Detroit began an experiment to enter the inner-city ghettos and hire hard-core unemployed black people on the spot, without bothering with the usual aptitude tests and application forms. Ford did more than simply recruit blacks; its representatives personally went to the ghetto to lead people by the hand into the factory and to jobs. This approach is certainly commendable in theory, but there are many practical disadvantages. A person who is considered hard-core unemployed is not going to adjust easily to the rules, regulations, and discipline of a structured workday. If he has no training for the job he is expected to do, he will either be fired quickly or become discouraged and quit. This is what happened at Ford. The experiment was a good idea, but the hard-core unemployed need orientation to the whole work atmosphere, and changes in self-concept are not always smoothly assimilated. Other companies will surely be prompted to follow Ford's example, and the more people who are absorbed into the labor force in a community, the better. The economy of an area improves with a decrease in unemployment.

However, even with federally funded affirmative action programs and with private industry's response to the programs, the liberal activities of the 1960s and 1970s have not accomplished their goal.

True, there are more members of minorities working now than there were 20 years ago, but the hard core unemployed have not been significantly helped, and women still earn only 59¢* to every dollar earned by men. The great liberal experiment was only partially successful which may be why the country took such a significant turn to the right in 1980.

The affluent unemployed

A large and ever-increasing group of unemployed people are those who are overeducated and overtrained for available jobs. The drastic decrease in space exploration has led to the joblessness of thousands of highly specialized people whose technological abilities are no longer needed. These are mostly white upper–middle class men who were supporting wives (most of whom did not work), children, and extremely expensive suburban lifestyles. They do not have the years of developed "street" knowledge of ghetto dwellers to help them cope with unemployment. Many do not even know how to apply for unemployment benefits or food stamps, and many are unable to because they cannot face what they perceive to be the humiliation of being on the "public dole." In some respects the impact of unemployment is harder on these people than it is on the hard-core unemployed because of the drastic change in circumstances. If one has never had three cars, a $125,000 home, expensive furniture, and a swimming pool, one cannot know what it is to have them repossessed. Not having a lifetime of experience with unemployment tends to lead to a lack of ability to cope with it when it occurs, and many upper–middle class men sink into depression and often turn to alcohol for solace. This is doubly defeating because one cannot go out to hunt for work when one is too depressed to get out of bed or too drunk to carry on a coherent interview. The plunge into poverty is so much more drastic from $80,000 a year than it is from the minimum wages of a grocery clerk that it is no wonder the affluent are less able

*Statistic from the National Organization for Women.

to cope with poverty than the poor. Not only space scientists are facing this problem. The military-industrial complex that was booming while we were involved in the Vietnam war for so many years has thrown many highly skilled and highly paid factory workers out of jobs. Teachers, because of decreases in school enrollment, are considering themselves lucky to find any job, and it is not uncommon to get into a taxi cab and find that the driver has a doctorate in philosophy or English literature. When asked, he will tell you that he is grateful to be working at all. "A substantial number of unemployed are those with research knowledge and talents who have developed the complex technology that is responsible for their unemployment."[11,p.107]

Unemployment and health

The way in which unemployment contributes to the health risk is twofold (Fig. 11-3). Unemployment is in itself unhealthy; it contributes to depression and all of its concomitant symptoms: drinking, sleeplessness, the lack of motivation to look for work, and even suicide. Unemployed people have no health insurance provided by an employer, and they are loath to pay (and frequently do not have the money for) the high cost of individual payment premiums. There is always the hope that next week they will find a job and that luck will hold and stave off illness during unemployment. Unemployed people are poor people and have all the problems of poverty. Women sometimes become pregnant while their husbands are unemployed (sex is free entertainment, and there may not be enough money for contraception) and then need to spend precious money either terminating the pregnancy or paying for prenatal care. The diets of people who suddenly find themselves unemployed usually change for the worse, and families who have no idea that other sources of protein exist besides meat, fish, and poultry become heir to all kinds of illnesses which are intensified by poor nutrition.

Unemployment breeds discontent, particularly if it goes on and on, and discontent breeds violent crime, which most assuredly is not healthy. People

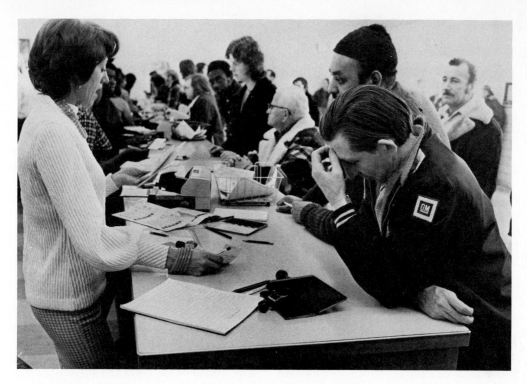

Fig. 11-3. Unemployment leads to a cycle of poverty and high health risks. (Photograph by Andrew Sacks; courtesy Editorial Photocolor Archives, Inc., New York.)

who are chronically unemployed have time on their hands to permit resentments to grow into bitterness and perhaps to violence. Armed robbery, assault and battery, and other violent personal crimes are usually not committed by people who have steady (legal) jobs. Younger and younger people are committing violent crimes. It is not uncommon for 12-year-olds to be brought repeatedly into juvenile court after they have violently attacked other people.[6] The person with a habitual criminal record cannot find work (even the Ford Motor Co. refused to hire people with criminal records judged to be incorrigible), becomes permanently unemployed, and may commit more frequent and more vicious crimes.

If economists consider "full" employment to include only 4% unemployed, that still means that 10 million people are out of work.[12] This conservative estimate does not include all the unemployed who do not register for (or are not eligible for) unemployment insurance and thus do not appear in the statistics. It also does not include those who have never been employed, are not known to Social Security, and thus "do not exist" in the eyes of the government. Having 10 million people who are not earning their own living when they are physically and mentally capable of doing so is not a healthy way to run a society. Simply giving people jobs that they do not want and cannot handle is not the answer; they will soon quit or be fired. Handing people money for an indefinite period of time that they have not earned merely fosters dependence and perpetuates the cycle of unemployment defeatism. The negative income tax has more disadvantages than advantages and is not supported by the electorate. On-the-job training is expensive and is practical in only a small number of instances. Formal education requires the motivation and foresight of a future-oriented philosophy, which is lacking in the chronically unemployed. Continued public support of those who do not work will place an unbearable strain on our capitalist economy. Continued high rates of unemployment lead to social unrest, crime, and riots. The eventual breakdown of social order has happened so frequently in world history that it is naive to think that it cannot happen here. What then is the solution? Aside from the alternatives already discussed, it seems that only the individual's own inner strength can help. It may be perfectly legitimate to blame social and economic conditions for the causes of unemployment, but this is of no practical help in getting a job. Only individual motivation, determination, and the need for personal gratification will make a person get up in the morning, wash his face, and pound the pavement every day until he finds work.

THE COMMUNITY NURSE

The community nurse can help, though in a limited way, by using her professional skills to help people motivate themselves. This is an enormous task and involves high levels of interpersonal communication.

In nursing the interpersonal relationship is a caring one. Caring is akin to warmth. It differs from warmth in that it is more enduring and more unconditional. Caring comes from a reverence for life; this general appreciation of humanity translates into concern for the cares of the individual. Caring creates a social climate that communicates feelings of goodwill and concern when feelings cannot be put into words. Human pain has many sources: the physical diseases that scourge man, as well as wounds of the mind and spirit. The challenge is to learn that care of the patient is inseparable from *caring* for him.[13,p.17]

The client must also be able to trust the nurse, which is sometimes difficult, particularly if he is not able to trust himself. A chronically unemployed person has learned to distrust the system, the social order, and probably most of the people with whom he associates. There is no reason for him to immediately trust the community nurse merely because of her good intentions. An atmosphere of

mutual trust, if it develops at all, takes time and a great deal of effort on the part of both the nurse and the client. It is a tremendous intellectual, as well as emotional, exercise for a community nurse to empathize with a client who is unable to get a job. How can she, whose professional skills are in demand all over the country and who can pick and choose among a wide variety of jobs, know what it *feels* like not to work? How can she feel the pain, humiliation, and degradation of having to depend on others for the fulfillment of even the most basic needs? How can she know what it is like to have an empty refrigerator and hungry children? There is no way to truly experience the pain of another human being, but the effort to mentally place oneself in another person's life may be worthwhile if empathy can be increased.

For the communication process to be helpful in getting the client to motivate himself, there must be a sense of mutual respect between the nurse and the client. It has become almost a cliché among health care workers that social and cultural differences between the client and the worker must be respected. Clichés are boring, but they are almost always based on truth.

Implicit in respect is the concept of acceptance of man in his totality: what he is and what he does; yet behavior that results from a patient's perceptions has a reality impact ethically, morally and legally. Thus *total* acceptance seems to be a difficult conceptual stance to take. Total acceptance of *all* behavior implies that the patient is able to control himself within the context of the situation.[13,p.24]

Perhaps total acceptance is not a reasonable or practical goal of the nurse working with the hard-core unemployed. Perhaps *changing* a person's perception of reality is a more logical approach than merely accepting it. If a person's perception of the world, or at least his part of it, is that it is a place in which he will never be able to earn a living, then he probably never will. If, however, he can be convinced that at least part of his reality is erroneous, then his perception of that reality may be altered. If a 30-year-old black man who cannot read or write can be shown direct and concrete evidence of other people in *his* situation who have become literate enough to obtain and hold a job, then he may be motivated to try also. If there is no evidence of a way out of his predicament, then there is no reason for him to believe that his situation could change. He must be shown "success stories" of people who are like himself and with whom he can relate. It does no good to use an example of a 15-year-old high school dropout who has returned to school. ("I'm twice his age; he has his whole life before him.") Neither does it help to show him a white man in a similar situation ("He's white and isn't discriminated against on the job") or a woman, a man with an education, or anyone else in a situation with which he cannot identify. Respect is an essential ingredient in communicating with people we wish to help, but its too-narrow definition can thwart some attempts at creative solutions to problems.

LACK OF EDUCATION
Problems

Education can sometimes counteract defeatism at home. The school is important mainly because every child must pass through the system. The quality of public education, particularly in metropolitan areas, is declining steadily and rapidly, and social and occupational skills that once could be learned in school are now nonexistent. "The schools in many cities have turned into criminal dens where the distraught teacher spends most of the time trying to keep order. The FBI reports that . . . 70,000 teachers were assaulted in U.S. schools and the cost of vandalism reached $600 million. Every school day an estimated 200,000 New York City kids are truant. At least some are fleeing the danger of the classroom."[6] There are still instances, though, when a child, almost always with the help of a teacher who cares, can have his eyes opened to the alternatives to poverty. Vocational education is an important way to prepare people for the job market. If children could be prevented from quitting school until they are old enough to be admitted to vocational high schools,

they would have an excellent chance of escaping poverty. But quitting school is almost endemic among poor people who cannot see the long-term value of an education. Again, attitudes learned at home are hard to change.

Adult training and education is another way to escape poverty. When unemployment is high, on-the-job training (OJT) is low because employers can take their pick of experienced workers, and unskilled laborers are not hired. People lucky enough to participate in OJT and apprenticeship programs learn valuable trades that can be taken from one employer to another. The military has been an excellent source of training for the unskilled. Military training itself (except insofar as self-discipline is concerned) is not very useful to civilian life, but most of the skills needed to run the machinery and bureaucracy of the military are also needed to run civilian businesses. A truck is a truck, whether it has army stars or a company logo painted on its side, and knowing how to keep it running is a highly marketable skill. And if one can drive a tank, one can surely drive a truck. The federal government has instituted a variety of OJT programs, notably the Manpower Development and Training Administration (MDTA) and Job Opportunities in the Business Sector (JOBS), which have been only moderately successful.

A lack of education leads to unemployment, which leads to poverty (money may be "the root of all evil," but the lack of it is certainly not a source of good) and greater than average health risks. Although free public education is mandatory in the United States until age 16, there are thousands of children who quit school well before their sixteenth birthday, or, if they do not formally quit, they are truant so frequently that they may as well not be enrolled at all. Functional illiteracy[14] is prevalent, even among high school graduates,[15] and absolute illiteracy suggests that the mandatory education laws are being flouted on a rather grand scale.

There are many reasons why students quit school. As was mentioned earlier, the acquisition of an education requires, at least to some degree, a future-oriented philosophy. The student must be convinced that the long hours he spends in a classroom, learning things which to him seem totally useless (after all, how many employers are actually impressed with the fact that we know when Christopher Columbus reached these shores?), will pay off with a job. He looks around and sees his friends and neighbors who did stay in school standing in the unemployment line, and he becomes discouraged. He hears on the radio that people with doctorates are driving trucks, and his discouragement lapses into cynicism. Then the poverty-stricken ghetto student takes another look around him and sees his buddies who quit school ahead of him making lots of money. They run numbers for the local "organization bosses"; they snatch purses from old ladies; they sell their bodies; they rob their corner grocer and druggist; they sell drugs. These buddies are wearing fine clothes and have the awed "respect" of the neighborhood. There is a great deal of fast tax-free money to be made on the streets, so the student wonders why he should sit in a stuffy and boring classroom.

These are some of the external reasons for quitting school. There are also internal ones: the nature of the school system itself. The physical plant of many inner-city schools leaves much to be desired. The meager facilities that the board of education can afford to provide are quickly destroyed, vandalized, or stolen. Bands of young toughs roam the halls, mugging students and teachers alike, sexually assaulting both men and women (and even young boys and girls) in the bathrooms, and generally making attendance at school risky. Schools are old and badly in need of maintenance. Space is often at a premium, and the overcrowding problem has become so severe that many schools are on double and even triple sessions. This creates grim conditions for the teachers, and it is no wonder that they are often portrayed as a humorless, disgruntled group of people. Teachers who have to fight for every piece of chalk and every inch of space do not have much energy left for creative caring in the classroom. By the same token, teachers burdened with the task of hall monitoring, ab-

sentee reports, lunch money distribution, and other nonteaching functions come to see their jobs as less than satisfying and consequently do a less than satisfactory job. The teaching load in public schools is burdensome: five different classes a day, preparation for these classes, reading homework and composition assignments, devising and correcting examinations, and keeping up with developments in one's field. These tasks, coupled with the unending clerical duties, are extremely time consuming, and soon the teacher begins to slack off by not reading homework assignments, by not updating lesson plans, or by taking unnecessary sick days and leaving the students to poorly prepared substitute teachers. And the quality of education declines.

The aura of hostility in many public schools is palpable. This is less true in suburban public schools, but there is also less unemployment in the suburbs than in the cities (although both crime in the schools and unemployment are on the rise in suburbia). Police, often with attack dogs, patrol the hallways and cafeteria, and there is always a teacher or an aide standing guard outside the bathrooms.

Under the circumstances, it is not difficult to understand why so many students react badly to school authority. If the student is not given any degree of free movement and if, in fact, the school does not provide a hospitable and suitable working and social environment, it does not seem likely that the student will view the system with any degree of charity.*

Why, then, should a student remain in such an atmosphere when he can have policemen, attack dogs, and general bedlam on the street? The desire to learn for the sheer joy of acquiring knowledge is a myth that has been perpetuated by academicians who have never set foot inside a ghetto school. If students do not see value in what they are being taught, they will not sit still for the les-

*From Lester, Jean: The teacher is also a victim. In Leacock, Eleanor B., editor: The culture of poverty, p. 114. Copyright © 1971 by Simon & Schuster, Inc. Reprinted by permission of Simon & Schuster, a Division of Gulf & Western Corporation.

sons. Gone are the days of politely folded hands and cherubic faces, gazing with respect and admiration at the teacher. Jean Lester, who spent several years teaching in the New York City school system, disagrees:

Contrary to popular educational mythology, it is surprisingly easy to motivate the shy, the backward, the recalcitrant, the underpriviledged or even the truant child. All it takes is a small dose of daily encouragement and a belief that the work that is being done is meaningful. I have often seen a small bit of faith in a child work great miracles. Children cannot resist a compliment, nor are they invulnerable to well-placed confidence in their intelligence. It fires their imaginations, expands their hopes, and opens up possibilities for their futures that they have never before envisaged or dreamed could be theirs.*

This may well be true, and Lester has had practical experience, but considering the dropout rate from public school, there most likely are not many encouraging words being passed from teachers to students.

Solving the problems

The problems of the public schools are almost impossible to solve, and most of them stem from a lack of money. City budgets all over the country are in acute crisis, and allocations for public schools are growing smaller. Teachers are being laid off, and "nonessential" curricula such as art, music, and sports are being eliminated. If there is no money for teachers, there is surely no money for maintenance of the physical plant. So solutions are going to have to come from places other than a checkbook. Parents are becoming increasingly interested in the operations—academic, fiscal, and general—of public schools and are demanding a greater voice in the decision-making process about what and how their children will be taught. Some groups, like the Amish in central Pennsylvania,

even refuse to send their children to public school at all. They believe that a public education will impinge on their own social and cultural mores; long and involved legal battles have been fought over this issue. A major reason that parents want increased participation in the schools is their view that in our society the school system is the entry point to the business and professional systems, and this view is well founded. Failure to do well in elementary school results in the child being placed in a nonacademic program in high school, which automatically precludes admission to college. The parents'

exclusion from involvement in the running of schools, combined with their children's educational failure, casts the schools in the light of denying to the poor equal access to economic and social success. The mutual distrust and fear between school and community which results leads at times to open hostility. In places such as New York City, where the overwhelming majority of the school staff is white and the school population more than 50 percent black, the conflict has become inextricably interwoven with the problem of race relations.*

Parental involvement in the school's organization and operation is a positive step forward, although this view may not be shared by teachers and school administrators. The principle of consumerism remains the same whether it is in the health care system or in the school system. The more a parent knows about what is happening inside the classroom and the more that is learned about educational philosophy in general, the more likely the parent is to motivate the youngster to stay in school, to help him with his homework, and to want to have a voice in the educational curriculum. Given the bureaucratic mess that typifies most big-city school systems, an ombudsman would definitely be an asset. Public schools are being supported by taxpayer money, are run by municipal governments, and should be held accountable to the citizens.

One of the major problems in the exercise of parental control over schools in areas where there is much poverty and unemployment is that there are few parents who have the knowledge, ability, and experience to know what they are doing when they try to institute changes. Change merely for its own sake is useless, and, unless the parents can offer some constructive suggestions for positive change, they might be better off waiting until they have learned more about education. The problem then arises of where the parents wil learn about learning. Parent education classes could be instituted, and it might well be the community nurse who initiates and coordinates the effort to do this.

Some forces operating within the public school systems are totally out of the control of either parents or school authorities: the dictation of standards and topics of subject matter. Business dictates to the universities what kinds of professional and technological programs it needs to prepare workers. Universities devise courses to meet the demand and then dictate to secondary schools what preparation is needed; thus there is little academic choice in high school if the student's goal is higher education. If the goal is an occupation or trade, the student must vie for a limited number of places in vocational/technical schools, and admission often depends on the degree of success achieved in elementary schools. Placement and aptitude examinations and college entrance boards are all standardized, and the results play a large role in the academic and occupational future of the student.[16] Parents, teachers, and even school administrators have almost nothing to say about whether these tests will be used.

Because parents of ghetto schoolchildren do not have the educational background necessary, it is difficult for them to make an informed impact on the school's organization and curriculum. One of the few alternatives open to them is to engage in social protest.

Much of the social protest has centered on the eradication of *de jure* and *de facto* school segregation. More

recent efforts have concentrated on the decentralization of city school systems and the substitution of local community control. It would appear that even if school districts were under the direct control of local parent and community groups, this form of organization would not preclude the disaffection of some groups from what would remain essentially a monopolistic, compulsory educational system. Such programs run the risk of being stillborn, strangled not only by the opposition of conservative forces supporting the traditional system, but also by internal factional disputes.*

It seems that not much can be done about the system itself, at least not in any large or permanent way. The solutions to the problems of the uneducated are similar to the solutions (if indeed there are any solutions) of the problems of the chronically unemployed. It again becomes a matter of individual choice and personal motivation, and the community nurse's role is important but limited to one-to-one relationships, which can include families as well as individuals. Role models must be found to convince children and adolescents to stay in school. The role models need not necessarily be positive ones. A 12-year-old whose older brother is in jail for armed robbery may have the negative example pointed out to him, although in a positive and nonthreatening way. It does little good to say, "Do you want to be locked up forever just like your brother?," when in fact the brother may be idolized as a hero or martyr. It might be better to emphasize the negative aspects of a life behind bars, in a way in which a 12-year-old can understand. Helping a child to expand his horizons, to think about what he could be, and to show him what options are open to him is the greatest gift that the community nurse can give a child who is on the verge of dropping out of school.

Maslow[17] has developed a sequential arrangement of need priorities (Fig. 11-4). The first level is physiological needs, which have to do with self-

*From Fuchs, Estelle: The Danish *friskoler* and community control. In Leacock, Eleanor B., editor: The culture of poverty, p. 188. Copyright © 1971 by Simon & Schuster, Inc. Reprinted by permission of Simon & Schuster, a Division of Gulf & Western Corporation.

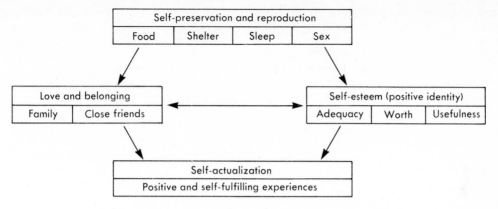

Fig. 11-4. Schematic representation of Maslow's need priorities.

preservation and reproduction. One must fulfill one's needs for food, shelter, sleep, and sex before one can be free to think about or take any action on the next level, which is the need for love and belonging. Everyone needs to be embraced by and have the interpersonal companionship of a family or a close group of friends who act as a family. Close emotional ties are essential for psychic survival. The need for security from physical and psychic harm and a sense of order and familiarity in one's life are equally essential. Only when these basic needs are met can the individual go to the next, more transcendent, level, which is the need for self-esteem. This is characterized by a positive identity: feelings of adequacy, worth, and usefulness. The higher one's self-regard, the better the ability to cope with life. Unless there is self-esteem, the last need of self-actualization cannot be met. Self-actualization can be described as the use of energy and capacities to create positive and self-fulfilling experiences for oneself. It is the ability to make dreams come true, or at least to make the effort. These needs must be met in the order in which Maslow listed them; if one is worried about whether there will be food on the table for the next meal, one will not have the energy left to plan a career. The community nurse needs to remember this first-things-first approach when she is working with families who are poor, uneducated, and unemployed. Given the social and economic conditions in which we live, society's tendency to main-

tain the status quo, people's need to have someone to discriminate against, and the defeatism (usually well founded) of people who have been mired in poverty for generations, it is easy to believe in the axiom, "The rich get richer and the poor get poorer."[18] A comparatively few poor people are able to lift themselves out of poverty, and few people who were born to affluent families ever sink to the levels of poverty discussed here.

Since little can be changed, why should the nurse bother at all? Because it is better to spend a year trying to help one person become independent than it is not to have tried at all. One human life salvaged is better than no human lives salvaged. It is a beneficial intellectual and professional exercise to understand the entire social and economic picture of poverty and its attendant unemployment and lack of education, but it is also possible to become paralyzed by the enormity of it all. It is much more practical to look at one family at a time and try to help that family within the context in which the members function.

A FAMILY SITUATION

The Kerper family lives in the shadow of the elevated railroad tracks in Harlem. Barbara Kerper is white, born in Appalachia, and is now 36 years old, although she appears to be closer to 45. She is a product of alcoholic parents who beat her, kept her out of school to work on the farm, and generally made her life miserable. When she was 17, she stole the few dollars cash her parents had in the house, packed a small bag, and went out to the main highway to hitch a ride to the "Big Apple" to a better life. If anything, life was worse. She had no skills, no friends, no money, and not even the sophistication to know how to seek public assistance. She got a few odd jobs that paid almost nothing, and she picked up men in order to go home with them and sleep between clean sheets. In due course she met a pimp, a black man named Arnie, who "professionalized" her and made her the star of his stable. Barbara worshiped Arnie, which is common in such working relationships, but what was unusual was that Arnie found himself falling in love with Barbara. He fought the feeling for as long as he could (Barbara was an important source of income to him), but finally his ego could no longer permit him to sell the woman he loved, his property, to other men. So Barbara moved into Arnie's apartment (there was no marriage), stopped taking birth control pills at his direction, and began having babies: five in all.

Arnie is a "revolving door jailbird," in and out of prison for a variety of offenses, almost all dealing with physical violence and the sale of illegal drugs. Three of the older children, ages 15, 13, and 12, have been in trouble with the police on a number of occasions, all for theft of one kind or another. The oldest has officially quit school; the next two are still registered but are truant so frequently that they are unable to follow the lessons when they do attend. The youngest, ages 7 and 9, are still in school, but they idolize their elder siblings, complain about having to go to school, and attend only because they still are afraid of the beatings they know they will receive at home if their mother finds out they are playing hooky. The 13-year-old girl, Connie, has been raped twice, once in the schoolyard by a gang of boys her own age and once by a "friend" of her father.

Arnie's stable of prostitutes deserted him, preferring to work the streets independently. Because he is a small-time hoodlum and not very bright, his drug profits are constantly being stolen or embezzled.

Barbara is in a trap. Her only source of money is what Arnie chooses to give her, which is very little very infrequently. When he is in jail, there is nothing at all. Every time Barbara suggests getting a job, Arnie smacks her across the mouth and says, "No woman of mine is gonna work." She feels a sense of responsibility toward her children, but at the same time she hates and resents them for keeping her at home. She sees no escape, so she relieves her anger, frustration, and boredom by beating them. Although she lives in an almost entirely black ghetto, Barbara is white, and her conjugal arrangement with a black man is disapproved of by the neighbors to the point of total social ostracism. Welfare is an inadequate source of income, and every now and then Barbara steals, usually food but sometimes a pretty little thing for herself. She does not like to steal and always feels guilty. Once she was caught by a grocer but managed to talk and cry her way out of a criminal prosecution. She stopped for a while, but the lure of good things to eat and pretty things to wear was too strong, so she resumed her occasional shoplifting.

Discussion

This family could certainly be considered to be a high health risk, although their mental and emotional health seems to be in greater jeopardy than their physical health, at least for the moment. Neither parent has any education, although both have "marketable skills." Barbara, however, is too old and worn to be a successful prostitute, and Arnie's arrest rate proves him to be a rather inept criminal. So their skills are not providing them with a dependable income, and they must be considered among the hard-core unemployed. There seems to be little motivation to find legal work with a future. The children are well on the way to following in their parents' footsteps, and unless intervention takes place immediately (it may even be too late for the older children), they too will be lost. Connie, who was raped, both times in particularly ugly circumstances, is just now going through puberty when her sexual needs and desires are coming to her conscious mind. Rape is a devastating experience for any woman, but in a preadolescent its consequences could be permanently damaging and could prevent her from forming any close sexual attachments. Neither of her parents seems to be the kind of person with whom she could talk out her feelings. It almost goes without saying that this family has no health maintenance, and, because the children attend school so infrequently, they cannot even take advantage of whatever screening programs there are. Barbara's stealing is a problem in three ways: her own emotional health is suffering because of her guilt; the next time she gets caught (and there *will* be a next time), it is likely that she will be prosecuted; and eventually she will be sent to prison. If her husband is also in jail, the children will become wards of the state and either be placed in foster homes or kept in juvenile houses in detention. Barbara is a battered wife and an abusing mother, but she does not drink or take drugs, and although she has no formal education, she is quite intelligent. The nutrition of this family is inadequate, but, aside from the usual colds, flu, and occasionally a child with a broken bone, there have been no major physical illnesses.

It is unlikely that this family would come to the attention of a community nurse. Hospital emergency rooms that the Kerpers use for their infrequent accidents do not think about the kind of follow-up care that this family needs. Except for Barbara's childbirths, no one has ever been hospitalized, so there has never been a request to a social service or home health agency. The prison system has its hands full simply keeping track of its parolees and cannot attend to the needs of the family. School authorities and teachers most likely do not know anything about the home situation of the Kerper children, and, if they did, the problems would be seen to be not much worse than or not much different from those of thousands of other children. The police have neither the time, the facilities, nor the inclination to help solve the problems of families like the Kerpers. So until they come to the attention of some social or health agency, they will remain "lost."

If the Kerper family, or one of its individual members, had come in contact with a nurse, perhaps the course of their health and life might have been altered. If Connie had had the advantage of being taken to a rape crisis center, one of the volunteers might have referred her to crisis intervention or some other kind of counseling. If there had been an alert and perceptive nurse in the emergency

room who might have had the time and inclination to interview the hurt family member in depth, there might have been a referral to a community nursing agency. When Barbara was in the hospital having her children, a nurse could have found out about some of the home problems. These are all instances in which the family could have been "found" and helped by a community nurse. But in actual fact, the health care environment for nonprivate clients in big cities is mostly cold and indifferent, and it is unlikely (although not impossible) that the Kerpers would come to the attention of a community nurse.

These are the realities of the situation, but what *if* the community nurse did have the opportunity to make a home visit? What would she do? What would be the best approach, after making her assessment and diagnosis, to help this family? With whom should she begin? Arnie's problems are so vast, so all pervasive and deep rooted that they would not be within the scope of the community nurse's abilities. Children can be helped only with the cooperation of the parents, or at least one of them, so Barbara is the most logical place to start. She is not stupid, only bored, untrained, and uneducated. She is not evil, only angry and resentful, and at age 36 she is old enough to see that life will not change unless she initiates change, but she is still young enough so the attempt to change her life could be worthwhile. Barbara is in crisis; she must first be helped to understand this, and then with concentrated nursing intervention she can begin to set some priorities for herself and take the action necessary to make changes. She had the independence of spirit to leave home and seek a better life when she was only 17 years old and to do what she felt was necessary to earn a living. That spirit is demonstrated in the way in which she steals (she is not a kleptomaniac or a hardened thief), and the fact that it is important to her that her two younger children continue to attend school. If the nursing intervention, and whatever other professional help the nurse thinks Barbara needs, can encourage and redirect that independent spirit, Barbara could learn to lead a more satisfying life.

PHYSICAL ILLNESS

It is not only physical illness that creates risk in families, but it is the way in which the family is affected by the fact of the illness. How they cope, what they do, and what strengths they find to deal with illness in themselves or in family members determines, to a large measure, the degree of risk.

Levels of wellness and the health-illness continuum have been discussed in Chapter 8; it is difficult to describe a "normal" way of coping with physical illness. There are so many variables involved, for example, how serious the illness is, whether one is expected to recover, how long the illness will last, how much of one's life has been disrupted, how much pain there is, whether the ability to earn a living is permanently in jeopardy, the degree of dependence on others, one's living arrangements, and one's previous experience with illness. Everyone is thrown into some degree of disequilibrium by even the most minor illness like the common cold or a sprained ankle. We may even continue to function with illness; we may go to work with a red stuffed-up nose or a bandaged ankle, but there *will* be a change because of the illness. Perhaps we will not be able to concentrate because of pain or we will not be able to speak clearly because of nasal stuffiness, and our co-workers might avoid us for a day or two because of our unpleasant mood. Consider the impact on you, your job, and your family when you are in bed for a week with a case of flu; then consider the impact on the client and his family when he is bedridden for a year in a body cast after an automobile accident.

Physicians concentrate on disease itself; it is the function of the community nurse to concentrate on the person, as well as his family, who has the disease. It is the impact of the illness that will be discussed here, not the illness itself. The field of somatopsychology deals with the psychological aspects of physical disability and handicaps and was developed as a result of all the permanent injuries arising out of World War II. The study, however, has expanded to include all physical illness that involves some change in the perception of one's physical body—loss of parts, the change in function of a part, alteration is size by a gain or loss of weight, or a change in the way one can use one's body (e.g., the need for absolute rest following a heart attack). Somatopsychology in conjunction with psychosomatic medicine can explain illness to clients and help them deal with it.

After a search of the literature, Schontz maintains that independence between body and behavior is implied by the lack of correlation between the two and that "systematically collected research evidence provides no convincing proof of direct causal relations between personality and physical illness or disability."[19,p.37] He may be right in that one cannot predict the personality of a person simply by knowing what disease he has; that is, there is no such thing as a "cancer person" or a "blind personality." But there is no mistaking the fact that behavior fluctuates with the degree of physical health. We, as people, know it about ourselves, and we, as nurses, see it in the clients we care for.

There are some interesting theoretical assumptions between the body and behavior. "Correspondence remains fairly close at the level of functional relations between physique and behavior, for example, at the level of the influence of illness or disability on ability to perform activities of daily living."[19,p.61] A person responds as much to the meaning of bodily events as he does to the events themselves. That is, for example, a pain may be perceived in two ways: as a condition that in itself causes suffering and as a condition that will affect the individual's ability to function. The degree of disruption of the life situation is an important index of the psychological impact of physical illness. Perception of illness can range all the way from total denial, which is called *anosognosia* and was first described by the French neurologist Joseph Babinski in 1914, to complete subjection to illness with resultant loss of will to function. There are, of course, many reactions between these two extremes. All body experiences have psychological functions, and it might be well to examine some of these functions so we can see how they are altered by physical illness.

1. The body is a sensory register that records and stores all incoming sensory data. This function is how we protect ourselves from harm (the sensation of intense heat will cause us to remove our finger from the stove) and how we learn about environmental stimuli.

2. The body is an instrument for action. Every action, from basic reflex to advanced thinking, requires operation of some group of body structures. Loss of the function of any structure reduces the capacity for action.

3. The body is a source of drives. Body functions impel us to take certain actions, such as eating, breathing, defecating, and having sex. Some of the drives are productive and maintain life and function. Some relieve tension, and others are defensive. Many of the drives are automatic, many are conditioned, and still others are learned. All the actions serve a purpose, and if body functions are impaired, the drives will also be impaired. In illness or disability, drives and motives may undergo modification as a result of somatic damage. Nevertheless, observations of people with long-term conditions reveal that stability rather than change of need structure is the rule. The adult paraplegic, for whom normal sexual activity is impossible, usually retains the need for sexual contact, despite his physical loss. A hostile person who suddenly experiences paralysis that prevents him from expressing aggression does not ordinarily lose his hostility; in fact, he becomes more angry because techniques for expressing hostile impulses are no longer available.

4. The body is a stimulus to the self. This concept is closely allied with self-perception, self-awareness, and a resultant self-esteem. Our own perceptions of our bodies may differ from others' perceptions of us, and this is also true of various losses of body function or changes in appearance. A pimple on one's face may seem to stand out like a beacon, whereas someone else hardly notices it.

5. The body is a stimulus to others. Behavioral expectations often result from what our appearance is or what our functional abilities are. A modification in appearance or ability can lead to changes in the expectations of others and consequently to changes in self-concept. As an example, a young girl with a leg amputation has a prosthesis that fits and functions well. She has been rehabilitated to the point where she participates in all sports and can even run. She knows what she can do and consequently functions well. At parties, though, her friends do not ask her to dance because they do not expect her to be able to. She is too shy to initiate dancing, so she does not dance, and soon even she is convinced that she is unable to. This, of course, affects her self-concept and interferes with her social development.

6. The body is an instrument of expression. The term "body language" is well integrated into our lexicon. We show love, hate, fear, anger, happiness, and every other emotion with our bodies, and, perhaps most important, we use our bodies for having sex.[20] Physical illness decreases our ability to express ourselves with our bodies. Even the simple "Don't kiss me, I have a cold" can be a disappointment to someone who is badly in need of a hug and a kiss. Think of what the loss of the use of one's arms could do to a person who could never again physically embrace another.

Reactions

People react in various ways to physical illness. One way is the adoption of the "sick role," which involves passive behavior, social and psychological regression, and submission to a variety of treatment regimens. There are varying degrees of this behavior; some are adaptive and beneficial, whereas some are maladaptive and harmful. Staying home from work for a few days and luxuriating in someone else serving you meals in bed and taking your temperature is physically beneficial for the treatment of flu. Turning oneself into a cardiac cripple and refusing to engage in any physical activity after the crisis of a heart attack has passed has damaging long-term effects for both the body and the spirit. Families have a great deal to do with the way the client adopts the sick role. Sickness and disability can be encouraged, and a client's family can quickly turn him into a nonfunctioning and helpless, dependent person. The family can also go to the other extreme of ignoring illness and pain to such an extent that the client receives no emotional support and sometimes not even the physical help he needs. The ability to strike a balance between sympathy, empathy, encouragement, support, and love is an ideal way for a family to relate to an individual who is ill.

People can react to physical illness by using it as a weapon to manipulate family members, to inflict guilt, and to keep them forever dependent. Turning oneself into a martyr not only impedes whatever rehabilitation could be possible, it can magnify the illness itself. Family members can be easily convinced that an individual is more ill than he really is, and their catering to his needs simply magnifies the whole process. This strategy (even though it may be unconscious) can backfire, however. Whining, complaining, laying on of guilt, and the trip down into dependency can cause the family members' anger and resentment to burn slowly until they become fed up and finally refuse to be manipulated. The care and attention that were lavished could suddenly be withdrawn, leaving the individual truly helpless. Whatever the outcome, this situation is never healthy for the sick person or his family. They are excellent candidates for crisis intervention.

Because illness is a modification of the ability to function, there is always a concomitant modification in behavior, no matter how slight. A certain amount of aggression is inevitable, but there is also the possibility of displays of extreme psychic strength and determination. People often grow and change because of physical illness, and it is not uncommon for people to say that, although they did not *enjoy* being sick, the situation taught them something about themselves, and they are glad to have had the experience. Behavior sometimes even changes for the better. Illness and the resultant physical inactivity gives time for restful contemplation and dialogues with the self. Relationships can be examined, plans made, and life goals reevaluated, and an individual can emerge from a physical illness a "new person." Illness, especially if

it is a serious one, gives one a sense of the finiteness of life, which can lead to productive contemplation.

The cultural and social background of the individual, as well as his previous experience with illness (his own and those of people he knows), can affect the way in which he reacts to it. People from cultures that give tacit approval to displays of emotion may easily permit themselves to "go to pieces" when they or family members become ill. More stoical cultures require more tight-lipped responses. The necessity for meeting the expectations of family members may put undue strain on the sick person. A man who wants and needs to bury his face in his pillow and sob may feel constrained from doing so because of his own concept of what his behavior "as a man" should be and because he fears other people's reactions to his behavior. But the effort to hold back his tears might be both physically and emotionally harmful. Tolerance to illness also varies from individual to individual. One person may be almost glad of the imposed restriction of activity of a broken leg, whereas another person's anxiety level and impatience with the inconvenience may cause him to do himself further harm as he hops about in an attempt not to be slowed down.

Dealing with the illness

In dealing with people's reactions to physical illness, the community nurse should consider a few guiding principles.

1. The nurse must seek a cause-and-effect relationship between the client's personality and situation and the behavior he is exhibiting. It is unlikely that there is a single or simple cause for any behavior, and it may take a good deal of careful probing for the nurse to figure out what is happening. The family may or may not be aware of why the client is behaving in a certain way, and they themselves may demonstrate varying degrees of cooperation in working with the nurse.

2. The nurse should determine how well integrated the family structure is, what kind of support they give each other, what they think and feel about

each other, and what the operant dynamics are in the interpersonal relationships. If a woman hates and resents her husband, it is usrealistic to expect her to give him much genuine support and sympathy. If a husband is out of town on business half the time and pays little attention to his wife when he is home, it is unreasonable to expect that he will be able to meet her dependency needs when she falls ill.

3. The nurse needs to find out how reality oriented the client and his family are. How do they perceive this illness, and how does their perception match reality? If they are the same, then there is no problem. If, however, the perception is different from the reality, the nurse must find out why and then try to increase the reality orientation of the family. For example, if the parents of a child with cystic fibrosis insist that the child merely has a temporary lung congestion that will disappear with some patent medicine cough syrup, there is a real problem with reality orientation. Not only will the parents be cruelly hurt when the reality finally sinks in, but the child will be deprived of badly needed medical attention. The nurse must gently but firmly make the family face the truth.

4. The nurse needs to know how the client anticipates the future. Will he be handicapped for the rest of his life? How is he reacting to that prospect? Does he think he will be handicapped when, in reality, he will regain full functioning? Does he *want* to be handicapped? Will the client be able to earn a living? If not, what financial provisions can be made? If the illness is a chronic one, how will the family cope with it? If they do not have the strengths and resources to cope with a permanently ill person, the community nurse can help to develop them.

These four principles are based on the nurse's ability to assess the family situation and work within the context of that situation to improve the coping mechanisms in the face of physical illness.

This chapter is concerned with conditions that lead to high-risk situations in families, and one of these conditions is the way in which individuals and families react to physical illness. The parameters of wellness and illness have been defined in Chapter 8. However:

> It is not enough to define illness as an experience manifested by aberrations in living organisms, for there are many individuals with aberrations who would say they are not ill. . . . How then shall we differentiate between a disabled well person and a disabled ill person? The author [Wu] suggests that the incorporation of the social dimensions of illness can be used to distinguish those individuals who are experiencing illness and those who are not. In the presence of an aberration or dysfunction outside the normal range, the criteria for illness shall be the feeling state of the person and his performance capacity.*

An individual frequently perceives the extent of his own disability in terms of his ability to perform his usual functions and to carry out the behaviors of the role he has chosen for himself. The individual's perceptions are easily transmitted to the family. When role behavior becomes impaired, for example, when a breadwinner becomes disabled and cannot engage in the activities that earn him a living, there are two main choices open to him: to give up the role or to modify the role to his changed abilities. For example, a man who is in a cash-and-carry retail business with much physical activity and a great deal of day-to-day stress and worry about customers, the weather, and his employees has a heart attack. He spends some time in the hospital and is told by his physician that he must change his life-style and subject himself to less anxiety and stress. He can give up his role as breadwinner, sell his business, retire to Florida or Arizona, and lead a life of inactive indolence. Or he can modify his role as breadwinner by changing the way he runs his business. Perhaps he can hire responsible people to deal with the everyday aggravations while he concerns himself with long-range planning or fiscal management, which has a different kind of stress (it is impossible to totally eliminate stress from one's life). He also has

*From Ruth Wu, Behavior and illness, © 1973, pp. 183-184. Reprinted by permission of Prentice-Hall, Inc., Englewood Cliffs, N.J.

choices about the way in which he relates to his family. He can state his decision and ask for their help and cooperation, or he can bend his will to theirs and let other people make the decisions about how he will spend the rest of his life.

Being ill implies some degree of dependence on others, and there are choices here, too. Some people find it almost impossible to ask for help of any kind, some people find it almost impossible to get through any day without help, and the vast majority fall in between. The choice comes in how one incorporates dependence into one's life-style. The act of asking for help can be fought all the way, which usually results in tremendous feelings of anger and self-loathing. Or the need to ask for help can be accepted in a philosophical way, and a healthy balance worked out between dependency and independency. This is much easier said than done, and it could well be the community nurse who works with the client and his family to achieve this balance. Some of the ways this can be done are to make the individual the manager of his own illness or disability; that is, he must make the decisions about what he will and will not do, how he will live his life, on whom he wishes to depend, and what the extent of this dependency will be. This, of course, will all have to be decided within the limits of his physical abilities, but the individual, if he is to maintain any mental health and self-esteem, must make his own decisions. One of the most important things the community nurse can do is to encourage the individual to be the master of his own fate, which is one of the hallmarks of a physically and mentally healthy person.

An ill or disabled person must learn a whole new set of rules of behavior, which can be difficult. He must incorporate what society expects of him into what he expects of himself. This is not to say that he must *do* what society expects of him, but it surely will be part of his thinking. He may find himself explaining his illness to others, and he may find in his interactions with other people that they are relating to his disability and not to him. To be sick is to be different and to be part of a minority group that is discriminated against in no less brutal ways than are other minority groups. Not only will an individual need to "learn" to be a sick person, he will need to learn to cope with other people's reactions, with decreased employability, with a set of erroneous stereotypes about his disability (e.g., paraplegics cannot have sex, or people with cerebral palsy are mentally retarded), and perhaps with a changed physical appearance. He must also be prepared for people to like him less, and this is perhaps the biggest blow of all. In a study done by Richardson et al.[21] in 1961, children ages 10 and 11 were shown pictures of variously handicapped and nonhandicapped children and were asked to rank them in the order of likability. The rank order of preference was (1) a child with no physical handicap, (2) a child with crutches and brace on the left leg, (3) a child sitting in a wheelchair, (4) a child with the left hand missing, (5) a child with a facial disfigurement on the left side, and (6) an obese child. A physical disability is more repugnant than a functional one, and the reaction to it does not improve as children become adults. Ugly people, deformed people, and handicapped people are not as well liked as "normal" and attractive people, and this is a bitter pill to swallow by a person whose physical status has changed from normal to ugly, deformed, or handicapped. He may see himself as the same person he was before, *as indeed he is,* but others do not, and, consequently, they expect his behavior to be modified. The comedienne Lily Tomlin does a most poignant character sketch of a quadriplegic named Crystal who is traveling west across the country in a motorized wheelchair to go hang gliding in the air currents of California's Big Sur. Crystal constantly meets people who are horrified that she is not conforming to the expected behavior of a quadriplegic, that is, sitting quietly somewhere out of the sight and thoughts of the people she calls "walkies." Crystal has enormous strength of character, but one can see tremendous anger and frustration behind the bravado. She is a fictional character, but there is not one person whose life has been changed by illness or disability who has not felt Crystal's feelings.

Wu[22] has suggested that adoption of new behaviors for a person who has impaired functioning is facilitated or hindered by several conditions:

1. If there is a congruence between the old behaviors and the new ones the disabled person is expected to learn
2. If the individual is capable of learning new behaviors
3. If he is motivated to adopt the new role
4. If he has had some preparation, through rehearsal, imagination, or actuality of the new behaviors
5. If the transition from a well or sick role to an impaired role is gradual rather than sudden

Wu goes on to say that "unfortunately the characteristics of most disabilities acquired late in life are accompanied by a sudden rapid onset, basic incongruence between the old and expected new behaviors, a lack of motivation to change (especially true for older persons), and inability or incapacity to perform the new and different behaviors."[22,p.196] This may be true of older people, but there are few instances in which there is *no* spark of hope or motivation; it is the community nurse's ability to find and recognize the spark that is as important as her capacity to do something about it.

Families can be helped to deal with physical illness in a positive way, and their strengths can be used to help themselves and the sick individual. One must first recognize and define the family strengths, and this involves looking at the internal and external psychic and material factors with which the family is dealing. These factors include the socioeconomic conditions, the living arrangements, and the relationship of the sick member to the rest of the family. The family may not recognize its own strengths and weaknesses, and in the face of physical illness they may lose sight of the "cosmic glue" that has held them together through other disasters. When the nurse assesses the family's ability to deal with the illness, it is essential that the family be viewed as a unit, as well as a collection of individual people. This is difficult to do because the strengths and weaknesses of each individual may be different from those of the family

as a whole. The family's success in meeting its developmental tasks affects its maturity and its ability to cope with the crisis of the illness of one of its members. Hill,[23] in research of black families, identified five characteristics that are indicative of family strength:

1. A concern for family unity, loyalty, and interfamily and intrafamily cooperation
2. An ability for self-help and the ability to accept help when appropriate
3. An ability to perform family roles flexibly
4. An ability to establish and maintain growth-producing relationships
5. The ability to provide for the physical, emotional, and spiritual needs of a family

The greater the abundance of these qualities and the more highly developed they are, the greater the family's ability to cope with the illness and the individual and to be of some constructive and positive help to him. Other areas of strength are the ability to use the resources available and to be resourceful in finding avenues of help that are not readily apparent. Learning about the illness and its causes, treatment, and prognosis is a sign of strength and shows the family's willingness to accept a problem and meet it head on. The more one knows about an illness, the better equipped one is to deal with it. The family's successful coping with previous crises is a strength because coping mechanisms and the development or enhancement of family solidarity have been learned. It is a strength to be able to adopt the roles and behaviors of other family members; that is, an adolescent "mothers" a sick mother, or a father performs the functions usually done by his wife. Hope is a strength, and the absence of hope is almost a guarantee of failure to deal with the illness. Hope should be based on the reality of the future, not on the occurrence of a miracle. To hope that a young man with multiple sclerosis will throw down his crutches and go back to jogging every morning is futile, useless, and an invitation to failure and depression. But to hope that physical therapy will retard the progress of the disease and even to hope that there will be a remission is positive, realistic, and practical because hope will lead to a redoubling of effort during physical therapy.

INABILITY TO BE A PRODUCTIVE PART OF THE COMMUNITY

What is meant by the phrase "a productive part of the community"? What is produced? By whom? In what amount? What are the characteristics of someone who is productive and someone who is not? Was Henry David Thoreau less productive than Henry Ford? How can the production of William Shakespeare be compared with the production of Wilbur and Orville Wright? One cannot, of course, make any objective comparisons. Everyone's production and contribution to society is important, both to society itself and to the individual. The value of different kinds of production also cannot be compared. Astronauts and garbage collectors are of *equal* value in this society but for different reasons. Each function meets different societal needs, and, ironically, we could *function* without space exploration, but we could not function if we were buried beneath mountains of garbage!

To define and to measure productivity or to itemize the characteristics of someone who is productive is difficult. It is not merely the ability to earn money, although that is a part of it. It is not merely the ability to see the results of one's efforts. It is not merely society's acknowledgement of the value of one's production. It is not merely the self-esteem gained by being productive. It is not merely the joy of accomplishment. Productivity is all of this and more. It is the self-knowledge of contributing *something* to the fabric of society, something that has value to oneself and to others. It is to put back into the stream of life a measure of what we take from it. It is to be not a parasite. It is to *do* something, no matter how seemingly insignificant. This does not necessarily mean that a person must be employed to be productive; much worthwhile activity is done for no money at all. Perhaps another way to define a productive person is one who has reason to get up in the morning, who sees a purpose to life (although all thinking people during various stages in their emotional development wonder what the purpose of their lives is).

Defining and identifying nonproductive persons

Who, then, is a nonproductive part of the community, and what makes him that way? He is characterized by qualities and behaviors that are opposite to what was just described, although the condition of nonproductivity may be temporary. Aside from the fact that a nonproductive person has value as a human being, just because he *is* a human being and has potential for productivity, the nonproductive person contributes nothing to the community, to society, or to his fellow human beings. He is a taker who does not give anything in return.

An example of a person who is nonproductive is a severe user of drugs, either alcohol or "hard" drugs such as heroin or amphetamines. For a drug user to be considered nonproductive in the context of this chapter, he must be so dependent on the drug that he is incapable of doing anything else: his whole being is devoted to the obtaining, taking, and "enjoyment" of the drug. He does not have a job, and all his human relationships revolve around his need for the drug and are secondary to that need. He is consumed by his need, and in addition to being a drug user, it might be accurate to say that he is *used by* the drugs.

The National Council on Alcoholism estimates that there are more than 10 million alcoholics in this country, and the Food and Drug Administration estimates about half a million heroin addicts. These statistics arise from sources of treatment (clinics, hospitals, and private physicians) and do not include all the drug users who never seek treatment. The total of 10.5 million people is a very conservative estimate. Alcoholics range in age from the very young to the very old, whereas heroin and amphetamine addicts tend to be younger: below 30. Although individual people are addicted to drugs, they are not the only ones affected. It is impossible for the family life of an addict[24] not to be disrupted, often to the point of turmoil and utter chaos. The addict cannot maintain satisfactory human relationships with anyone, is always psychologically abusive because of his own tremendous self-hatred, and sometimes is physically abusive. Few marriages can survive this strain, employers will not tolerate the irresponsible behavior, and friends leave quickly. As his life falls apart, the addict takes refuge from reality in more drugs, compounds the problem, and causes his life to become even more hopeless. It is a vicious circle from which it is extremely difficult to emerge. The cure rate for drug addiction is depressingly low.

The definition of alcoholism proposed by Mark Keller of the Center for Alcohol Studies at Rutgers University and adopted by the World Health Organization is "a chronic disease, or disorder of behavior, characterized by the repeated drinking of alcoholic beverages to an extent that exceeds customary dietary use or ordinary compliance with the social drinking customs of the community, and which interferes with the drinker's health, interpersonal relations or economic functioning."[25,p.6] A slight change in the wording of this definition could make it apply equally well to people who are addicted to other drugs. Various theories exist about what causes people to become addicted to alcohol or drugs, but it is impossible to pinpoint a single or specific cause. There are so many variables in people's lives that one must consider all the psychological, physiological, and sociological factors when trying to get to the root of why one becomes addicted. Following are some of the theories:

1. Nutritional or endocrine theory. Although there is no proof, it is thought that some people simply cannot physiologically tolerate some substances, but the body, in a perverse sort of way, craves these substances.

2. Heredity theory. This may be a predisposing factor, but it is not an exclusive one.

3. The desire to alter consciousness by distorting it in order to gain new insights or different perceptions of reality.

4. The seeking of new experiences, to explore the unknown, to be "high" or "out of one's head,"

and to explore new physical and psychic sensations. The claims of great euphoria or sensuality (many of them exaggerated) or even of physical ecstasy can lead people to want to add a new dimension to the same old life.

5. Parental and societal example. Young people see their parents and other adults drinking and taking drugs and follow the example in an effort to be grown up. Adults are affected strongly by the behavior of their friends and often can become addicted in the effort to keep up with the group. We have all had the experience of arriving late at a party and being urged to have several drinks quickly in order to "catch up" with the people who are already there.

6. An escape mechanism, which is self-explanatory. When one is under the influence of drugs, one is oblivious to one's surroundings and can escape the reality of life, which, for one reason or another, is intolerable.

7. Rebellion and the display of hostility. One of the best ways to express contempt for one's friends or employers or for society in general is simply to remove oneself by not being able to function. The need for rebellion is most common in adolescents but is certainly not limited to that age-group. Adults often find that they have "had it" with their lives and are unable to make constructive and positive changes in a life that has become unsatisfactory.

There are three stages of drug addiction. The first is the knowledge that the ingestion of the drug leads to relief of tension or the obliteration of stress. A pattern is established that leads to the second stage, which is the deliberate repetition of the behavior and gradual dependence on the drug to produce the desired loss of sensation. At this point the person is unable to meet stress without the drug but is not yet a true addict. If the behavior continues, physiological dependence develops, the tissues of the body begin to adjust to the presence of the drug, and more of it is required to create the desired effect. This is known as tolerance, which is the hallmark of an addict and the third stage. Other signs of addiction are loss of control when taking the drug; a craving, psychological and physiological, for the drug; and the inability to be without it. There is also a withdrawal syndrome when the intake of the drug is decreased or stopped. The syndrome is a series of symptoms in which the entire body and mind scream out for the drug; behavior ranges all the way from mild tremulousness to full-blown delerium tremens. During the third stage of addiction, the person has no choice of whether he will take the drug; he needs it, cannot exist without it, and will do *whatever* he feels necessary to obtain it. He will kill for it.

Helping individuals become productive

Treatment for addiction is long, painful, expensive, and not often successful. Again, there are a myriad of theories about the best way to treat addicts; none of them work in all instances, and the decision of what kind of treatment might be best for the individual can be made only after thorough evaluation of the causes of the addiction and all the other variables that make up the individual's functioning. Following are some of the treatment approaches that are currently popular:

1. Learning theories such as aversive conditioning, reinforcement techniques, and behavior modification. Use of emetic drugs is sometimes successful.

2. Group therapies like Alcoholics Anonymous where addicts share experiences, learn from each other, and reinforce each other's positive behavior. There is emphasis on the sharing of common problems, and group members are highly supportive of each other.

3. Psychoanalytic treatment, which may focus on character disorders; arrests in personality development; or a variety of other psychological approaches.

4. Rehabilitation programs, which are usually community based and which concentrate on the reestablishment of personal and social relationships. The programs are often in halfway houses and employ a variety of treatment modalities and professional personnel. Reintroduction to the world

of employment and responsibility is a part of the rehabilitation process. Moreover, many industries are taking an active interest in the alcohol addiction problems of their employees. Companies are engaging in case finding and the encouragement of treatment. They try not to fire the alcoholic employee if he shows indications of rehabilitative efforts.

5. Family therapy, which can be informal and done in groups with other families, or it can be part of an intensive psychotherapeutic process.

6. Methadone maintenance for heroin addicts. This has been extremely controversial and is becoming more so now that it is known that methadone is as addictive as heroin and has appeared as a street drug. The theory is that the effects of heroin are blocked when an individual is taking methadone. Consequently, the addict should feel no high when he takes heroin. There has, however, been a transfer of abuse from heroin to methadone, and many people feel that addicts are "falling out of the frying pan and into the fire." However, methadone maintenance had been successful in many instances, and people have remained off heroin long enough to get their lives back in order.

The general goals of treatment for drug addiction are to stop the physical and psychological craving for the drug and the consequent physical complications (e.g., liver and kidney damage and malnutrition), to stop criminal activity that is caused by the need to get money to buy drugs, to achieve an understanding of why there was addiction, to improve the individual's self-concept sufficiently so that he can function without the use of drugs, to teach new ways of reacting to stress and tension, to get and maintain a job, and to become a contributing member of society. Treatment often takes years, and there is frequently much backsliding along with the progress. Not only does the addict have to contend with his own self-image, he must deal with the damage and pain he has caused others: the members of his family whom he cares about and perhaps strangers whom he has robbed or hurt. His life is a mess, and the strength and perseverance that is necessary to straighten it out is often not available to the addict. The condition of his life is a source of stress to which he may well react by crawling deeper into his addiction. Previously learned patterns of coping behavior are hard to break, particularly if they are complicated by a physical craving.

The community nurse can play a role in the care of the addict and his family. One of her most important functions may simply be the identification of the addict. Sometimes during a home visit a mother will let it be known that she thinks her child is taking drugs, or she describes behavior that the nurse associates with possible addiction. Sometimes the nurse herself will observe signs of addiction: the physical appearance or behavior of a family member or an unusual number of empty liquor bottles. Addicts try for as long as possible to hide and deny their addiction, so identification may not be easy. An even more difficult task for the nurse is to persuade the addict to seek treatment. In addition to denial of the problem, there is the attitude of "I can lick this myself" and the refusal to seek professional help. Many times the addict is too sick to care whether he receives help, and even if he does care, he lacks the strength and motivation to do anything about it. In this case all the talking and persuasion in the world will do no good. An alternative is to let the family member know what resources are available on an emergency, as well as an ongoing, basis. The family should be prepared in case there are bouts of violence or in case the addict becomes ill because of withdrawal. There are almost always financial problems, especially if the addict was the breadwinner; the family needs to know where to go for emergency funds. Sooner or later the addict will become involved with the police and the courts and will find himself in jail. The family then needs to know where to go for reputable legal help and what to do when the telephone call from the police station comes. Treatment of the addict himself is beyond the ability of the average community nurse, but she is equipped to give supportive family counseling, to be a lis-

tener, to offer alternative ways of dealing with the problem, to help establish new roles and new ways of behaving toward the addict, and perhaps even to help the family begin a new life without him.

Drug addiction is probably the most frustrating community health problem because it is so incurable. The vast majority of alcoholics fall "off the wagon" and climb back on countless times during their lives, and the people who are addicted to hard drugs almost always remain that way. The life span of addicts is shorter than normal both because of the physical complications associated with addiction and also because of the violent nature of their life-styles. A skid-row alcoholic is as likely to be killed by a car as he stumbles across the street at night as he is to die of cirrhosis of the liver. A heroin addict is as likely to be stabbed by a fellow addict for his supply of drugs as he is to die of an abscess at the site of injection.

A drug addict cannot possibly be a productive part of the community. He cannot think clearly enough to hold a job, to establish any kind of effective personal or social relationships, or even to function beyond obtaining his next drink or his next "fix." He is a user of social services, although not by his own conscious choosing, and he is a doer of harm to others. He contributes nothing but trouble, and the only remotely positive thing that can be said for his existence if that he provides work for others, for example, police, nurses, physicians, and drug rehabilitation experts. Reams of articles and books are published about his problems and their causes, solutions, and effects on society, but the fact remains that he is a negative force, both to himself and to everyone else.

MATERNAL AND CHILD HEALTH PROBLEMS

Some of the greatest sources of high health risks revolve around mothers and children and the childbearing and child-rearing processes. There is no aspect that does not entail risk, and the facts of poverty, unemployment, lack of education, and physical illness simply compound the risks.

Nutrition

An excellent example is poor nutrition. It is not true that only poor people are not well nourished, but it is more likely that the nonpoor will have better diets.

Scientific research has identified the nutrient needs for optimal body function, growth, development, maintenance of body tissues, prevention of disease, and repair. Foods and their preparation to retain or enrich their nutrient value command a significant share of the scientific technology in North America. Yet many people are malnourished, undernourished or obese. Dysfunctional nutrition prior to pregnancy may have long-term effects on the physical and mental development of the child and the subsequent health of the mother.[26,p.91]

If good nutrition is important all the time, then it is absolutely essential during pregnancy, childhood, and adolescence.

So many things influence the way we eat. Personal likes and dislikes are probably the most potent force, but so are cultural and traditional habits. Our wallets strongly affect our nutritional status. It is unreasonable to expect a person to buy a bottle of orange juice when for about a third the price he can get a can of some artificially flavored orange drink that has only about 10% real juice, a great deal of sugar, and not much else. A poor person might not care that the orange juice is good for him and that the orange drink is a nutritional waste of money. It tastes good and is cheap, and that is what matters. It is also unreasonable to expect that a family of six in which no adult has a job will be able to eat much protein. They will eat bread, potatoes, other carbohydrates, and whatever else takes away the feeling of hunger. Psychic needs also influence what we eat. We eat what will satisfy us emotionally, even though it might not be good for us physically. It is a rare person who does not find a hunk of chocolate cake more desirable than a bowl of vegetables, even though the vegetables have badly needed vitamins and minerals and far fewer calories. Food habits are extremely hard to change; an addiction to Coca-Cola may be as hard to break as an addiction to cigarettes.

The specific nutritional needs of pregnant women, children, and adolescents will not be discussed here; the reader is referred to maternal and child health texts for that information. But there are some things that the community nurse should be aware of so she knows why and how to motivate the families she sees to improve their nutrition. Many pregnant women feel that they should "eat for two," and consequently they double their caloric intake. This is not true; a pregnant woman needs only about 200 calories more than her usual intake, and a weight gain of more than about 24 pounds* is one of the greatest factors contributing to the development of toxemia. There is also an established correlation between the nutritional status of the woman during pregnancy and the birth weight of her child. A lack of adequate nutrition leads to low–birth weight infants who have a higher risk of all neonatal illnesses, including brain damage and retardation in growth and development.

Jensen, Benson, and Bobak[27] list several groups of pregnant women who could be considered nutritionally at risk and who need special attention and counseling from the community nurse and the nutritionist:

1. Adolescents ages 13 to 18 who may be deficient in iron and other nutrients. Their lack of musculoskeletal maturation and undeveloped independence makes them prone to poor nutritional status.
2. Women who are experiencing rapid successive pregnancies (grand multiparas) and whose nutritional stores are being quickly depleted.
3. Those who were underweight before pregnancy have a higher than average incidence of toxemia and an increased incidence of prematurity.
4. Those who have much less than average weight gain during pregnancy often have low–birth weight infants.
5. Those who were overweight before preg-

---

*Obstetric texts differ about the range of allowable weight gain, but most fall somewhere in the 20- to 30-pound range.

nancy often have poor nutritional status and eat a lot of ''empty calories'': foods that are high in carbohydrates but low in essential proteins, vitamins, and minerals. Weight-reduction diets during pregnancy can lead to metabolic disturbances such as ketosis and resultant neurophysiological problems in the infant.

6. Those who have low income and cannot afford to buy foods that are high in the needed nutrients. These women have a high incidence of infant mortality and prematurity.
7. Those who have concurrent medical problems with pregnancy such as diabetes; systemic disorders involving the heart, liver, or kidneys; and infections such as tuberculosis.
8. Those who, for various cultural and religious reasons, have eliminated certain groups of foods from their diets, for example, vegetarians or fruitarians. Nutritional counseling is needed and must be given within the religious and cultural framework of the individual.
9. Those who have a lack of correct information about nutrition.
10. Those who smoke to excess or who are dependent on alcohol or drugs.

The community nurse can try to alleviate some of these problems. The first step is to assess the family's eating habits and find out the reasons behind the habits. The approach to correcting poor eating habits will depend on why the habits were formed in the first place. The more the nurse can actually observe the way the family eats, the more accurate her assessment will be. She needs to talk with the person who is responsible for buying and preparing the food, and she must learn what the family's attitudes about food are and how much they know about nutrition. The religious, racial, ethnic, and economic status of the family must be taken into consideration, as well as how they have been acculturated by society. Is the larder filled with expensive prepared snack foods instead of lower-cost and more nutritionally sound natural

foods? How much television advertising does the family believe, and how influenced are they by nutritional information? Does the family indulge in fad foods often? When the assessment has been made, the community nurse will need to use all her skills to try to change some of the family's worst nutritional habits. If any member of the family has been seen at a clinic or at a neighborhood health center, the nutritionist can be called in as a consultant. The nurse might even go grocery shopping with the person in the family who is responsible for buying food, and she could teach the person how to comparison shop, how to take advantage of bargains, how to read the nutritional information on the labels, how to make a shopping list, and how to avoid impulse buying.

When there are children in the home, nutritional risks becomes greater.

From infancy onward, food and closeness are associated with love and security. Food and eating, in and of themselves, are looked upon as symbolizing interpersonal acceptance, warmth and sociability. . . . It is easy to see why food has become associated with the symbolism of motherliness. Feeding is not only kindly and warm in its emotional meaning to those who receive food, but it is also essential to growth and well-being; hence, it has become bound up with the idea of the mother, the one who originally nurtured, loved and supported.[28.p.189]

Mothers, in an effort to please their children and to be loved by them, give food as an offer of love, as a placating gesture, and to quiet a screaming child. They also use food as a substitute for physical affection: a cookie instead of a hug. Food is used as a system of rewards or punishment; an ice cream cone is given as a prize for being good at the dentist, or dessert is withheld from dinner to punish misbehavior. It is almost always carbohydrates that are used in this way (no one ever says, ''If you stop crying, I'll give you a carrot''!); consequently children associate sweets with pleasure, which can lead to poor nutritional habits.

Again, the nutritional needs of children can be found in pediatric texts, and the community nurse faces the same assessment and implementation problems in dealing with poor nutrition of children as she does with that of pregnant women. An added problem is that as soon as the child is old enough to leave the house, either to be taken to a day-care center or to be sent to school, his parent can no longer control everything he eats. Children will eat what they want, whether or not it is good for them. There is also the problem of what the child does not eat, for example, his dinner when he has stuffed himself with candy and potato chips on the way home from school. The nurse will also run across the problem of the irresponsible parent who, for a variety of reasons, does not provide the child with an adequate diet. This may be conscious or unconscious cruelty, or it may simply be a result of ignorance. There may be literally not enough money to feed some of the family, although most parents will feed their children before they eat. Whatever the reason, it is the obligation of the community nurse to take some action about the starvation or malnutrition of children. Education and counseling may be sufficient, but it may also be necessary to call in the juvenile authorities. Child abuse includes starvation. Childhood and adolescence is a time of rapid growth and development, and inadequate nutrition can cause irreparable damage.

Prematurity

Another high-risk health problem is prematurity.

By far the greatest number of premature infants enter their life in an environment of poverty. Premature infants from middle-class and upper-middle-class families usually have the advantage of better care as they are growing up. Their mothers are often better educated than those of the poor. The nonstimulating environments found in ghettos contribute to slower physical and intellectual growth of high-risk infants.*

The incidence of prematurity is highest among low socioeconomic groups, which are characterized by

*From Vulnerable infants, edited by Schwartz, Jane L., and Schwartz, Lawrence H., p. 5. Copyright 1977 by McGraw-Hill, Inc. Used with permission of McGraw-Hill Book Co.

poverty, poor nutrition, and lack of adequate health care. Many women in this group receive only sporadic prenatal care, if they receive any at all, and sometimes their first contact with an obstetrician is in the labor room. The greatest single "cause" of prematurity[29] is inadequate prenatal care and poor maternal nutrition. A woman who is poor and not eating correctly has a greater than average chance of delivering a premature infant. The irony is that women in these circumstances are not likely to be aware of the statistics and are mostly ignorant of the ways to remedy the situation.

The premature infant who survives until he has reached 5 pounds and can be sent home from the hospital still has formidable handicaps to overcome. The reader is again referred to pediatric texts for the physiological needs of the newborn, but it is obvious that less than ideal conditions in the home will increase the infant's risk, both of its normal growth and development and even of its actual survival. The impoverished family will not be able to provide for the infant's needs. Formulae are expensive (even the old-fashioned do-it-yourself formula of evaporated milk, corn syrup, and water required time, effort, and money, as well as a knowledge of terminal sterilization), and in many homes there is not enough heat. The added burden of a premature infant may be too much to bear for a family already saddled with a myriad of other problems. A measure of knowledge and expertise is needed that goes beyond ordinary child care. This is often lacking in the poor, uneducated family.

There are also parental problems caused by the arrival of a premature infant that are not related to socioeconomic status. The mother faces emotional trauma and loss because she cannot have immediate and continuing body contact with her child. She may even precede him home from the hospital by several days or weeks and may be feeling some vague, undefined guilt that she is the cause of the prematurity. The hustle-bustle of an intensive care nursery can make a person who is not familiar with hospital procedures even more shy and reticent about asking questions, so fears grow, and frightening fantasies about the baby develop. "The loneliness continues when the parents go home without their infant, and because of the continued separation, the task of integrating the new member into the household is delayed."[28,p.577] The community nurse can be of help in these areas by visiting the mother and the baby as soon as possible, preferably in the hospital before the mother is discharged. Anticipatory guidance and crisis intervention are two essential nursing functions.

Growth and development of the premature is dependent primarily on the degree of immaturity at birth, but special care at home is essential if he is to catch up. With adequate care most premature babies make the growth and development adjustment within a year. Proper nutrition is the most important part of the care of a premature baby. Malnutrition will lead to a reduction in the quantity of brain cells with consequent permanent intellectual impairment. This impairment can range all the way from minimal brain dysfunction to profound mental retardation. Correcting the child's diet later in life will be of no use.

Birth defects

A family who has a child with a birth defect with long-term implications has a high health risk. An example of this kind of birth defect is mental retardation, which is a particularly cruel kind of affliction because there is no cure. Although the child may be trained to make full use of what capacities he has, his innate ability to learn cannot be changed. Health authorities have difficulty agreeing on a definition, but the one Marlow[30,p.588] uses seems to sum it up best: "Mental retardation is any interference with intelligence that causes a limitation in the way in which the child is able to adapt to his environment." Mentally retarded people can be grouped into three classifications:

1. Those with an IQ of 51 to 75 are considered mildly retarded but educable.
2. Those with an IQ of 21 and 50 are moderately retarded but trainable.
3. Those with an IQ of 1 to 20 are severely retarded and are completely dependent on others for their care.[31]

Those who have an IQ of 76 to 95 or 100, which is the national average, are not considered to be retarded, but they most definitely are not able to keep up intellectually with their normal peers. They are sometimes called "slow learners" or "minimally retarded" and are not usually given any special medical or educational consideration even though they are handicapped in the competition for jobs, basic schooling, and the ordinary survival techniques needed for life.

Diagnosis of mental retardation (unless there are accompanying physical symptoms, as in Down's syndrome) is usually not made until it has become all too obvious that the child is not reaching developmental landmarks when he should. In a family in which the parents do not know the normal growth and development process, the retardation may not be detected until much later. In any family, regardless of its educational level, denial of the fact of retardation is not uncommon. It is easy to rationalize away the lateness or absence of developmental tasks. Families who are not receiving well-child care tend to recognize the retardation later because there are no developmental tests being applied. There comes a time, however, when realization can no longer be postponed, and the family must face the enormity of the problem. Accurate diagnosis is essential for the ultimate development of the child's abilities, and in this, as in all other health problems, the affluent have the resources to have the child evaluated, whereas the poor and ignorant do not.

The entire family may be thrown into turmoil by the presence of a mentally retarded child; an example in Chapter 8 shows what can happen. The needs of the retarded child are enormous, but other family members cannot be expected to give up their own lives for the retarded one.

There are only two basic things that can be done with the child; he can be institutionalized, or he can be kept at home. Private institutions for the mentally retarded are few and far between; they are tremendously expensive, and they often have long waiting lists. Some state institutions are overcrowded and understaffed. Others, particularly small ones that are relatively new, make an effort to provide progressive and humane care. Others are absolutely unbearable. Most are so lacking in funds and professional personnel that the care provided is mainly custodial, and the child becomes more and more dependent. If the family chooses to keep the child at home, all kinds of problems arise. Many states provide special day education for retarded children, but sometimes long-distance busing is required, and the fact that there are special classes is not widely publicized; many parents do not know they exist. There are also private day schools for the mentally retarded, but they share most of the expensive characteristics of live-in institutions.

The function of the community nurse in a family with a mentally retarded child, aside from providing information about educational resources, is mainly that of family counselor and coordinator of care. The parent who is at home with the child will need support, both emotional and practical. The other children still need love and attention; it is easy for them not to receive their share and consequently begin to resent and hate the retarded sibling. Financial resources will be strained, and the nurse may be able to suggest avenues of help. It is likely that marriage counseling will be needed; the nurse can also refer the family to support groups of parents of retarded children.

A mentally retarded child who has the misfortune to be born into a poor family is sometimes at a double disadvantage. Sometimes, however, he is more readily accepted than he would be if he were born into a wealthy family who might view him as a "shameful" burden. Whatever potential he might have, however, is more likely to be left undeveloped than it would be in a child of affluent parents because the poor are less likely to be aware of the resources available. "Poor, culturally deprived children comprise the majority of the retarded."[32,p.72] Poor women who have inadequate prenatal care and insufficient nutrition during pregnancy are more likely to have retarded children:

To eradicate this type of retardation it will be necessary to attack every aspect of poverty. Contrary to the mode of thinking illustrated by medical research, no spectacular breakthrough can be made until the whole structure of the culture of poverty is destroyed. . . . No amount of research will ameliorate the conditions and human sufferings of poverty as long as poverty itself remains. Research in fact can reveal only the obvious, for as long as civilization has existed man has known that severe poverty degrades and debilitates man. We do not need a more sophisticated, academic understanding of the exact way poverty breaks the human spirit. We need to eliminate poverty.[32,p.73]

INABILITY TO CONTROL REPRODUCTION

DOLORES T. MAZURKEWICZ

Implicit in the term *family planning* is the active decision to have or not to have children, and some form of contraception must be used. The task of planning one's family, along with the choice and use of a suitable contraceptive method, involves a decision-making process. It is not a *simple,* dichotomous issue, that is, one of use or nonuse of contraception or having children or not having them. Like any decision-making issue, it is complex and requires time, communication, and understanding of all related issues and concerns.

Some families have difficulty controlling their reproductive capabilities for several reasons: (1) the various conscious and unconscious motivations for childbearing that are operative at different times; (2) the contraceptive method itself, that is, how it is obtained and used, its side effects, etc.; and (3) the dynamics of the man-woman relationship.

MOTIVATIONS FOR CHILDBEARING

Rejection or failure of contraception may be related to several little-known, yet still present, motives for having a child. For some women, getting pregnant is a sign of femininity and proof of reproductive capability. For some men, impregnating a woman is a sign of virility and proof of potency. Becoming pregnant might be perceived as a way of getting even with a man or ensnaring him in a permanent trap. "Coital gamesmanship," that is, a power struggle between the man and woman regarding who will take responsibility for the use of contraception, may prove that one is more powerful than the other. Pregnancy might be seen as something easy to do, and having a child is socially rewarded. On the other hand, to some, having a baby is a gift of love to the partner.[36]

Some people may have narcissistic, fatalistic, or instrumental reasons for having a child.[37,38] There may be a need to have ''a little me'' who will bring glory to and immortalize the parent, and there is the desire to continue the family lines or traditions. The belief that pregnancy and childbirth are natural, right, and fated occurrences may highly motivate some people to have children. The life situation of the couple also has an effect on the decision to have a child. If a couple finds themselves in a marital situation they perceive as being tenuous and less than ideal, they may either hope that having a child will improve the faltering relationship, or they may fear that a child would make it more difficult or impossible to escape from a negative situation. On the other hand, if the relationship is mutually gratifying, the couple can either want a child to bring additional satisfaction into the marriage or not want a child to interfere with the good situation.[39]

Preferences regarding timing, spacing, number, and sex of the child, as well as considerations regarding the effect the child will have on the couple, all affect motivation for parenthood.[40] Motivations for the first child may be different from motivations for another child. Some couples may want to try out the parent role and will therefore be motivated to have a first child.[41] Hoffmann and Wyatt[42] suggest that the desire for another child stems from an attempt to recapture the good, gratifying experiences of having the first child. So wanting another child depends, to a great extent, on the effect the first child had on the couple's life.

Characteristics of contraceptive methods

Birth control pills, intrauterine devices (IUDs), diaphragms, condoms, rhythm, withdrawal, assorted spermicides (foams, jellies, and suppositories), and sterilization are among the present contraceptive options. Each of these coital-related con-

traceptive methods has certain characteristics that interact with the personality and behavioral style of the individuals who use them. It is easier to obtain information about and have access to some methods than others. The ease with which the method can be obtained, how the method works, and the feelings that are engendered by use of the method are three prominent factors in birth control use or nonuse. For example, condoms and spermicides can be purchased in a variety of places, particularly drugstores, at varying prices, with no prescription needed. However, they do tend to interrupt lovemaking, since they must be used immediately before coitus. This may be a problem, depending on the people involved and the kind of sexual relationship they have. If spontaneity is highly valued, or if one or both people want to be swept off their feet with passion, these methods will be neither appropriate nor effective. Some people maintain that condoms reduce sensitivity, and because they are the only method which sometimes protects against venereal disease, this association may create conflicts over their use. Furthermore, neither condoms nor spermicides are among the most effective methods. Rhythm and withdrawal require nothing but self-control; however, the effectiveness and desirability of these methods is questionable, to say the least.

Pills, diaphragms, and IUDs are more effective methods, but they require a physical examination and periodic checkups. Some people are resistant to methods requiring physical examinations or a physician's intervention. Yet, for some, the fact that a physician does intervene increases the chances that the method will be chosen. The IUD, for example, must be inserted by a physician. It may reflect a woman's desire to shift responsibility for avoiding pregnancy onto an outside source.[43] Once inserted, the IUD need not be dealt with except for periodic checks on the presence of the attached string. However, certain side effects such as intermenstrual bleeding, cramps, or expulsion of the IUD must be tolerated.

Pills, on the other hand, must be taken every day by the woman herself. This implies forethought and responsibility. In addition, women must be willing to accept the side effects of the pill (nausea, breast tenderness, and some that are more serious) and be able to deal with the uncertainties of the long-range effects. Ziegler et al.[44] suggest that if the sexual relationship is mutually satisfying, the pill and its side effects will be tolerated. If not, the woman will not continue to endure its discomforts. Bardwick[45] found that certain women taking the pill have ''prostitution anxieties'' or feelings that they are at the mercy of the sexual demands of their partners. However, these feelings, and the resolution of them, depend on the relationship of the people involved.

A diaphragm is a highly effective contraceptive method, although it may interfere with spontaneity to a certain extent. It also involves planning for sex, which may not be appealing. The diaphragm, with a spermicidal jelly or cream, may be inserted up to 4 hours prior to intercourse, but for best results, a new application of jelly or cream is needed each time there is coitus. This jelly or cream is not pleasant to taste, for some, and may therefore preclude or discourage oral-genital relations. In addition, the diaphragm involves self-insertion, which means touching oneself. This is looked at unfavorably by some men and women. In certain ethnic groups, touching oneself is rarely, if ever, desirable or done. Some men are perplexed, confused, and disturbed about the diaphragm having to be inserted into the woman's vagina. Some contraceptive methods create certain tensions, conflicts, and negative reactions that do not make for positive, regular, and effective use.

Male and female sterilization (vasectomy and tubal ligation) have become increasingly popular contraceptive options. Several factors need to be taken into consideration when discussing voluntary sterilization. Although both vasectomy and tubal ligation can be reversed, the effects of the reversal procedure are by no means certain; therefore, for practical purposes the operations should be considered permanent. This may be a potential hindrance to choosing it as a method of contraception. For men, the idea of permanent sterility has great emotional impact in some cases. Studies of men who have had vasectomies showed increased emotional disturbance, such as defensiveness and compensatory masculine behavior.[46,47] Another factor involved is the psychological effect of an operation performed on one person for the benefit of another,[48] as well as the whole issue of whose responsibility contraception should be. The study by Rodgers et al.[46] showed that men who had vasectomies acted as if they had made a great sacrifice for the marriage and no longer needed to be considerate of their wives. For a woman, the sterilization procedure may mean loss of femininity. However, faced with the dilemma of too many children and a husband who might be in conflict about his sterilization, a woman must assume the responsibility for contraception.

Man-woman interaction

Since contraception is so intricately and directly related to sexual relations, attitudes toward sexuality are an important determinant of contraceptive use or nonuse and success or failure. If one already holds a negative attitude toward sexual intercourse, effective contraceptive use is not likely. Depending on circumstance and/or the type of relationship, a possible reason for contraceptive failure is the woman's complaint that her partner could demand sex at any time. Of course, this is more likely to occur if a woman is in conflict about the act of intercourse. In such cases, the freedom that contraception gives increases the conflict. When contraception is used, the excuse for not having sexual relations is no longer tenable. If this is too threatening, discontinuance of contraception occurs. It is also possible that a man may feel threatened by a woman's ability to control the occurrence of sexual intercourse simply because she is the one who takes responsibility for contraception. Whether such threat is felt also depends on the man's personality, his sexual attitudes, and the kind of sexual relationship that exists.

How women and men feel about the particular contraceptive method is also a most important factor in whether it will be used effectively. If a particular method makes one or both people fearful, anxious, or disgusted, these feelings will interfere with the use of the contraceptive and possibly with the sexual relationship, as well. For most effective contraceptive use, both people should discuss the issues involved, decide on a method that is mutually satisfactory, and *cooperate* in its use. It is important not to downplay the role of a man in the choice and use of contraception. Some men, particularly nontraditional and modern men, want to know and understand the implications of the method. Unfortunately, there are some men who may not, and it is this lack of caring that is another factor in contraceptive failure, as well as an indication that the relationship is not optimum. Bakker and Dightman[49] report that women who forget to take their pills are more often than not involved in discordant relationships with their partners regarding attitudes toward sexualtiy.

Other factors

A variety of other social, religious, and cultural factors affect successful or unsuccessful contraceptive use. The physician's way of dealing with the client, the values of certain people regarding virility and reproduction, and beliefs among certain ethnic groups that widespread contraception is genocide all constitute resistances to contraceptive use. Another related issue is how family planning is verbally conceptualized. The term *birth control* implies a kind of self-mastery that, for some people who believe they are the masters of their fate, is very appealing. The term *contraception,* on the other hand, implies something that goes against conception (*contra-* means against). If conception is highly valued, doing something that goes against it may elicit negative reactions and responses. If one is dealing with the problem of how to go about changing people's attitudes and reproductive behaviors, knowing how one conceptualizes these issues is extremely important. People will selectively attend to those things which are not too threatening and will disregard those which are.

As age increases, so do the number of deaths because of various contraceptive methods, particularly the pill, and because of pregnancies that result from contraceptive failures.[50] There is little positive assurance about the safety of any contraceptive method. Our sexual natures are still bombarded with violations, prohibitions, and inhibitions resulting from faulty means of preventing pregnancies. Unreliable methods and inadequate teaching and dissemination of information necessary to change attitudes and behaviors make more and more of a challenge of something that should be relaxed, joyful, and beautiful. Furthermore, some people's attitudes about fertility and pregnancy include the need to believe that ''it won't happen to me.'' Imitating an ostrich with its head in the sand is not dealing with one's sexuality in a responsible way. Perhaps, if we can reduce or eliminate the shame, guilt, ignorance, and anxiety associated with sexuality, we will be better able to deal with contraception and the other issues related to our sexuality.

Even though the contraceptive methods we have are far from perfect, this is not an excuse for deliberate dismissal or denial of the fact of life that sexual intercourse can and does result in pregnancy. We owe it to ourselves to keep on trying to find a personally appropriate fit between the dynamics and demands of our current life situation and our sexual and contraceptive needs.

MENTAL ILLNESS
DOLORES T. MAZURKEWICZ

Within any family, there is bound to be some amount of stress, dissatisfaction, unhappiness, and complication. Some families, however, have such an inordinate amount of negativity that emotional instability and illness are the norms rather than the exceptions.

The causative factors for emotional instability in families may be divided into biological, psychological, and sociological categories. However, no one factor accounts for all of the explanations; all interact with each other at various times.

How to define mental illness is a difficult and controversial area in contemporary psychology and psychiatry. Some people believe there can be no such thing as mental illness because only the body can get ill. Therefore, mental illness is a metaphor, and psychiatric labels serve only to stigmatize and victimize individuals.[51]

However, for those who believe that mental illness is real and can be categorized, the various mental disorders are generally classified as being either organic, that is, based on some type of brain pathology, as in senility or mental retardation, or functional, in which no brain pathology exists, and the disorder is a result of some kind of faulty psychological functioning. The disorders that are considered functional include neuroses, certain kinds of psychoses, character or personality disorders, alcoholism, and drug addiction.

Genetic factors probably play some part in certain kinds of psychopathology. How to define these different pathologies and to what extent they are attributed to faulty biological development are moot issues. The most controversial issue centers around the topic of schizophrenia. Studies have shown that the incidence of schizophrenia increases as the degree of blood relationship increases.[52] However, early environmental influences cannot be neglected when studying family histories. Therefore a more efficient way of understanding inherited illness is to talk of an inherited predisposition to certain illness. This predisposition is activated or not, depending on the individual's social situation. It is the social situation in which each family member finds himself that influences psychological development and contributes to emotional ease or disease.

The interrelationship among family members determines the kind and amount of satisfaction or dissatisfaction that each person will feel through his life stages.

Faulty parent-child relationships

Neurotic households generally produce neurotic individuals; through imitative learning, the same dramatic scenes, behaviors, and patterns are perpetuated. The spoiled, inadequate, awkward, anxious, closed-minded parent teaches these same behaviors to the children.

Innumerable factors may contribute to what are called functional or psychogenic neurotic (and perhaps psychotic) disorders. Early maternal deprivations resulting from separation from the mother and placement in institutions or lack of adequate mothering within the home contribute heavily to emotional and social disturbances later in life as well as during infancy. Institutional care contributes to such disorders as retardation, isolation, withdrawal, and marasmus, which is a kind of wasting away despite adequate physical care. Inadequate mothering in the home either because of selfishness or immaturity seems to produce tense, irritable, and negativistic infants, exhibiting feeding problems, bed-wetting, and aggressiveness later in life.[53-55]

Another contributing factor centers around the lack of sufficient sensory or environmental stimulation. There are certain critical periods during which stimulation, learning experiences, and need gratifications are essential for adequate emotional, social, and intellectual development.

As the infant grows, so too do his interaction experiences. Faulty parent-child relationships contribute immensely to maladjustment, not only within the family setting but with other interpersonal interaction patterns. A rejected child feels insecure, seeks attention, engages in negative, hostile behaviors, and has difficulties with giving and receiving affection. A smothered, overprotected child is unsure, feels inadequate, behaves passively, and is overly dependent on others. Overindulgence, on the other hand, teaches selfish and demanding behaviors. Some parents, by overassuring their children, create a situation in which the child mistakenly believes that he can do or have anything he wants without expending effort. Such an individual is bound for some kind of sadness and disappointment when the world does not kowtow to his whims.

If a parent expects too much from the child and has unrealistic and perfectionistic ambitions for him, failure is inevitable, and with it come frustration, guilt, and shame. Marital discord, broken homes, and faulty and inconsistent discipline all lead to a lack of stable values, anxiety, tension, insecurity, and perhaps socially unsanctioned behaviors. Parents who do not relate harmoniously to each other as spouses rarely relate harmoniously and appropriately with their children, who, in turn, learn faulty interaction styles. Parents' interactions with each other give the child his first glimpses of the dynamics of interpersonal relations, as well as male-female relationships. In many cases, these first impressions are long-lasting ones, difficult to modify.

Neuroses

Learned maladaptive behaviors; excessive, continual stress; severe conflict situations; immaturity; and guilt increase the probability of what is called neurosis: a condition characterized by anxiety, phobias, obsessions, compulsions, depression, and many other symptoms.

The neurotic personality is never quite satisfied with things as they are, yearns for "something else," believes "if only I had or was or could be such-and-such," things would be better. He has disturbed interpersonal relationships and is wrapped up in his own needs, feelings, and hopes. This kind of person makes unrealistic demands on others and engages in defensive, self-defeating, and nonadaptive behaviors. More often than not, he is tense, anxiety ridden, irritable, not self-actualized, and manifests somatic symptoms such as fatigue, indigestion, insomnia, heart palpitations, headaches, and an assortment of other organic disturbances.

Some believe that so-called neurotic individuals recover on their own and adjust their maladaptive behaviors to create joy for themselves and others instead of doom and misery. Perhaps because of new insights, more pleasant experiences, taking responsibility for their own lives, or exerting more or less self-control, "spontaneous" recovery occurs. The prognosis is that between 40% and 60% of neurotics recover without professional therapeutic intervention.[56]

For those who enter therapy, the recovery rate goes up to about 90%, but it depends on the kind of treatment, the type and intensity of the problem, and the particular person's own degree of receptiveness to treatment. Some people are extremely willing to talk avidly about their problems, but when it comes down to changing the maladaptive behaviors, the willingness declines. Some even drop out of therapy; the problems continue, and the personality continues to decompensate further.

Psychoses

Schizophrenic reactions are psychotic disorders, characterized by a retreat from reality; disturbed thought processes, including delusions and hallucinations; emotional shallowness; and withdrawal. Schizophrenia is the most common of the functional psychotic reactions. Others include paranoid reactions, manic-depressive reactions, and involutional psychotic reactions, which include abnormal depressions, agitation, and anxiety.

The symptoms of childhood schizophrenia are a lack of relatedness to others, low frustration tolerance, obsessive desires for sameness, delayed and disturbed language development, and almost continual rocking movements. Self-identity development is difficult, as is identification with parents as role models. Effective and adaptive behavior is not adequately developed.

Family situations in which parents place the child in a double-bind, that is, make contradictory demands on the child, or continuously disqualify his statements increase the probability of schizophrenia. Other kinds of miserable, intricately tangled family situations might be equally responsible catalysts in schizophrenia-type life-styles.

The degree to which genetic factors, social and family factors, or the interaction of all these are precipitating causes of schizophrenia is still within the realm of speculation. The prognosis for schizophrenia has, in the past, been unfavorable. With modern chemotherapy, however, symptoms are significantly alleviated, and with psychotherapeutic interventions, more integration is achieved. Sociotherapy directed toward the family as a unit attempts to reduce pathological family interactions and conditions.

A big part of rehabilitation is gaining acceptance back into the workings of the community and once again becoming a functioning member of that community. If the client has a favorable home situation to which to return, and if the prescribed medication is taken, the prognosis for recovery is better than if the home environment is not supportive and co-operative in the recovery process. Unfortunately, however, the incidence of schizophrenia is higher for lower-class individuals who come from homes in which they experience rejection, isolation, and less than ideal social-emotional treatment.

Antisocial reactions

A most fascinating and rapidly growing social-personality dynamic is that of psychopathic or sociopathic character structure. These individuals are most charming on first meeting them. They appear to be ethical, principled, interesting, stimulating, and optimistic. Studies suggest that underlying their seemingly calm outward appearance, they are actually experiencing a ''nervous high'' more often than not,[58] which would explain their craving for change and excitement. They are self-indulgent, callous to the needs and feelings of others, unable to give or understand love or loyalty, impulsive, manipulative, rebellious, hostile, sometimes criminally violent, incorrigible, and feel a large discrepancy between desired goals and actual attained goals.[59]

Antisocial personalities act out their conflicts, as opposed to brooding or worrying over them. Certain studies reveal that the home situation was within a middle- to upper-class level and seemed to be one of keeping up a good appearance within the neighborhood and community. So illusion replaced actuality, and it was necessary to charm and please those from whom approval was important. Usually the father was definitely the feared head of the household, stern and remote, whereas the mother was indulgent and pleasure loving and openly expressed contempt for the father.[60] The prognosis for such ingratiating, charming, manipulative souls is that sometimes after forty years of accumulated social conditioning, the ''burned out'' psychopath improves somewhat. Improvement, however, does not mean suddenly developing a social conscience; in fact, conscience development always seems to remain arrested.

Alcoholism, drug addiction, criminal sexual deviations, and murderous aggressive assaults are some other extremely complicated behavioral dynamics that can hardly be accounted for by a simple analytical explanation. Environment, personality or character structure, genetics, opportunity, and other socioeconomic conditions may all interact as causative factors.

A fascinating yet frustrating aspect of human behavior is its fluidity. This is why speaking of a predisposition to certain behaviors is more valuable than giving a hard and fast thumb rule. Person A may share the same deleterious background as person B, yet retain normal functioning within the society. Of course, what is considered normal functioning is endlessly debatable.

Alleviating problems

All kinds of therapies exist: behavior modification, chemotherapy, psychosurgery, shock therapy, psychoanalytic therapy, psychodrama, client-centered therapy, occupational and recreational therapy, rational emotive therapy, and environmental therapy, all of which may be group, individual, or family oriented.

Whatever the name of the therapy, the goal is to explore and change the faulty assumptions and maladaptive behaviors of the individual(s) involved. The one who takes responsibility for the change differs among the different therapeutic procedures. For example, Rogerian client-centered therapy is just that: the client decides his moves, as opposed to traditional Freudian psychoanalytic therapy in which years may be spent by the therapist exposing the patient to himself. Seeking the appropriate type of counsel may be time consuming and expensive. However, if one is already committed to the idea of going into therapy, one might conceivably also be willing to spend the necessary time and money to interview several therapists to find the right one.

Sometimes a human and natural response is to either deny or ignore the problems, fear the shame and humiliation of therapy, and hope it will ''go away.'' The emotional difficulties of one family member, whether they require hospitalization or not, place strain and additional responsibilities on other family members. A psychiatric social worker, a medical doctor, and a psychologist may often team up to assist in the handling of these additional strains, particularly when young children are involved. In addition, when hospitalization is required, the return to the community and to the family is a big step, not only for the client but also for the family. Follow-up of the client is essential. So often, the recidivism rate of hospitalization for emotional problems is high because the client does not take the prescribed medication, and the family slips back into old behavior patterns.

Mental health requires a certain set of attitudes and behaviors. It means living in the present and taking joy in that living, integrating the various parts of the self and ultimately accepting that self, with its limitations as well as its strengths.

The role of the community health nurse in dealing with clients who are mentally ill is difficult to define. Most community nurses are not specifically trained in mental health work; therefore their most important function is referral of the disturbed individual or family to a mental health professional as well as ongoing support and care.

SUMMARY

This chapter has dealt with conditions that result in increased health risks. It has shown that poverty causes some health problems and compounds all of them. It is often not the amount of income but what is done with it that is an accurate measure of whether a family is poor. Certain groups of people are more likely than others to be poor: the elderly, women, nonwhites, and the uneducated. These are groups who are often discriminated against simply because they are who they are, and thus poverty becomes a vicious circle.

Poverty is also perpetuated by the economic system in which we function. Welfare has, in many cases, become the sole means of survival for some people because they cannot *afford* to get off welfare and have no means of escape. Dependence on charity, whether public or private, perpetuates itself, most often through no fault of the person receiving the charity.

Providing jobs is the most obvious way to help poor people to become nonpoor. The development of human potential by providing education and job training, plus a certain intangible motivation, is necessary for people to *want* to work.

Poverty increases people's health risks mainly because of the lack of health maintenance and health education. Chronic illness is much higher among poor people than among the affluent, mostly because the poor could not afford to treat the illness before it became chronic. The poor also are sick more because of the conditions in which they are forced to live and because health services are not as available to them for a variety of reasons.

If poverty affects health, then so does unemployment that causes poverty. In the past ten or fifteen years, government and big business have yielded somewhat to the demands, some of them quite militant, of minority groups and chronically unemployed people to find jobs for them. Various projects to train people have been successful, but a large-scale solution has not yet been found for the overall problem of unemployment. Unemployment contributes to the health risk both because it creates poverty and because in and of itself it is an unhealthy situation. Helping people to motivate themselves is probably the best way in which the community nurse can make a contribution to the unemployment problem.

Poverty and unemployment are often caused by a lack of education, and the number of people in the United States who are illiterate and who do not have a high school diploma is staggering and contributes greatly to the high number of unemployed people. The desire to get an education requires at least a semblance of a future-oriented philosophy, and it is easy to see why this is difficult for people who are products of generations of poverty and ghetto life. The public school system in most large metropolitan areas does not encourage students to stay there, and the prevailing attitude toward students seems to be tolerance at best and outright hostility at worst. The community nurse's contribution to the problem of a lack of education can be the establishment of a one-to-one relationship with families to try to increase personal motivation to stay in school.

The way in which a family reacts to the physical illness of one of its members is a factor that influences its health risk. How they cope, what they do, and what strengths they find to deal with illness in themselves or in family members determines, to a large measure, the degree of risk. Community nurses, in dealing with reactions to physical illness, need to consider a few guiding principles:

1. They should seek a cause-and-effect relationship between the client's situation and the behavior he is exhibiting.
2. They should assess the integration of the family structure and what kinds of support each member gives to the others.
3. They should find out how reality oriented the client and his family are.
4. They must know how the client and his family anticipate the future.

The inability to be a productive part of the community increases one's health risk tremendously. The nonproductive person has been defined as one who contributes nothing to the community, to society, or to his fellow human beings. He is a taker without being able to give anything in return. An example of a nonproductive person is a drug or alcohol addict. There are many theories about why people sink into drug addiction and as many theories on how to get them out of it, most of them not very successful. The community nurse can be a source of positive emotional and practical support for the family as they either try to live with the problem of addiction or try to make a new start by themselves. Sometimes the nurse's greatest contribution is the identification of the addict and the referral to an appropriate treatment facility.

Various maternal and child health problems cause families to become high health risks. Poor nutrition not only causes physical illness, it magnifies whatever illness already exists. The most important function of the community nurse is to assess, by a variety of means, the family's eating patterns. A premature infant is a high-risk infant, and poor people have a much higher incidence of prematurity than do affluent people. The greatest single cause of prematurity is the lack of adequate prenatal care that is prevalent among poor people. Another example of a maternal and child health problem is a family who has a child with a birth defect with long-range implications, such as mental retardation. Early and accurate diagnosis is essential if the child is to be able to develop to his maximum potential.

The inability to control reproduction is definitely a health risk. The decision to use or not to use contraception is as complex as are the personalities of the people who must make the decision. The major factors that determine success or failure of contraception are (1) the conscious and unconscious motivations to become pregnant, (2) the contraceptive method itself and how it is used or not used, and (3) the dynamics of the man-woman relationship. The socioeconomic status of the couple, their feelings about their own and each other's sexuality, their cultural and religious backgrounds, their education, the side effects of the various contraceptive methods, and their feelings about femininity and masculinity all combine to make contraception a much more complicated social and psychological issue than it would appear to be.

Mental illness makes someone a high health risk and is generally categorized as organic (based on some type of brain pathology) or functional (resulting from faulty psychological functioning). The latter includes neuroses, psychoses, character or personality disorders, alcoholism, and drug addiction. There are several contributory factors in the development of mental illness, including heredity, and individual's social situation, interrelationships among family members, and infancy and childhood experiences.

Various kinds of therapy are used to treat the mentally ill. The goal of all of them is to change the individual's (or family's) faulty assumptions and maladaptive behaviors. Sometimes hospitalization is necessary, but more often it is not.

NOTES

1. Hanlon, John J., and Pickett, George E.: Public health: administration and practice, ed. 7, St. Louis, 1979, The C.V. Mosby Co., p. 499.
2. Batchelder, Alan B.: The economics of poverty, New York, 1971, John Wiley & Sons, Inc.
3. No-fault divorce is a development that has abolished the

concept of the "guilty party" and assumes that blame for the failure of the marriage rests with both partners. Since in the past guilt and blame determined the size and duration of alimony payments, no-fault divorce has changed the nature of alimony.

4. Williams, Roger: Alimony: the short goodbye, Psychology Today, p. 75, July, 1977.

5. Ben Maimon, Moses. Quoted in Minkin, Jacob S.: The world of Moses Maimonides, New York, 1957, Thomas Yoseloff, Inc., Publisher.

6. Time, p. 20, July 11, 1977.

7. Roemer, Milton, and Kisch, Arnold I.: Health, poverty, and the medical mainstream. In Bloomberg, Warner, and Schmandt, Henry J., editors: Urban poverty: its social and political dimensions, Beverly Hills, Calif., 1970, Sage Publications, Inc.

8. Keynes, John Maynard: The general theory of employment, interest and money. In Ginsburg, Helen: Poverty, economics and society, Boston, 1972, Little, Brown & Co.

9. Baran, Paul A., and Sweezy, Paul M.: Capitalism and persistent poverty. In Ginsburg, Helen: Poverty, economics and society, Boston, 1972, Little, Brown & Co.

10. Friedman, Milton: The alleviation of poverty. In Ginsburg, Helen: Poverty, economics and society, Boston, 1972, Little, Brown & Co.

11. Tinkham, Catherine W., and Voorhies, Eleanor F.: Community health nursing, New York, 1972, Appleton-Century-Crofts.

12. This is based on a population of 250 million, which will be reached by the turn of the century.

13. Collins, Mattie: Communication in health care: understanding and implementing effective human relations, St. Louis, 1977, The C.V. Mosby Co.

14. Functional illiteracy is the ability to read and write at such a low level that for all practical purposes it might as well be nonexistent. A functional illiterate cannot read a classified ad and cannot spell well enough to fill out a job application; consequently, his minimal skills are of no real use to him.

15. A 1976 survey of Philadelphia high schools showed that over 25% of students in the graduating classes were not able to master fourth-grade reading skills.

16. The validity of these standardized tests as accurate measures and predictors of intelligence or academic ability has been called into question in the last decade or so. The emphasis on verbal and mathematical ability has been labeled as discriminatory against children whose verbal and mathematical expertise has not been developed.

17. Maslow, Abraham H.: Toward a psychology of being, New York, 1968, Van Nostrand Reinhold Co.

18. A variation on this is "The rich get richer and the poor get children."

19. Schontz, Franklin C.: The psychological aspects of physical illness and disability, New York, 1975, The Macmillan Co.

20. This is not to imply that having sex is the most important thing we do. It is well understood that the mental activity involved in sex very much directs the physical activity. But it is also true that sex without the use of one's body is impossible.

21. Richardson, Stephen A., et al.: Cultural uniformity in reaction to physical disabilities, American Sociological Review **26:**241-247, 1961.

22. Wu, Ruth: Behavior and illness, Englewood Cliffs, N.J., 1973, Prentice-Hall, Inc.

23. Hill, R.B.: The strengths of black families. In Reinhardt, Adina M., and Quinn, Mildred D., editors: Current practice in family-centered community nursing, vol. 1, St. Louis, 1977, The C.V. Mosby Co.

24. The term *addict* in this chapter will refer to anyone who is dependent on any kind of drug: alcohol, heroin, or whatever.

25. National Institute of Mental Health: Alcohol and alcoholism, Public Health Service Pub. No. 1640, Washington, D.C., 1968, U.S. Government Printing Office.

26. Benson, Evelyn R., and McDevitt, Joan Q.: Community health nursing practice, ed. 2, Englewood Cliffs, N.J., 1980, Prentice-Hall, Inc.

27. Jensen, Margaret Duncan, Benson, Ralph C., and Bobak, Irene M.: Maternity care: the nurse and the family, ed. 2, St. Louis, 1981, The C.V. Mosby Co.

28. Reeder, Sharon R., et al.: Maternity nursing, Philadelphia, 1976, J.B. Lippincott Co.

29. The exact reason why a uterus begins premature contractions is not known, just as the stimulus that triggers labor at term is not fully understood. But correlations between certain prenatal circumstances and the incidence of prematurity have been proved.

30. Marlow, Dorothy R.: Textbook of pediatric nursing, ed. 2, Philadelphia, 1978, W.B. Saunders Co.

31. Fletcher (see Chapter 5 on biomedical ethics) and others would consider an individual with an IQ of 20 and below not to be a human being.

32. Hurley, Roger L.: Poverty and mental retardation, New York, 1969, Random House, Inc.

33. Time, pp. 18-28, October 10, 1977.

34. Butler, Robert N., and Lewis, Myrna I.: Aging and mental health: positive psychosocial approaches, ed. 2, St. Louis, 1977, The C.V. Mosby Co.

35. Cousins, Norman: The right to die, Saturday Review, p. 4, June 14, 1975.

36. Sandberg, E., and Jacobs, R.: Psychology of the misuse and rejection of contraception, American Journal of Obstetrics and Gynecology **110:**227-237, 1971.

37. Rabin, A.I., and Greene, R.J.: Assessing motivation for parenthood, Journal of Psychology **69:**39-46, 1968.

38. MacDonald, A.P.: Internal-external locus of control and the practice of birth control, Psychological Reports **27:**206, 1970.

39. Flapan, M.: A paradigm for the analysis of childbearing motivations of married women prior to the birth of the first child, American Journal of Orthopsychiatry **39:**402-417, 1969.
40. Wood, Roberta, Campbell, F., Townes, Brenda, and Beach, Lee: Birth planning decisions, American Journal of Public Health **67:**563-565, 1977.
41. Wyatt, F.: Clinical notes on the motives of reproduction, Journal of Social Issues **23:**29-56, 1967.
42. Hoffmann, Lois, and Wyatt, F.: Social change and motivations for having larger families: some theoretical considerations, Merrill-Palmer Quarterly **6:**235-244, 1960.
43. Kutner, S.J., and Duffy, T.S.: A psychological analysis of oral contraceptives and the intrauterine device, Contraception **2:**289-296, 1970.
44. Ziegler, F., Rodgers, D.A., Kriegsman, S.A., and Martin, P.A.: Ovulation suppressors, psychological functioning, and marital adjustment, Journal of the American Medical Association **204:**849-853, 1968.
45. Bardwick, Judith: Psychology of women, New York, 1971, Harper & Row, Publishers.
46. Rodgers, D., Ziegler, F., Altrocchi, J., and Levy, N.: A longitudinal study of the psycho-social effects of vasectomy, Journal of Marriage and the Family **27:**59-64, 1965.
47. Ziegler, R., Rodgers, D., and Kriegsman, S.: Effect of vasectomy on psychological functioning, Psychosomatic Medicine **28:**50-63, 1966.
48. Wolfers, Helen: Psychological aspects of vasectomy, British Medical Journal **4:**297-300, 1970.
49. Bakker, C.B., and Dightman, C.R.: Psychological factors in fertility control, Fertility and Sterility **15:**559-567, 1964.
50. Birth control deaths, Newsweek, p. 60, March 1, 1976.
51. Szasz, T.S.: The myth of mental illness, New York, 1974, Harper & Row, Publishers.
52. Kallman, F.J.: The use of genetics in psychiatry, Journal of Mental Science **104:**542-549, 1958.
53. Sears, Robert R., et al.: Patterns of child rearing, Evanston, Ill., 1957, Row, Peterson & Co.
54. Bowlby, J.: Maternal care and mental health, World Health Organization Monograph Series, No. 2, 1952.
55. Rebble, Margaretha: Infantile experiences in relation to personality development. In Hunt, J., editor: Personality and the behavior disorders, vol. 2, New York, 1944, The Ronald Press Co.
56. Eysenck, H.: Behavior therapy, spontaneous remission and transference in neurotics, American Journal of Psychiatry **119:**867-871, 1963.
57. Laing, Ronald D.: The politics of the family, New York, 1972, Pantheon Books.
58. Schacter, S.: The interaction of cognitive and physiological determinants of emotional state. In Berkowitz, L.: Advances in experimental social psychology, New York, 1964, Academic Press, Inc.
59. Harrington, A.: Psychopaths, New York, 1972, Simon & Schuster, Inc.
60. Greenacre, Phyllis: Conscience in the psychopath, American Journal of Orthopsychiatry **15:**495-509, 1945.

BIBLIOGRAPHY

American Journal of Maternal and Child Nursing **2**(2), 1977. Entire issue.

Barbieri, Winnie: No pity, American Journal of Nursing **76:**1482, 1976.

Batchelder, Alan B.: The economics of poverty, New York, 1971, John Wiley & Sons, Inc.

Benson, Evelyn R., and McDevitt, Joan Q.: Community health and nursing practice, ed. 2, Englewood Cliffs, N.J., 1980, Prentice-Hall, Inc.

Bloomberg, Warner, and Schmandt, Henry J., editors: Urban poverty: its social and political dimensions, Beverly Hills, Calif., 1970, Sage Publications, Inc.

Bowlby, J.: Maternal care and mental health, World Health Organization Monograph Series, No. 2, 1952.

Burkhalter, Pamela K.: Nursing care of the alcoholic and drug abuser, New York, 1975, McGraw-Hill Book Co.

Butler, Robert N., and Lewis, Myrna I.: Aging and mental health: positive psychosocial approaches, ed. 2, St. Louis, 1977, The C.V. Mosby Co.

Chopoorian, Teresa, and Craig, Margaret M.: PL 93-641, nursing and health care delivery, American Journal of Nursing **76:**1988-1991, 1976.

Collins, Mattie: Communication in health care: understanding and implementing effective human relations, St. Louis, 1977, The C.V. Mosby Co.

Davis, Kenneth S.: The paradox of poverty in America, New York, 1969, The H.W. Wilson Co.

Ditzler, Joyce M.: Rehabilitation for alcoholics, American Journal of Nursing **76:**1311-1313, 1976.

Freeman, Ruth B.: Community health nursing practice, Philadelphia, 1970, W.B. Saunders Co.

Fuhrer, Lois, and Bernstein, Ronnie: Making patient education a part of patient care, American Journal of Nursing **76:**1798-1799, 1976.

Ginsburg, Helen: Poverty, economics and society, Boston, 1972, Little, Brown & Co.

Gladwin, Thomas: Poverty, U.S.A., Boston, 1967, Little, Brown & Co.

Hanlon, John J., and Pickett, George E.: Public health: administration and practice, ed. 7, St. Louis, 1979, The C.V. Mosby Co.

Harrington, A.: Psychopaths, New York, 1972, Simon & Schuster, Inc.

Hurley, Rodger L.: Poverty and mental retardation, New York, 1969, Random House, Inc.

Jensen, Margaret Duncan, Benson, Ralph C., and Bobak, Irene M.: Maternity care: the nurse and the family, ed. 2, St. Louis, 1981, The C.V. Mosby Co.

Laing, Ronald D.: The politics of the family, New York, 1972, Pantheon Books.

Leacock, Eleanor B., editor: The culture of poverty, New York, 1971, Simon & Schuster, Inc.

Leahy, Kathleen M., et al.: Community health nursing, New York, 1977, McGraw-Hill Book Co.

Marlow, Dorothy R.: Textbook of pediatric nursing, Philadelphia, 1978, W.B. Saunders Co.

Maslow, Abraham H.: Toward a psychology of being, New York, 1968, Van Nostrand Reinhold Co.

McGrath, Barbara: Nursing in area health education centers, American Journal of Nursing **76:**1605-1607, 1976.

Milio, Nancy: The care of health in communities, New York, 1975, The Macmillan Co.

Murray, Ruth, and Zentner, Judith: Nursing assessment and health promotion through the life span, Englewood Cliffs, N.J., 1975, Prentice-Hall, Inc.

Rebble, Margaretha: Infantile experiences in relation to personality development. In Hunt, J., editor: Personality and the behavior disorders, vol. 2, New York, 1944, The Ronald Press Co.

Reeder, Sharon R., et al.: Maternity nursing, Philadelphia, 1976, J.B. Lippincott Co.

Reinhardt, Adina M., and Quinn, Mildred D., editors: Current practice in family-centered community nursing, vol. 1, St. Louis, 1977, The C.V. Mosby Co.

Schontz, Franklin C.: The psychological aspects of physical illness and disability, New York, 1975, Macmillan, Inc.

Schwartz, Jane L., and Schwartz, Lawrence H.: Vulnerable infants, New York, 1977, McGraw-Hill Book Co.

Schwartz, Lawrence H., and Schwartz, Jane L.: The psychodynamics of patient care, Englewood Cliffs, N.J., 1972, Prentice-Hall, Inc.

Shaw, Dale, et al.: Multiple impact therapy, American Journal of Nursing **77:**246-248, 1977.

Tinkham, Catherine W., and Voorhies, Eleanor P.: Community health nursing, New York, 1972, Appleton-Century-Crofts.

Weaver, Jerry L.: National health policy and the underserved: ethnic minorities, women, and the elderly, St. Louis, 1976, The C.V. Mosby Co.

Williams, Roger: Alimony: the short goodbye, Psychology Today, p. 75, July, 1977.

Wu, Ruth: Behavior and illness, Englewood Cliffs, N.J., 1973, Prentice-Hall, Inc.

Ziegel, Erna, and VanBlarcom, Carolyn: Obstetric nursing, New York, 1972, The Macmillan Co.

12

MATURATIONAL AND SITUATIONAL CRISES

DEFINITIONS AND GENERAL THEORIES OF ANXIETY REACTION TO CRISIS

A person in crisis is at a turning point. He faces a problem that he cannot readily solve by using the coping mechanisms that have worked for him before. As a result, his tension and anxiety increase, and he becomes less able to find a solution. A person in this situation feels helpless—he is caught in a state of great emotional upset and feels unable to take action *on his own* to solve his problem.[1,p.1]

Almost every client whom the community nurse sees can, to one degree or another, fits this description of a person in crisis. The nature of our health care system almost ensures that the nurse will not see her clients until they are well enmeshed in crisis. The exception is the practitioner doing primary nursing who can be a crisis prevention agent. This nursing function will be discussed at the end of the chapter. The rest of the chapter will deal with the kinds of crises the community nurse will encounter most often and the ways in which the nurse might be able to intervene to achieve a positive result for the client.

It must be remembered that a client can view *any* situation as a crisis; an event that one person can take in stride may be totally devastating to another. This phenomenon is easily seen in outpatient abortion clinics. All the women are in approximately the same stage of pregnancy (first trimester), and all are having the same vacuum aspiration procedure performed. But the emotional reactions are as varied as the number of women there. It is the function of the professional community nurse to see each person's crisis as a unique entity and to deal with it accordingly.

Definition of crisis

Crisis can be defined in many ways. It is most often an acute situation with which an individual is unable to cope.[2] There is usually an extreme degree of stress, manifested by high anxiety, a decreased level of day-to-day functioning, and, most important, the failure of previously workable coping mechanisms. The realization that familiar ways of dealing with anxiety and stress are no longer workable can, and often does, lead to panic and an increase in the amount of anxiety and stress perceived. This, of course, leads to a decreased ability to function and the worsening of the crisis. A vicious circle ensues, and the client can find himself paralyzed and impotent while faced with a situation with which it is imperative that he deal.

Fink[3] has described a framework of changes through which an individual in crisis moves. He describes the various behaviors that the nurse might be expected to observe and what feelings the individual in crisis might be experiencing.

1. The shock or impact phase is the one in which the individual realizes that something has hap-

pened, but the enormity and future implications of the crisis are not yet apparent. There is a feeling of depersonalization (''Something terrible has happened, but it can't possibly be me to whom it has happened'') and a general lack of subjective feeling. If the crisis is a physical one, there may not yet be pain. The individual is in profound emotional shock and often is incapable of planning a course of action to resolve the crisis. He is sometimes passive and malleable, and at this stage almost all his help must come from other people. The shock phase is relatively short, but exact time parameters cannot be given because of the individual nature of reactions to crisis. Emotional shock from an emotional crisis is generally more long lasting than emotional shock from a physical crisis.

2. During the realization phase, panic begins to set in. The reality of the situation may appear to be overwhelming and hopeless, and anxiety soars. The degree of anxiety may be so great that the individual still is unable to think clearly and to plan a logical course of action. There may be a breakdown of the individual's usual social controls with a resultant exhibition of bizarre or irrational behavior. He is still much in need of outside help, and it is usually during this phase that the individual enters the health care system, although the community nurse might not see him until some time later.

3. The defensive retreat phase of a crisis is the one in which reality emerges from shock. The individual can feel attacked by the reality he perceives and often makes a great effort to avoid or to deny that reality. He has a choice of three basic courses of action: withdrawing entirely from the situation and retreating into fantasy, expressing his anger and despair with verbal and nonverbal behavior, or yielding to the disorganization he feels and permitting his life to continue in a disrupted manner. Many behaviors are exhibited during this stage: indifference or euphoria; expressions of hostility and anger by lashing out at family, friends, or health workers; hysteria; and sometimes passive stoicism. The responses by health workers to the individual in crisis during this phase can have a great bearing on how he is ultimately able to resolve the crisis.

4. The phase of acknowledgment is when reality imposes itself to such an extent that it must be dealt with. The person must face the situation, assess its implications, and make plans to resolve the crisis. There may be great depression, remorse, pain, and bitterness, but out of these feelings, and with professional intervention, comes a reorganization and restructuring of coping mechanisms. Sometimes there is even a reevaluation of one's entire life-style. It is also during this phase that an individual may choose *not* to deal constructively with the crisis. This is the time when the person may opt for suicide or for a permanent retreat into fantasy and nonreality. Community nurses, in their roles as crisis intervention therapists, can be instrumental in helping clients to work through crises.

5. The adaptation or change phase is a time of reorganization and stabilization during which the person acquires new insights and new ways of dealing with problems. Anxiety decreases, and self-worth increases. Sometimes there is even a repatterning of modes of behavior that will prove useful in preventing or dealing with future crises.

The five stages of crisis are similar to the five stages of dying (shock, denial, bargaining, depression, and acceptance) described by Elisabeth Kübler-Ross in her book, *On Death and Dying*.[4] Death, either one's own or that of someone else, is perhaps the biggest crisis we will ever have to face. The five stages have been described because community nurses must recognize the kinds of behavior they may encounter so they will be able to deal with them in a therapeutic manner.

Symptoms of anxiety

Because many degrees of anxiety and panic are almost always present in a person in crisis, the nurse should be able to recognize the physical and psychological symptoms of anxiety. Gebbie and Lavin[5] characterize the symptoms of moderate and severe anxiety as the absence of a concrete object of anxiety, the narrowing of the perceptual field (i.e., the inability to pay attention to many things for long periods of time and to be oblivious to many of the things going on around oneself), unusual attention to detail, muscle tension, perspiration, the need for help to focus on problem solving, scattering of attention, decreased ability to conceptualize, trembling, nausea, headache, a feeling of dread, and rapid pulse. The symptoms of panic are also an absence of an object of anxiety, distortion of reality, extremely narrow mental focus, difficulty in verbalizing feelings, bizarre behavior, dilated pupils, increased pulse and respiration, and ashen color. If the client is fortunate, he may seek or be referred to a crisis intervention counselor while he is still in phase one, two, or three of the crisis. The community nurse then has an opportunity to observe these symptoms. It is more likely, however, that the nurse will not see the client until he has reached phase four and may already have dealt with these symptoms alone or with the help of people close to him.

It is often helpful during crisis intervention to ask the client to describe the feelings he experienced during the acute phase of the crisis. Learning how the client dealt with those feelings could provide valuable clues for the planning of therapy. During crisis intervention therapy, anxiety should persist because if there is no anxiety, the learning process is impaired. Without anxiety the client will have a false sense of security, and his perceived need for therapy will be decreased. Severe anxiety can be tolerated for only certain periods of time; then the level must be reduced so that the cognitive process can continue to function.

Caplan[6] sees crisis as a transitional period that presents an individual with a chance for personal growth or with an equal chance for an increased vulnerability to mental disorder. The way in which the person handles the situation usully determines the direction his future life will take. It is not so much the nature of the crisis but the reaction to it that is the indicator of future growth or the lack of it. The community nurse as a crisis intervention therapist and as a researcher can contribute to the growing body of knowledge about dealing with crisis. The nurse is also the person who is in the best position to interpret this body of knowledge to the client and help him see how his particular crisis fits into the general theoretical framework.

These ideas about crisis as a turning point toward or away from mental disorder also offer the hope that we may learn enough about the current situational factors which determine the outcome during the disequilibrium of the crisis so that we may intervene at that time and increase the possibility of a healthy outcome.*

This places great responsibility on the community nurse, whether or not she is a practitioner of crisis intervention therapy. During the course of her routine activities, she will see many clients and their families who are in crisis. If she is able to recognize this fact, the client will most likely receive appropriate help. Even if the nurse is not giving direct therapy, she can play an important supportive role in helping the client and his family, and she can refer them to the appropriate professional health workers.

According to Caplan, individuals maintain their equilibrium by operating in consistent patterns and by using habitual mechanisms and reactions to solve problems. What makes a crisis a crisis is its difference from these habitual patterns. The problem stimulus or precipitating event is larger or more exaggerated than those which the client has been accustomed to handling; thus the forces that had been previously used to maintain equilibrium are no longer effective. The period of disequilibrium is usually longer, and behavior inconsistency is more pronounced and of longer duration. When equilibrium is finally achieved, behavior patterns may be quite different from previous ones.

The essential factor influencing the occurence of crisis is an imbalance between the difficulty and importance of the problem and the resources immediately available

*From Principles of preventive psychiatry, pp. 37 and 39, by Gerald Caplan, © 1964 by Basic Books, Inc., Publishers, New York.

to deal with it. The usual homeostatic, direct problem-solving mechanisms do not work, and the problem is such that other methods which might be used to sidestep it also cannot be used.*

During crisis, people become more open to suggestion and more amenable to receiving help. Methods of dealing with previous crises can be explored and examined, and it is often a time of flux and behavioral change for family relationships. The individual in crisis needs the understanding and support of his family more than he ever has before. Family counseling and therapy is often the most appropriate mode of treatment and will be discussed more fully later in the chapter.

Cadden,[7] in an article first published in *Redbook,* lists seven ways in which one can be of help to a person in crisis. Although the advise was directed toward lay people, it incorporates the elements of professional nursing:

1. Help the person to confront the crisis by talking about the danger, pain, trouble, and real elements of the crisis. Help him to verbalize his unspoken fears, to grieve, and even to cry.

2. Help the person to confront the crisis in manageable doses. The individual occasionally needs to have his mind taken off the crisis from time to time as a respite or as a brief mental vacation from the continuing tension and anxiety.

3. Help the person to find the facts. Fantasies and fear of the unknown are infinitely more frightening than reality. Seeking and finding the truths about a situation is the healthy way to deal with crisis.

4. Do not give the person false reassurance. "There, there, everything will be all right" is an approach that fosters dependence and encourages weakness and childlike behavior rather than the strength and maturity that are needed. The person in crisis needs faith that he will be strong enough to master the problem, and relegating him to the role of a child by giving him false reassurance

*From Principles of preventive psychiatry, pp. 37 and 39, by Gerald Caplan, © 1964 by Basic Books, Inc., Publishers, New York.

simply undermines his own sense of self-worth and ego strength.

5. Do not encourage the person to blame others. Blaming is a way of avoiding truth and avoiding facing the problem at hand. Blaming others may feel reassuring for a while, but in the long run it encourages weakness rather than strength.

6. Help the person to accept help. Asking for and actively seeking help dispels the fantasy that nothing is wrong and contributes to the acceptance of reality; it is usually the first step toward healthy and positive resolution of the crisis.

7. Help the person with everyday tasks. A crisis disorganizes and disorients an individual, and he needs all his energy to maintain whatever equilibrium remains. He often does not have sufficient energy left over to manage the routine day-to-day tasks that must be accomplished.

Murray and Zentner[8,p.207] define crisis in a slightly different way: "Crisis is any transient situation that necessitates reorganization of one's psychological structure and behavior, that causes a sudden alteration in the person's expectation of himself, and that cannot be handled with the person's usual coping mechanisms." Although the basic elements of the definition have been previously discussed, the implication here is that not only do previous coping mechanisms fail, but a certain amount of revamping of the psyche needs to be instituted. If there is no positive adaptive resolution to the crisis, then maladaptive behavior is the result. This maladaptation may not be evident at the time of the present crisis (by the same token, the current crisis may be the result of a past failure to resolve a crisis in a productive manner) but may manifest itself in future behavior. Maladaptation can include prolonged expressions of hostility, sadness, apathy, lack of initiative, irritability, and withdrawal. Suicide attempts may be precipitated by feelings of hopelessness, isolation, worthlessness, and guilt. The individual who has not coped successfully with a crisis may become extremely ritualistic or indulge in excesses of food, drugs, or alcohol. Some of these behaviors begin early in the crisis and are not necessarily delayed reactions. The nurse can be effective in making the client aware of his behavior so it does not become maladaptive or habitual. For instance, the nurse who notices a client suddenly eating a great many candy bars and other sweets after the sudden death of his mother should discuss this new behavior with the client, perhaps even explaining the relationships of mothering, nurturing, and food intake, especially sweets. This discussion and analysis, as well as understanding, of the behavior might prevent a maladaptive pattern of compulsive eating.

MATURATIONAL AND SITUATIONAL CRISES

Crises generally fall into two categories: maturational (also called developmental) and situational (also called accidental).

Definitions

Maturational crises are changes or transition points that every person experiences during the process of physical, social, psychological, and intellectual growth. "They usually evolve over an extended period of time, . . . and they frequently require that the individual make many characterological changes. There may be an awareness of increased feelings of disequilibrium, but intellectual understanding of any correlation with normal developmental change may be inadequate."[1,p.132]

A situational crisis is an external event, usually sudden and unexpected, that is not part of everyday living and with which the individual is unable to deal by using his usual coping mechanisms. It is frequently characterized by high degrees of anxiety and tension and throws the individual into a state of disequilibrium.

Often it is impossible to make a discrete classification of crises. Some fall into both maturational and situational categories (Fig. 12-1). Early marriage (prior to age 21) is an excellent example. There are the maturational crises of adolescence and marriage, both of which are among the most turbulent of the life cycle. On top of this are the continuing crises of school, trying to earn a living,

and coping with the new roles of husband and wife. This combination generally results in a situational crisis to which is sometimes added a pregnancy (in many cases unwanted and unplanned). The added role of parenthood is then suddenly thrust on people who have not fully completed and given up their roles as adolescents. This is a difficult set of conditions to survive and grow from, and it is easy to see why so many early marriages end in divorce.

Maturational crises

The process of growth can be viewed as the process of mastering a series of tasks in a reasonable semblance of order. During the course of the mastery of these tasks, new relationships are formed and old ones broken off; new interests and abilities are developed, and old ones are discarded. New perceptions and a sense of awareness replace old ones. This is a gradual and inexorable process that continues from birth to death and is influenced by every variable that can affect human development. One of the important measures of the change and growth process is the assumption of new roles as life proceeds. A role is a set of behaviors that is learned within one's sociocultural situation and which is carried out by an individual because it is expected of him, either by himself and/or by others. One individual's role or roles exist with and are enmeshed by the roles of the people around him, like the pieces of a puzzle fitting together to form a complete picture. Maturational crises most often develop when a person is unable or unwilling to take on a new role. Pressure to accept certain roles, which society deems natural and unavoidable, is great in today's world; the person who cannot or who will not accept the role or who has difficulty growing into the role, will face a maturational crisis. Murray and Zentner[8] list three reasons why a person may be unable to make the role changes necessary to prevent a maturational crisis:

1. An adequate model from whom to learn a role may be absent. Consequently the person is unable to picture himself in a certain role.
2. Inadequate intrapersonal resources may make a person unable to make role changes. There

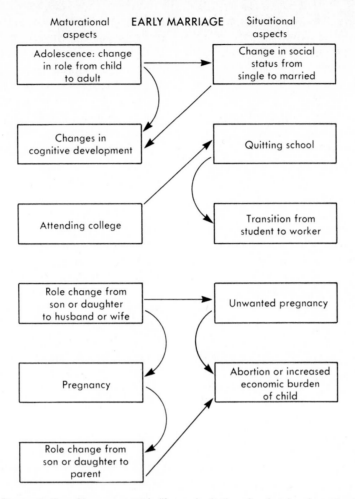

Fig. 12-1. Demonstration of how an event in life can be both a situational and a maturational crisis.

may be a lack of certain skills or the realization that some of life's goals will not be achieved. There may be an inability to create alternatives to an unwanted life-style.

3. Others in the social system may refuse to see the person in a different role. For example, when the adolescent tries to move from childhood to the adult role, the parent may persist in keeping him in the child role.

Erik Erikson conceives of maturational crisis as a time of necessary change. His eight stages of the life cycle are (1) integrity versus despair, (2) gen-

erativity versus stagnation, (3) intimacy versus isolation, (4) identity versus diffusion, (5) industry versus inferiority, (6) initiative versus guilt, (7) autonomy versus shame, and (8) trust versus mistrust. These stages represent a synthesis of developmental and social tasks with growth taking place from the constant interaction of learning and maturation.

The crises during growth and development, as Erikson uses the term, connote a heightened potential for development (or change) accompanied by greater vulnerability. Crisis is not necessarily a negative state of affairs, but rather an unavoidable occasion requiring coping of some variety. In Erikson's view the crises occur at their proper time out of the organism's maturation and society's expectations. The outcome (not *resolution* necessarily) is dependent upon the personality resources the individual has accrued up to that point *and* the opportunities and resources available in his social situation.[9,p.121]

The last phrase in the preceding quotation should be the key one for community nurses. In working with clients in crisis, they will have the opportunity to make appropriate resources available to the clients. So many community health centers, with therapists who specialize in crisis intervention, are unknown to (and consequently unavailable to) the general public. Community nurses, in their roles as resource people and referral agents, can bring these resources to the clients.

INFANCY

Maturational crises begin in infancy and continue through old age. The infant must learn to trust the maternal figure, and he must begin to develop a confidence in the consistency and continuity of his environment. In order for the infant to develop this trust that is basic to all other developmental tasks, the maternal figure (it need not necessarily be the mother; it could be the father, grandparent, aunt, or anyone as long as the person is a constant and enduring figure in the infant's life) must be available to satisfy his needs and to provide love, warmth, and security. If the maternal figure is dependable, the infant will learn dependability and trust; if the maternal figure is not dependable and there is a general absence of mothering, the infant can develop symptoms of insecurity (crying, depression, withdrawal, and even death in extreme cases) and a resultant maturational crisis. If this kind of emotional insecurity persists, it can lead to the retardation of sensorimotor and intellectual development *even though* there is no inherent physical or mental reason for retardation. A maturational crisis this early in life, unless it is success-

fully dealt with, has far-reaching, even lifetime, implications. The infant often develops into an adult who is chronically mistrustful, dependent, depressed, withdrawn, and incapable of developing deep interpersonal relationships.

During late infancy a struggle for autonomy begins. The infant ventures from his mother's arms out into the world. His need to explore and learn is almost unlimited, and he starts to recognize the difference between himself and others. It is during this time that a sense of independence can be fostered, and power struggles between the child, who wants to let go, and the parent, who wants to keep him in, are common. During this phase, cognitive development, particularly in the area of abstraction and communication, is rapid, and the major psychosocial task is the achievement of self-esteem and self-control. If an infant is repeatedly thwarted in his attempts to reach out and grow, a crisis will develop. If he is not able to achieve mastery of the tasks of infancy, a sense of independence will not be established, and he may become an adult unable to function effectively on his own.

SCHOOL YEARS

The preschool and prepuberty years are concerned with the development of initiative, autonomy, cognitive skills, and a sense of usefulness and self-esteem. The time is fraught with crises. The child begins to peep out into the adult world that he can see at a distance, but he always scurries back to the safety of childhood. Beginning school is a major step into independence, and in the eyes of the child there is constant excitement, stimulation, and danger. Peer acceptance is of prime importance. Who among us cannot recall the intense anxiety we felt when the grammar school softball team captain chose sides, and we prayed not to be the last chosen? Preschool and school-age children are also heirs to a variety of physical illnesses, which, if they are severe or prolonged, can lead to developmental retardation and a maturational crisis. The loss of parents (through death, divorce, or even through emotional distance) and the guidance they give almost always leads to a maturational crisis. The loss of a parent can be said also to be a situational crisis. If childhood can be viewed as preparation for adulthood, and if there are insurmountable crises that prevent the acquisition of skills needed as an adult, then there will be maturational crises in subsequent phases of life.

ADOLESCENCE

Adolescence is the phase during which the most serious and long-lasting (both in duration and in aftereffects) maturational crises occur (Fig. 12-2). Bodily changes are drastic and rapid, and the adolescent is often uncomfortable with the strangeness of his own body. The need to be accepted by one's peers and to be "like the rest of the kids" is often in conflict with the need for independence and the need for what the adolescent might consider daring radical behavior. The crisis of sexual development is enormous. The dichotomy between feelings and accepted modes of behavior is strong, and lack of accurate knowledge about sex often leads to guilt and misunderstanding.

In about 90% of adolescents sexual development is heterosexual. But for the 10% who are beginning to realize that they are homosexual, the maturational crisis has profound implications. Most parents and school personnel are not equipped to deal with homosexual adolescents, so the adolescents are often forced to think of themselves as shameful and sick. The guilt arising from this situation can last a lifetime and is often emotionally crippling.

Having to choose a career and a future life-style at age 17 or 18 is a crisis in itself. Adolescents have done so little living, and there is such a wide variety of careers to choose from, that it is no wonder adolescents vacillate from week to week and sometimes succumb to the pressure of having to make so important a choice with inadequate preparation. Adolescents are being constantly torn between the demands of an independent adulthood and the security of childhood; they feel "betwixt and be-tween," and it is a constant source of wonder that so many adolescents survive to become reasonably independent and fulfilled adults.

YOUNG ADULTHOOD

The maturational crises during young adulthood are legion. This is the time when people leave childhood and enter roles, many of which they will fill for a lifetime. Most of the crises occur as a result of society's expectations that roles *will* be chosen and settled into. Up until ten or fifteen years ago there was almost no choice. Men got jobs, married, and provided for their families. Women married, bore children, and kept house. These roles were expected of everyone (with slight sociocultural variations); the majority of people acquiesced, and if they were dissatisfied, restless, or unhappy, there was little to be done about it. Maturational crises existed but were mostly ignored. Now the choice of life-styles for both men and women is almost unlimited, and many young adults go through agonies of indecision. The pull of tradition (marriage, a family, and "security") is strong. So is the need to seek out and explore other modes of living and behavior. Parental pressure to "settle down and make something of yourself" is often at war with the young adult's wanderlust and need for adventure. Maturational crises are abundant and severe. Decisions made as a young adult are less easily reversed than those of an adolescent. An employer looking at the résumé of a 20-year-old and finding frequent job changes will be more likely to accept this behavior than he would the same behavior in a 30-year-old. An adolescent girl has time to make up her mind about whether she wants to bear children. A woman in her late twenties begins to experience the pressure of "It's now or never." The need to develop intimate (both sexual and nonsexual) relationships with other people is extremely important during young adulthood, and the inability to do so, perhaps because of previous maturational or situational crises, can lead to a crisis. Feelings of alienation and of not belonging to someone special also produce crises.

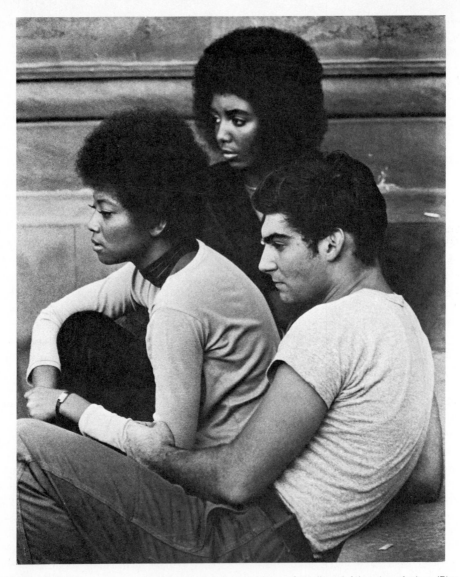

Fig. 12-2. Adolescence is a maturational crisis that can be profoundly painful and confusing. (Photograph by Jan Lukas; courtesy Editorial Photocolor Archives, Inc., New York.)

The greatest crises of adulthood again arise from chosen roles. If an individual is happy in and satisfied with his chosen role, there is usually no sense or feeling of crisis. However, it is a human experience, more common than not, that a person has doubts about his chosen role, becomes dissatisfied with it, and often feels he cannot continue to act out a role in which he no longer wishes to be. This is how maturational crises occur in adulthood. Every now and then we hear about a man or a woman who "goes out for a pack of cigarettes" and is never heard from again. This is crisis resolution at its most drastic, but there are thousands of adults who feel trapped in roles and desperately long to be released.

MIDDLE AGE

The crises of middle age result mainly from physical, cultural, economic, and psychological stresses. Encroaching baldness, sagging of once-firm body tissues, irregular menses, and occasional impotence are all signs that the flesh will not last forever and that death is in sight—far away, perhaps, but definitely in sight. The impact of the realization that one's body may no longer be functioning perfectly and that as time goes on the functioning will become even less dependable can become a maturational crisis of the first magnitude. American culture reveres youth, or at least a youthful appearance, and the shock of being no longer young is a profound one. "Oh, Daddy, you're such and old fogy" heard from adolescent children is a constant reminder of the crisis of middle age. Economic stresses of a rising cost of living and the feeling of responsibility to educate one's children also can lead to maturational crisis. Psychological stresses, however, are the greatest cause of crisis during middle age. Nearness of death, feelings of failure in not having achieved a hoped-for measure of success in business, realization that marriage was not what it was expected to be, regret of having not followed through with plans laid in youth, growing independence of children, loss of hope that life-styles can always be changed if the dissatisfaction becomes too great—all of these contribute in great measure to the maturational crises of middle age. Marmor[10] has described four factors on which the method the individual uses to cope with these crises is dependent:

1. The individual's basic capacity for flexible adaptation to change, in contrast to emotional rigidity
2. The nature of his interpersonal relationships: the character of his marriage and his relationship to his children, other relatives, and friends
3. His sense of continuing usefulness, which depends on the extent of his functional relationships and the degree of fulfillment they afford
4. The breadth of his interest in the outside world

OLD AGE

The maturational crises of old age revolve almost totally around four things: retirement, physical illness, economic problems, and the increasing nearness of death. In our culture, where work and productivity are considered essential for a worthwhile life, the rejection experienced in retirement (often at the height of an individual's creative ability) becomes a crisis. Those additional 8 or 10 hours a day are difficult to fill, and many elderly people are bored and "at loose ends." They sometimes think that there is no longer a reason to get up in the morning, and in almost no time, severe depression sets in. The suicide rate for the elderly has been increasing steadily over the past ten years. It is not easy to make activities that had formerly been reserved for leisure time a central part of one's existence. A person who is accustomed to tending his garden on Saturday and Sunday mornings may not want to make it a full-time occupation.

Although elderly people have fewer acute illnesses than younger people, they are prone to chronic diseases that are often costly, debilitating, and psychologically depressing. There is no cure for many of the diseases of old age; in addition to knowing that one will be ill, to some degree, for the rest of one's life, there is the added fear of dependency and further rejection by being placed in a nursing home by one's family. The death of a spouse also leads to loneliness and feelings of rejection.

Economic burdens are often a source of crisis. Living on a fixed income in a time of rapid inflation is a paradox that is hard to bear. The sudden decrease in income from a salary to a pension often makes drastic changes in life-style imperative. Most people who have worked all their lives dream about and plan for a retirement of relative ease and comfort. To find their hopes shattered is a blow that can cause a serious maturational crisis.

As elderly people live their lives, each day brings them closer to death and the realization that many of their hopes, fantasies, plans, and ambitions have gone unfulfilled and that now there is no chance. Often there is an acceptance of the inevitability of the end of the life cycle, and with it a kind of resigned sadness. But just as often, there is pain, depression, and bitterness about the coming of death. Not long ago on a television program about death, the interviewer asked an elderly woman if she was afraid of or sorry to be dying. The woman replied that she was tremendously sorry to be dying because she felt that she had not given herself a chance to really live the way she wanted to live. Chapter 17 discusses the crisis of aging in greater detail.

Situational crises

The community nurse will encounter situational crises of such a wide variety that it is impossible to discuss them all here. Any situation that is not part of a person's everyday activity can become a crisis, and all situatinal crises are not necessarily negative experiences. Falling in love is an experience which comes immediately to mind as an example of a situation that (luckily) does not happen every day and that many people interpret as a crisis, although an oftentimes pleasant one. Falling out of love or being rejected by the object of one's love is also a crisis, this time an unpleasant one. The loss of love through rejection can be as painful and can have as many attendant physical and psychological symptoms as the loss of love through death. The pain the individual experiences is real and should not be treated lightly.

PREGNANCY

Although the community nurse may not always be aware of the love status of her clients, she is aware of their reproductive status. Normal pregnancy and childbearing may be considered by some authorities to be a maturational crisis. It will, for two major reasons, in this text be considered a situational crisis. First, pregnancy is not a common human experience; that is, it does not happen to everyone, not even to every woman. Second, it is not an everyday experience when it does happen. Although pregnancy can certainly be said to be normal in the physiological sense, the life changes and disruption it causes in all family members make it an extraordinary experience. Thus there are the beginnings of a situational crisis. First pregnancies tend to develop into crises more frequently than do succeeding ones. A couple's life will be totally and forever changed when a child is born, and the realization of this can precipitate an enormous crisis. Feelings of anxiety during pregnancy or shortly after childbirth are not uncommon, and postpartum depression is seen frequently. Having to be completely responsible for another human being (who is totally dependent for the first several years) for *at least* eighteen years is a sober and even frightening thought. The fantasized image of a cute, pudgy, and perpetually smiling baby is replaced by the reality of a red-faced shrieking infant who has a diaper full of feces and refuses to be soothed by any means. This is a difficult situation with which to deal, and many women do not realize that they are unwilling or unable to do so until *after* they have had the baby. Even a woman who wants and has planned for the baby may find herself in crisis because the shock or reality is a difficult one. Both the mother and father worry about so many things: Will the baby grow up normally? Will they be able to support it? Will they be good parents? Will they ever have any time alone again? Will they love the child?

When the pregnancy is unwanted, it is a different kind of crisis. The marital status of the woman may be a central issue, as are the woman's philosophy and feelings about abortion. Because the pregnancy is unwanted, it may be ignored or denied, sometimes for so long that abortion becomes too risky. The decision of what to do about the pregnancy can be a difficult one. Even a woman whose political views are extremely proabortion can have mixed feelings about terminating the life she personally is carrying. There may be differences of opinion with the father of the baby, and, if the woman is young and living at home with her parents, she faces possible parental anger and lack of understanding. An abortion is a crisis in any woman's life, no matter how calm she appears to be. Many abortion clinics offer excellent professional counseling for the pregnant woman. These same clinics, however, do not extend their counseling services to the woman after she has had an abortion and needs to talk about her feelings.

Another situational crisis of pregnancy with even longer-lasting implications is making a decision to give up the baby for adoption and carrying through that decision. The feelings of loss, shame, sadness, and guilt can be overwhelming for any woman, but for an adolescent it can be a disaster. It is the policy of many hospitals that a woman who wishes to give up her baby must herself give the infant to an attorney or adoption caseworker. The philosophy of whether she should see and hold her baby prior to releasing it forever can be debated endlessly. However, there is no doubt that the emotional impact of this action results in a crisis. Even though the woman may display no outward feelings, it is essential that she receive counseling for as long as she needs it.

PREMATURE BIRTH

The situational crisis of pregnancy is often compounded by prematurity. Then, in addition to all the feelings described previously, there is shock, guilt, fear, grief, and heightened anxiety. Most mothers of premature infants feel somehow to blame and often see themselves as failures for not being able to carry a pregnancy to term. The mother's need to hold, cuddle, and feed her newborn baby is thwarted, and grief over separation from her child becomes a problem. Another problem that is not often acknowledged is the reuniting of the mother and baby when it comes home from the hospital. The longer the period of separation, the more of a stranger the baby will seem, and the

more problems of adjustment there will be. The mother has fears about the physical care of the baby: "He's so tiny; I'm afraid I'll break him if I pick him up." And there is often constant anxiety that the baby will die at any moment. Hospital costs for premature care can be astronomical, and, if there is no insurance coverage, a financial crisis compounds the problem. Caplan[6] has shown that women who chose not to face the reality of prematurity—the danger that their babies could die—demonstrated more symptoms of crisis and stress than did women who dealt with the facts in a realistic way.

UNEMPLOYMENT

The loss of a job is a situational crisis that may affect people other than oneself. This is a society where the ability to get a job and to earn a living is so important that it is almost the whole measure of the success of an individual. The ego identity of most men, as well as increasing numbers of women, revolves solely around the kind of work done and the success and status achieved doing that work. When this identity is suddenly lost, feelings of grief, loss, despair, and depression go with the crisis of unemployment. Added to that is the practical consideration of a loss of income; unemployment insurance does not go far in feeding a family of four or five people. The need to find another job is paramount in most people's minds. Yet it is at this time, during the throes of severe anxiety, that many people cannot function effectively in the task of job hunting, which is a highly stressful activity in the best of circumstances.

PHYSICAL ILLNESS

Physical illness, especially when there is a course of hospitalization, is always a situational crisis for both the individual and the family. There is often pain, sometimes severe and prolonged, a period of inactivity, and a loss of one's sense of autonomy that is heightened if the person is in the hospital. Sometimes there is long-term disability, which results in a reduced capacity to earn a living or to carry out one's usual activities. Feelings of helplessness and dependence on others create anxiety, especially in a person who cannot easily give up independence. Sickness in a household creates a different and unpleasant atmosphere. A husband or wife may suddenly have to assume the role of nurse and maid; rambunctious children must be constantly admonished to make less noise and perhaps not to bring their playmates home. Irritability and anger often become the prevailing feelings, and it is sometimes difficult to express these feelings in a positive and constructive way. It is not easy to say, "I'm angry at you for having broken your leg and for being dependent on me." Every person has his own way of coping with physical illness, but depression, regression, aggression, and hostility are common. Every hospitalized client who has ever been labeled "uncooperative" by the nursing staff has probably merely been employing one or several of these coping mechanisms. Denial of the severity of the illness is also a frequently used method of coping with it. If the illness is a terminal one, no matter how far in the future death will occur, a whole new set of problems will arise. There will be anticipatory grieving, intense emotinal (and often physical) pain, anger, and an entire range of other feelings that are among the most difficult with which to deal.

DIVORCE

Divorce is a crisis that is occurring more and more frequently. According to the Marriage Council of Philadelphia, almost 50% of all marriages eventually end in divorce. Marriage is generally viewed as a full-time and lifetime relationship, with constant work and effort needed by both partners to make it a success (Fig. 12-3). There is no other "job" in the world (with the possible exception of parenthood) that is so demanding and for which there is so little preparation. Two people, who are relative strangers, promise each other eternal love and fidelity and in essence vow to meet all of each other's needs: expectations and promises that are impossible to keep. When one looks at all the couples who wish they were divorced but feel compelled to stay together for one reason or another, plus all the couples who are divorced, it seems that

there is something drastically wrong with the institution of marriage, either in the institution itself or in the preparation for it. There are several major causes for divorce: communication problems; lack of sexual harmony; the age at which people marry; mixed racial, religious, ethnic, or cultural backgrounds; unhappy parental marriages that result in poor role models; too short a courtship; economic difficulties; lack of love; different growth and change patterns of each partner; and a general lack of readiness for marriage. No matter how long a couple has been married, there is always a feeling of being wrenched apart when divorce occurs. Living alone (even though the children may be present) is a difficult adjustment. There are often strong feelings of hate, anger, and bitterness between the husband and wife, and custody battles for the children can be painful and demoralizing. Changing one's role and self-perception from a married person to a single one is difficult and lonely, and in many parts of the country divorced people are still looked on as pariahs. Although it is still usually the woman who is granted custody of the children and the man who must pay alimony and child support, these practices are slowly beginning to change, and divorce courts are now trying to seek solutions that are more equitable than traditional. The rate of remarriage for divorced people is high. Women feel a great pressure to find a new husband, and men who have been used to the comforts and convenience of marriage also feel a need to return to that role.

CRISIS INTERVENTION
General theories and the role of the community nurse

Crisis intervention is becoming an increasingly used and effective technique in dealing with life's problems. A person in crisis may not need, want, or be able to afford years of intensive psychotherapy or psychoanalysis. Caplan[6] has described various factors that influence the outcome of a crisis and that can affect the course of crisis intervention therapy:

1. The symbolic linkages of the present situation with similar problems in the past and how ade-

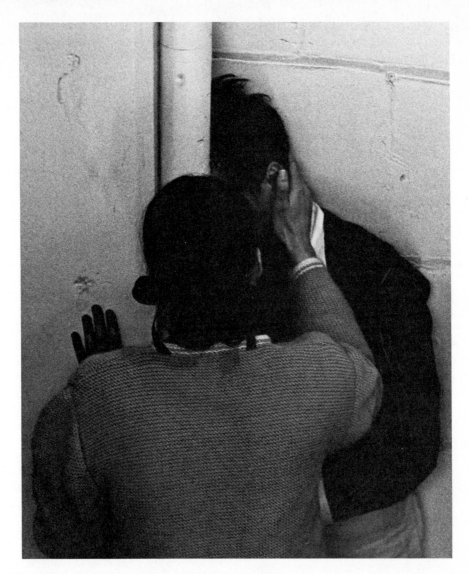

Fig. 12-3. A marital argument is a situational crisis that frequently requires professional intervention. (Photograph by Marion Bernstein; courtesy Editorial Photocolor Archives, Inc., New York.)

quately the past problems were dealt with. The therapist can help the client find positive problem-solving techniques in his past and help him apply them to the current situation.

2. The way in which the client perceives the situation and how stressful and problematic he finds it to be. The therapist must find out how much disequilibrium the client is experiencing.

3. Sociocultural influences and the milieu in which the client functions. An individual is helped or hindered in crisis resolution by people with whom he works and lives.

4. The way in which the client relates to his family, how they perceive the crisis, and how much positive support he can realistically expect from them. ''If any member of a family or other primary

group bound by close personal ties faces a problem involving a threat to need satisfaction, the group as a whole is inevitably involved in one way or another and to differing degrees according to whether the problem impinges on the need relevant to the individual's duties toward or demands from the group."[6,pp.44-45] The important thing for the therapist to remember is to encourage the family to help the person in crisis to deal directly with the problem, rather than making it easy for him to avoid it.

5. The influence of key members of the community. During the period of disequilibrium the individual is more susceptible to influence by others (e.g., friends and co-workers) than he is when he is in a stable emotional state. A relatively minor force can tip his emotional balance one way or another, so relationships with others can be extremely helpful or harmful during a crisis.

6. The influence of professional workers. The health worker who first becomes aware that an individual is in crisis plays an important role in the outcome of that crisis. "Crisis therefore presents care-giving persons with a remarkable opportunity to deploy their efforts to maximum advantage in influencing the mental health of others."[6,p.54]

The nurse is the health worker who most frequently discovers the existence of a crisis. The hospital nurse sees illness and its ramifications, but the community nurse, who visits in the home, sees this and everything else. Her first task is the recognition that a crisis is indeed taking place. The next step is to talk with the individual about his perceptions and feelings and how he thinks the crisis is affecting his life. She can then explore with him the various kinds of crisis intervention therapy and can either become the therapist herself or make an appropriate referral. If the client chooses to see someone else, or if the community nurse is not a therapist, it is important that she maintain contact with the client and his family during the course of the therapy and for as long afterward as they both feel is necessary.

The nursing process is an especially appropriate tool for crisis intervention therapy. Aguilera and Messick's[1] description of the process of crisis intervention follows the steps of the nursing process, as does the analysis and solution of any problem. The attitude of the nurse therapist and her relationship to the client are extremely important. The nurse must be skilled at assessment, and it is essential that she develop her sensitivity and perception so she can be empathetic as well as sympathetic. Reading and research are neither the only nor the best roads to increased sensitivity. No book can help the nurse to completely understand another person's anguish. She can do this only by permitting herself to feel and to open herself and her own life to as many human experiences as possible. She must be aware of the differences between her value system and that of the client; although she need not personally approve of his behavior, she must be able to accept it. If she is truly unable to do so, then she cannot continue as therapist for that client.

In effective crisis intervention, Caplan[11] believes that the essential aspects of mental health are the state of the ego, the stage of its maturity, and the quality of its structure. The therapist can assess the client's ego by looking at three major areas:

1. The capacity of the person to withstand stress and anxiety and to still maintain ego equilibrium
2. The degree of reality recognized and faced in solving problems
3. The repertoire of effective coping mechanisms available to the individual to help him maintain his ego balance

According to Aguilera and Messick[1,p.6]:

Caplan believes that all the elements that compose the total emotional milieu of the person must be assessed in an approach to preventive mental health. The material, physical, and social demands of reality, as well as the needs, instincts, and impulses of the individual, must all be considered as important behavioral determinants.

Crisis intervention is primarily aimed at resolving the individual's immediate crisis and restoring him to at least the level of functioning that existed prior to the crisis. A secondary goal, which usually takes longer, is to improve the level of functioning and to try to prevent further crises of a similar nature that arise from similar conditions. Crises are usually self-limiting, and crisis intervention usually lasts from six to eight weeks. The two approaches, generic and individual, to crisis intervention will be more fully discussed later in the chapter. There are, however, specific steps that are followed in any kind of crisis intervention. Aguilera and Messick[1] describe them:

1. Assessment of the individual and his problem. The therapist must assess the degree of severity of the problem and the risk of danger that the client might pose to himself or to others.

2. Planning the therapeutic intervention. The therapist must know the extent to which the client's life has been disrupted because of the crisis, what level of functioning he is able to maintain, what strengths and coping skills he has, to whom he can turn for emotional and practical support, and how long the therapy is likely to take.

3. Intervention with some or all of the following techniques:
   a. Help the individual to intellectually understand his crisis. Often the therapist can point out relationships between modes of functioning and life situations that the client has been unable to see.
   b. Help the client to bring his feelings into the open. Denial and suppression of feelings that "we are not supposed to have" is very common, and the tension and anxiety that results from their suppression can block or slow down the progress of therapy.
   c. Exploration of coping mechanisms. There are almost always alternate ways of coping with problems, and sometimes all the therapist need do is to point them out.
   d. Reopening of the social world. People in crisis often retreat into themselves, especially if the crisis is a result of the loss or death of a loved one.

4. Resolution of the crisis and anticipatory planning. Adaptive coping mechanisms are reinforced, and help is given in making realistic plans for the future.

Each stressful life situation that results in a crisis poses a coping task for the individual involved. He moves from a state of relative security to the danger of the unknown. The individual is threatened with the loss of need satisfaction, and there is a challenge of one's coping abilities. When faced with certain crises, notably death, religion provides ritual or a rite of passage to help manage the crisis. Most religious rituals have some aspects of crisis intervention. They provide a support person: a cleric. They offer psychological supports by keeping the individual close to reality, and they maintain a focus on the crisis. They involve the individual in organized activity such as praying and singing, and familiar and specific symbols are used.

An excellent example of this is the Jewish custom of sitting *shiva* (from the Hebrew word for the number seven) for a week after the death of a close relative. The bereaved family members stay at home, receive the condolences of friends and relatives, and engage in prescribed prayers. Talking about the dead one is encouraged, and open displays of grief are responded to with support and understanding. The purpose is to disregard one's life for a week and to give oneself over to grief and mourning: to "let it all out" while the pain of grief is still fresh.

Generic approach

The generic approach focuses on the characteristic course of the *particular kind of crisis* rather than on the psychodynamics of each individual in crisis. A treatment plan is directed toward an adaptive resolution of the crisis. Specific intervention measures are designed to be effective for all members of a given group rather than for the unique differences of one individual.[1,p.22]

In this approach each member of the group has the *nature of the crisis* in common with every other member, and all members of the group are experiencing a similar kind of crisis. They may all be victims of a disaster, grieving spouses, or recently divorced women. This can lead to an increased sensitivity toward the feelings and experiences of fellow group members. The intervention is geared toward the crisis related to the events themselves and is usually carried out by nonmental health professionals. This is of particular interest to community health nurses who have always done much crisis intervention on an informal basis but who may not have felt qualified as therapists. Because a mastery of the knowledge of the intrapsychic processes of the individual in crisis is not necessary in the generic approach, the nurse is able to focus on the crisis itself and to use all her creative processes in helping the client to find his way out of crisis.

Much of generic crisis intervention is done in groups because it is the crisis and not the individual that receives the bulk of the focus. The two major categories of groups are therapy groups and crisis groups. There are so many types of therapy groups that a definition becomes impossible. It is far more practical for the reader to understand the function of several different kinds of therapy groups.

1. *Social groups.* The purpose is to achieve a common group goal with the help of a leader. Socialization is the result of a project or activity that is designed to unite all the group members. The leader must be skilled in understanding group actions and cultural patterns. In crisis intervention this kind of group might be useful for adolescent maturational problems or for the crisis of retirement.

2. *Counseling.* This approach focuses on solving specific problems, and the group leader takes an active role in finding solutions that are agreeable to the clients and toward which they can work.

3. *Guidance.* This is similar to counseling, but there is greater emphasis on exploring feelings and emotions and on reducing anxiety and tension to tolerable levels so solutions to problems can be sought. This approach is especially effective in family therapy where there may be one or more maturational crises, perhaps compounded by a situational one. An adolescent who is failing in school and then drops out is an example of a situation that could benefit from a guidance group.

4. *Group psychotherapy.* This approach requires the use of a group leader who is trained in psychodynamics, and it is intended to make basic personality and behavior changes and to look at underlying emotional problems that cause crisis. Unless the community nurse is also a psychiatric

nurse practitioner, it is unlikely that she will find herself leading this type of group.

In crisis groups the goal is to return the individual members to levels of functioning they had achieved before the crisis and even to improve their level of functioning.

> The focus of treatment . . . is oriented [sic] to the present and to the problem that is of concern at the time the individuals request help. It deals with the stresses and balancing factors that are either absent or ineffective in the present crisis situation and is directed toward assisting the members to achieve a resolution of their crises.[1,p.35]

The group usually becomes cohesive quickly, and each member supports and receives support from the others in exploring events that led to the crisis. They discuss what their past coping skills were, what kind of external support they can expect, and why they were able to solve their present problem.

> The use of therapeutic groups in nursing practice is probably the result of at least three important factors: (1) nurses' involvement with social workers in groups of this kind, (2) the growing attention of all nurses to the psychosocial factors of illness and growth and development, and (3) the increased interest in mental health nursing in group work with a variety of nonpsychiatric patient populations.[12,p.23]

At the initial interview, the therapist determines whether the client could benefit from a crisis group. Sometimes a group with similar problems cannot be found, although the therapist frequently feels that membership in a group is more important than the existence of a common problem. This may be the case with people who have difficulty with interpersonal relationships or whose major contributing problem is social isolation. The group leader takes an active and direct role, focusing the discussion on the problem at hand and discouraging general conversation and social chitchat. The leader also acts as a facilitator, encouraging everyone to participate and to control overebullient monopolizers of the discussion. Translating nonverbal behavior into verbal conversation is also a function of the group leader. ''You seem very tense this evening, Ken. Will you tell us what you're feeling?'' Or, ''You have such a sad expression on your face. Are you feeling sad?''

There are advantages and disadvantages to crisis groups. The advantages are the group support for individual members and the amount of peer help and reassurance that can be given to particularly distraught members. Sometimes social relationships develop, and group members often suggest to each other effective coping mechanisms that can be quite original. The group is an excellent vehicle for the expression of feelings; as each member encourages others to speak out, he is more likely to follow the set example. On the other hand, it is often difficult to keep each person's crisis in focus, and reassessment of a problem is difficult in a group. Group members sometimes make suggestions for maladaptive coping mechanisms; the leader must then take time to point out the error of the suggestion and seek a new one. Many professionals think this process of client trial and error wastes time.

Special problem groups are closely related to crisis groups. They address problems that are of concern to all members of the group, and, although individuals may not be in acute crisis, the problem is such that crisis is always imminent. Special problems that are amenable to these groups are adolescence, alcoholism, narcotics addiction, and homosexuality. While homosexuality is no longer considered by the American Psychiatric Association to be sick or maladaptive behavior, and many homosexuals have no wish or need to become heterosexual, they often have difficulty adjusting to a gay role in a straight world. Persecution and oppression of homosexuals is still common, and a special problem group (some call them consciousness-raising groups) can be an important source of emotional support and practical help.

Similarity of problems creates a climate of acceptance and can encourage the serious discussion of problems without the fear of possible discrimination, rejection, and social isolation that might be elicited in a group where there is no such similarity. Because all members of the group have already experienced or will experience similar crises (e.g., loss of a job because of alcoholism or eviction from one's apartment when homosexuality is discovered), each individual can relate the success or failure of his various coping mechanisms, and other individuals can adapt them to their own particular needs.

Rogers[13] has identified and defined the phases of encounter groups that can be observed in almost any therapy or crisis group:

1. *Milling around.* This is a period of initial confusion, awkward silence, ''cocktail party chatter,'' a lack of purpose, and some degree of frustration.
2. *Resistance to personal expression or exploration.* Members who reveal personal attitudes are likely to provoke ambivalent reactions from other group members.
3. *Description of past feelings.* Expression of feelings begins to assume a larger proportion of the discussion.
4. *Expression of negative feelings.* Negative attitudes expressed toward other group members or toward the leader are an excellent way to test the freedom and trustworthiness of the group. Positive feelings are more difficult and dangerous to express.
5. *Expression and exploration of personally meaningful material.* Some member will begin ''a journey to the center of self,'' and the group may not be receptive to such personal revelations.
6. *The expression of immediate interpersonal feelings in the group.* Group members have direct confrontations among themselves concerning how they feel about each other's behavior and personality.
7. *The development of a healing capacity in the group.* A number of group members begin to show a capacity for dealing in a helpful and therapeutic way with the pain and suffering of other members.
8. *Self-acceptance and the beginning of change.* Group members bring to the surface the reality of their feelings and problems.

9. *The cracking of facades.* The group demands (sometimes gently, sometimes not so gently) that each group member be himself.
10. *The individual receives feedback.* Group members verbalize their perceptions of other members.

BEHAVIOR MODIFICATION

The behavior modification process is used sometimes in crisis intervention by practioners who are skilled in the art. Crises, especially recurring ones, often develop as the result of a certain behavior pattern. For example, an individual may be fired from a succession of jobs because his behavior pattern of responding with aggression and hostility to criticism from his superiors makes him difficult to work with. Crisis intervention with each loss of job will be useless unless the underlying behavior that caused the crisis is changed. This is where behavior modification has value. There are three stages of behavior modification: (1) assessment, during which problem behavior and the events leading to that behavior are observed, defined, and recorded; (2) intervention, which involves the application of behavior modification techniques; and (3) evaluation, in which changes in behavior during the intervention are observed, and there is a decision about whether the changes are positive ones. There should also be long-term follow-up to see how long the changes last.

Goals for the treatment process are formulated by the therapist and the client as a result of discussion of what kind of behavior the client would like to exhibit and what kinds of behavior he feels comfortable with. There should also be agreement about which behaviors the client wishes to eliminate. The theory of behavior modification is based on the assumption

that behavior problems are learned and—what is becoming less of an assumption and more of an established fact—that such difficulties can be rectified through planned changes in the current external environment of the individual. When carefully planned and systemati-

cally executed alterations in an individual's environment are instituted, his behavior problems (i.e., his excesses and deficiencies in specific behaviors or objectionable behaviors *per se*) can be remedied.*

All behavior is controlled by its consequences in the external environment. If a behavior is regularly followed by a positive consequence, an individual will repeat the behavior. If a behavior is followed by a negative consequence, an individual will not repeat the behavior. Behavior modification therapy is based on reinforcing desired behaviors and punishing negative ones. This can range all the way from using moderately painful electrical shocks in order to control some forms of unwanted behavior (punishment or negative reinforcement) to permitting a reward for refraining from smoking cigarettes for an entire day (positive reinforcement). Some of the problems that are being successfully treated with behavior modification are smoking, overeating, bed-wetting, extreme hyperactivity (e.g., pacing, screaming, scratching, and twitching), fire setting, and anorexia nervosa. Some clients can be successfully treated in behavior modification groups; others need to be hospitalized.

It is not within the scope of this chapter to describe all intervention techniques currently in use by behavior therapists. Suffice it to say that when the community nurse encounters a client whose crisis was precipitated by persistent behavior that was negative to the client, she might want to consider discussing behavior modification therapy with the client.

Individual approach

The individual approach to crisis intervention therapy emphasizes assessment, by a professional, of the interpersonal and intrapsychic processes of the person in crisis. This approach is used mostly with people who, for some reason, do not respond

*From Michael D. LeBow, Behavior modification: a significant method in nursing practice, © 1973, pp. 3-4. Reprinted by permission of Prentice-Hall, Inc., Englewood Cliffs, N.J.

to the generic approach or with people whose underlying problems are so severe that short-term crisis therapy will not suffice. Emphasis is on the unique needs of the individual and on the circumstances that precipitated the crisis rather than on only the crisis itself. There is not much concern with the developmental past of the individual (as there is in psychotherapy and psychoanalysis) except as it directly relates to the immediate cause of disturbed equilibrium. Even then, emphasis is placed on restoring or improving functioning and behavior rather than on restructuring the personality. Individual crisis intervention therapy should be done only by mental health professionals.

Therapy process

Accurate assessment of the existing problem is the key to the effectiveness of therapy, and, because of strict time limitations, the energies of both the client and the therapist should be directed toward the resolution of the problem at hand; digression to other developmental or life problems is not appropriate. It is the function of the professional mental health worker to help the client to choose healthy coping mechanisms. This can be done by enlarging the client's understanding and perception of the situation, by supporting the client in expression of both positive and negative feelings, and by opening channels of communication with other people, for example, family, friends, and other health professionals. Results are usually achieved in a relatively short time because people who are in crisis are usually amenable to help and to suggestion and because there is no need to uncover the underlying reasons for the poor coping mechanisms. Rather, emphasis is placed on the behavior itself, which can frequently be quickly changed.

If the client is unable to resolve the crisis or to attain equilibrium in the allotted time, or if the same kinds of crisis occur repeatedly, he may be a candidate for brief psychotherapy or even for psychoanalysis.

Brief psychotherapy has its roots in psychoanalytic theory but differs from psychoanalysis in terms of goals and other factors. It is limited to removing or alleviating specific symptoms when possible. Intervention may lead to some reconstruction of personality, although it is not considered as the primary goal. As in more traditional forms of psychotherapy, the therapy must be guided by an orderly series of concepts directed toward beneficial change in the patient. It is concerned with the degree of abatement of the symptoms presented and the return to or maintenance of the individual's ability to function adequately.*

A CASE HISTORY OF CRISIS

Louise is 38 years old and has been through enough physical and psychic pain to last a lifetime. She and Robert were married when they graduated from college. He had been to West Point and decided to make the army his career. Robert was a brilliant tactician, and, as he received promotions and increasingly more complex assignments, he moved emotionally further and further from his family and closer and closer to the army. Three children were born at "appropriate" intervals; they are now ages 10, 13, and 17. Until two years ago, Louise had never held a job outside her home. She was genuinely happy to be an army wife; she made friends easily and took their frequent household moves in stride. Her children were healthy and did well in school. Most of her friends' husbands seemed to behave as Robert did, so she saw his emotional withdrawal as a regrettable but inevitable situation rather than a serious marital problem.

Five years ago while she was bathing, Louise noticed a lump in her breast and within a week had a radical mastectomy. The shock, grief, and mourning she experienced were extremely severe, but, with the help of other women who had also undergone mastectomies, she worked through her grief and recovered her sense of self-esteem and self-worth. She gradually returned to her usual life except in one area. Robert refused to look at her scar, to discuss any aspect of her surgery, and to listen

*From Michael D. LeBow, Behavior modification: a significant method in nursing practice, © 1973, p. 14. Reprinted by permission of Prentice-Hall, Inc., Englewood Cliffs, N.J.

to her feelings; moreover, although they still slept in the same bed, he refused to make love to her. Louise was devastated, not so much by the lack of sex (although that was a large part of it), but by Robert's total rejection of her as a woman and as a human being with feelings and needs. She decided to fight to save this rapidly deteriorating situation and persuaded Robert to join her in marriage counseling.

They worked hard together with the therapist (Louise and Robert loved each other very much) and eventually achieved a happiness even greater than they had when they were first married. It seemed ironic, but Louise credited the "rediscovery" of her husband to the loss of her breast, so that loss became less and less important to her. Life was happy, prosperous, and filled with contentment. Then two years ago, Robert dropped dead when an aortic aneurysm ruptured.

Louise did not think she would survive the depths to which she had fallen. But she did. Extremely slowly and with enormous pain she struggled to go on with her life. After the initial shock eased, she moved to a new community, found a sales job at a local boutique, and enrolled in evening business courses at the community college. Her social life was limited, but she was beginning to feel an interest in meeting people again. Her children seemed to survive all these traumas with no evident ill effects.

The community nurse's first meeting with Louise was at her home a few days after she had signed herself out of the hospital against medical advice. She had been admitted with suspected metastasis of the cancer to her lower colon. Tests confirmed the diagnosis, and it was recommended that she have surgery—removal of her lower colon and rectum with a resultant colostomy—as soon as possible. As the nurse sat and talked with her, Louise said that she had no intention of having her body "further mutilated" and that in fact as soon as she could arrange for the permanent care of her children, she intended to kill herself. She told the nurse all this in a clear and decisive (although not unemotional) manner, and the nurse had the impression that Louise had given the whole situation much intelligent thought. She appears to be a bright woman who knows what she wants. She said that she "has been through too much already" and cannot face more suffering. That she is suffering a great deal now is evident to the nurse.

Discussion

Louise's two major present crises are severe depression and impending death. The surgery may postpone death for a few years, but the prognosis for metastatic cancer of the colon is extremely poor; barring a miracle, Louise will shortly be in the terminal phase of her illness. Each of these crises is both the cause and the result of the other. In crisis intervention therapy, the first step is always assessment of the situation; the nurse will need to know how Louise assesses her own problem and exactly *why* she has chosen suicide as the way to solve it. At first glance the nurse might agree with Louise that this seems to be the only alternative, but, because death is so final, it is a decision that should be arrived at only after the most careful analysis of all the other alternatives. It may possibly be that Louise will decide to kill herself, and the nurse, whatever her own feelings and values on the subject are, must respect the client's right to make the decision.

Louise has survived and been strengthened by so many past crises that it would seem that she might have the inner strength and learned experience to deal with this one. Her coping mechanisms are excellent, and she has demonstrated extremely adaptive behavior in the past. Louise has dealt with body mutilation and death. Although the two impending experiences will not be the same, there are similarities in the coping mechanisms involved. The loss of a breast is not the same as the loss of the ability to defecate normally, and dealing with the death of another person, no matter how close or how dearly loved, is not the same as dealing with one's own death. So these crises are new and old at the same time, and this fact may be causing Louise a tremendous amount of conflict and ambivalence.

There is also the problem of the children. At ages 10, 13, and 17, they are not yet independent, and, although they seem to have faced all the previous crises with equanimity, there must have been some psychoemotional effects. It is difficult to predict what effect the suicide of their mother may have on their future lives. The only certainty is that whatever the effect, it will be profound. If Louise does choose to kill herself, she will need to decide whether to discuss it with her children first. This would be an incredibly difficult thing for anyone to do, and one could certainly argue logically both for and against the advisability of doing it at all. After Louise's death (either by her own hand or by the cancer), where will the children live? Who will care for them? Is there any money to rear and educate them? Louise must deal with all these problems, and she will need help.

During the first few meetings between Louise and the community nurse, there may be no specific action taken. Ideally it should be a time of expression of feelings, of sharing perceptions of the problems, of sorting out needs and desires, of verbalizing fears, of assessing strengths and weaknesses, and, finally, deciding whether crisis intervention therapy would be appropriate. If Louise chooses to enter therapy, plans should be made. Either the nurse herself, if she is qualified, will be the therapist, or Louise will be referred to one. She might be a good candidate for generic therapy because some of her problems are shared by so many people. In addition to therapy she might want to seek out the local Ostomy Club[14] so she can at least meet people who are living with colostomies. Members are often frank in the revelation of their feelings and give much emotional support and practical help to people who are facing or who have recently had surgery. Even if Louise decides not to go through with the operation, she will see what a colostomy looks like and will have spoken with people who are living with one. Her therapy may take place at the office of a private practitioner (nurse, psychologist, or psychiatrist) or at one of the many community mental health centers. The crisis intervention therapy may also take place in Louise's home. If she and the community health nurse who visits develop a trusting relationship, the visits become therapeutic. The community nurse may not see herself as a trained crisis intervention therapist, but if she can help Louise to look at her problems and the various alternative solutions, and if Louise resolves the crisis in an adaptive way, the nurse is indeed providing crisis intervention therapy. The usual course of crisis therapy is six to eight weeks, and, given Louise's strengths, her intelligence, and all the thought she has already given to the problem, it seems likely that she will be able to complete the course of treatment in the allotted time.

If a nurse practitioner is doing the crisis intervention therapy, she might keep in mind the following nursing and humanistic concepts and principles:

1. Certain basic human rights belong to all people entering the health care system. The denial of these rights is most frequently the result of ignorance, apathy, and cruelty.
2. Clients exhibit varying degrees of mental health and a varying ability to verbalize their thoughts and feelings. The professional nurse must assess and understand every client's mental health status and help him to communicate.
3. Professional nurses are assuming autonomous roles and are making independent judgments and nursing diagnoses. They are responsible for *all* their professional actions.
4. Clients come from varying sociocultural groups with varying standards of ethical, social, and moral behavior, and these differences may or may not conform to what the nurse believes to be appropriate, ''good,'' or proper behavior.
5. No nurse can meet all the needs of every client. Neither can any human being meet all the needs of any other human being. The community nurse must know and use resources (e.g., people and agencies) to help the client meet his needs.
6. The professional nurse uses the five steps of the nursing process in order to meet clients' needs. She also uses nursing research in planning and carrying out nursing care.
7. In the past biomedical ethics was a matter of

concern only to people doing clinical research. Professional nurses need to become involved in ethical issues for their own sakes and for the sake of their clients.

8. The health-illness continuum[15] is an abstraction of real-life situations of which the nurse must constantly be aware.

CRISIS PREVENTION AND PRIMARY CARE

Preventing crisis is an important function of professional community nurses. As has been previously mentioned, they are the health professionals who see the client most frequently and in the widest variety of circumstances. They are in the client's home where he is apt to behave naturally rather than being on his "best behavior" in the clinic or physician's office. Community nurses often can see problems arising or can recognize situations that could turn into crises.

Crises can sometimes be prevented by helping the client to recognize and work through the developmental period of a crisis or difficult situations. The community nurse can also teach the client the recognition process so that he can learn to ward off crises alone. If an individual thinks through or worries about a potential crisis before it occurs, he has a greater chance of adequate adjustment and adaptive behavior. He will also be less vulnerable to physical and mental illness. Of course, there is a point beyond which the thinking and worrying become ineffective, and the individual becomes so tense and full of anxiety that he is unable to think clearly and make logical and effective plans. Groups can be effective in primary prevention in several ways:

1. Premarital counseling to recognize and avoid some of the stressful pitfalls of marriage
2. Prenatal classes to understand the mechanics of labor and to learn the basics of child care
3. Preretirement counseling to help plan for the drastic change of life-style and the sudden increase of leisure time
4. Counseling of a terminally ill client and his family to help with the anticipatory guidance of grief and mourning

5. Preoperative teaching for someone who is undergoing major surgery that will result in a change in body image and/or functional ability, such as amputation or mastectomy

Secondary prevention involves early identification of the crisis so the individual can work through it effectively and can avoid maladaptive behavior. This is basically the intervention or therapy stage and has already been discussed.

"Tertiary prevention is aimed at preventing further decompensation or impairment, after the person has partially resolved a crisis, so that he can continue to lead a useful role in the community."[8,p.218] This is essentially a rehabilitative procedure and depends strongly on the continuity of the nurse-client relationship *even if* the community nurse has not been the crisis intervention therapist. Ideally the nurse will have followed the progress of the therapy. She can then help to strengthen and reinforce coping mechanisms learned in therapy so that the client becomes behaviorally more effective.

Caplan's program for the primary prevention of mental disorder[11] can be adapted to the primary prevention of maturational and situational crises. His program is divided into two basic units, social action and interpersonal action, and consists of the following major points:

1. *Social action* is the effort to modify political and social policies and legislative action in the fields of health, education, and welfare to provide certain basic supplies and services to help people cope with crisis.

   a. *Physical supplies.* The provision of the physical needs of people, for example, safe shelter, uncontaminated food, and reasonable safety on the streets. Starvation, homelessness, and accidents are all crises of major import, and many could be prevented by simply providing the physical requisites that are needed by all human beings.

   b. *Psychosocial supplies.* The most important ones are provided through family relationships, and a major aim of primary prevention is the safeguarding of family integrity. Employment regulations, welfare laws, and divorce and custody laws are all excellent vehicles for primary prevention.

c. *Sociocultural supplies.* In this regard there should be a focus on altering legislation and policies so that community attitudes and practices are influenced. An example is modifying retirement policies and extending the provision of services for the elderly. There are other high-risk groups of people, for example, the young, the unemployed, the alcoholic, and the unmarried mother, who would benefit from primary prevention at a community level.

d. *Social action in crisis.* The goal of a program of primary prevention is "to identify the commonly occurring hazardous circumstances in a community and to modify them so that their impact on the population is less severe, which means that people will have a better chance to find healthy adaptive and adjustive ways of handling them."[11,p. 68] In addition to the attenuation of hazardous circumstances, the provision of services to foster healthy crisis coping is an essential social action. This means that there should be competent professional health workers available.

2. *Interpersonal action* involves face-to-face interactions between professional caregivers and individuals and groups. Crisis can often be prevented by observing interpersonal interactions in the home, clinic, or community center. Disturbed relationships can often be prevented from becoming crises or even pathological behavior problems. The care-givers, whether or not they are mental health professionals, need the support of professional consultation that can best be provided by community-based agencies, many of which should be funded through public money.

Anticipatory guidance

Anticipatory guidance is an important feature of crisis prevention. An example of a maturational crisis that might be averted through effective anticipatory guidance by the community nurse is childbearing. When the nurse first meets the pregnant woman, as well as during succeeding meetings, she has the opportunity to assess the client's life-style, her feelings about being pregnant, her relationship with the father of the baby and his feelings about the pregnancy, her knowledge of anatomy and physiology, what misconceptions she has and what "old wives' tales" she believes, what her nutritional habits are, and what she perceives her needs to be. The nurse can then sort out her impressions of the client and compare what she thinks the client needs with what the client thinks she needs, and a logical program can be embarked on. As the pregnancy progresses, further discussion can take place, and needs can be reassessed. Ideally the father and other children, if there are any, should be involved in the anticipatory guidance because they would surely be involved in the crisis if there was to be one. During pregnancy and immediately thereafter mood swings occur that are often frightening to both new parents. If these moods can be discussed and the reasons for them understood, the resultant behavior need not precipitate crisis.

SUMMARY

Crisis intervention therapy, or the referral of clients to those services, is becoming an increasingly large part of the community nurse's function. She must be able to recognize when the client is in crisis—when his previous coping mechanisms have failed, when he is in a period of disequilibrium, and when the increase in anxiety and tension has reached an intolerable level, and she must know what she can do for him. The nurse must also be able to recognize maladaptive behavior that may precipitate a crisis but which also may be a result of the unsuccessful coping with a previous crisis.

There are maturational and situational crises. A maturational crisis is a change or transition point that every human being experiences during the process of physical and nonphysical growth. It usually evolves over a long period of time, but the cognitive awareness of the problem has little to do with the amount of disequilibrium experienced. A situational crisis is an external event that is not part of everyday life and that is usually sudden and unexpected. There is a sharp rise in tension and anxiety with a resultant disequilibrium. Many crises cannot be classified as either maturational or situational but have the characteristics of both.

Crisis intervention therapy is generally of short duration (approximately six weeks), is specifically goal oriented, focuses on the situation at hand rather than on the individual's developmental processes, and takes place either in a group (the generic approach) or on an individual basis. The therapy is influenced by many variables: the ways in which the individual has coped with previous crises, what sociocultural and emotional factors are extant in his life, and the quality of his relationships with the people he lives and works with and the kind of support he can expect from them. Crisis intervention is aimed primarily at resolving the individual's immediate crisis and restoring him to at least the level of functioning that existed prior to the crisis. If the level of functioning can be improved, so much the better. The steps in crisis intervention therapy closely resemble the steps of the nursing process itself. It is the function of the therapist, who may or may not be a professional mental health worker, to help the client choose healthy coping mechanisms.

Crisis prevention is within the province of community nurses. They are the health workers who are most likely to see crises as they are brewing, and they have access to a great many sources of referral. Crisis prevention is also very much a function of the community, and it is the nurse who can be an activist on social, cultural, and political levels.

NOTES

1. Aguilera, Donna C., and Messick, Janice M.: Crisis intervention: theory and methodology, ed. 4, St. Louis, 1982, The C.V. Mosby Co.
2. Maturational or developmental crises arise over a longer period of time (and will be discussed later in the chapter), but it is still usually one event that sets off the acute phase of the crises and with which the individual is unable to cope.
3. Fink, S.L.: Crisis and motivation: a theoretical model, Archives of Physical Medicine and Rehabilitation **48**:592-597, 1967.

4. Kübler-Ross, Elisabeth: On death and dying, New York, 1969, The Macmillan Co.
5. Gebbie, Kristine M., and Lavin, Mary Ann, editors: Classification of nursing diagnoses, St. Louis, 1975, The C.V. Mosby Co.
6. Caplan, Gerald: Principles of preventive psychiatry, New York, 1964, Basic Books, Inc., Publishers.
7. Cadden, Vivian: Crisis in the family. In Caplan, Gerald: Principles of preventive psychiatry, New York, 1964, Basic Books, Inc., Publishers.
8. Murray, Ruth, and Zentner, Judith: Nursing concepts for health promotion, Englewood Cliffs, N.J., 1975, Prentice-Hall, Inc.
9. Anderson, Ralph E., and Carter, Irl E.: Human behavior in the social environment, Chicago, 1974, Aldine Publishing Co.
10. Marmer, Judd: The crisis of middle age. In Schwartz, Lawrence H., and Schwartz, Jane L.: The psychodynamics of patient care, Englewood Cliffs, N.J., 1972, Prentice-Hall, Inc.
11. Caplan, Gerald: An approach to community mental health, New York, 1961, Grune & Stratton, Inc.
12. Marram, Gwen D.: The group approach in nursing practice, ed. 2, St. Louis, 1978, The C.V. Mosby Co.
13. Rogers, Carl: Carl Rogers on encounter groups, New York, 1970, Harper & Row, Publishers, Inc.
14. An Ostomy Club is a group of people, all volunteers, who have had colostomies, ileostomies, or ureterostomies. Their function is to provide education about the surgery and to give emotional support and practical help to other people. They hold regular meetings, have information about various ostomy appliances, and visit people in the hospital and at home who have recently had surgery. They also provide speakers for audiences who express an interest. They can usually be found in the telephone book or always through the local chapter of the American Cancer Society.
15. See Chapter 8 for a detailed discussion of health, illness, and wellness.

BIBLIOGRAPHY

Aguilera, Donna C., and Messick, Janice M.: Crisis intervention: theory and methodology, ed. 4, St. Louis, 1982, The C.V. Mosby Co.

Anderson, Ralph E., and Carter, Irl E.: Human behavior in the social environment, Chicago, 1974, Aldine Publishing Co.

Berni, Rosemarian, and Fordyce, Wilbert E.: Behavior modification and the nursing process, ed. 2, St. Louis, 1977, The C.V. Mosby Co.

Cadden, Vivian: Crisis in the family. In Caplan, Gerald: Principles of preventive psychiatry, New York, 1964, Basic Books, Inc., Publishers.

Caplan, Gerald: An approach to community mental health, New York, 1961, Grune & Stratton, Inc.

Caplan, Gerald: Principles of preventive psychiatry, New York, 1964, Basic Books, Inc., Publishers.

Carruth, Beatrice: Modifying behavior through social learning, American Journal of Nursing **76:**1804-1806, 1976.

Clark, Terri: Counseling victims of rape, American Journal of Nursing **76:**1964-1966, 1976.

Collins, Mattie: Communication in health care: understanding and implementing effective human relations, St. Louis, 1977, The C.V. Mosby Co.

Epstein, Charlotte: Effective interaction in contemporary nursing, Englewood Cliffs, N.J., 1974, Prentice-Hall, Inc.

Fink, S.L.: Crisis and motivation: a theoretical model, Archives of Physical Medicine and Rehabilitation **48:**592-597, 1967.

Gebbie, Kristine M., and Lavin, Mary Ann, editors: Classification of nursing diagnoses, St. Louis, 1975, The C.V. Mosby Co.

Gentry, W. Doyle, editor: Applied behavior modification, St. Louis, 1975, The C.V. Mosby Co.

Hott, Jacqueline: The crisis of expectant fatherhood, American Journal of Nursing **76:**1436-1440, 1976.

Hymovich, Debra P., and Bernard, Martha: Family health care, ed. 2, New York, 1978, McGraw-Hill Book Co.

LeBow, Michael: Behavior modification, Englewood Cliffs, N.J., 1973, Prentice-Hall, Inc.

Marks, Mary Jo: The grieving patient and family, American Journal of Nursing **76:**1488-1491, 1976.

Marmer, Judd: The crisis of middle age. In Schwartz, Lawrence H., and Schwartz, Jane L.: The psychodynamics of patient care, Englewood Cliffs, N.J., 1972, Prentice-Hall, Inc.

Marram, Gwen D., Schlegel, Margaret W., and Bevis, Em O.: Primary nursing: a model for individualized care, ed. 2, St. Louis, 1979, The C.V. Mosby Co.

Marram, Gwen D.: The group approach in nursing practice, ed. 2, 1978, St. Louis, The C.V. Mosby Co.

Marriner, Ann: The nursing process: a scientific approach to nursing care, ed. 2, 1979, The C.V. Mosby Co.

Murray, Ruth, and Zentner, Judith: Nursing concepts for health promotion, Englewood Cliffs, N.J., 1975, Prentice-Hall, Inc.

Nakushian, Janet: Restoring parents' equilibrium after sudden infant death, American Journal of Nursing **76:**1600-1604, 1976.

O'Brien, Maureen J.: Communication and relationships in nursing, ed. 2, St. Louis, 1978, The C.V. Mosby Co.

Peplau, Hildegard E.: Interpersonal relations in nursing, New York, 1952, G.P. Putnam's Sons.

Rogers, Carl R.: Counseling and psychotherapy, Boston, 1942, Houghton Mifflin Co.

Rogers, Carl R.: Carl Rogers on encounter groups, New York, 1970, Harper & Row, Publishers.

Schwartz, Lawrence H., and Schwartz, Jane L.: The psychodynamics of patient care, Englewood Cliffs, N.J., 1972, Prentice-Hall, Inc.

Schoenberg, Bernard, et al., editors: Anticipatory grief, New York, 1974, Columbia University Press.

Simmons, Janet A.: The nurse-client relationship in mental health nursing, Philadelphia, 1976, W.B. Saunders Co.

13

THE NURSING PROCESS AS IT APPLIES TO COMMUNITY NURSING

The nursing student or practitioner is by now familiar with the nursing process. This method of doing professional nursing is particularly well suited to community health because the community nurse is required to use all her independent judgment skills. Because the nursing process is nothing more than a tool or guide for the provision of excellent nursing care, a community nurse, who must rely on her own judgment a good deal of the time, needs the most effective guidelines available. The nursing process, if it is used appropriately, can be just that. There is also no end to the kind of ingenuity and professional judgment the community nurse will be required to bring to her job.

DATA COLLECTION

The first and most important part of the nursing process is data collection; this is why investigative skill is fundamental to nursing. Auger[1] stresses this as she describes the many external and internal stimuli that affect the client. Without sound, accurate, detailed data, a nurse cannot set goals or determine problems accurately. Data collection involves the nurse's cerebral cortex and all the senses in an intricate process of assimilating, coordinating, and abstracting from the given universe in order to describe the client's health problem. Nurses are continually collecting data, but only

when they are consciously aware of this process can an accurate detailed history be developed.

Gathering data begins when the nurse first contacts the client, or perhaps even before when she receives the client referral. Data gathering continues throughout the entire association with the client and family, but it is especially important when forming a hypothesis about what seems to be the problem. Every conceivable hypothesis should be noted and investigated. The proof or disproof becomes the motivating force for further inquiry. The following example illustrates how a nursing hypothesis is made:

Ms. Aimes was recently discharged from the hospital, and the visiting nurse agency was notified because the hospital nurses were aware of her extreme distress following a bilateral radical mastectomy. The client is 37 years old, has two children ages 4 and 7, and had planned to have another baby. Ms. Aimes has made several remarks stating that she does not think her husband will ever look at her again.

On hearing this history, the community nurse thought of several hypotheses about the client's psychological, emotional, and physical state. The first speculation is that Ms. Aimes believes her husband will withdraw his love as a result of the

336

surgery, and the second is that Ms. Aimes feels mutilated and dehumanized. It appears that the major emphasis of nursing care will be emotional support. The nurse, however, realizes that she must visit the client to make an accurate assessment of the situation.

There is a systematic approach to gathering data,[2] and it is best to follow it step by step, particularly if the nurse is inexperienced. This chapter employs the systems approach of data collection; each system is assessed as to why and how it interacts with a variety of stimuli.

The physical person

The physiological systems deal with the client as a physical and chemical organism trying to maintain homeostasis. To collect data about the physical person, inspection should begin from the head and proceed down. It is important to be inclusive and accurate when describing an abnormal or peculiar finding. Accurate description of the physical person includes both quantitative and qualitative factors. As the body is inspected, the nurse has the opportunity to practice observational skills. These skills are necessary, not only for physical inspection, but for the psychological assessment that will follow or that is going on at the same time.

The data collection process is described by the example of the assessment of the head, which includes hair, eyes, nose, oral cavity, ears, and the overall appearance of the skin. Each organ system that can be described in this way is noted. The nervous system is described by the integrity and functioning of the sensory organs; the integumentary system is assessed by the condition of the skin and hair; even the circulatory system is assessed by describing skin color, turgor and degree of warmth, and the level of orbital edema.

As the assessment is done, information about the external environment should also be included to make the data relevant and to maintain perspective. For instance, the head does not exist as a separate entity in space; it is connected to the body with which it interacts. Including information about how the client is affected by or affects external stimuli

provides data about the degree of homeostasis; it also gives more complete information about why the client is at a particular place on the health-illness continuum. Thus the information that the eyes are of normal shape, size, and placement and that they are clear and react to light is incomplete data. Can the client see? Is there a corneal reflex to touch? Do the eyes tear when external allergens are present? To state that skin is cold, clammy, and diaphoretic would also be insufficient data if the nurse failed to include the presence of a stimulus that might cause the client to be fearful or nervous. This might be done by simple observation, or the nurse might also want to ask the client what he is feeling. This process of relating findings to stimuli is important. Without the notation of the relationship, data collection is incomplete. Although at times this added information may be merely superficial, only professional judgment can distinguish between what is important to note and what is not. In the community this data about external stimuli is important because the client is seen surrounded by everyday stimuli, as opposed to "artificial" ones in the hospital.

We return to Ms. Aimes. On the first visit the nurse will establish an initial rapport with the client through the process of introduction and begin data collection. The nurse is not certain what she will find when she arrives in the home, but she has made the following assumptions based on the history she has received:

1. There will be a primary client, Ms. Aimes.
2. There will be secondary clients who live with Ms. Aimes or those who do not live with her but who are close to her.
3. There is a physical environment that acts as a stimulus for the primary client and which is also to some degree the external molder of the client's behavior, character, and value system.

The environment will be a material representation of Ms. Aimes' life: her likes, dislikes, feelings, and goals.

Data collection is the foundation of the nursing process. As the nurse becomes increasingly skilled in assessment, she will be able to decide which systems need to be assessed in greater detail. It is essential to make at least a cursory assessment of all physical systems. In this way the unintentional elimination of pertinent information can be avoided. When the nurse becomes experienced, she will learn which physical systems require the most detail. There are many references available for a review of physical assessment.

General appearance is also a part of data collection. It serves to validate subjectively inferred data, and it helps the nurse to make an accurate diagnosis. One observation is the care the client takes of his body, clothing, and home. These data may tell the nurse more about how the client feels about himself than he is willing or able to verbalize. A meticulous housekeeper who neglects herself may indicate two totally different pictures of the client and may have some personality significance. This added dimension of the client's profile helps to expand the data base, and it can add congruity to seemingly unrelated data.

The nonphysical person

The second part of the data collection process concerns the mental and emotional systems. Data should be collected with all available tools because overlapping findings (data that were collected by different methods but which yield the same results) validate data. It is important to assess mental and emotional status with the most objective approach possible. One cannot totally avoid subjectivity, but a conscious effort should be made to do so. Important areas to include are speech and behavioral gestures: repetitive physical gestures that are either congruent or incongruent with the verbal message being communicated. Behavioral gestures are sometimes difficult to notice during verbal communication, but with practice the active listener can become adept at noticing behavioral patterns, the stimuli that provoke them, and the people in the environment who elicit them most frequently. Often the client is completely unaware of his own behavioral gestures; pointing out those which are incongruent with the simultaneous verbal message can result in important feedback for the client.

The community nurse saw that Ms. Aimes exhibited behavioral patterns that indicated her difficulty in adapting to her changed body appearance: the client often crossed her arms over her chest, particularly when her husband entered the room or when any male was present. She also looked at the floor when she talked about the mastectomy. Mostly she sat in the chair, arms crossed, in a rather listless position.

Data regarding mental, emotional, and social status should be collected and recorded every time the nurse sees the client. Behavioral patterns can indicate underlying problems, and changes in behavior can then be noted by comparing new behaviors with what was observed on the previous visit. Overall attitude, temperament, activity level, and coping mechanisms of the client should be noted, and including examples of behavior would be helpful. For instance, it could be recorded that every time her children come home from school, a client takes an alcoholic drink. Or the nurse might note that every time the father enters the room, his adolescent daughter gets up and leaves. When this is done at the outset, comparative changes can be measured and described. Data collected for this purpose would be validated to an even greater extent if they involved observing the client in a number of settings to determine regularity, intent, and any causes of various behaviors. Noting family interactions provides clues as to defense mechanisms and other behaviors employed by the client and other family members.

Data collection of mental and emotional systems should include information about the primary client and the ways he has adjusted to his environment and to circumstances. The nurse needs to assess the level of functioning the client has attained in need fulfillment, cognitive, emotional, social, and sexual development. She may use Freud's, Erikson's, or Kohlberg's scale of physical/psychosexual development[3] to validate the data. What the nurse essentially wants to know about the client is how he is meeting his needs and how dependent he is on the defense mechanisms he uses to suppress or repress them. The nurse needs to know what the client's fears are. Does he accept his medical and nursing diagnosis? How much does he know about the diagnoses, and how much input has he had in their formulation? How motivated is he to change or modify the behaviors that may be causing his health problem? What is his maximum level of independent functioning?

The nurse must be able to use the appropriate interviewing techniques (details on interview methods follow) to collect data about the mental and emotional status of the client. The first step in this process is the establishment of a basic rapport between client and nurse. This involves honesty, sincerity, and openness; the purpose of the visit should be frankly explained. Data collection is also directed toward assessing how the client adapts to his environment and how he acts on his environment to change it. The nurse must therefore always question the meaning of an action, a gesture, or a particular verbal statement in order to understand how the behavior or statement is used by the client as a means of achieving a desired outcome. For instance, the nurse may wonder why Ms. Aimes laughs every time her husband glances at her; it seems an awkward grimace. The nurse hypothesizes that the client is fearful of having her husband look at her flat chest. She investigates the hypothesis, and after some gentle prodding, Ms. Aimes admits that she believes that her husband now thinks she is repulsive looking and by her laughing at him, she can pretend that her husband's opinion and her own feelings about his opinion do not matter. The nurse has now proved the hypothesis and can go on to decide what the best course of action will be.

The social person

Assessment of the social system(s) is the third part of the data collection base. The family is the social system that has the greatest impact on the client. Information recorded about the family can be critical to the nursing problem list and diagnosis. It includes general information about the family: age of each member, sex, marital status, a brief past and present health history, religion and the extent of participation in religious activities, and the role of each family member in the functioning of the family unit. Additional data will specify which member in the unit is the primary character at any given time. Of course, this could be a matter of inference on the part of the nurse, even though she has detailed descriptive data about how each member exerts some positive and negative control over the rest of the family.

In the case of a five-member family with one hyperkinetic child, that child will most likely be observed as exerting an important influence on the entire family; in this case the child is the primary client. Yet the nurse may further observe that it will be impossible to intervene in this situation unless she works closely with the mother, who is the main influence on the child. The mother-child dyad then becomes the primary client. The data base should include information about how each family member has adjusted to this situation and which family members are most affected by the stressful stimuli and in what ways. To what degree has the family maintained its ability to cope with the external world in spite of its internal problems? Which family member is strongest in independent functioning abilities, and what are those abilities?

To assess the family as a social institution, the nurse will require information about its cultural history, present practices, and rules for acceptable behavior. Economic status is important to know because income has a direct effect on family behavior and activities. It is helpful to note the number of working and nonworking adults with a brief description of each one's employment. It is not always the father or the head of the household who is primarily responsible for the family's income. Are there any working children in the home? How does this affect their family role? It is not unethical to ask the working adults to give an estimation of the family's overall income. This is an important piece of data, particularly since so many family crises center around money. How does the family spend its money? Is there a system by which they pay bills and divide the money to provide for necessities, or is one person completely responsible for household expenses? What items does the family save for? It is wise to also include information about the family's attitude toward money: how it should be spent, who should have control over it and why, and for what reasons children should receive an allowance. These questions may seem trite, or even presumptuous, but experience has shown that money is an underlying problem in many families. In fact, it often means the difference between a family that practices preventive health care and one which does not.

Another area that helps the nurse to understand the family as a social system is the assessment of its activity. The way in which a family spends its leisure time—together as a family and separately as individuals—is indicative of the way it functions in other areas. Can the family plan and take a vacation together? Or can they not stand each other's company for concentrated periods of time? Do the family members like each other enough to *want* to spend time together? What is the usual outcome of a planned project or activity? Do the children take part in deciding how leisure time will be spent?

How the family members interact with and function in the outside world—the neighborhood and the larger community—and the extent of participation in this environment is also a part of the activity assessment. The way the family functions within the larger social community is a good index of its ability to maintain a dynamic equilibrium. If interacting with the community causes additional stress, it is added to the data base as a present or potential problem. The lack of family interaction outside the home is also an indicator of a present or potential problem. The nurse might want to find out why the family does not interact with the community. Do they prefer to be alone, or are they being ostracized for some reason? Assessment of community interaction includes club memberships, sports involvements, church group activities, and the like.

The type of reinforcement family members give each other for accomplishments or failures should be noted. What is the system of rewards and punishments? How are children disciplined? The noise level in the home may be a significant clue about the emotional tone of the family. It tells the objective observer something about the organizational structure. Blasting televisions, screaming children, arguing adults, and frustrated family members are symptomatic of an eroded communication system. On the other hand, laughter, smiles, listening, talking, and caring are indicative of a working system.

The leadership pattern of the family system can indicate a great deal about its dynamics. How are the tasks and chores divided? Which member is the chief decision maker, or is the decision-making process based on equal participation? How do family members arrange themselves in the nurse's presence? Who seems to control the conversation? This kind of information can best be collected by observation and by talking with family members. The absence of any observable leadership pattern is also important to note because it can be indicative of the erosion of the entire family system. A disorganized family cannot solve problems, withstand crises, accomplish tasks, or identify and work toward a goal.

What is the general temperament of the family? Is it an easygoing, nonabusive one? Or is it a neurotic, compulsive family? Perhaps it is highly aggressive, abusive, combative, and disorganized. The personality of the family has a great deal to do with its success as a working system.

Assessment of interacting systems

Several interacting systems in the community must be assessed: the family, peer groups, the extended family when present, the local community, schools, and any other social group that has an influence on the client. The nurse needs to know as much as possible about these groups and should note communication patterns, culture, and behaviors that have an influence on the client and on surrounding nongroup members. The nurse would also like to know why the client is part of a particular group and how it meets his needs. How much of a client's socialization is involved in groups, and how is he accepted by them? This kind of data could be useful when the nurse formulates the care plan, and it gives an added dimension to the total picture of the client.

Assessment of all the systems that affect the client involves all the nurse's observational skills, and it also uses the process of analysis, inference, interpretation, and further research in order to form the data into a meaningful statement about the client. Data collection is perhaps the most fascinating, complex undertaking in the problem-solving task because the nurse is assessing the client in his natural habitat, not in the artificial environment of a hospital. *All* the aspects of his life and personality—in essence, his reason for being—should be a part of the data collected. A basic question that the nurse explores during data collection is to what degree the client himself understands his emotional and psychological self.

VALIDATION OF DATA

Validation of data is essential; without it there can be no assurance that the nursing care plan will be based on what is true about the client. One of the best ways to validate data is to compare it with other data: either that collected by someone else or data collected by the nurse during a previous contact with the client. Changes in data usually indicate either inaccuracy or a real health problem. Again, professional judgment is needed to distinguish between these two alternatives.

For instance, in the case of Ms. Aimes it was considered necessary by the nurse that a sexual history about the client be included in the data base. The nurse realized that this area was an extremely sensitive one in the client's life, so she jotted down a few statements during their discussion and relied on her memory for most of the interview. She thought the client might be uncomfortable to see the nurse with a long written form.

The goal of every nurse is accurate data. Trying to fill in all the blanks on a history form may appear to be the only way to obtain complete information. But filling in blanks on a form often interferes with the more important purpose of finding out what really happened, what the actual underlying problem is, or what is really on the client's mind. Also, when a form is taken to the interview or used at the clinic as the sole means of assessing a particular area, the client often tries to give what he thinks is the proper or best answer, and sometimes the truth is lost.

Preparation needed to validate data

Working in the community requires preparation, and a sound knowledge of nursing theory is basic. A nurse must keep up with disease etiology and clinical symptomology so she can recognize health problems as they appear. A working knowledge of epidemiology (Chapter 9) is essential for the community nurse. This information gives the nurse an understanding of the reasons for certain community-wide health problems. In order to better understand the client, the nurse assesses the neighborhood even before she arrives at his door.

The nurse assesses internal systems when recording data about the external systems. Messages are being continually transmitted from the external environment to the person and back again to the environment or to the external system. When a dysfunctional balance occurs during this process, the nurse observes patterns which indicate that a need is unfilled or that a behavior is nonfunctional. An example of this is the sleep-rest cycle of the body. The internal environment provides stimuli to tell the body when rest is needed; if the body does not properly compute this message or chooses to ignore it, then there is a break in the equilibrium, and symptoms appear. Thus it is important to include information about the living patterns and to note in detail the patterns that lead the client to disharmony with his external environment.

RECORDING OF DATA

Recording information about symptoms or patterns of behavior is one of the most difficult, but most essential, aspects of the data collection process. Chapter 14 provides details on how to record the various aspects of the nursing care plan and the nursing process. In an effort to always use correct methodology and to include all details, the nurse may lose sight of the overall picture; she may become lost in a morass of detail and forget the client as a human being. The community setting may not be the environment to which the nurse is accustomed, and she will have to take into consideration all the external stimuli. One of the most distressing factors is that the nurse does not have complete control over the situation. She should rely on her senses to develop an awareness of the external systems that are a part of the client's everyday life. If the client lives in an urban ghetto, there is an environment of noise, confusion, and danger. If he lives on a farm, the stimuli are different. External stimuli are often not what they appear to be, as illustrated by the following example:

Ms. Baile is a 38-year-old mother of five children. She lives in a low-income neighborhood, and her husband is well known for his frequent disappearances from home. Ms. Baile was referred to the Camden Visiting Nurses Association following Billy's discharge from the hospital, where he was treated for multiple contusions of the face and legs. Billy is her youngest child and is 2 months old. Child abuse was highly suspected. When the visiting nurse entered the home for the first time, she was confronted with the following situation: Karen, age 3, was listlessly sucking her thumb in a far-off corner of a dingy and cluttered room. The nurse heard an infant's cry in the distance that seemed to be coming from upstairs. She heard the blaring television and the screaming, shrieky voices of small children fighting as they attempted to play a game of darts in the middle of what appeared to be the living room. The children were shabbily dressed, and the older girl was noticeably obese.

It would be difficult to assess this family with a ready-made interviewing guide. For the nurse it was most helpful simply to look around and notice the different external stimuli interacting with and affecting the behavior of the children. She found it useful to jot down key word descriptions to characterize each child and to describe briefly the room and its atmosphere, as well as the physical outlay. Also, the communication system between the children was noted. Karen's behavior was precisely described for later reference.

In the preceding example Ms. Baile is the primary client. The nurse believes that in order to make positive changes in this family system she will have to establish rapport with Ms. Baile first. Recording the behavioral patterns of the children in relation to each other and to their mother gives the nurse insight into their mother's belief and value system and her educational level. If Ms. Baile and the nurse can agree on a nursing diagnosis and work together on the care plan, it is likely that intervention will be effective. This makes it essential that the data is collected and recorded accurately. The client's childhood development and present personality characteristics will have a direct bearing on the nursing care plan. Understanding Ms. Baile's needs will help the nurse to know why she interacts with her children the way she does. The nurse will also want to understand Ms. Baile's self-concept, since changing the outward behavior toward her children may begin with changing or modifying her own level of self-acceptance.

Describing the people who relate to the client

The significant people who directly influence the life of the client are also important. Their roles in relation to the client must be understood so that effective intervention can be based on a family or group process if necessary. The nurse needs to know how all the "secondary" people relate to and interact with the client. Is the primary client emotionally dependent on the relationship? Some relationship patterns commonly described are symbiotic, mutual, or parasitic. A symbiotic relationship is characterized by two people living in a mutually dependent way; each cannot (or think they cannot) exist without the other. A mutual relationship is when two people give equally, but neither is actually dependent on the other. A parasitic one is when one person takes from the other and actually causes harm to the other in so doing. Some relationships are further described as masochistic, sadistic, or a combination of the two. The Baile family is actually a conglomerate of relationship patterns: a relationship network.

Data collection of interpersonal patterns of living is especially necessary when the relationship is in a situational or maturational crisis. The nurse needs to know what the crisis is so she can assess the situation and begin crisis intervention therapy (see Chapter 12 for details). The more data she collects about the special people in a client's life, the more accurate the nursing diagnosis will be. It is usually not difficult for the observant nurse to pick up key clues signaling that a crisis is at hand. Many times the client himself will give the signal: ''I just can't cope with it anymore''; or, ''I feel like I hate my mother more each day; she just refuses to understand me.'' It is not really significant whether the crisis is situational or maturational; what is important are the resources available to the client to enable him to cope. Probably the most significant data are the subjective clues offered by the client or someone very close to him. It is essential that the nurse be particularly aware of key statements indicating an impending crisis. It is at this time that these statements or behaviors can be brought to the attention of the client so he can learn to recognize what the behaviors mean in terms of adaptation to external events. However, in some instances objective data are all that are needed. Returning to the Baile home, when the nurse observed two small quarreling children playing darts, her immediate thought was the possible disaster that could develop from a badly aimed dart. Sometimes data are right in front of the nurse's nose, but she is so accustomed to digging for hidden meanings that she misses the obvious, like a dart in the eye.

DATA COLLECTION ABOUT THE COMMUNITY

Community data collection does not focus on one client; rather the nurse uses her skills to identify community health problems and implement change. The initial assessment should be a general profile of the community population. Then a specific area of health behavior, level of health knowledge, or scope of an identified health problem is investigated by the nurse. The investigative tools

are the same as those in assessing individual clients, as is the process of data collection. The area from which data is collected is wider, but the method and process remain the same. The nurse still needs all her observational and interpretive skills. Thus in the case of a defined population group, the entire group is the client, and the health problem of the group is the reference point from which the population is studied.

Depending on the nature of the community and the area in which it is located, any number of health problems can surface at any time. Health problems that the community nurse sees are not always the result of hunger and deprivation. Sometimes the opposite is true, and the health problem is the result of affluence. A good example is the type A and type B personalities that have been recently discussed in medical literature. The type A personality is a compulsive, aggressive, and competitive one often seen in the upper echelons of business and industry. The person with a type A personality is almost always a man, and he lives in an affluent community. Some symptoms that have been associated with this character type are a variety of common gastrointestinal disturbances and heart disease. He also tends to work long and hard, often neglects the emotional needs of his family, and seems obsessed by success. He is a ''workaholic.'' The individual with a type B personality tends to be more placid and does not suffer from so many stress diseases. Type A personalities are likely to suffer from stress diseases. These health problems when they appear in a Type A personality much more often reflect success and affluence than poverty and hunger. It is easy to ignore or trivialize the health problems of the wealthy because they do not come to the attention of the community nurse as frequently as those of the poor.

Intervention in the community is a tremendous undertaking, and one nurse cannot do it alone. She needs to function as part of the community health team and may also become the overseer of nursing care in a community. Whatever roles the nurse assumes, she has a responsibility to learn all she can about the population she is serving. The nurse's long-range objective is health maintenance, and as she examines the extent, scope, and range of a particular problem, she can also function as an epidemiologist. The community nurse must know what resources are available to a community for various health needs, as well as the level of effectiveness of those resources. This is part of community assessment.

Collecting data for a specific problem

An example of team data collection is participation in a community project. A nurse joined a newly forming committee on the battered child that was an extension of DHHS efforts established to describe the extent and nature of child abuse in Camden County, New Jersey. Another objective was to increase the county's efficiency in dealing with the problem. The committee was joined at its initial stage of development, which meant that there was a chance to take part in outlining and collecting data to describe the extent and pattern of child abuse in the community. In order for the data collected to be as objective as possible, the process began with a definition. It was decided what a battered child was and what the specific characteristics of the community were that contributed to the problem. Because the constituents of the committee were from a variety of backgrounds, each member contributed toward broadening the data base by suggesting a range of possible causes. The nurse's function was to research case histories, to interview medical professionals who had dealt with the problem, and to assist in diagnosing the problem once the information was collected.

The Committee on the Battered Child never left the data collection stage, but the process continued and increased throughout an entire year. Apparently the extent and scope of the problem was far more extensive than the committee had thought. As the investigation continued, more professionals and lay people entered the data collection effort, including business people, police, clergy, medical records personnel, physicians, community nurses, social workers, teachers, probation officers, and interested parents. The processes of data collection and intervention eventually became inseparable, and the interest of lay people added a momentum to the community that served as an abuse deterrent. The problem became public, the law was clarified, and, as time went by, citizens were made aware of their responsibility to the problem. This team effort to define, prevent, and intervene in a community problem was not a complete success, and there are still many battered children in Camden County. It would be too much to expect that the problem of child abuse could be solved in only a year. However, the process of systematic, comprehensive data collection validated many hypotheses about the nature of the problem and suggested ways to intervene. The key element was all-out interest and involvement.

The problem of child abuse was described as widely distributed and not specific to any income group or educational level. The data indicated that low-income areas were characterized by an abuse problem that was primarily related to financial frustration. In the higher-income areas, neglect was more prevalent than abuse, and the battered child syndrome was particularly noted in high-tension families in which divorce, alcoholism, and poor family communication patterns existed. Because data was collected by a variety of health professionals and lay people, the data was validated, and the foundation for intervention was laid. The tools for research were varied, depending on who was interviewed or what characteristic of the population was to be studied.

TOOLS FOR DATA COLLECTION
The interview

The most basic and essential tool the nurse uses to collect data is the interview. The purposes of the interview are to (1) establish the relationship needed to effectively work with the client, (2) to start the process of finding out about the client as a whole individual, and (3) to outline the client's predominant needs, motives, and conflicts. The interview precedes the formulation of the nursing care plan because it is the necessary starting point of the nurse-client relationship; without it the nurse cannot understand the client or interpret his needs. There is no such thing as nursing care without an interview, which might be formal or informal in structure, of long or short duration, planned or spontaneous. A 5-minute conversation with a client while standing in line at the bank is as much an interview as a formal discussion in the clinic. In fact, it is likely that more "straight talk" will take place in the bank than in the clinic, and the data collected can be among the most valuable the nurse receives.

There are many interview techniques. Even before the interview begins, the nurse must decide what she wants to know about the client, what her hypotheses are, and what she wants the client to understand about her. To establish a trusting relationship, the nurse must *actively* explain the purpose of the interview and find out whether the client has understood the explanation. The best way to do this is to have the client repeat in his own words what the nurse has said. The word 'actively' means that the nurse uses as many ways as are necessary to communicate the message in order that it be accurately perceived by the client.

Another important characteristic of the interview is that it has and maintains direction. Maintaining direction and purpose is often the most difficult aspect of the entire process. It may be useful to write down the data that are to be gathered and the hypotheses which will be explored and refer to them when the interview seems to be going off course. When communication becomes social chit-chat, it may no longer be a therapeutic data collection event, although it does have use as a tension-relieving device and as a transition between "serious" topics. Losing control of the interview is common because the client or the nurse may have a need to distract the process or divert it when it becomes uncomfortable. It is usually obvious when the interview has become hopelessly mired in trivial conversation, and the nurse must then take hold of the situation. Saying "I'd like to get back to what we were talking about a few minutes ago" is a technique that usually works. There may be times when the nurse will allow the direction of

the interview to change. In this case it may be that the client's expressed (either verbal or nonverbal) need not to continue is more important than the interview. Allowing the client this freedom does not mean that the nurse has lost control of the situation; she has merely acknowledged her understanding of the client as a person with needs and discomforts.

The most widely used interview is the open-ended one. It is best described by comparison with the closed interview. A closed interview is composed of questions that are easily answered by simple, brief statements such as "Yes," "No," "I don't know," or "Sometimes." Closed questions are useful in the interviewing process when a direct answer is most suitable or when they serve as a technique to direct the evasive, easily distracted client. In the case of a severely depressed client, the closed interview may be the only way to stimulate the client to talk, and sometimes it can be used to head a client into a more open conversation. Often the nurse-directed closed interview is used at the beginning to put the client at ease or to obtain straightforward information such as name and address. The closed interview has several excellent purposes, but used alone it does not give nurses the kind of broad data base they need to develop effective nursing diagnoses. Uninhibited free-flowing dialogue is necessary for the client to express the kinds of feelings that can give the nurse some insight into his needs.

In comparison with the easily answered questions which require a nod of the head at the very least, the open-ended interview employs questions that require descriptive, detailed, and at times complex answers. The types of questions presented in the open-ended interview require reflection and often elicit the expression of emotion from the client. The conversation has momentum as nurse and client explore feelings, attitudes, and goals together. Questions are always focused on the client, as the nurse guides him toward reflecting on what has been expressed and what must still be explored. During the open-ended interview the nurse can maintain her role as a supportive, caring person, but she can also function as an educator by supplying health information and correcting misconceptions. The following example of an open-ended interview conducted on a visit to a family suspected of child abuse will clarify the method.

The nurse had received a call from the Division of Youth and Family Services (DYFS) about Ms. Lane, who is known to the agency and suspected of child abuse. The nurse questioned the social worker at DYFS about the extent of abuse, past history, and the community environment. She learned that Ms. Lane's childhood was characterized by family discord and that she had spent several years in boarding schools, foster homes, and with neighbors when her mother "just couldn't stand her any longer." Ms. Lane is a high school graduate and lives in a middle-income area. The nurse hypothesized that the client has an inadequate concept of the mothering role, but only a home visit could prove or disprove the hypothesis. She used an open-ended interview because it allows free discussion.

INTERVIEW ONE

Nurse: Hello, Ms. Lane, how are you? *(Nonverbal gesturing, voice intonation, and frequent eye contact communicates to the client that the nurse is interested in her.)* I was told by DYFS about what happened to Johnny. *(Nurse specifically leaves out the details; this allows the client the freedom to describe the situation without being defensive.)*

Client: Yes, well you see, Johnny fell down . . . the stairs. *(Pause; the nurse gives no cue that she will comment about this. Silence will encourage the client to continue.)* Well, you see, Johnny is very clumsy; he's always falling down and breaking something. *(The nurse moves closer, looking the client directly in the eye, demonstrating interest and concern and yet maintaining a nonjudgmental attitude. The client begins to shake as she stoops down to pick up her son.)* I don't know why I told you that, he didn't fall. *(The client clutches her son.)* Johnny, I need you. I'm sorry.

Nurse: You know, Ms. Lane, I came here today because I care about you and Johnny. I'm not sure what happened yesterday, but we can talk about it. *(The nurse reaches out to take the client's hand as if to communicate that she knows how hard it must be to talk about this. She tries to imagine how difficult it is for*

this mother to know how to love her child when she herself had such an unhappy childhood.)

Client: I swore I would never treat my own child like this. I really don't know what comes over me. It's that feeling of hate or getting back, but then I look down at him and just burst into tears. *(She bursts into tears.)* Please help me. . . .

The nurse saw what she thought was an unresolved love-hate conflict between the mother and child. She also noted that the mother has strong guilt feelings about her inability to control some of her emotion or behavior. Some of the external environment was also noted; the house was in perfect order, and there were no toys or baby things in view. The baby did not cry during the interview but merely stared into space. There seemed to be stimulational neglect of the child, but this hypothesis will have to be proved, and further data are needed. The mother sometimes seemed to be "not there," and at other times she seemed to concentrate very hard. She appeared to be aware of her inability to understand her feelings about herself and her child, but this also requires further data.

INTERVIEW TWO

Client: Why can't I be like other mothers?

Nurse: Ms. Lane, being a mother is a difficult job, and there is no set way of behaving. Can you explain what you mean?

Client: Other mothers don't hit their babies for no reason. They. . . . *(The nurse notes that the client is having difficulty verbalizing what she is feeling. She waits as the client gropes for the words.)* I really don't know who I am sometimes. I forget that Johnny is my baby and that he won't leave me.

Nurse: He won't leave you? *(She observes that the client is in a trancelike state with no facial expression. This repetition of her remark startles her, and she laughs nervously.)*

Client: Well, everybody else has left me, haven't they? I thought marriage would have changed things, but he left me too. I just feel empty inside, like nobody cares about me. So why should I care about them?

When the nurse wrote an abstract of the interview, she included the following: the hypothesis that the client has a decreased affect is validated by the client stating that she feels empty inside.

Her husband has left her, and she does not know of anyone who cares about her. She is having a problem in socialization, in establishing close ties with others, and in understanding past experience. She forgets that her child is a baby and has difficulty relating to him as such; she was not observed talking to her child. The plan is to make a referral to a psychologist or a community mental health center, and the nurse will visit to try to find ways to help the client relate to her child and to other people.

This excerpt illustrates the many techniques that the nurse used to gather significant data. She listened, reflected the client's own expressions back to her, touched, empathized, and expressed honesty in communicating with Ms. Lane. By trying to empathize with the client, the nurse can increase her level of awareness of what the client may be feeling and her own reactions to the client. The nurse directed the conversation by focusing on key statements and feelings and by exploring possible situations that will aid in diagnosis and intervention. As demonstrated in the two examples, the interview is therapeutic while at the same time is used for collection of data. The nurse was able to permit the client to express her feelings in a free and open way, which is therapeutic. The nurse did not conduct the interview merely to validate hypotheses; she also wanted to help the client resolve her problems. It is the aim of the nurse, then, to remain continuously aware of how her behaviors and attitudes affect the client; even the most pertinent data go uncollected if the nurse feels that questioning in that area will have a harmful effect on the client. The nurse should be able to tell by the client's nonverbal behavior that he is uncomfortable, and the subject could be changed. Pressing on with a topic when the client obviously does not want to discuss it will only create antagonism and make the client less willing to talk in the future. Data might then be gathered from other sources until the client feels able to discuss the matter.

The nurse is director, planner, and organizer of the therapeutically conducted interview. Her role as a health professional is to remain objective and to record the interview from the client's point of view. Interviewing is a process by which questions are answered and information is exchanged. As the nurse makes observations and validates hypotheses, she is sometimes led to more data, or she reaches a dead end and must change her technique if she needs more data.

Suggested data record outline form

1. General description
   a. Age, sex, race, religion, and marital status
   b. Present status: current crises and the way in which they are being handled, chief complaints, and understanding of medical diagnosis
   c. Present social status: educational achievements, work, socialization, insurance and retirement plans, and social goals
2. Physical health: past health and name of family physician or clinic
   a. Statement from client about health history and attitudes, as well as subjective statements
   b. Prostheses, activities of daily living, and prognosis if it is limited
   c. Medications
   d. Growth and development: subjective and objective data and summary of developmental tests
3. Family system
   a. General health history of the family
   b. Relationship of the client to other family members, the client's description of his family role, attitudes toward his family, communication patterns, and maladaptive coping patterns
   c. Family profile: general temperament, safety, economic status, condition of home, and kinds of demonstrations of physical touching and affection
4. Psychological system: summary statement on each visit about the client's general mood and coping ability, how he meets his own needs, his emotional depth, and his ability to relate to others
5. Social system: cultural, ethical, and behavioral practices of the client and amount and kind of socialization in community activities
6. Safety and health maintenance: sanitary facilities, condition of the neighborhood, degree of health maintenance and primary care, and adequacy and use of health facilites

This outline is merely a guide. The questions will change depending on the client, environment, and nurse. The most important goal of the data collection process is that it be purposeful and directly related to the formulation of a nursing diagnosis. Data must be validated by subjective and objective information so there will be a rationale for the diagnosis and the care plan. The data are analogous to the cement foundation on which a home must stand. If the foundation is faulty, the entire house is at risk.

Throughout the process of data collection, the nurse should discuss her findings with other health professionals. This is important because different viewpoints lead to further speculation, which leads to increased data collection and a more comprehensive care plan. What one nurse views as a problem, another may easily overlook. Every possible hypothesis must be explored before a diagnosis is made. Hypotheses will be proved (and form the basis of the nursing diagnosis) or discarded and new ones formulated. At this point the problem list can be drawn up and a diagnosis made.

NURSING DIAGNOSIS

The nursing diagnosis is the nurse's concluding statement about the client's health problem, or it could be termed a definition of the problem. An accurate diagnosis is fundamental to the nursing care plan; an incorrect diagnosis is most often the product of an inaccurate data base or a poorly analyzed one. The nurse plays detective, searching for the statement(s) that best summarizes the overall problem. The diagnosis can be seen as subjective because it is the nurse's assessment of the client's problem, but because it is formulated in a scientific way and is based on both subjective and objective data, it can be considered objective and logically deduced.

The community nurse's diagnosis is not easily arrived at, simply because the facts do not lie immediately before her; she must search them out. It is her diagnosis that will communicate to the rest of the health professionals what the client's needs and resources are. With an accurate data base and a perceptive diagnosis, the nurse can be the initiator of an entire team process of intervention. Thus the diagnosis is the core message of the care plan.

Diagnosis is a common word in medical terminology. The nursing diagnosis can best be defined as a statement of the client's central or focal problems. The word focal means that the main portion of the data tends to point to a group of needs, deficits, or nonactualized capabilities of the client. The foci of problems recorded in a brief summary form are the core of the diagnosis and serve as a basis for the nursing care plan. There can be several diagnoses, or there can be several subdiagnoses that are part of the larger one. Fig. 13-1 illustrates the process.

Demonstration of nursing process from data collection to diagnosis

1. Data base: mental and emotional system
   a. *Subjective data.* "I feel like my life is worthless. I just sit and daydream all the time. If it weren't for television soap operas, I don't know what I'd do with myself."

   ↓

   b. *Objective data.* Client stares past nurse in a nonfocused way; asks no questions and does not respond to those asked by the nurse; demonstrates poorly developed communication skills; talks to herself frequently.

   ↓

   c. *Analysis.* Client sits most of the day, getting inadequate exercise and socialization; lacks self-motivation. Inadequate communication skills most likely because client is usually alone and does not have a need to communicate.

   ↓

   d. *Diagnosis.* Inadequate communication skills; present problem of inactivity; potential problem of complete isolation as client separates herself from the real world. Further validation needed.

2. Data base: social systems. *Subjective data.* "The people around here are just not my type. All my friends moved away. I don't enjoy group activity."

   ↓

   b. *Objective data.* Client from low-income rural area; claims no involvement with any community group; does not socialize with neighbors; does not

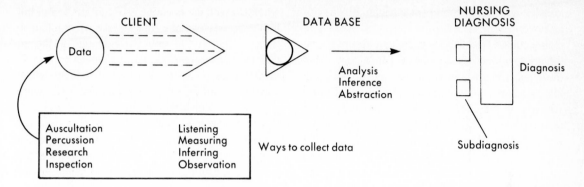

Fig. 13-1. Process of data collection. Formulation of a data base leads to the nursing diagnosis.

work and claims no working skills; completed high school education; claims that all her close friends moved away. When client is encouraged to make new friends, she looks away from nurse and drifts off into thoughts of her own.

↓

c. *Analysis*. Data further support hypothesis that client does not socialize and lacks skill in this ability; the motivation to socialize is absent. Client lacks friends or any support system in the community; has a tendency to use isolation as a defense mechanism to avoid discussion of social systems.

↓

d. *Diagnosis*. Present problem of inadequate socialization; potential problem of total isolation from others and eventual psychosis; needs motivation to socialize and practice communication skills.

The diagnosis is an essential tool for the continuity of care because the community nurse will have to make the decision to do the nursing intervention herself or to make a referral to another agency. The spectrum of problems that the nurse will find in a community is limitless, and there is no end to the kind of nursing diagnoses that can be made.

The initial diagnosis is an inclusive statement that will be updated and completed on further data collection, and a note should be made to this effect on the diagnosis. Examples of a tentative diagnosis are disorganized family system, nonsupportive parenting, or family in state of conflict concerning change in role. In each case the nurse has not validated the diagnosis but has perceived the situation on an initial assessment. The reason tentative diagnoses are made is that the sooner the diagnostic process is begun, the sooner intervention can begin. The initial diagnosis leads immediately to collection of further data to validate and to elaborate on it.

The clearest way to write the diagnosis is to state the objective and subjective data on which it is based (see the preceding examples) and include at least an initial plan of care, either as part of the diagnosis or separately. The planning stage is then indicated as the next step in the nursing process. What the diagnosis should immediately communicate to all members of the health team is the level of wellness of the client, what his problems are, and what resources he has to solve them. The diagnosis should be written in terms of the client as a whole person and should not make him sound like a disease entity. The diagnosis is usually stated as a summary of the health problems, but it is easy to become too negative when writing the diagnosis. It is true that health problems usually *are* negative, but the client's personal and commmunity resources should also be included to avoid unintentionally reinforcing the client's negative behavior and overlooking the positive.

A second reason the diagnosis should summarize the actual or potential resources of the client is that the client should take an active role in assessing his problems and formulating his care plan (Fig. 13-2). It is the client who must ultimately agree on the behaviors he wishes to change or the health problems that affect his wellness. Having the client participate in the formulation of his diagnosis can motivate him to continue to function even in the absence of the nurse. The client is not then over-whelmed with the negative aspect of his being, but rather he can examine the disease or problem in light of his positive self. For example, in the diagnosis of a disorganized family, whatever positive elements exist, such as trust or independence, should be stated so the client and nurse can work together to resolve the conflict.

The problem list is a result of the data base and nursing diagnosis, and the client will participate in ranking the priority of the problems and in delineating the actual, possible, and potential ones.[4] There should be a differentiation between problems

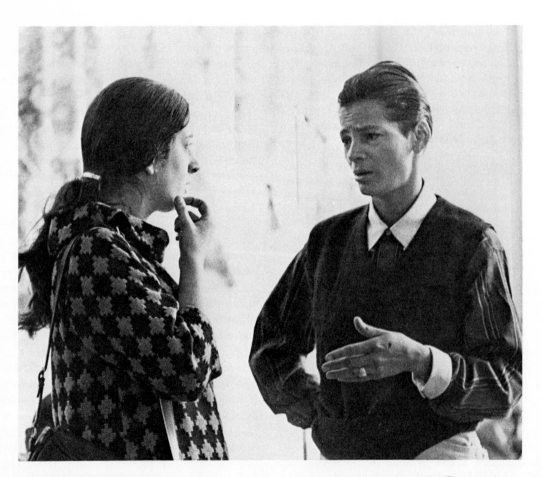

Fig. 13-2. The client must be an integral part of the formulation of the nursing diagnosis. (Photograph by Marion Bernstein; courtesy Editorial Photocolor Archives, Inc., New York.)

that are solvable and those which are beyond the scope of nursing practice. Shindell[5] emphasizes the importance of knowing the resources and characteristics of the client prior to the impairment or health problem. In this way the nurse can use comparison to predict the problems that will respond to intervention.

NURSING CARE PLAN

A nursing care plan that can be documented with scientific principles and theory is far superior to one which overlooks the rationale behind the plan. This can be accomplished by using the results of formal nursing research as well as by doing informal anecdotal nursing research of one's own. However, it is more likely that the community nurse will do the former rather than the latter. Research in this context means reading and studying what other nurses have found to be effective in similar situations. A problem that is not researched in the literature can lead to an inaccurate and unimaginative care plan and an unmotivated nurse. One that is based on research will most likely be more effective than one which is not, and it is one in which the client is more likely to participate. Research should begin in the data collection stage and continue throughout the nursing process. Too often the planning stage is the point at which objectivity ceases and professional judgment goes out the window, and the nurse bases her intervention on her past experience alone.

An example of a poorly researched care plan is the one that Mr. Yorker, the nurse, made for the Spearos, an elderly couple:

Mr. Spearo had a stroke a year ago and has been rehabilitated since then only to a minimal degree. The couple live in a one-bedroom middle-income apartment, and Ms. Spearo provides all the care for her husband. She does quite well because she was lucky to find the hospital rehabilitation nurses to be excellent teachers. Mr. Yorker assessed the situation using his past experience with stroke clients, those he had seen in the hospital, as his sole criterion. The care plan that he and Ms. Spearo developed was effective in prescribing progressive physical stimulation and exercise for Mr. Spearo. However, Mr. Yorker failed to include a vital component in the care plan. He realized this several months later as he read a journal article about stroke clients in the community. His plan had totally disregarded sexuality and rehabilitation toward improving the couple's intimate experiences, which is an important component in their ability to continue a satisfying relationship. Mr. Yorker should have picked up the many clues that Ms. Spearo gave indicating that she was sexually and emotionally frustrated. He vividly recalled that she made several remarks about never being able to sleep with her husband again.

The problem list may or may not be ranked by severity, depending on the policy of the agency, but the problems are always numbered and dated, and the plan of intervention is listed by coordinating the numbers with the problem list, as is the validation and rationale for the plan. Goals and objectives should be stated in precise and measurable terms when possible or in behavioral terms when that is more appropriate. The expected date of outcome, if this is feasible, will aid in evaluation, as will a description of expected behavior that will occur as a result of the intervention. For example, a goal for Spearos could be stated: Mr. and Ms. Spearo will express sexual awareness of each other by the end of next month by holding hands, touching, verbally expressing love, sharing the same bed, and decreasing the wife's behavior that indicates a mothering role. She will stop referring to her husband as "my baby." Of course, this is not a quantifiable goal, but it is sufficiently qualified and descriptive so that it can be observed and discussed.

The community setting usually calls for intervention on an interval schedule: daily, weekly, or biweekly visits. Behavioral changes are evaluated on a continuum as the client advances from step to step in an effort to attain the goal. Goals can be stated with a main objective and subgoals, with expected dates of outcome for each. The subgoals give the nurse and the client the opportunity to evaluate progress toward the main goal. The client is often the best one to determine his own progress, and he should always be given a copy of the nursing care plan so he can have a constant reminder of the goals. Including the client as a collaborator reinforces the fact that he is responsible for his progress and that only he can be the cause for change in his life.

Example of a nursing care plan

Problem

Ms. Spearo does not regard her husband as a person with sexual needs or as a person able to satisfy her sexual needs.

Validation

Wife refers to husband as "baby." States she can no longer sleep with him. She also makes frequent statements that her husband no longer regards her in a sexual way. "All he cares about is eating and sleeping."

Resources

Couple lives and spends many hours together. Ms. Spearo is a very affectionate person and is willing to try new approaches to caring for her husband. Mr. Spearo is responsive to others and reacts to touch and kindness in an emotional way; cries, looks into eyes, etc.

Goal

By the end of a three-week period, Mr. and Ms. Spearo will interact as husband and wife, demonstrating their love with an expression of sexuality.[6]

Subgoals

Week one

1. Ms. Spearo will hold her husband's hand when feeding him and when speaking to him and will kiss him whenever she wants.
2. Ms. Spearo will refrain from referring to her husband as her baby and will use the words of endearment that she used before his stroke.

Week two

3. Mr. and Ms. Spearo will sleep in the same bed with safety adjustments for Mr. Spearo. All "sick room supplies" will be kept outside the bedroom.
4. Ms. Spearo will take a half hour of each day (not necessarily all at the same time) to sit and talk with her husband about how she feels toward him sexually and what her desires are.

Week three

5. Couple openly touch each other, sleep together, and express an awareness of each other's sexuality.

"The identification of a problem requires an analytical approach, careful attention to detail and an ability to determine which information is relevant."[7,p. 296] Ongoing descriptions of changes in health status or behavior make the evaluation process easier. If the evaluation is done on a continuing basis, the ultimate success or failure of nursing intervention will be evident.

Another way of stating problems is in terms of primary and secondary problems.[8] This is actually a hypothetical relationship of problems that is deduced from the data and from the nurse's professional judgment; the secondary problem is stated as the result of the primary one. The *way* in which the problem is stated allows the receiver of the message (anyone reading the record) to understand the thought processes of the communicator (the person who wrote the record). This relationship of primary and secondary problems may be proved invalid by further data collection, but it is a beginning.

Example of primary and secondary problem recording

Primary problem

Mr. Spearo is dependent on his wife for assistance in all activities of daily living and in need fulfillment: love, entertainment, play, physical care, safety and protection, socialization, etc.

Secondary problems

1. Ms. Spearo is overtired, hyperactive, and has difficulty controlling her energy levels.
2. Ms. Spearo has much suppressed and repressed guilt about her desire to spend time away from her husband doing things that are pleasurable to her.
3. Mr. Spearo uses inappropriate coping mechanisms when he cannot accomplish a task, such as crying, yelling, and temper tantrums, to gain his wife's sympathy and reinforce her guilt. This leads to a vicious circle of inappropriate coping mechanisms, guilt, and reinforcement of his babylike behavior.

The way in which the nurse chooses to state the problem list may vary with the client, the nurse-client relationship, and the setting of the interview. The important elements of every problem list are conciseness, documentation, completeness, and accuracy. Mayers[8] substitutes the phrase "expected outcome" for the terms "goals" and "objectives." She believes this phrase emphasizes the centrality of the client in the goal-setting process. Mayers states, "An expected outcome is a statement of the intended, or realistically expected, correction of the patient's problem by a certain point in time."[8,p.57] The expected outcome is stated as the change in behavior that will be the result of the nursing intervention. The present behavior or condition is the problem or the indicator of a potential problem. It does not really matter what terminology is used as long as the goals are stated in behavioral terms that are as precise as is humanly possible; this is the only way the care can be realistically evaluated.

PROGRESS NOTES AND EVALUATION

The evaluation process actually begins with the first intervention and will continue throughout the entire nursing process. It is most covenient for the nurse to write progress notes during or after each client contact to document the progress and objectively evaluate the success of the intervention. The nurse can then make changes in the intervention plan based on the intervention that has already taken place and which serves as a rationale for the new plan. The notes then become the core of the care plan because they indicate what level of change the client has achieved to date.

INTERVENTION AND EVALUATION

Intervention can be considered the third part of the nursing process, and evaluation is the last. A well-done nursing care plan will include evaluation as an ongoing part of intervention. The plan is the provision of nursing care to meet the stated objectives; it is the process of actively stepping into a human system to resolve the needs of that malfunctioning system. The nurse takes on many functions as part of intervention: referral agent, consumer advocate, teacher, nurturer, member of the community health team, and several others. (See Chapter 6 for a full description of the functions of the community health nurse.) Whatever her role, her primary function is the resolution of a defined nursing problem; she is intervening to meet the needs of the client. In the community, intervention usually takes place over a longer period of time than it does in institutionalized settings because community problems deal with an open system that is continuously affected by changing stimuli. For this reason the nursing care plan is particularly important: it provides for the systematic supply of nursing care and for the continuous evaluation process.

The purpose for the evaluation is to find out if the goals and objectives were accomplished. If so, what behavioral changes is the client exhibiting? If he is showing no changes, why not? There are usually only a few reasons for the failure to accomplish the goals:

1. The data base was incorrect or incomplete.
2. The problem list was based on faulty data.
3. The client did not participate in the formulation of the nursing care plan.
4. The goals were unrealistic.
5. Intervention was ineffective.
6. The client, for some reason, thwarted the achievement of the goals.

The nurse must first decide which one of the reasons caused the failure; to do this she needs to be honest with herself, and she must be a good detective. Then it is simply a matter of reassessing the point at which the failure occurred and going on from there.

The plans for intervention and evaluation must be written so the rest of the community health team can understand them; this is especially important if the person writing the care plan will not be the person who provides the intervention or does the evaluation.

The nursing process will always be no more than what the professional nurse makes it. There is no *one* way of systematically providing care; each nurse must develop a style of using the nursing process that will be most useful and meaningful to her. The nursing process remains no more than another tool in the provision of professional nursing care, and its productivity is always contingent on the resourcefulness of the practitioner.

CASE STUDY

Peggy was recently released from a state mental hospital; she will be maintained on an outpatient basis with frequent visits from the community health nurse, periodic evaluations by the psychiatrist, and a program of chemotherapy. She has been diagnosed as schizophrenic and has a history of maladaptive behavior patterns stemming from an extremely unhappy childhood. Ms. Evans is a beginning community nurse, and this is her first assignment.

Peggy lives with her parents in a two-bedroom home. She dresses inappropriately at times, sometimes in a very masculine style and other times in old ragged clothes with heavy makeup. When the temperature is cold, she sometimes forgets to dress warmly but appears not to notice. She is 28 years old and had been married for four months when her husband left her. She had a stillborn child shortly before her husband left, although she often refers to her baby as though it were alive. She takes no part in community activities and stays home watching television all day.

Discussion

Ms. Evans, before seeing Peggy for the first time, talked with the psychiatrist and reviewed the literature about schizophrenia. Her starting hypothesis is that she would be able to guide Peggy toward a higher level of community functioning, but she would not be able to change Peggy's behavior patterns or do anything about her schizophrenia. She formulated the following problem list after the second visit:

1. Peggy: inappropriate affect; disturbances in thought patterns and conversational abilities; needs assistance in self-expression and other communication techniques.
2. Peggy: self-isolation from society; spends most of the day fantasizing; needs to be motivated to socialize.
3. Peggy: inadequate understanding of sexuality; spends many hours masturbating and discusses it openly; needs education regarding sexuality, birth control, and care of her body.
4. Peggy: does not understand what schizophrenia is and how it affects her life.

5. Mother: does not talk to Peggy other than to tell her what to do; unable to express affection.
6. Father: very apathetic and quiet; needs to be motivated to take part in family activities. Examine relationship between Peggy and her father.
7. Family: need to examine roles and relationships. They do not take part in any activities together.

These were the primary problems Ms. Evans saw, but there were also many secondary ones, mostly relating to Peggy's socialization and the lack of spending money she needed for beginning independence. The care plan helped the nurse to organize her observations and to stimulate her creativity in devising intervention plans. Behavior modification seemed essential, and she thought that every visit should include some type of nurse-client therapy. The eventual goal was to teach Peggy to become a thinking, feeling, and caring person: one that would take a long time, if ever, to achieve. Ms. Evans made the following intervention plans:

1. Inappropriate affect. Will converse with client in a way that requires expression of her feelings; reflexive technique and open-ended interviewing; teach client how to verbalize what she is feeling; give her exercises to increase her nonverbal communication skills, such as eye-following exercises, body movements to music, touching to express warmth, and smiling only when happy. The goal is to demonstrate an increase in appropriate verbal and nonverbal communication.

2. Isolation. Will try to teach client how things can be done with another person; will discuss with client how she spends her time and will suggest desirable activities; set time limits for activities that tend to reinforce isolation; motivate client to attend socialization sessions at outpatient clinic. The goal is to understand the concept of friend and to interact with some of the people at the clinic.

3. Sexuality. Need to collect further data about client's concept of sexuality; will use topic of masturbation as starting point. The goal is to under-

stand herself and to verbally express her sexual feelings in an appropriate manner.

4. Mother and father. Will suggest that parents seek psychological evaluation and consultation to help them develop communication skills. They need to be able to talk about their feelings in regard to Peggy's illness and how it affects their own lives. All intervention plans for Peggy will be discussed with her parents. The goal is the parents' understanding of Peggy's illness and their reaction to it.

5. Family interaction. An hour twice a week will be set aside for family group discussions, which the nurse will lead. Topics discussed will be specific to the entire family or to the needs of an individual family member as related to the family process. The goal is better family communication.

Ms. Evans used the nursing care plan as a guide for the weekly evaluation, and she employed behavioral contracts, which made Peggy take part in the planning and prevented further alienation. Sometimes they would decide on simple changes of routine such as a walk for half an hour just to concentrate on feelings. Evaluation was a team process. Peggy was the first to decide what she considered to be an achievement, a setback, or a goal obstacle. If the intervention plan was a failure, it was Peggy who first judged it as such. The nurse was motivated by Peggy's excitement and positive self-reinforcement. She did the exercises with a sincere effort, even though her progress was not as fast as Ms. Evans had hoped. Her expressed enthusiasm was reason to continue the exercises, and they seemed to give her pleasure. New plans were developed as old goals were achieved, and the progress notes were used to indicate the evaluation and new implementation techniques.

SUMMARY

Planning, evaluation, and replanning are what makes the nursing process dynamic. It changes, grows, and adapts to whatever the situation warrants, although the form remains the same. Its very form and function provide for adaptation to the needs of individual clients. The process, used to its ultimate degree, will offer the nursing profession new and exciting ways of dealing with problems in the family and community. The innovative community nurse will find the application of the nursing process effective in many untried areas. It is the nurse's way of approaching a problem in order to achieve a maximum level of change toward the expected healthy outcome. In other words, the components of the nursing process are assessment, planning, implementation, and evaluation, and the word *process* indicates that it is not a static system.

NOTES

1. Auger, Jenine Roose: Behavioral systems and nursing, Englewood Cliffs. N.J., 1976, Prentice-Hall, Inc.
2. Kraegel, Janet, Mousseau, Virginia, Goldsmith, Charles, and Arora, Rajeev: Patient care systems, Philadelphia, 1974, J.B. Lippincott Co.
3. Sutterley, Doris C., and Donnelly, Gloria F.: Perspectives in human development: nursing throughout the life cycle, Philadelphia, 1973, J.B. Lippincott Co.
4. Crow, Jean: The nursing process. III. A nursing history questionnaire for two patients, Nursing Times **73**(26):978-982, 1977.
5. Shindell, Sidney, Salloway, Jeffrey C., and Oberembt, Colette M.: A course book in health care delivery, New York, 1976, Appleton-Century-Crofts.
6. Sexuality does not mean sexual intercourse.
7. Benson, Evelyn Rose, and McDevitt, Joan Quinn: Community health and nursing practice, ed. 2, Englewood Cliffs, N.J., 1979, Prentice-Hall, Inc.
8. Mayers, Marlene G.: A systematic approach to the nursing care plan, New York, 1972, Appleton-Century-Crofts.

BIBLIOGRAPHY

Aeschleman, D.D.: A strategy for change . . . the nurse practitioner must develop a workable solution, gain acceptance for the solution, acquire negotiation skills and develop a reputation as a successful innovator, Nurse Practitioner **1**:121-124, January-February, 1976.

Auger, Jeanine Roose: Behavioral systems and nursing, Englewood Cliffs, N.J., 1976, Prentice-Hall, Inc.

Backman, H.A., et al.: Camp nursing: an opportunity for independent practice in a miniature community, M.C.N.: The American Journal of Maternal Child Nursing **1**(2):88-92, 1978.

Becknell, Eileen Pearlman, and Smith, Dorothy M.: System of nursing practice: a clinical nursing assessment tool, Philadelphia, 1975, F.A. Davis Co.

Benson, Evelyn Rose, and McDevitt, Joan Quinn: Community health and nursing practice, ed. 2, Englewood Cliffs, N.J., 1979, Prentice-Hall, Inc.

Browning, Mary H.: Nursing process in practice, New York, 1974, American Journal of Nursing Co.

Burton, Genevieve: Personal, impersonal, and interpersonal relations: a guide for nurses, ed. 3, New York, 1970, Springer Publishing Co., Inc.

Carter, Joan, Hilliard, M., et al.: Standard of nursing care: A guide for evaluation, ed. 2, New York, 1976, Springer Publishing Co.

Commission on Chronic Illness: Chronic illness in the U.S., vol. 2., Care of the long term patient, Cambridge, Mass., 1956, Commonwealth Fund/Harvard University Press.

Crow, Jean: The nursing process. III. A nursing history questionnaire for two patients, Nursing Times 73(26):978-982, 1977.

Dressler, Forrest G.: Patient care assessment in extended health care facilities. In Connecticut Health Services research series, no. 1, New Haven, Conn., 1971, Connecticut Health Services.

Eckstein, K.: Initial rapid assessment, Journal of Emergency Nursing 2(3):29-30, 1976.

Epstein, Charlotte: Effective interaction in contemporary nursing, Englewood Cliffs, N.J., 1974, Prentice-Hall, Inc.

Fowkes, William C., Jr., and Hunn, Virginia K.: Clinical assessment for the nurse practitioner, St. Louis, 1973, The C.V. Mosby Co.

Gellus, Su Ann: Patient assessment and management by the nurse practitioner, Philadelphia, 1976, W.B. Saunders Co.

Gordon, M.: Nursing diagnosis and the diagnostic process, American Journal of Nursing 76:1232-1234, 1976.

Gorman, M.L.: Conscious repatterning of human behavior, American Journal of Nursing 75:1752-1754+, 1975.

Harnish, Yvonne: Patient care guides; practical information for public health nurses, League Exchange (111):1-354,1976.

Hayakawa, K.: On nursing plans—impressions on "Technics in Formulating Nursing Plans" by D.E. Little and on "Systematic Approach in Nursing Plans," by M.G. Meyers, Japanese Journal of Nursing 39:1191-1198, 1975.

Heinemann, E., et al.: Assessing alcoholic patients, American Journal of Nursing 76:785-789, 1976.

Hoole, Axalla, J., editor: Patient care guidelines for family nurse practitioners, Boston, 1976, Little, Brown & Co.

Jimenez, E.S.: Theoretical framework of the nursing process, The A.N.P.H.I. Papers 10(2-3):7-14, 1975.

Koehne-Kaplan, N.S., et al.: The process of clinical judgment in nursing practice: the component of personality, Nursing Research 25(4):268-272, 1976.

Kraegel, Janet, Mousseau, Virginia, Goldsmith, Charles, and Arora, Rajeev: Patient care systems, Philadelphia, 1974, J.B. Lippincott Co.

Lidz, C.G.: Changing the methodology of learning, N.L.N. Publication (23-1618):27-31, 1976.

Little, Dolores, E., and Carnevali, Doris L.: Nursing care planning, ed. 2, Philadelphia, 1976, J.B. Lippincott Co.

Luker, K.A.: Adjusting to being a health visitor, Nursing Times 72(39):Suppl. 22, 24, 26, 30, 1976.

Malloy, J.L.: Taking exception to problem-oriented nursing care, American Journal of Nursing 76:582-583, 1976.

Marriner, Ann: The nursing process: a scientific approach to nursing care, ed. 2, St. Louis, 1979, The C.V. Mosby Co.

Mayers, Marlene G.: A systematic approach to the nursing care plan, New York, 1972, Appleton-Century-Crofts.

McCloskey, J.C.: The nursing care plan: past, present, and uncertain future—a review of the literature, Nursing Forum 14(4):364-382, 1975.

O'Brien, Maureen: Communications and relationships in nursing, ed. 2, St. Louis, 1978, The C.V. Mosby Co.

Pareja, C.: Clinical assessment, The A.N.P.H.I. Papers 10(2-3):15-16, 1975.

Pearson, L.B.: Protocols: how to develop and implement within the nurse practitioners setting, Nurse Practitioner 2(1):9-11, September-October, 1976.

Price, F.: Initiation and development of individual patient care plans, Journal of Gerontological Nursing 2(4):24-26, 1976.

Problem-oriented systems of patient care, Department of Home Health Agencies and Community Health Services, Pub. No. A74, New York, 1973-1974 workshop, National League for Nursing.

Records system guide for a community health service, Department of Public Health Nursing, New York, 1970, National League for Nursing.

Rehman, Jean E.: Writing patient care plans: a reference guide for nurses, San Diego, 1976, Professional Lecture Series, Inc.

Rubel, M.: Coming to grips with the nursing process, Supervisor Nurse 7(2):30-32+, 1976.

Scutchfield, F.D.: Alternate methods for health priority assessment, Journal of Community Health 1:29-38, Fall, 1975.

Serafini, P.: Nursing assessment in industry, American Journal of American Public Health 66:755-760, 1976.

Shindell, Sidney, Salloway, Jeffrey C., and Oberembt, Colette M.: A coursebook in health care delivery, New York, 1976, Appleton-Century-Crofts.

Suraria, M.C.: Theoretical framework for goal setting and evaluation, The A.N.P.H.I. Papers 10(2-3):38-41, 1975.

Sutterley, Doris C., and Donnelly, Gloria F.: Perspectives in human development: nursing throughout the life cycle, Philadelphia, 1973, J.B. Lippincott Co.

Taylor, Deane B.: Systematic nursing assessment: a step toward automation, U.S. Department of Health, Education, and Welfare, Public Health Service, Health Resources Administration Bureau of Health Research and Development, Division of Nursing, Washington, D.C., 1976, U.S. Government Printing Office.

Vincent, P.A., et al.: Developing a mental health assessment form, Journal of Nursing Administration 6(4):25-28, May, 1976.

The problem-oriented system in a home health agency—a training manual. Visiting Nurse Association, Inc., Burlington, Vermont, League Exchange 103:1-27, 1975.

Walter, Judith Bloom, editor: Dynamics of problem-oriented approaches: patient care and documentation, Philadelphia, 1976, J.B. Lippincott Co.

Wandelt, M.A., et al.: Quality assurance: models for nursing education tools for measuring quality of nursing care, Pub. no. 15-1611, New York, 1976, National League for Nursing.

Yura, Helen, and Walsh, Mary B., editors: The nursing process: assessing, planning, implementing, and evaluating, Washington, D.C., 1967, The Catholic University of America Press.

14

RECORDS AND THE NURSING AUDIT

PURPOSE OF RECORDS

Nurses grumble and groan about the volume of written material they are required to produce as the result of every nursing interaction. One community nurse remarked that she felt obligated to write a report in triplicate if she said good morning to a client on the street! Things have not yet reached that point, but there is no doubt that the amount of paperwork required is steadily increasing. Many of the reports are necessary and vital; many are useless and a waste of paper; most fall somewhere in between.

Records are here to stay. They are a necessary and important tool in the provision of health care; without reports health professionals would have almost no way of communicating with each other about the care and services provided to and required by clients. This chapter will explore some of the purposes for keeping records, will suggest some criteria for the record-keeping process, and will look at some of the trends and developments in written communication about health care.

Documentation of care rendered

The client's record is a type of accounting system that provides a written statement of exactly what has been done for the client and his family. The kinds of care provided are recorded for several reasons:

1. Other health workers who read the record may base their intervention on what has and has not already been done.

2. The agency must know what charges are to be made to a client or to a third party.
3. Periodic evaluations are not possible unless it is known what kind of intervention has been tried and what the results were.
4. If the client's record should ever be subpoenaed, an accurate account of all care rendered may be vital to the case.
5. The documentation of all care rendered provides additional and continuing information about the client's health status.

Health problems that were thought to be major may turn out not to be, and, unless the community nurse records her actions and observations, she and other members of the professional staff may not be able to recognize changes. An example of this situation is the family of a premature infant. The health problems were originally thought to be centered on the growth and development needs of the new baby, but after several home visits the nurse began to observe some unusual behavior in a 3-year-old sister. The stronger and healthier the premature baby became, the more regressed the 3-year-old became. This process developed rapidly over a period of a few months, but the mother made no comment about the changes in her older daughter. As a result of the continued home visits, a change in the emphasis was instituted, and eventually the nurse was successful in persuading the mother to have the little girl psychologically evaluated. A diagnosis of childhood schizophrenia was made, and the child began treatment.

A nurse caring for a client or a family for the first time will need to know exactly what health care intervention has gone before so she will know how to proceed. Reading the anecdotal comments should give her an idea of what to expect on a first meeting. It should be emphasized, however, that the client's reaction to nursing intervention differs widely depending on which nurse is giving the care. Even if there is no change in personnel, documentation of care rendered is important.

This documentation provides the nurse caring for the family, as well as other health workers, with a picture of how the client and family are reacting to nursing intervention. The method of recording these reactions will be discussed later in the chapter; it is essential to record not only the care given but also the circumstances surrounding the care. If an elderly client is receiving help with his personal hygiene and food preparation three times a week, the nurse (or home health aide) should record not only that she gave him a bath and helped him make a pot of stew, she must also record the other facets of his life: what he does for socialization, the condition of his home, his general appearance and health, and what his mood is. In this way, other people reading the record have a more accurate idea of what is really going on in the client's life.

Staffing patterns can frequently be determined by the kinds of care that are rendered by an agency, and this kind of information can be gathered only if accurate and complete recording has been done. It may be that in a given period of time there has been an increase in a specific kind of nursing intervention which would indicate that a certain kind of health worker should be brought in, as either a full-time employee or as a consultant. It may also be that an agency would want to reevaluate the composition of its professional and nonprofessional staff as the result of the documentation of care.

Written record of nursing history as basis for prescribed therapy

A description of how to take a nursing history and how to formulate a nursing diagnosis has been detailed in Chapter 13, but writing the information in a clear and logical fashion can be a different task. If there is no nursing history, there can be no diagnosis, and if there is no diagnosis, then nursing care planning will be haphazard and fragmented rather than well planned and directed. If there is no written record of the history and diagnosis, the people providing care will have no basis for what they are doing. The written record should flow from the history to the diagnosis to the goals to the implementation to the evaluation and then perhaps back to the implementation. Fig. 14-1 illustrates the direction of flow.

NURSING ORDER

Some community health agencies use the concept of the nursing order, which is a written direction that prescribes certain behaviors by which nursing care objectives are to be achieved. The objectives arise directly from the nursing diagnosis and are designed to help the nurse to achieve the stated goals. Specific behaviors are called for, and a correctly written nursing order gives precise directions. For example, a nursing diagnosis of chronic constipation resulting from decreased physical activity might require any one of a number of nursing orders. The orders based on this diagnosis can be written correctly or incorrectly:

Incorrect	Correct
1. Ensure proper ambulation.	1. Take client on a 15-minute walk every day.
2. Ensure proper diet.	2. Give client raw fruit or vegetable to eat every day.
3. Maintain adequate bowel movements.	3. Give a 2-quart soap-suds enema if client has no bowel movements two days in a row.

The difference in clarity is readily apparent, and there is much less room for error when the orders are written explicitly. The nursing order is particularly effective when nonprofessional nursing personnel (home health aides, LPNs, or physician's assistants) are caring for clients. The nursing order ensures that the judgment needed will come from

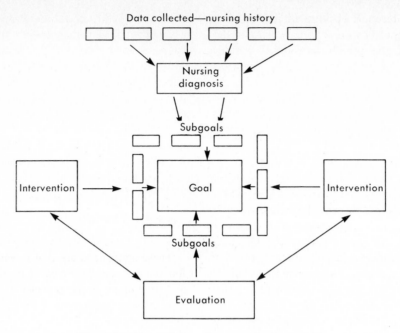

Fig. 14-1. Flow of information on a client's record.

a professional, whereas the intervention itself may be done by a nonprofessional.

Regardless of whether specific orders are written, and it may not be practical in all instances, a written nursing history and nursing diagnosis is essential. Whoever is planning the care needs a base from which to begin, as well as a reference to justify whatever intervention is planned. The evaluators need to know exactly what they are evaluating. Goals cannot be made if reasons are not known. A written record of the nursing history and diagnosis *is* a basis for all prescribed therapy, and there can be no professional functioning without it.

Communication among health professionals

The trend in recent years in community health agencies, as well as in hospitals, is for all health workers to record their observations and interventions on a single client record. This can present logistical problems in a large and diversified com-munity health agency, but it is also an extremely effective way for all members of the team to communicate with each other. The record can eliminate a tremendous amount of duplication of services. If a nurse is planning to discuss a particular problem with her client, she has only to look through progress notes to see whether the social worker or the home health aide has had any conversations on that particular subject and what the outcome was. This can save time and avoid frustration for both the nurse and the client, and it leads to the promotion of better interpersonal relationships among health workers.

The problem-oriented record as well as the SOAP method of writing progress notes will be discussed in detail later in the chapter. For the moment we are concerned with how the act of recording can promote better communication among health professionals. In addition to showing what implementation has already taken place, reading the record can reveal the necessity for a conference between various members of the team or perhaps for the entire team. By paying attention to what other team members write on the record, each individual coming in contact with the client has a better idea of the goals and thought processes of each other individual. In addition to encouraging conferences and other forms of spoken communication among health workers, the interdisciplinary record can ensure that plans and goals are not formulated at cross-purposes with each other. In other words, the goals of the social worker should not defeat the plans of the nurse, and the physician's assistant should not engage in any intervention that will interfere with what the home health aide is doing. The object of the interdisciplinary record is to aid in providing professional health care as efficiently and productively as possible. The more communication there is between health workers, the more likely the client is to benefit.

Material for research

The community health agency's family record is an excellent source of material for research. Included in the record are most of the demographic data that researchers need: age, race, sex, type of living environment, income, occupation, education, and many of the other variables that affect both people's health and the research studies that are conducted about their health. Also on the record is much information about the nature and progress of the health problems themselves. A study of the records, in addition to providing familiarity with clients, can give the observant nurse much information about areas of health that might warrant a full-scale research study. This research can be epidemiological or medical in nature, but it can also be research on nursing needs of clients. Every community health agency will provide dozens of interesting research topics, such as the following:

1. The determination of why children do not receive recommended immunizations, despite encouragement by physicians and nurses.

2. What kinds of motivations are involved in families following up on prescribed or recommended treatment or other therapy in the instance of chronic health problems? For example, what causes one family to provide physical therapy on a regular basis for an adult with multiple sclerosis and another family to fail to provide the therapy?

3. A study of the outcomes of families with children who have been accidentally poisoned in the home by medicine, a household cleaning product, or some other substance around the house. This study could include conditions in the home, parental attitudes, and the effect of health teaching.

4. The kinds of home care referrals made by acute care facilities: what the health problem was, what intervention was required, and whether the intervention was useful and successful. This kind of study would be beneficial to the hospital as well as to the community health agency.

These are general areas of research that can be found in any part of the country in urban, suburban, and rural areas. Some agencies have a large percentage of one segment of the population, for example, Orientals, factory workers who are exposed to certain pollutants, or the elderly living in high-rise retirement communities. The health record can provide essential background data for more specific research studies. When the nursing audit, which will be discussed in detail later in the chapter, is done, a properly recorded nursing history and diagnosis and informative progress notes can point out areas of health care that require further study. The auditor frequently can suggest areas for research.

STATISTICS

The record also provides statistical information for official counts of one kind or another. It is important to know how many of various kinds of clients are seen, how many cases of certain kinds of health problems were referred to an agency, what the incidence of a certain type of health problem is in a specific population group, and various other health problem statistics. The statistics are used for a variety of purposes, such as planning future health services, evaluating staffing patterns, determining what charges should be made for what services, budget planning, and requesting consultative help. There is no doubt that statistics can be misused with as much imagination and creativity as they are used, but they are vital to the overall running of any community health agency.

In most cases, statistical data are more useful if they contain an element of *comparison*. For example, the number of home visits made on behalf of school children during one year has much more meaning if it is shown in comparison with visits made during the previous year or with the number that would have been made if need were the only criterion for making the visit.[1,p.298]

Comparisons might also be made between visits to the child only and visits to the entire family as well. One might compare visits between public schoolchildren and those who attend private and parochial schools. The ages of children with similar health problems might be compared, as might several family variables such as economic status, whether both parents are working, number of siblings, and the kind of living environment.

Kinds of records
SERVICE RECORD

The service record is the health record on which the history, diagnosis, progress notes, and all information pertinent to the health care of the family are written. It is the record that traditionally has been called ''the chart'' and the one which is used most frequently by nurses, physicians, and other health workers.

ACCOUNTING RECORD

Included in the accounting record are such data as the number of times a client or family is seen, the number of home visits made, the amount and kind of supplies used, the amount of service time spent with the family, and the person who actually saw the client. The information is usually tabulated on a weekly basis and is also used for planning, staffing, and budgeting. It is the way in which the agency administration keeps track of who is doing what, how much time is spent on various activities, and how much each health care activity costs the agency in terms of both money and personnel time.

The accounting record is also a means by which to record expenses for supplies and equipment, agency automobile maintenance, and mileage for personal travel.

CONTROL RECORD

A control record determines whether agency commitments are being met. There is usually some type of central index system which separates the various records into categories, such as requests for service, active families for whom health care is currently being provided, and inactive families, that may be further subdivided into files which were closed within a given period of time (usually a year) or before that. The system may also be indexed in another set of ways: geographically, by specific health problem, or by the nurse who is responsible for the care. It does not really matter *how* the control system is organized as long as one exists and everyone in the agency understands its operation and cooperates in contributing to its maintenance. Usually a clerical worker maintains the file, but it is up to the professional health workers to ensure the accuracy of the data in the file. Without an effective case control system, the functioning of the agency would shortly become chaotic.

ANNUAL REPORT

The annual report communicates to the administration and other employees and interested people exactly what the agency has done during the past year, the significance of its activities, and what it plans to do in the future. The budget is included in the report, as are the reasons for the success or failure of last year's plans. Major health and population trends of the agency's service area are usually included, as well as any special or outstanding accomplishments of the past year. The annual report usually contains qualitative as well as quantitative information: how well the agency has met the health needs of the community as well as the number of clients seen or home visits made. The annual report is also a public relations tool; it can be an effective means of requesting funds from charitable organizations such as the United Fund. It is also a way to communicate the purpose and functions of the agency to others, including other agencies and the public.

PLANNING RECORD

A planning record is a composite of several of the other records and is used for both long- and short-term planning. It can be seen as an elaboration or continuation of the accounting record and usually includes a statement of the community health needs and problems as seen by the health workers, a list of objectives for a specified period of time, an interim report on the status of the objectives, the procedures being used to meet the objectives, and various evaluation tools. The planning record is usually quite detailed and is the basis for supervisory and administrative conferences at which decisions will be made about the operation of the agency.

An annual or quarterly review and plan for each service district, or program, may be required, in which the responsible individual indicates what has been done, what is in process, and what the plans are for the coming year. This differs from the annual report in that it places greater emphasis on the coming period as it relates to what has gone before.[2,p.253]

POLICY AND PROCEDURE MANUAL

Another written record, although different in function from what has already been discussed, is important to the community health nurse: the policy and procedure manual. This is a tool that can save time, prevent errors, and serve as a guide to the professional nurse and to several other members of the community health team. The manual should contain the official policies of the agency that pertain to the functioning of all members of the agency. It should include an organizational chart with lines of authority, as well as the job description for each classification of employee. If the agency requires that certain procedures, whether they are physical tasks, written reports, or other procedural matters, be done in a specified way, it should be

clearly defined in the procedure manual. The manual should also include reference sources and policies of other health agencies that might be useful or necessary for effective functioning. The policy and procedure manual is a reference guide and should become an integral part of every health worker's activities. In many agencies it is referred to as ''the bible,'' a somewhat irreverent expression but one that expresses the importance of the manual well.

Educational tool for students

Every nurse remembers what she did as a student when first assigned to a new client: she ran for the record and read every word before even saying hello to the client. At times students seem to be taking refuge in the record, and sometimes the instructor must pry them away from their reading and force them to come face-to-face with the client. But the client or family record *is* a valuable source of information for the medical and nursing student. The student can learn what comprises a history, how to state a diagnosis, and what does and does not belong in a progress note. She can familiarize herself with the legality of the recording process, and it is an excellent opportunity for her to organize her own thinking about the client's needs. She can decide what nursing interventions will best meet these needs. Sometimes the learning is negative; that is, the student learns what *not* to write or how *not* to state a particular piece of information. The hindrance of a poorly written record becomes glaringly obvious to the student, and these kinds of negative lessons are often long remembered.

The record can provide the student with pertinent data about the client and his family that she might need before meeting them. She might want to learn more about a specific health problem or read a bit about a religion with which she is not familiar. She may want to make an informal and loosely structured plan of action prior to meeting the family, or she may find gaps in the already recorded data that she thinks it would be necessary to have. After meeting with the client, it is always important to compare one's observations with those previously recorded and perhaps even to discuss major differences with the instructor or the person who did the recording. The opposite side of the coin, however, is that reading the record prior to visiting the client or family can create negative biases or judgments on the part of the student. The best way to minimize or prevent this is by means of effective preclinical conferences with the instructor and student peer group.

The student can also familiarize herself with medical terminology, abbreviations, and jargon, although a well-written record uses a minimum amount of jargon. It is usually desirable to have a medical dictionary at one's elbow while reading a record.

The record as a baseline and evaluation tool

Every agency has a number of clients and families who are on active status for long periods of time, sometimes for many years. Their records become thicker and thicker with little pieces of paper inserted here and there. The number of health workers contributing to the record grows until the whole thing becomes an unreadable jungle of paperwork. People hesitate to read it for the same reasons they hesitate to begin *War and Peace:* it looms as an impossible task.

For this reason the record should function as a periodic evaluation tool in which baseline data can be recorded and changed as necessary and in which interdisciplinary evaluations can be made on a periodic basis. These summaries should cover a specific time period. In this way someone reading the chart for the first time can have an overview of the family situation; she can see what has changed and what has remained the same over the months or years, how the goals and objectives have changed, and what the result of the health care intervention has been. She can read the entire record when she has the time. The necessity for writing a periodic evaluation will force the health workers to look at what they are doing and determine what the effectiveness of their intervention has been. The sum-

mary promotes communication among team members and improved health care. Form A (p. 365) illustrates how major events and problems in a family's life are highlighted briefly, and the reader is referred to other sections of the record for details of what was emphasized in the summary. The summary is essential for any record that is to be kept active for more than a few months.

CRITERIA FOR RECORD KEEPING

The purposes just discussed for keeping a record will be accomplished only if everyone contributing to it follows certain procedures and meets the criteria for accurate and readable records.

The degree to which the information is effective—the degree to which it accomplishes the purposes just described—is determined by 1) accuracy, 2) timeliness, 3) completeness, and 4) relevancy to the problem. The patient and his environment are the source of information, and the chart format is where the information is collected and integrated into usable form. Placing the chart format as close to the patient as possible will allow the above criteria to be met effectively. When an observation of a patient can be put directly in the chart without time, distance, written transcription, or verbal transfer intercepting, patient information will be available to all members of the health team the moment it is collected, and will be as free from loss, distortion, or error as is humanly possible.[3,p.25]

This statement, although it was written about hospital charts, is particularly valid for the community health nurse, as shown in the following example. The nurse sets out on a day of home visits and sees six or seven client families by 4 P.M. If she waits until she returns to the office at the end of the day to do her recording, she will have forgotten many of the important things that transpired in the clients' homes. If, however, she records right in the home or perhaps sitting in the car immediately after she has left, what she writes will be much more accurate. She will remember what the client has said and the tone with which he said it, and she will still have a vivid picture of the "flavor" of the visit; the client's mood and feelings will be fresh in her mind. This is the kind of observation that

Family name ____Jackson____   Family members __Andrew (father)__
                                                       __Tonia (mother)__
Address ____811 N. 10 St. – Central City 00031____   __Lucy Thomas (Tonia's mother)__
                                                       __Lester (age 4)__
        ____42 Elbow Lane – Maplewood 00100____   __Jennifer (age 2)__
                                                       __Michelle (10/4/80)__

Phone ____555-6248____   Physician/clinic __Robert Lock__

      ____555-1117____   Date first seen __8/14/80__   School __Central__

Referred by ____Dr. Lock____

Original health problems ① Tonia — toxemia of pregnancy – 7½ months;

② Andrew — unemployed aerospace technician; ③ Lucy Thomas —

growing senile; ? placement in nursing home

Major family events	Periodic status evaluation and problem resolution
10/4/80 – baby girl born – Michelle – healthy	1/8/81 ① Toxemia controlled by medication until birth of Michelle; ② Andrew still unemployed; actively seeking work but becoming depressed and drinking heavily; ③ Mrs. Thomas – no action; family decided to postpone decision.
5/1/81 – applied for welfare and were accepted	
8/18/81 – Andrew employed as technical manager of civil engineering firm – salary $25,000	6/10/81 ② Andrew still unemployed; cannot find work in aerospace and refuses to look elsewhere; referred to University depression clinic; ③ Mrs. Thomas – no action.
9/4/81 – Lester started school	12/11/81 ② Andrew employed and not depressed but is continuing private psychotherapy; ③ family is looking at nursing homes but without much enthusiasm; ④ Lester has a temper tantrum qd before going to school (see consult c̄ school nurse in record); still goes to school but tantrums increasing (see referral to Maplewood Child Guidance Clinic)
10/16/81 – moved to house in suburbs	
3/27/82 – Andrew vasectomy	

Form A. Periodic evaluation sheet and problem summary.

is so important to record, but in a few hours the ability to transform this elusive flavor into words can be lost.

General criteria

Some general criteria for the record system itself should be discussed before detailing criteria for the actual writing of the record. The system should be designed so that it is *easy* to use. The uniformity of the order of the various parts of the record is essential; each client's record should be identical in form to every other record in the agency. There should be sufficient space for recording all the pertinent data, and each piece of information should be recorded a minimum number of times on each record. For instance, the client's medical and nursing diagnosis should be written *once*. There is no need to repeat it on the progress notes, in the physician's or nurse's orders, or in any place other than that specifically designed for it.

The storage and retrieval system should be designed for ease, accessibility, and the saving of time. The records should be kept in a specified place, and their whereabouts should always be known. The ideal way to record most of the progress data is for the health workers to dictate their reports into portable tape recorders and hand them in to a clerical worker to by typed onto the record. The cost of the tape recorders and the clerk's salary more than pays for itself in terms of professional time saved. Many community health nurses say that they could make one or two more home visits in the time it takes to write down the day's activities. The major disadvantage of dictation is that it tends to encourage excessively long progress notes. Health workers can, however, consciously guard against this tendency and practice conciseness. If progress notes are dictated, there is no reason why the entire record should ever be removed from the central storage area for a long period of time. Thus all health workers will have constant access to the records, and the chance of them becoming lost or falling apart will be minimized. The confidentiality of the records must be assured. The larger the

agency and the more health workers with access to the records, the easier it is to lose this confidentiality. Besides the professional ethics of the health workers and having a system of knowing who has a record at any given time, it is difficult to counteract or prevent the unauthorized discussion of the contents of client records. Therefore the agency should have specific policies and rules about record maintenance and handling of conferences about clients.

Focus on the recipient of care

The focus of every written statement on the record should be on the client and his health problem. This may seem like an obvious or superfluous statement, but in reviewing nursing comments and notes, there is frequently emphasis on agency policy, a physical procedure (with no mention of the client's reaction to it), or a note that was obviously written for the convenience of the nurse. In the next section of this chapter there will be a detailed discussion of how to state health problems and how the statements refer to the progress notes. The nurse's subjective feelings about the client's behavior or his statements have no place on the record. Judgments about a client's behavior are also not to be written. For example, if a client is beating his wife, the problem and suggestions for its resolution should be stated as behavior that is detrimental to both people, not in terms of moral judgments. Words like "sick," "bad," "wrong," and "evil" have no place in the evaluation of the husband's problem. These words describe how the *nurse* feels about the behavior, not how the client feels. It is the *client* who is being cared for, and it is the *client* who should be written about. All notations should be written in terms of the client's behaviors and actions. Several examples of this appear on p. 369.

Writing: comprehensive, concise, and explicit

"Clutter is the disease of American writing. We are a society strangling in unnecessary words, circular construction, pompous frills and meaningless jargon.''[4,p.6] Zinsser made this statement in his book, *On Writing Well,* and gave a short example of "governmentese" about a blackout order of 1942.

Such preparations shall be made as will completely obsure all Federal buildings and nonFederal buildings occupied by the Federal government during an air raid for any period of time from visibility by reason of internal or external illumination.[4,p.7]

Such pomposity makes us laugh, but when we look at the kinds of things we write in clients' records, that laughter should choke us. Zinsser has a few cardinal rules about writing well, and they are all applicable to professional recording:

1. Simplify. Say what has to be said in the fewest possible words. The expression "at this point in time" is ludicrous when the temporal concept could be expressed by the single word "now".

2. Fight clutter by thinking about every adjective and descriptive phrase. Does it add to the clarity of the thought, or does it merely obscure the sense of what one is trying to say? Double-talk and jargon have no place in the client's record. Do not say "Ms. M.'s epidermis lacked its customary erythematous appearance, and the nurse observed an uncharacteristic pallor today," when "Ms. M. looked pale" is what the nurse observed and should record.

3. Consider the audience. The record is being read by other health workers who need facts and observations. Their time is valuable, and it is unfair to make them wade through dozens of flowery and superfluous descriptive phases to get to the meat of the problem. The more words that are used, the greater the chance of misinterpretation, which can be more than simply annoying in a health record; it can be dangerous.

4. Use words correctly. Accuracy in written communication is always important; it is essential in health records. Do not use a word unless you are certain of its precise meaning and unless it is the best word to describe what you wish to communicate.

5. Use correct grammar, syntax, and spelling. True, one is not writing an English composition, but the rules of grammar were designed to facilitate the ease and accuracy of written communication. To follow these rules is to make what is written more readable. Misspelled words and grammatical errors are unprofessional.

STYLE

The style of writing on a record is different from almost everything else the health worker writes: personal correspondence, professional articles, or business letters. It is more concise and compact and frequently employs phrases instead of complete sentences. Because the style is more terse does not mean that it is less informative than other writing styles. One of the cardinal rules for record writing is to *be informative*. The ability to *describe* what happened is essential. Incidences, observations, and verbal statements all must be described accurately. Following are some common examples of incorrect ways to describe things, as well as the way in which they could be corrected.

Incorrect	Correct
1. SSE with good results.	1. SSE with client on left side. 10 minutes later client had BM of approximately 4 cups dark brown solid stool.
2. Heavy postpartum bleeding. Doctor notified.	2. Client saturated 2 peripads in half hour. Fundus firm. Client instructed to remain in bed. Dr. Ben Gazi notified by phone. Said he would arrive within an hour.
3. Client depressed and suicidal.	3. Client sat in chair during entire visit, wringing hands and sighing heavily. When asked what she was feeling, replied with several statements. "I can't take it much longer." "I don't want to live any more." "Life is too much for me." Aside from these remarks,

Incorrect	Correct
3. Client depressed and suicidal—cont'd	3. (cont'd) client said almost nothing and appeared uninterested in her surroundings.

Descriptive data can come from a variety of sources: the nurse's own observations, statements made by or behavior exhibited by the client and his family, reports and observations from other members of the health team, and data from objective sources such as a physical examination or laboratory tests. All the data might not agree, and this is why professional interpretation and judgment are so important. This is also why it is essential to record exactly what the *client* said and did and not the health worker's analysis of what was said and done. The circumstances surrounding a statement of grave importance should also be described. The remark, "I wish I were dead," can be made for a variety of reasons. A woman who is acutely depressed after an unwanted divorce gives the statement one meaning, while a man who has just spilled a bowl of soup in the lap of his dinner partner means something entirely different.

The question of *when* to write something on the record has never been entirely resolved. Some community health agencies have specific rules about when and what to record, but these regulations usually cannot be applied in all instances. A good rule of thumb about when to record something is if the occurrence has a direct bearing on the outcome of the health problem or if the occurrence is such that other people should know about it. A man saying to the nurse that he had gotten drunk at a party the night before would be extremely important to note if the man's health problem was alcoholism, but if he merely mentioned it in passing and it has little bearing on his life or health, there would be no reason to record it. However, this kind of statement, made on several different occasions, might indicate an incipient health problem.

Goals and objectives of care should be clearly defined

All nursing intervention is based on a plan of care, and this plan is based on goals and objectives that derive from the nursing history and diagnosis. Without clearly stated goals and objectives, the nurse who cares for the client will not know what is required of her, and she will waste time going back over previous progress notes, often written over a period of months by several different nurses, to see what the health problems are and what has already been done about them. If the goals are stated in a specified place on the record, she will know how to proceed. This does not mean that there can never be any change in the goals; on the contrary, this is what periodic evaluations are for. But as long as a certain goal or objective has not been changed or already accomplished, it should be stated on the record. Not only will this save the nurse's time, the client's time will be saved and his health problems solved sooner.

Reactions and responses to care given

It is not sufficient to record only what was done for or said to the client; the client's responses and reactions must also be noted. If this is not done, anyone reading the record would see only half a picture, and they would have the frustration of "waiting for the other shoe to drop."

Every nursing intervention will elicit some kind of reaction or response from the client, although it may not always be verbalized, apparent, or immediate. Just because there is no overt behavior change on the part of the client does not mean that the intervention has had no effect. Many people need time to think about or assimilate what has been said to or done for them. We have all had the experience, in both our personal and professional lives, of having someone say, "I've been thinking about what you said to me a while ago, and I've come to the conclusion that. . . ."

This does not mean that all reactions are delayed. Some are immediate and quite obvious and should be recorded. In all instances, the client's words and behavior should be described, not the nurses' interpretation of the behavior. Following are examples:

Incorrect	Correct
1. Client was surprised and angry at being removed from the welfare rolls.	1. Client stated, "How dare they do this to me; I deserve to have welfare, and if I have to tear the building down brick by brick, I'm gonna get what's due me."
2. Untoward reaction to penicillin.	2. Penicillin V 600,000 units IM given at 2:45 P.M. At 3 P.M. client had large red hives on all body surfaces. 10 minutes later developed severe dyspnea and SOB.
3. Does not seem interested in new baby.	3. During the hour I spent in the home, Ms. B. did not look at Maria (age 1 week) or touch her. Maria was in a bassinet in the same room. Ms. B. would not initiate a conversation about Maria, and when I mentioned her name, Ms. B. looked away from me or changed the subject at the earliest possible time. There was no one else home at the time.
4. Harold (age 7) is a hyperactive child and is driving his mother to drink.	4. Harold (age 7) demonstrates his extreme energy by racing around the house, yelling at the top of his voice, and throwing his possessions across the room. Ms. A. made several unsuccessful attempts to quiet him, but Harold ignored her. Ms. A. sighed heavily and said, "The only way I can tolerate Harold is with a glass of whiskey in my hand."

The interpretation of the client's response should be discussed with other members of the health team. There may be a new or changed health problem, but the interpretation does not belong in a descriptive note *unless* it is clearly stated as such. In example three it would be easy to jump to the conclusion that Maria is an unwanted child, and Ms. B. is a potentially neglectful parent. This may or may not be true and certainly warrants further investigation, but this kind of value judgment does not belong in a progress note. In example four Ms. A. may be an actual or potential alcoholic, and Harold may be a hyperactive child. On the other hand, both behaviors may be temporary or result from some household crisis. Again, interpretation and judgment should be withheld until further and more conclusive data can be obtained.

PROCESS RECORDING

The process recording is a tool to sharpen the interviewing skills of the nurse (or any other health worker) by examining the responses and reactions of the client to what the nurse says and does. It is a verbatim recording of all verbal and nonverbal communication that took place between the nurse, client, and other people who were present. The process recording begins with an introductory statement about the history and health problems of the family, then procedes with the dialogue and nonverbal communication (it is written in drama form), with a concluding statement and analysis of the interaction. There are short examples of process recording in Chapter 13. It must be done during or *immediately* after the interaction and is extremely time consuming if done accurately. Obviously it is not a tool that the community nurse will use as a routine part of her professional activities, but it can be useful in instances in which she is having difficulty communicating with a client or if she is unable to meet her objectives and cannot figure out why. A well-done process recording is effective in pointing out errors in communication skills or areas of intervention that have been inadvertently neglected. It is a perfect tool to help students develop their interviewing techniques and to make them more aware of the ways in which people react and respond to them. It takes practice to do an effective process recording that will be useful as a self-teaching device.

Periodic summaries on long-term families

The purpose of the periodic summary was discussed in the previous section, and one example of how it can be done was given. In addition to a list of major family events and the status of health problems, the periodic summary should include what nursing intervention was done, how successful it was, and how much effect it had on the health problem. These summaries should be done at specific intervals, depending on the severity and complexity of the health problems, how often the client is seen, and how many other members of the health team are involved in the care. All the general criteria for recording and reporting should be applied to the summary.

SOAP

SOAP is an acronym to describe a format for progress notes, written by any health worker who ordinarily contributes to the client's record. The letters of the acronym spell out the kinds of data relevant to the progress note:

*S*ubjective data
*O*bjective data
*A*ssessment
*P*lan

Each SOAP note refers to a specific problem and is labeled as such. Subjective data are those obtained from the client. Objective data are those observed by the nurse or other health worker, as well as the data gathered from other objective sources such as laboratory or x-ray studies. The assessment is the interpretation of the subjective and objective data, or it can be a diagnosis. The plan is the kind of intervention that will take place to attempt to alleviate or solve the problem. Form B (p. 371) illustrates some examples of progress notes using the SOAP format.

The notes are simple, informative, clear, and precise. Occasionally one would want to record greater detail on a progress note, but the nurse should ask herself exactly what it is that further verbiage will contribute to anyone else's understanding of the problem or the planned intervention. Only if greater detail provides more information or clarity should it be included. If it merely provides embellishment on what has already been said, it should not be included. The purpose of using the SOAP format is to save time and paper and to ensure that what is written on the record will be purposeful, informative, and directly relevant to the care of the client. If the SOAP format is used as it should be, one would not see a hospital night nurse writing "Slept well" on everyone's chart at 6 A.M. when in fact half the clients may have been tossing and turning or pacing the halls all night. So too one would not see a nurse at a well-baby clinic writing "Discussed proper nutrition" on the record of every infant. Also obsolete is the community health nurse's note, "Gave reassurance and assistance with A.M. care," on the records of clients she visited at home. None of these common comments provides any real information about the client, and there is no effort to address the health problem itself.

The SOAP format forces us to think about what we are writing, which will force us to think about what we are doing.

PROBLEM-ORIENTED RECORDS

The problem-oriented record (POR) was first described by Weed in 1970 and is based on the problem-solving process. The basis for the system is clear and precise identification of health problems. A health problem can be defined as any condition or situation with which the client needs help.

The purpose of the POR is to construct a detailed model of health care problem solving and recording that, once implemented, will be improved on and expanded by all health care personnel, a model that is a behavioral analysis system engineered to become a health care audit.[5,p.3]

Date	Problem

8/12/82   #1   Toxemia of pregnancy (Tonia)

S - Complains of headache, extreme fatigue, and o "bloated feeling."

O - BP 180/100; albuminuria 2+; fingers and facial features very puffy; wedding ring too tight; ankles 2x usual size.

A - Moderate pre-eclampsia; severe anxiety.

P - Complete bed rest at home for 1 week; if no improvement then hospitalization; teach husband to take BP; low Na diet; home visit qd.

#2   Andrew unemployed and drinking heavily

S - States "There's no one who wants me," "My talents are wasted"; collecting unemployment; has 3-4 job interviews per week.

O - Wife says he comes home from interviews drunk frequently; drinks a 6 pack of beer qd; talks much less than usual; frequently stares off into space for long periods.

A - Depression as a result of unemployment.

P - Refer to University depression clinic; suggest he read employment opportunities in Sunday New York Times.

#3   Lucy's reddened areas on buttocks

S - States she has decreased sensation in buttocks.

O - Reddened area approximately the size of 50¢ piece just above buttocks cleavage.

A - Development of pressure sore.

P - Teach daughter how to give back rub and how to keep client off the area; visit q week; request water bed from Medicare.

D. Jonathan, RN

Form B. SOAP format in progress notes.

The goals of the POR system are consumer oriented and employ a system of accountability to the health care consumer as well as a system of reinforcement of health care personnel as they are needed by the consumer. The POR consists of four components: the data base, the problem list, the initial plan or orders, and the progress notes.

Data base

The data base is simply a total (which can always be added to) of information about the client. This includes socioeconomic, educational, and psychological as well as physical data. It comes from a variety of sources: the client and his family, the observations of health workers, and laboratory and x-ray reports. Special forms are designed for the collection of data; "the data base should be so constructed that the guidelines built into the system demonstrate explicitly what is to be included and what is to be omitted."[5,p.5] A different problem list can arise if each health worker is permitted to create his own standards and objectives about what information is to be included in the data base. The problem list should arise directly from the data base. A nursing history is also part of the data base.

Problem list

The problem list should serve as an index for the rest of the client's record and consequently should be placed at the beginning of that record. The problem list is simply that: a list. It does not include any editorial comment for the solving of the problem. The problems are simply numbered and dated and then placed on inactive or resolved status when appropriate. As long as the client's record is open, new problems are added to the list as they arise. In community health agencies in which a family health record is kept, it is a good idea to have a separate problem list for each member of the family. This avoids confusion and keeps the record easy to read. Form C (p. 373) illustrates one way to organize a problem list.

Psychological problems should be defined in terms of behavior such as "Will not speak with any other members of the family" or "Laughs and cries at inappropriate times," and they should not be stated as diagnostic guesses. It is better to simply define a behavior than to run the risk of misdiagnosing it. To ensure accuracy, problems should be updated frequently to keep track of the client's progress. For example, for a 2-month-old baby who has the problems of listlessness, lethargy, and decreased appetite, there should be, within a very short time, either a notion on the problem list that the problems have been solved or a definite medical diagnosis. Otherwise a health worker reading the record will be at a loss to know what is being done for that infant.

Initial plan

The initial plan should be stated in terms of diagnostic considerations, therapeutic plans, and client education. This is a summary or statement of intention of what the health worker plans to do about a given health problem. Following are some examples of the statement of initial plans:

Problem: Pain in left wrist.
Diagnosis: R/O arthritis or other inflammatory process (x ray); R/O trauma (x-ray).
Therapy: Hold until films are read.
Education: Nature and progress of arthritis explained to client; explained why x-ray film was taken; will show x-ray film to client and discuss findings.

Problem: John (age 13) quit school.
Diagnosis: Evaluate relationships with other members of family; find out from John why he quit school; investigate school record from teacher, school nurse, principal, etc.
Therapy: Convince John to return to school (methods used will be determined by diagnostic data).
Education: See therapy; explain the consequences of a lack of education; use negative examples from among people in the community.

Problem: Diabetic living at home with blind husband.
Diagnosis: Home visit to evaluate what client can do for herself and in what areas she needs help.
Therapy: Provide home visits prn until client can be self-sufficient.
Education: Routine diabetic teaching.[6]

Progress notes

The progress notes should be written in the SOAP format, which has already been described. All the health workers who care for a client should contribute to the progress notes to assure integration of care and to avoid duplication of information and service.

Disciplines other than the medical profession contribute at their own level of understanding and should not attempt to state assessments that are not substantiated by evidence. In fact, the documentation of evidence that leads you to your decision clearly spells out for all concerned the reason why you said what you did.[5,p.12]

Name of hospital _____

Name of client _____

ADDRESSOGRAPH STAMP

Problem list

Date of onset	Active problems	Date resolved	Inactive or resolved problems

Form C. Example of a problem list. (Modified from Berni, Rosemarian, and Readey, Helen: Problem-oriented medical record implementation: allied health peer review, ed. 2, St. Louis, 1978, The C.V. Mosby Co.)

Flow sheet

A flow sheet can sometimes be used as a substitute for some (but not all) progress notes. It is usually employed for a problem which is being frequently monitored or for health problems that are similar for many clients.

The flow sheet serves as an excellent guide to ascertaining the source of a pathological process or to revealing relationships among many variables. When isolated parameters must be observed frequently, the flow sheet may be the only progress note necessary. The flow sheet often serves to eliminate a multitude of narrative notes and indicates the patient's progress at a glance.[5,p.15]

One of the most familiar kinds of flow sheets is the one used by obstetrical departments of many hospitals. The condition of the client, including that of her fundus, lochia, episiotomy, and breasts is recorded by a series of check marks on a form designed for that purpose. This way the nurse does not have to waste time writing the same information every 2 to 4 hours. Form D (p. 375) illustrates a flow sheet used by the community health nurse for a frequently seen health problem: the assessment of a home into which a premature infant will be arriving. Specific and definite kinds of information are needed, but a great deal of narrative is not required for this kind of assessment. If a health problem needs to be solved, the SOAP format can be used.

There are several definite advantages to using the POR system in a community health setting. It encourages a multidisciplinary approach to the solving of the client's problems and establishes mutual goals and plans of action. The care for certain types of problems will be standardized with a resultant increase in the quality of care, but there is enough flexibility incorporated into the format so that individualized care is not lost to standardization.

The POR emphasizes the client and not the health care personnel. This is done by relating everything written to the problem list, which focuses attention on the client. The system requires that all action planned and taken be written on the record. This protects the client, gives the people reviewing the record a chance to compare what was done with a previously established standard, and facilitates communication. The POR saves time and space; needless verbiage is not permitted, and everyone is saved from having to read such inane remarks as "Having a good day" or "Condition improved." Periodic summaries, which are an integral part of the system, also lead to ease of readability. Continuity of care is more likely to occur as a result of the existence of the problem list and because of the multidisciplinary approach to the record. Flow sheets greatly enhance the continuity of care because of their "at-a-glance" readability and the ease with which progress can be assessed. Flow sheets can be designed to accommodate any health problem or group of variables. The POR is

an educational tool for everyone using the record because it encourages—insists on—excellent recording techniques.

The POR lends itself to research pursuits because patient problems are organized into a meaningful whole, and feedback regarding the management of each problem is evident in chronological sequence in the progress notes. Striking similarities between problem lists of various patients become readily evident, enabling us to deal more intelligently with the problems in terms of available resources and the way that these problems respond to prescribed procedures.[5,p.20]

A nurse or a physician who has been absent from the care of a client for a period of time will be able to look at the POR and become fully acclimated and caught up in a matter of minutes. The health professional will also be able to evaluate what his colleagues are doing, and he can be the recipient of valuable suggestions because everyone reads what everyone else has written on the record.

Students using the POR have a positive role model for learning how to record. The POR emphasizes creative planning in solving clients' problems rather than relying on a memorized approach or falling back on the old "we've-always-done-it-this-way" kind of behavior. It encourages thinking and individual planning rather than resorting to conformity, and it reinforces the process of questioning and inquiry. The POR system lends itself readily to the audit process, as well as giving the agency a much more efficient record retrieval system. Since everything is documented in writing, any possible litigation will be simplified. Documentation for insurance companies, Medicare, and Medicaid will also be more readily available. Costs of health care should decrease because all diagnostic tests and treatment modalities would have to be justified on the basis of a particular health problem, and unnecessary or wasteful procedures could be at least partially eliminated.

NURSING AUDIT

The purpose of a nursing audit is to assess the quality of care by the analysis of records over a

Mother's name _____ Address _____

Baby's name _____ EDC _____ Birth date _____ Weight _____

Hospital _____ Date of expected discharge _____

Initial evaluative home visit   Date _____

Physical condition of mother	Comments
Satisfactory ____	
Unsatisfactory ____	
Preparation for baby	Comments
Physical space	
Own room ____	
Share with sibling ____	
No space provided ____	
Furniture for baby	
Satisfactory ____	
Unsatisfactory ____	
Clothes for baby	
Sufficient ____	
Insufficient ____	
Ability of mother to care for baby	Comments
Excellent knowledge ____	
Needs some teaching ____	
Needs concentrated teaching ____	

Subsequent home visits

Date _____ Progress _____

_____

Date _____ Progress _____

_____

Date _____ Progress _____

_____

Date _____ Progress _____

_____

Form D. Example of a flow sheet for the evaluation of a premature infant's home.

given period of time. The objectives of the concept of the nursing audit are to provide a measure or standard against which actual performance can be compared and to do this on a continuing basis so that there is always feedback to provide a basis for corrective action. The audit is also used to establish staffing patterns based on needs shown by the audit.

Statistical quality control should be used in the nursing audit. The principles are based on the probability that if a large enough random sample is taken from all the agency's records, a pattern of care will emerge that will apply to all the records as well as to the sample chosen. Following are three rules to be observed in doing a statistical quality control:

1. The sample must be selected at random.
2. A sufficient number of records must be used for the sample.
3. A decision regarding the attribute being observed must truly represent the immediate condition.

Any and all aspects of care provided may be audited, but the audit will be useless unless goals and guidelines are clearly established before the audit is begun. What is the purpose of the audit? What criteria are to be measured? What is the standard against which they will be measured? How many records constitute a large enough sample? What will be asked on the questionnaire? Unless these questions are answered, the audit will have no coherent form and will not accomplish a purpose. One can measure and evaluate almost anything, but the appropriate instrument must be devised. If one wishes to find out whether the health needs of postcardiac clients are being met, one must first decide what the needs are and then find a way, by looking at the record, to determine whether they are being met.

The audit is designed to measure the quality of care as it is reflected by what is written on the record. It cannot measure care given, or the quality of that care, unless it was accurately and precisely recorded. The audit can point out deficiencies in the care, and it can assess the effectiveness of action taken to correct these deficiencies. As an ex-

ample, an agency wishes to determine whether accurate and workable nursing diagnoses are being formulated for new clients. Listed here is a guideline for the procedures to be followed:

1. Determine the parameters of the audit and define the terms. If the focal point of the audit is nursing diagnosis, it is essential that everyone working on the audit use the same agreed-on definition of a nursing diagnosis.
2. Decide what will be considered a diagnosis and what will not. If there is a question or a borderline case, one person should be designated as the official arbitrator.
3. Choose a number that will be a sufficiently large sample; 15% of the total is generally considered adequate. Define what is meant by "new clients."
4. Devise a questionnaire or a checklist that will determine which of the records do and which do not have the required nursing diagnosis. Include both positive and negative examples.
5. Tabulate the results using correct statistical methods.

Form E (p. 377) shows one example of a way in which a checklist can be devised. Each item is given a numerical, qualitative weight (some items are more important than others); the "yes" scores are added up, and the record is given a "grade." There are several variations of this kind of checklist, but a determination of whether criteria are met must always be made.

The POR system lends itself particularly well to the audit process because there is a continuous surveillance of client progress and because record retrieval is so easy. The physical design of the POR, with its flow sheets, problem lists, and the SOAP format, makes finding a particular piece of data quick and easy. Problems are numbered and listed chronologically, so any one health problem can be followed for any length of time. Form F (pp. 378-379) is an example of the POR audit.

It is important to understand that formal audits, although they are facilitated by the problem-oriented record, are secondary to the continuous feedback provided

	Yes	No
Health history		
Reason for contact	_____	_____
Biographical data	_____	_____
Current health status	_____	_____
Past health history	_____	_____
Family history	_____	_____
Social history	_____	_____
Review of systems	_____	_____
Physical examination	_____	_____
Current problem		
Client's description of problem	_____	_____
Nurse's observations	_____	_____
Interaction with family	_____	_____
Record of physical functioning	_____	_____
Assessment		
What actions already taken	_____	_____
Client's goal	_____	_____
Nurse's goal	_____	_____
Health care plan	_____	_____
Nursing diagnosis stated	_____	_____
Comments		

Form E. Example of a checklist to determine the existence of a nursing diagnosis on a record.

by the record to the team delivering care. In the problem-oriented system auditing shifts from an evaluation of an individual provider to that of total patient care as delivered by the entire patient care team. A problem-oriented audit does away with nursing or physician audits and institutes total patient care evaluation. This represents a major step toward evaluation. This represents a major step toward evaluating actual quality of patient care.[7, pp. 302, 305]

Kinds of audits

There are two distinct kinds of nursing audits: the retrospective process audit and the performance and process-of-care audit. The former was developed by the Joint Commission on the Accreditation of Hospitals and is a review that is done by looking at the records of discharged clients. It identifies deficiencies in the client's condition or care and is composed of the following six steps[8]:

1. Establishment of criteria for client care
2. Comparison of criteria and actual practices
3. Analysis of actual practice findings
4. Corrective action
5. Follow-up studies to determine whether the corrective action was effective
6. Report of the results of audit activity to those to whom one is accountable

Data from the record are compared with preestablished standards; thus deficiencies in care are uncovered, and corrective action can be recommended. Further audits will determine whether the corrective action was effective. The retrospective

Patient _____ Chart No. _____ Date _____

Resident _____ Staff _____ Reviewer _____

	Yes	No	Comments
1. Chart			
a. Is the problem list properly prepared?			
b. Does the problem list appear to have been used?			
c. Are progress notes problem oriented?			
d. Are the progress notes indexed to the problem list?			
e. Is attending signature and/or note present?			
2. Screening data base			
a. Does past history include:			
Significant past illness?			
Childhood diseases?			
Surgery?			
Hospitalization?			
Allergies?			
Review of systems?			
Personal and social history?			
Family history?			
b. Is screening physical examination complete?			

Form F. Problem-oriented record audit for outpatient charts. (From Woolley, F. Ross, and Kane, Robert L.: Improving patient care through the interdisciplinary record. In Reinhardt, Adina, and Quinn, Mildred D., editors: Current practice in family-centered community nursing, vol. 1, St. Louis, 1977, The C.V. Mosby Co.)

process audit measures only what has already occurred, and using it alone will not give an accurate picture of the quality of nursing care. It should be combined with the performance and process-of-care audit, which measures current nursing performance and has six measurement categories[8]:

1. Action directed toward meeting the psychosocial needs of the client
2. Activities directed toward meeting the psychosocial needs of clients as members of a group
3. Operations directed toward meeting the physical needs of clients
4. Proceedings directed toward meeting both the physical and psychosocial needs of clients
5. Communications on behalf of clients
6. Measures directed toward fulfilling professional responsibilities

Each nursing activity is assigned to a category and then given a numerical score. The sum of points earned estimates the quality of care given.

In this manner the audit indirectly results in achieving quality assurance. The audit is one means of exercising accountability by nurses for nursing service. The audit requires that practioners of nursing care move away from an assumption of quality care to an evaluation of care.[8,p.78]

Another type of audit is the appraisal of the outcome of care. This is done on the basis of a health or wellness state of an individual after he has received care. Practitioners can determine whether

	Yes	No	Comments
3. Clinical care			
a. Data collection:			
Is data base complete for problems listed?			
Are lab and x rays used appropriately?			
Are they overutilized?			
b. Data processing:			
Are all problems summarized?			
Is there a plan for each?			
Is data used to arrive at an appropriate assessment?			
Are all problems recognized?			
Are the flow charts used to display data where appropriate?			
Do progress notes clearly relate patient's clinical course?			
c. Treatment:			
Is therapy appropriate to patient's problems?			
Are the number of patient visits and/or length of hospitalization appropriate for patient's problems?			
Are consultants used where appropriate?			
Is there a recorded plan for patient education?			
Does the chart list the medications the patient is sent home with, including dose?			
Are all procedures listed and described?			

General comments

Overall quality of care: _____ Excellent (4) _____ Good (3) _____ Satisfactory (2) _____ Poor (1) _____ Unacceptable (0)

Form F.—cont'd.

their objectives have been achieved. The audit is usually done by means of a retrospective study, but it focuses on the health of an individual rather than on whether certain procedures were done. The criteria to determine the quality of care depend on the nature of the health problem, but all records of clients with a specific health problem should be measured against the same criteria.

In addition to assessing the quality of care, the nursing audit has several practical uses. It can be an indicator of needed staffing patterns, and it can be used as a justification, at least in part, for the personnel budget. Personnel performance can be evaluated by means of the nursing audit, which documents outstanding (either in a positive or a negative sense) nursing care. It can be used as a basis for staff development and in-service education, on either an individual or a group basis.

SUMMARY

Record keeping *is* necessary. If the purpose for keeping the record is properly understood, the service to clients is enhanced, and nurses can more readily evaluate their efforts. Following are several important reasons for keeping records:

1. Documentation of care rendered. This is a recounting of what was done with the client, who did what, and the client's responses and reactions. There are administrative as well as professional reasons to document care, and it is necessary from a legal point of view.

2. A written nursing history as a basis for prescribed therapy. A written history and diagnosis is absolutely essential because whatever the plan of care, there must be a base from which to begin and a reference to justify planned intervention.

3. Communication among various health professionals. Duplication of service can be greatly reduced if health professionals can read each other's progress notes. Each member of the community health team can have a better understanding of the plans and goals of each other member if everyone reads and contributes to the record.

4. Material for research. All the demographic data that researchers need is on the record, as is information about dozens of areas which need to be researched. The record also provides statistical information for various official counts and agency analyses.

5. An educational tool for students. The student learns how to research background information on the client and also sees positive and negative examples of recording techniques.

6. The record as a baseline and evaluation tool. Periodic evaluative progress notes should be written on clients and families who are kept on active status for long periods of time. In this way intervention can be evaluated and plans and goals changed as needed.

There are four major criteria for record keeping: accuracy, timeliness, completeness, and relevancy to the problem. The record system itself should be easy to use and as uncomplicated as possible, and there should always be immediate access to the record. In the actual writing of the record, the focus should be on the recipient of care, not on the person doing the writing. It is the client's response and behaviors that should be noted, not the nurse's. The writing should be comprehensive, concise, and explicit. The nurse should make a conscious effort to simplify her writing by avoiding clutter, by considering who will read the record, and by using the correct words and grammar. The goals and objectives of care should be clearly defined and based on a plan of care, which is in turn based on a history and diagnosis. This method should be consistent throughout the agency. The client's reactions and responses are clearly identified, using the client's exact words where appropriate. It must be emphasized that the nurses's judgmental reaction to the client has no place on the record.

The SOAP method of writing progress notes has come into popular use in the past decade. SOAP is an acronym: *S* for subjective data; *O* for objective data; *A* for assessment; and *P* for plan. The assessment is the interpretation of the subjective and objective data and is the basis for the plan. The advantages of using the SOAP format for progress notes are that it is simple, informative, clear, and precise. Embellishments are eliminated, and whatever is written is directly relevant to the care of the client.

The problem-oriented record (POR) is based on an identification and listing of health problems. The problem-solving approach is used, and the POR system is consumer oriented. There are four components of the POR:

1. The data base is simply a total of information about the client.

2. The problem list is an index for the rest of the client's record and is based on an assessment and interpretation of the data base. Nonphysical problems are stated in behavioral terms, not diagnostic guesses. The problem list should be updated whenever necessary, and the resolution of a problem should also be noted.

3. The initial plan is stated in terms of diagnostic considerations, therapeutic plans, and client edu-

cation. It is merely a statement of what one intends to do about each problem.

4. Progress notes are written in the SOAP format, and flow sheets can sometimes be used as a substitute for some progress notes.

There are several advantages to using the POR system. It encourages a multidisciplinary approach to the solving of problems, and the care for certain types of problems can be standardized without losing individuality. The POR emphasizes the client and not the health care personnel, and it should save time and space in the recording process. It lends itself to research, and evaluation processes are much easier because of the way in which the record is organized.

The purpose of a nursing audit is to assess the quality of care given by the analysis of a sample of records. One sets a standard against which actual performance is measured to provide feedback for corrective action. The three cardinal rules for doing statistical quality control are:

1. The sample must be selected at random.
2. A sufficient number of records must be used for the sample.
3. A decision regarding the attribute being observed must truly represent the condition.

Any aspect of care can be audited, but it is essential that goals and guidelines be clearly established before the audit is begun. This is the procedure to be followed:

1. Determine the parameters of the audit and define the terms.
2. Choose a number of records that will be a large enough sample.
3. Devise a questionnaire or checklist that will measure what is desired.
4. Tabulate the results.

There are two different kinds of nursing audits. The retrospective process audit is a review that is done by looking at the records of discharged or inactive clients. Data are compared with preestablished standards, and deficiencies in the care are identified. The performance and process-of-care audit measures current nursing performance and is designed to increase the quality of care given while it is still being provided. Another kind of audit, which is not specifically a nursing one, is an appraisal of the outcome of care. This is done by determining the level of health or wellness of an individual after he has received care. It is usually done by means of a retrospective audit, but it focuses on health rather than on procedures.

The nursing audit assesses the quality of care; it can indicate staffing patterns, and it can be used in budget preparation. Because care is documented, the audit can be used as a basis for staff evaluation and in-service education.

NOTES

1. Freeman, Ruth B.: Community health nursing practice, Philadelphia, 1970, W.B. Saunders Co.
2. Freeman, Ruth B., and Holmes, Edward M.: Administration of public health services, Philadelphia, 1960, W.B. Saunders Co.
3. Kraegel, Janet M., et al.: Patient care systems, Philadelphia, 1974, J.B. Lippincott Co.
4. Zinsser, William: On writing well, New York, 1976, Harper & Row, Publishers.
5. Berni, Rosemarian, and Readey, Helen: Problem-oriented medical record implementation: allied health peer review, ed. 2, St. Louis, 1978, The C.V. Mosby Co.
6. In this instance the blind husband may have as many or more problems than the diabetic client. His problems should be listed and evaluated on a separate sheet to avoid confusion.
7. Woolley, F. Ross, and Kane, Robert L.: Improving patient care through the interdisciplinary record. In Reinhardt, Adina, and Quinn, Mildred D., editors: Current practice in family-centered community nursing, vol. 1, St. Louis, 1979, The C.V. Mosby Co.
8. Froebe, Doris J., and Bain, R. Joyce: Quality assurance programs and controls in nursing, St. Louis, 1976, The C.V. Mosby Co.

BIBLIOGRAPHY

Archer, Sarah, and Fleshman, Ruth: Community health nursing: patterns and practice, ed. 2, N. Scituate, Mass., 1979, Duxbury Press.

Becknell, Eileen Pearlman, and Smith, Dorothy M.: System of nursing practice, Philadelphia, 1975, F.A. Davis Co.

Benson, Evelyn Rose, and McDevitt, Joan Quinn: Community health and nursing practice, ed. 2, Englewood Cliffs, N.J., 1979, Prentice-Hall, Inc.

Berni, Rosemarian, and Readey, Helen: Problem-oriented medical record implementation: allied health peer review, ed. 2, St. Louis, 1978, The C.V. Mosby Co.

Carter, Joan H., et al.: Standards of nursing care, New York, 1976, Springer Publishing Co.

Davidson, Sharon Van Sell: PSRO: utilization and audit in patient care, St. Louis, 1976, The C.V. Mosby Co.

Durbin, Richard L., and Springall, W. Herbert: Organization and administration of health care: theory, practice, environment, ed. 2, St. Louis, 1974, The C.V. Mosby Co.

Freeman, Ruth B.: Community health nursing practice, Philadelphia, 1970, W.B. Saunders Co.

Freeman, Ruth B., and Holmes, Edward M.: Administration of public health nuring services, Philadelphia, 1960, W.B. Saunders Co.

Froebe, Doris J., and Bain, R. Joyce: Quality assurance programs and controls in nursing, St. Louis, 1976, The C.V. Mosby Co.

Kraegel, Janet M., et al.: Patient care systems, Philadelphia, 1974, J.B. Lippincott Co.

Kramer, Lou Ann: The audit and I, American Journal of Nursing **76:**1130-1141, 1976.

Leahy, Kathleen M., et al.: Community health nursing, New York, 1977, McGraw-Hill Book Co.

Mahoney, Elizabeth A., et al.: How to collect and record a health history, Philadelphia, 1976, J.B. Lippincott Co.

Phaneuf, Maria: The nursing audit, New York, 1972, Appleton-Century-Crofts.

Reinhardt, Adina M., and Quinn, Mildred D., Current practice in family-centered community nursing, vol. 1, St. Louis, 1979, The C.V. Mosby Co.

Rinaldi, Leena A., and Kelly, Barbara: What to do after the audit is done, American Journal of Nursing **77:**268-269, 1977.

Weed, Lawrence L.: Medical records, medical education and patient care, Chicago, 1970, Year Book Medical Publishers, Inc.

15

SCHOOL NURSING

GEORGIA P. MacDONOUGH

As our nation entered the twentieth century, America was compelled to begin a new phase of community health. Communicable diseases forced many children to be absent from school, and a majority of them roamed the streets rather than stay home. Searching for a solution that would allow them to get back to the learning environment, Lillian Wald of the Henry Street Nursing Association in New York demonstrated the importance of nursing care for school-age children. Lina Rogers, the public health nurse assigned to the project, was soon able to prove that with nursing follow-up these excluded children were back in school within a short period of time. As a result, several other nurses were assigned to work in the New York schools, and a new nursing specialty was born.[1] The basic principles of community health formed the foundation for the new school nursing practice; sound principles were adapted to a new setting. The primary function of professional school nurses has remained the same throughout the century: to keep students in school.

Although many professionals in the schools are expected to make important contributions to a successful health program, it is the purpose of this chapter to concentrate on the activities of the school nurse. The responsibilities of a school nurse obligate her to make a careful self-assessment of preparation and personal capabilities. Not all states have specific certification requirements that seek to ensure minimal entry qualifications, and this lack of formal guidelines places the burden on each nurse, who must set her own preparation standards. States that do not have certification requirements must rely on school nurses who may not be adequately prepared.

The controlling agency for schools in all states is the state education department. State legislatures pass laws and appropriate money in support of public education, including school health services. These funds are then distributed through the state education department. In its operation of the school health program this agency may be assisted by the state health department. The two departments should work closely during planning and implementation of services, and key people in each department usually communicate regularly and frequently with each other. The role of the state government includes development of programs, establishment of minimum standards, distribution of printed guidelines, training and in-service education, and giving direct service to communities when necessary.

Local control is frequently difficult to assess, and the actual political forces of control are diffuse and hard to identify. The responsibility of running the school district falls on the local superintendent of schools, who receives direction from the board

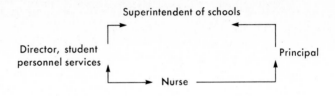

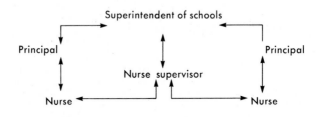

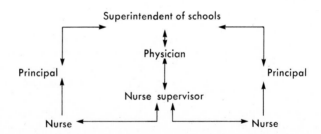

Fig. 15-1. Examples of the nurse position in the school hierarchy.

of education. Members of the board are usually citizens elected from those who live within the boundary of the district. In many states large cities have centralized districts that have some system-wide coordination of policies and procedures. In other states there are many small independent districts, jealously guarded by the local power group. Most school systems are arranged in a hierarchy with the higher offices supervising the work of the lower ones. Power and authority are distributed by policies and rules. A powerful element of control often is exercised from the top down, and differences of opinion arise because of factors such as

goals and methods, curriculum, level, student body, public support, cultural environment, and the local lineup of political forces.

A career in school nursing affords a remarkable degree of independent, self-directed practice. Yet along with this increased scope comes the much greater personal responsibility for judging one's own proficiency. Professional nurses are legally accountable for their decisions and actions. Although some school systems provide a nursing supervisor to whom the staff nurse can go for guidance and advice, in the majority of school nursing positions, the nurse will find herself the sole health-oriented faculty member, responsible for herself and her practice. At the same time she is administratively accountable to both the principal and the director of student personnel services. A similar situation exists for school physicians, whether the district has full-time or part-time coverage. Many districts have no physician at all. (Fig. 15-1 illustrates several possible organizational themes.) In many schools the nurse may be administratively responsible to a nonmedical person, but she cannot take medical direction from anyone but a physician or nurse supervisor. When no supervisor is available, the nurse must determine the proper course of action for herself. Sometimes a state consultant is available.

Basic preparation for the school nurse should be a baccalaureate degree, but in addition to general nursing education, the preparation should include courses in sociology, particularly those dealing with cultural mores prevalent in the geographical area in which the nurse works; psychology, both normal and abnormal; advanced pediatrics; emergency preparedness (emergency medical technician training is good); and community health nursing. To understand the method of operation of schools, the nurse needs courses dealing with theory of education, curriculum planning, health education methods, and counseling. A course in audiovisual methods is highly valuable because a school nurse will frequently be using equipment such as overhead, filmstrip, and movie projectors. Along with this theory, work experience is necessary, especially in schools where no nursing supervision is available. Some universities offer a master's degree in school nursing. Nurses with master's degrees are usually well equipped to handle most eventualities. Other nurses come to the job with work experience in pediatrics, emergency rooms, community health agencies, or as substitute or volunteer school nurses.

REVIEW OF LEGAL PROVISIONS

In our present legally oriented culture, nurses are well advised to review all laws relevant to their practices. This information is readily available from state boards of nursing. In particular, nurses should acquaint themselves with the state's nurse practice act; this is particularly important for school nurses who function independently. The provisions, rules, and regulations of this law help protect the public from harm and, at the same time, delineate the legal scope of nursing practice in each state. Perhaps the most important limitation of which the school nurse should be aware concerns the administration of medications and delegation of allowable nursing duties to nonlicensed personnel. The school nurse needs to be certain which areas of practice are within the realm of the professional nurse and which belong to the practical nurse. Most states stipulate that the practical nurse can function only under the direction of a professional nurse. The nurse will probably want to know how much time she will be spending supervising others, and it is well to find this out before she accepts the position.

Each school nurse should also have medical guidelines. These may be developed with the appointed school physician or the medical director of the health department or local medical society. The public health nursing division of the state health department or the school nurse consultant of the department of public instruction, sometimes called the state education department, has suggested guidelines for developing these medical-nursing responsibilities and relationships.

In several states proof of continuing education is necessary for relicensure. Whether mandated or not, professionally responsible practitioners periodically update their knowledge and skills.

The Pharmacy Act, along with the rules and regulations of the board of pharmacy, will clarify for school nurses their responsibilities regarding the administration, storage, and accountability for prescription and over-the-counter medications. In some states specific provisions are made for medical facilities other than licensed pharmacies. Particular attention should be paid to the definition of terms. *Administration* is defined as the giving of a unit dose of medication to a client as the result of the order of a physician or other authorized medical practitioner. Administration affects only the person receiving the drug. A registered nurse is licensed to administer medication, and, in some states after proper training, licensed practical nurses may also administer medications.

Dispensing is the issuing of one or more doses of medication from an original package in a suitable container with appropriate labeling for subsequent administration to, or use by, a client. Dispensing affects one or more people. In most states only pharmacists are educated and licensed to dispense medications.

Supplying is defined as the issuing of one or more doses of a proprietary drug in the original container of a manufacturer for subsequent use by the client. Some industrial medical stations supply such medications as cold remedies, analgesics, antacids, laxatives, antidiarrheics, and antihistamines in this manner. Some schools also purchase these prepackaged medications for administration to students and faculty.

Proprietary medicines are those identified by and sold under a trademark, trade name, or other trade symbol. They are sold without a prescription to the general public.

Large numbers of youngsters receive doses of medication during the school day in order to remain in school. Most states require the school nurse to obtain the physician's written order and written permission of the parent or guardian to legally administer the prescribed dose. An additional responsibility of the school nurse is to gather information regarding the efficacy of the prescribed medication. An example would be to sit in a classroom to observe the behavior of a student receiving methylphenidate (Ritalin). His activities for a half-hour period and the teacher's overall impressions of behavior change could be written in a concise report that is shared with the parents and physician. This may assist the physician in the decision to increase, decrease, or discontinue a specific drug. The local health department or board of education

usually makes rules about the variety and quantity of medications that are allowed to be kept in the health office, as well as any specifications regarding the security of drugs. It is also important to consider any limitations of acts permitted registered nurses regarding medications, such as assigning a school secretary to administer medications in her absence.

Every state's education code delineates the requirements for hiring of school personnel, including special provisions for periodic physical examinations, testing for tuberculosis, immunization demands, and compulsory health education. This group of statutes will determine whether the school nursing position is mandated. In some states the law specifies that a school nurse ''shall'' be available for every 1,000 to 1,500 students. In others, the statutes are permissive, stating that the local school districts ''may'' provide funds for the salary of nurses, physicians, dentists, and other employees necessary for the succeeding year. In this instance, the local board of trustees has the option to hire or not hire a nurse. In addition, there are other state and federal regulations regarding the way that school ''business'' is conducted. For example, Title IX of the 1972 Education Amendments prohibits sex discrimination in schools and colleges receiving federal financial assistance. Three years later regulations implementing Title IX's mandate went into effect. The regulations contain several provisions that are especially relevant to health services, such as sports medicine, insurance, marital status, pregnancy, access to service, and victims of domestic violence and incest. Although Title IX has decreased the incidence of sex discrimination in school health services, it is by no means nonexistent.

Special education

The Special Education Act of 1975, Public Law 94-142, ensures free equal educational opportunity for *all* youngsters. Part 84, nondiscrimination on the basis of handicaps, further instructs all school districts receiving federal funds. Subpart D applies to preschool, elementary, secondary, and adult education. It requires the following of schools:

1. To identify and locate every qualified handicapped person within the jurisdiction who is not receiving a public education.
2. To notify persons and their parents of the school's duty to provide the education.
3. To provide free appropriate public education regardless of the nature or severity of the handicap. This can be regular or special education or referral to other programs.
4. To provide educational and related services free except for fees that are imposed on the nonhandicapped. Funds available from any public or private agency may be used to meet these requirements.

Other subpart D stipulations are the following:

5. If the student is placed in another agency for education, transportation shall be provided at no greater cost than would be incurred if the student were attending a program operated by the recipient (the school receiving federal funds).
6. If residential placement is necessary, it shall be free.
7. If parents desire to place the student in a private school, there is no requirement for the recipient to pay.

Public Law 94-142 further states that nonacademic services, including meals, be appropriate to the needs of the handicapped and that services can include counseling, physical recreation, athletics, health services, and recreational activities.

Also important to school nurses are school bus safety regulations, Occupational Safety and Health (OSHA) standards, and local sanitation laws. A general working knowledge of the most important laws related to school health is essential to the quality of school nursing practice.

PLANNING FOR SCHOOL HEALTH SERVICES

School health services are provided in several different ways. In many cities the local board of education hires one or several nurses to conduct the program. The nurse may be assigned to cover one school or may be responsible for the health service program in several. In other areas the school health program is the responsibility of the local health department, which may either assign a community health nurse to provide school health services exclusively to one or more schools, or it may assign several community health nurses to cover the schools located within their regular districts as part of their case load. The United States Public Health Service provides school nurses to serve the boarding schools of the Bureau of Indian Affairs and the armed forces. School health service is even provided in the schools for American dependents overseas. All schools—public, private, and parochial—should have access to some school health program. The local health department is responsible for the health of the entire population, including schoolchildren.

Setting the broad goal of the school health program is usually an administrative responsibility performed by the superintendent or his assignee. This person may choose to involve a committee of district employees, including school nurses, or he may form an advisory committee of community representatives. A school nurse should always be involved in setting the goals of the health program. Whatever the source of these broad goals, the nurse then plans her program to accomplish them. If the goals need to be revised, it is imperative that nursing have a voice in this redirection. Each year the nurse will begin the term by setting specific goals for her own school(s) that should refine and concentrate the broader district goals. In addition to the general goals of the district and the nurse's professional ones, the school nurse will have to consider the goals of the student and his family. The student/family complex can be considered the school nurse's client. Occasionally, all these goals will not be compatible with one another, and the nurse will find it necessary to clarify and negotiate the goals with the district, with her principal, or with the student and his family in order for all to work together to accomplish them. Goals for nursing service cannot be vague; they must be realistic in view of the schools' and the students' specific needs. The goals must also be measurable so they can be evaluated.

The task of setting priorities can be accomplished after consideration of all aspects of the job at hand. The nurse will have to take into account the ratio of available nursing time to student load as well as the location for service. A nurse who is assigned to one school of 1,200 students will have different goals than the nurse who is assigned to three different schools all located a few miles from each other.

All state-mandated programs should be reviewed to determine if there is an exact time period during which screening such as that for vision and hearing must be done. Each school population may have different needs. It may be urgent to test kindergarten students immediately because most of them have never had previous exposure to vision and hearing screening. These kindergarten students might have been previously screened through the Early Periodic Screening, Diagnosis, and Treatment program under Medicaid, and they could benefit from a "waiting" period to become accustomed to their new school, teacher, and nurse. The longer a defect remains undetected, the longer the student is unable to take full advantage of the learning opportunities presented to him. It is important to do a health appraisal early in the school year on kindergarten children and other students who may be new to the school system. Freeman, in her book, *Community Health Nursing Practice,* states, "Priorities are established by ordering the various aspects of care in terms of urgency or impact in order to define those that warrant the earliest and most inclusive attention."[2,p.68]

It is a good idea for the school nurse to have a close working relationship with the state health department and its school health consultant. In some states all students must be immunized before they are permitted to enroll, and some states have policies regarding vision and hearing screening. The

school nurse must, of course, be aware of all state laws pertaining to the health of schoolchildren.

In the school system, priorities are set primarily according to the impact on the potential learning capacity of the student. In addition, the nurse considers such things as the urgency of an impending outbreak of a communicable disease that can be controlled by early action on her part or by the urgency of prompt and accurate treatment of accidental injuries.

The ultimate success of any school health program depends in large part on the nurse: her professional capabilities, knack in coordinating the health programs with other school activities in an unobtrusive manner, and flair for public relations.

Excellent sources of support for high-quality health services are the parents of the students. These citizens learn to appreciate and rely heavily on the services of a well-prepared school nurse. Many nurses depend on parent volunteers to relieve them of nonprofessional duties. The American Red Cross has a well-rounded training program for volunteer school health assistants that prepares these interested parents to work in the school health center. Through exposure to the daily occurrences in the health office, the parents become advocates for the nurse and the health program. The nurse should have a close working relationship with organizations such as the P.T.A. and student councils because these groups can provide valuable input in establishing health priorities.

Voluntary health agencies also assist the nurse in organizing community support and in cementing good relationships. Most voluntary health agencies supply high-quality health education materials, including films. They appreciate the exposure that occurs when the school nurse uses their services.

The most important endorsement and support can come from the official health agencies in the nurse's area. Official health agencies help determine school health programs. If the school nurse cooperates with and coordinates programs such as immunization clinics, epidemiological investigations, early periodic (Medicaid) screening and tracking, and research projects, local and state health departments can be outspoken in their praise and support of school health services. The nurse can also use official health agencies as a source of consultation and continuing education.

Private physicians and dentists appreciate nurses who identify problems early and refer students to them for prompt treatment. If nurses are prepared to offer physical assessments to their students, they can pass their findings of illness or abnormalities along to physicians. More important, they can save students' families time and expense. Most important, they can detect abnormalities while they are still in an early, and most likely treatable, stage.

In times of budget limitations, the school health program seems to be expendable in some areas of the United States where school and community relationships have been haphazard or nonexistent. In these instances school nurses need all their public relations skills to convince the boards of education that nursing service is essential.

In order for nurses to intelligently approach the task of choosing priorities, an overview of the many facets of the school health program will assist them. The program is frequently divided into three areas: school health services, health education, and the provision of a safe and healthy school environment. All are integral parts of the total program.

HEALTH EDUCATION

The health education role of the school nurse may be viewed as either direct or indirect. Direct health education occurs in every interaction the nurse has with a student or group of students. Teaching about one's body and its functions, health practices, prevention of injury, and disease control can be accomplished during every student contact (Fig. 15-2). Nurses in the school also find themselves in the role of teacher when they discuss health matters with faculty members and when they hold conferences with parents. Because it is necessary for all of us to be informed consumers in today's society, school nurses are urged to prepare their students to become knowledgeable consumers

of health services. The students need to know what health care facilities are available in the community, how to use them, and how to evaluate the services they receive at these facilities. Each student needs to learn how to participate in his own health care, how to ask intelligent questions about what is suggested for treatment, and how to make wise decisions regarding his health.

Indirect health education may be accomplished in a variety of ways. The nurse could plan a program with new teachers each year to review guidelines for determining which youngsters within a class need to be sent to the nurse's office for evaluation. Sometimes the approach is to review pertinent observations to be made of each body system, such as the following:

Eyes: redness, discharge, or inability to see the book or chalkboard

Nose: bleeding, running, or stopped up

Ears: aches, inability to hear

Nurses should be involved in health curriculum planning and review of textbooks, films, posters, or pamphlets that are to be used in the formal health education program. They are considered resource persons for the health teacher. Nurses can be guest speakers in health classes, where they contribute a nursing dimension. An example of this would be a discussion of the ''good'' uses of drugs, the ''miracle medicines,'' and some of the results accomplished through the proper use of medications. In such a discussion, the nurse can demonstrate the care with which she measures the correct dose and ensures the safe administration of medications to the proper person. In many schools the nurse keeps an updated file of reference materials for both the students and faculty to use for teaching or for writing reports.

Nurses in the school need to become informed about all community resources that may prove valuable for their students. If no directory is available in the community, they are well advised to compile one. Information contained therein should include name, address, phone number, and hours of business for each agency. The directory should

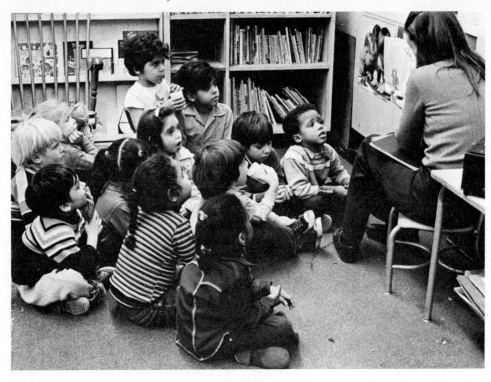

Fig. 15-2. The school nurse as teacher of health maintenance concepts is one of her most important functions. (Photograph by Marion Bernstein; courtesy Editorial Photocolor Archives, Inc., New York.)

also note eligibility criteria and intake methods. Nurses can often pave the way for inexperienced family members by a discussion of what they may expect when they apply for service. It also helps for the nurse to become personally familiar with the workings of the agency and to know some of the key administrative personnel, which can be valuable for future referrals.

The nurse should be a member of the safety committee of her school and in this capacity help review accident reports of students and faculty. She can inform fellow members of the committee about the possible long-range effects of specific injuries. She can also arrange for the training or retraining of selected personnel in the area of first aid. It is also the nurse who usually observes safety hazards in the school building that should be reported to the committee for action.

If the nurse is invited to be a guest speaker in one of the classrooms, it is important that she plan exactly what her lesson will incorporate. The nurse and the classroom teacher could engage in joint lesson planning and could share observations about the children's growth and development as well as the group's interest in the lesson. After assignment of the topic, the nurse should consider the grade level to whom she will be speaking and the developmental tasks of that age group. An example is this description of a 10-year-old:

Prefers silent reading

Meets situations head on with little embarrassment

Sense of fairness and being a good sport important

Evaluations deeper and more discriminating

More diplomatic, fewer fights with friends

Taking these traits into consideration, the nurse can begin to formulate a lesson plan that will appeal to youngsters of this age. Consideration may be given to such learning experiences as group problem solving, experiments, demonstrations, skits, role playing, or the use of puppets. Teaching aids can enhance the learning experience. These may be printed materials such as books or pamphlets, graphs, flip charts, cartoons, or overhead transparencies, and they may also include movies, photographs, tapes, records, or specimens. The formulation of behavioral objectives is important so the nurse can evaluate the learning that has taken place.

A lesson plan for 10-year-olds on the digestive system follows:

Topic: Digestive system.
Grade level: 5
Outcome: Students know parts, locations, and functions of the digestive system.
Content: Name each part of the digestive system and its location and function.
Learning experience: Use a balloon to conceptualize stomach action. Put a slice of bread and some water into the balloon, using fingers to stimulate muscle action to partially digest contents.
Key words: New vocabulary associated with topic.
Evaluation: Have students write stories pretending they are one part of the digestive system. Explain what happens when the food comes in.

The nurse can provide valuable assistance when decisions are to be made in choosing a particular school accident policy for the student body. Such insurance policies are offered by many school districts at low cost to help parents defray medical costs in case of accidental injury. Two options are available: "school time only" or "24-hour coverage." The nurse can help to determine which company offers the best coverage at the least cost. Although the school nurse is not expected to have great expertise in the area of insurance, she can act as a resource person when the school is developing or revising its accident and safety program, of which the selection of insurance may be a part.

SCHOOL ENVIRONMENT

All parents have a right to assume that the children they send to school will be provided with protected, uncontaminated surroundings. Although sanitation statutes require such items as warm water and soap, sewage and solid waste disposal, and adequate heating and lighting, there are still problems in implementing the laws. Maintenance personnel whose job is to keep the school clean are many times ill prepared for this work. For the most part they are people who have never been taught to clean and have no understanding of germ theory or principles of infection control. In addition, there is often not enough money to purchase supplies and equipment. It is not surprising to be told that soap is no longer available because the allocated amount is used up and no funds are left to buy more. The nurse must insist, of course, that funds be found, and they usually are. Occasionally there is a personality conflict between the nurse and other school personnel who feel she is "stepping on their turf." Several examples are the bus driver who resents being asked if the first-aid kit is well supplied, the kitchen worker who may have been admonished for serving food with bare hands instead of using tongs or plastic gloves, or the custodian who is told the bathrooms or showers are not properly cleaned and are a hazard. If such things interfere with practices that the nurse values as important for safeguarding the health and well-being of the students, she must attempt to resolve the difficulties. Often it is the principal who mediates and settles such problems.

The lines of authority within a school system should be investigated before a nurse decides to accept a position in that system. This becomes extremely important if a disagreement arises in an area outside the nurse's direct jurisdiction. The outcome of the disagreement can be influential on the physical and mental health of the students in the nurse's care. A common example of such a conflict is a situation that results in the removal of soap and paper towels from the lavatory because the students are stuffing the paper towels down the toilets and painting the walls with the soap. The nurse, in this instance, advocates handwashing for control of diseases such as pinworm infestation or hepatitis and for teaching positive health habits, whereas the custodian is concerned with plumbing problems. The nurse and the custodian might be able to resolve the conflict over a friendly cup of coffee without having to go to administrators.

The state or county sanitarian will be helpful in reviewing the regulations for school sanitation. Inspections are done periodically to check on the number and type of water fountains, the number of students per toilet, shower facilities, rest areas for faculty members, and kitchen and serving areas. The sanitary inspection of the kitchen is probably the most time consuming and significant and includes examination of food storage, food preparation, serving and handling techniques, and cleanup methods.

Fire drills are required at every school, and the nurse should plan in advance what her role will be in the event of an actual fire. A well-stocked first-aid case should be readily available to bring along when the school buildings are evacuated. The nurse should have a prearranged area away from all buildings in which she can ''set up shop.'' In sections of the country where hurricanes, tornadoes, severe snowstorms, or other natural disasters occur, the nurse should ensure that a disaster plan is established. The school should be prepared to go into action to protect employees and students. After such a plan is organized, training is held, and periodic practice is given to ensure that key personnel know exactly what to do when an actual disaster occurs.

The wellness of teachers and other school employees can sometimes become a touchy issue within the school system. It is wise to have a written policy established that outlines what steps will be taken in case of physical or mental illness of an employee. The procedure must protect the students, of course, but it should also ensure the employee due process before being sent home. Perhaps a physical examination or evaluation for emotional stability should be required. In many schools the nurse is given the responsibility to determine

when a teacher is contagious or sick enough to be sent home. If, for example, a teacher has vomiting and diarrhea but decides to remain on duty for the day, the nurse can insist that the teacher be sent home to keep the illness from being spread to the children in the classroom. Although the health of employees is usually not the direct responsibility of the school nurse, she will find herself giving counsel on health matters. She can provide some services such as first aid and weight and blood pressure surveillance, and can set an example of positive health habits through her own actions.

The open classroom concept and tight scheduling of subjects could be blamed for many psychosomatic problems in the schoolage youngster such as, ulcers, tics, nail biting, bedwetting, headaches, and stomachaches. It does little good for a student to take a stimulant in order for him to attend to the lesson if he is being bombarded with a variety of visual and auditory stimuli in a large classroom holding nearly a hundred students. The nurse has a responsibility to give suggestions to the principal in regard to placement and planning for students who are under a physician's care or who are handicapped in one way or another.

The school grounds and play areas should be periodically inspected for safety hazards. If this is done in connection with the review of accident reports, it has been found that repairs are made with little delay. Since busing of students is an integral part of the school program these days, it goes without saying that a safe school environment also includes the bus ride. School bus evacuation drills should be held throughout the school year in addition to the more familiar fire drills. These bus evacuation drills must include all students, not just regular riders, since many field trips throughout the school year include every student in a given grade.

It is becoming more common for schools to provide learning experiences away from the school site. An example of this is a camping trip to learn about nature and ecology. It is necessary to arrange for someone to scout the proposed area of the campout to assess its safety, water supply, and toilet facilities. It is also essential to review with the teacher in charge what arrangements have been made for food storage, serving, cleanup, and emergencies.

The inspection and maintenance of the buildings, grounds, kitchens, buses, and so forth are certainly not the responsibility of the nurse but are done by personnel assigned to the particular department. The nurse's task is to be aware of what occurs in the school in all departments as it affects the health and well-being of the students and faculty under her care. However, poor performance in the kitchen area could result in an outbreak of food-borne disease, and the nurse must know in advance what steps to take to deal with such a situation. She must be primed for immediate response in case of a bus accident. She must be prepared to defend a request for removal of a particular piece of playground equipment when she can prove that it is a safety hazard and thus a liability to the school.

SCHOOL HEALTH SERVICES

Within the services component of the school health program, nursing skills are used in more traditional ways. The school nurse will need to arrange for periodic appraisal of each student. Sometimes this is done because the state requires a physical examination for school entry (Fig. 15-3). If, however, the state in which the school nurse works has no such requirement, she should plan to do an assessment of new students by whatever method her education and professional ingenuity can help her to develop. The assessment if accomplished by a history, a physical examination, and other testing; if there are no state-mandated guidelines or requirements, the assessment can be as thorough as the nurse chooses to make it.

The school health center, as in all systems providing health care, must establish and maintain records on every student. The information contained in these records needs to be accessible and easily retrievable. For example, during a measles outbreak, it is important that the school nurse be able to identify students "at risk" within hours of the outbreak in order to begin control measures. The nurse should also be building linkages with other health care providers to ensure continuity of care without duplication of efforts.

Assessment and testing of students includes screening for physiological disorders such as vision, hearing, dental, or orthopedic problems; metabolic disorders such as diabetes; neurological disorders such as convulsive problems, petit mal episodes, and poor visual motor performance; communicable diseases such as pediculosis, impetigo, or tinea capitis; and psychosocial problems such as enuresis or school phobia. Nursing assessments are done to some degree on most children attending the school within any given year. In many states the timing of vision and hearing screening is mandated; in other states guidelines are provided that suggest specific grades to screen.

After the health appraisal of the student is completed, the nurse should talk with the student and parent regarding the findings. In many instances the school nurse will resort to sending a written notice home in the event that something is wrong. Her responsibility for follow-up, however, does not end with the notice. She must ensure that the discovery of a defect results in action being taken to alleviate the problem. In cases in which the problem can be remedied, it may be necessary to direct the family to the appropriate community resources. In cases in which medical follow-up has shown that remediation is impossible, the nurse, along with the student and parents, makes plans to maintain and/or restore health. The goal in all cases is to assist the students to attain their maximum potential.

With increasing numbers of handicapped youngsters enrolled in school, the nurse is well advised to review the skills necessary to care for these young people. Some students will need training in eating; the use of special utensils and modified school lunches might have to be arranged. Other students might need special chairs, mats, or tilt boards to ensure good positioning and frequent change of position. A physical or occupational therapist is a valuable resource for this. Arrangements will need to be made for special toileting needs, perhaps changing collection bags for urine

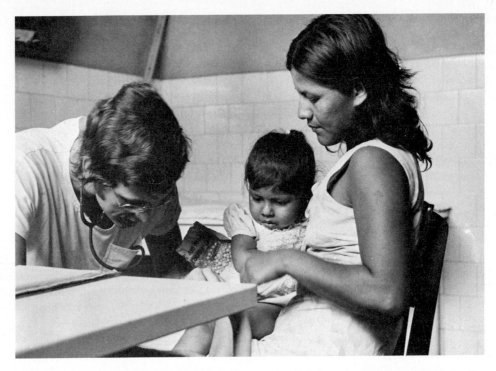

Fig. 15-3. Periodic physical examinations are one way in which the school nurse can identify health problems. (Photograph by Alain Keller; courtesy Editorial Photocolor Archives, Inc., New York.)

and/or feces, which creates the need for adequate skin care. Privacy and control of cross-infection is always of prime concern. Modified physical education should be organized for every handicapped student. Specific programs are usually worked out by a team composed of the physical education teacher, nurse, and physical or occupational therapist. Family or clinic physicians may write orders for certain exercises to be incorporated into these school programs. Safe transportation is a critical issue with handicapped students. At times these youngsters are transported in their wheelchairs, which are hoisted into vans and strapped into place. Many other handicapped students ride the regular bus along with the nonhandicapped.

Another facet of the school nurse's responsibilities is to prevent and control communicable disease among the school population, which means that the nurse must be well versed in the principles of epidemiology. Provisions should be made for initial immunizations or necessary boosters through school clinics, neighborhood public health clinics, or referral to private physicians. Whatever method is used, it is imperative that health records show which students are underimmunized in case of an outbreak.

The school nurse must always be alert, viewing signs and symptoms, evaluating each student carefully, and remaining ever suspicious that communicable disease may be present. She must be familiar with the usual rate of absenteeism and the "normal" incidence of contagious diseases in order to suspect the beginning of an epidemic. To establish the existence of an epidemic, she should consider the reliability of the reporting sources. Are the parents certain that the children have a contagious disease; have they taken them to a physician for a definite diagnosis? Have laboratory tests been performed for verification? Does the local health department offer this service to ensure correct diagnosis and institution of control procedures? When the nurse is convinced that she has an impending epidemic on her hands, she should immediately contact the local health department to ask for its assistance. She needs to be ready to help establish the time of onset, place, and person responsible for the outbreak. She should have some idea about the mode of transmission and should do a rapid preliminary analysis of the population at risk. She can also work with the school administration to facilitate measures to care for the sick, prevent further spread, and arrange resources to aid in investigation.

Emergency care for students and school personnel is necessary in case they become sick or injured. First-aid kits should be strategically located in all buildings, and some assigned personnel should have valid first-aid certificates. Written procedures must be established, along with a line of command and emergency phone numbers for rescue units, paramedics, or ambulance services easily located in case the school nurse is unavailable when an emergency occurs. These emergency functions are what people ordinarily think of when they think of school nursing, and they probably take up a great bulk of the nurse's time. However, the role of the school nurse has developed and expanded so dramatically in the past decade that the emergency functions are no longer theoretically the most important.

The other major function of the school nurse is that of health counseling. Often the nurse will find that families have not established a "medical home." These families do not practice preventive health care but instead seek medical care only when a crisis occurs. The nurse in this situation has unlimited opportunities to teach the youngsters and, through them, other family members about the value of preventive and early care and health promotion. Occasionally the nurse will have to assume a child advocacy role in order to intercede in a situation before it becomes critical. The child–protective service worker assists when children are

medically neglected as well as when cases of child abuse are suspected.

School nurse practitioner

Since 1970, when Henry K. Silver developed the School Nurse Practitioner Educational and Training Program at the University of Colorado Medical Center Schools of Medicine and Nursing, many school nurses have chosen to expand their role by such preparation. This program includes four months and intensive theory and practice in child care and school health. In addition, nine months of practice under the preceptorship of a qualified physician prepares these practitioners to assume basic responsibility for identifying and managing many of the health problems of children. This clinical specialist program is intended for nurses who already have a baccalaureate degree and who want advanced preparation in school nursing.

The concept of providing primary health care to schoolchildren using nurse practitioners with physician backup has been tested in Cambridge, Massachusetts. In 1968 efforts were made by the pediatric staff of the city hospital to consolidate resources from programs such as school health, city health departments, federal funds, and Head Start, a program for disadvantaged children that helps to prepare them medically and socially for school. The purpose was to demonstrate that by integrating these resources in comprehensive health centers located in schools, child health care costs could be contained and actually reduced without sacrificing the quality of care. Five health centers provided comprehensive health services to all Cambridge children ages 0 through 16.[3] The school nurse practitioners provided periodic physical assessments, including testing for anemia and dipstick urine testing for mental retardation. If any health problem was uncovered, the child was referred to the physician. This innovative approach to providing health care to children is just one within the school setting.

The goals of the school nurse practitioner program in Denver are twofold: (1) to prepare school nurses to deliver comprehensive health care to school-age children who do not use traditional health facilities except for emergency care and (2) to deliver health services to any child complaining of illness or injury at school. Courses include history taking, physical diagnosis, neurological appraisal, common pediatric problems, and many others. This School Nurse Practitioner Program is held at the University of Colorado at Denver. Classes are given at the College of Nursing, the College of Medicine, and some community agencies. The program is offered for eight weeks during two consecutive summers, thus allowing the school nurse to keep her job and continue her education during her vacation time. After the initial eight-week course there is an interim session during which the practitioner must work at least 4 hours a week with a medical preceptor in her home community. In addition there are other assignments such as readings and case study reports to be completed. Most of the students pay for the program themselves, but occasionally the members of a school district are so convinced of the value of the nurse in this expanded role that they provide some financial support.

Bellaire and Fine,[4] in an article in *Pediatric Nursing,* review the problem of the changing role of the school nurse. They describe the nurses who formerly were concerned only about the health needs of their students as now having to deal with a myriad of records, schedules, and meetings. The nurses are cheated of time that in the past was used for treating, caring, and listening. Although they are still concerned about these things, they tend to spend more time doing paperwork than giving nursing care. Bellaire and Fine caution, "The profession of school nursing is at a crossroad. It must dynamically grow to meet the health demands of school-aged children, or it will become obsolete."[4] School nurses must concentrate their efforts on *nursing* the students in their care and arrange for clerical assistance through the employment of nursing clerks or through the use of student or parent volunteers.

In comparing the differences in the functions of traditional school nurses and practitioners, studies[5,6] have found that practitioners (1) spend more time in provision of direct client care, (2) send fewer children home, (3) make infrequent inappropriate referrals, and (4) have a higher percentage of successful referrals for health problems. Not every school nurse can consider postgraduate education to become a practitioner. We must, however, heed the warning to keep the profession vital and essential, and the major way to do this is for each nurse to constantly improve her professional skills.

NURSING PROCESS IN THE SCHOOL

When discussing the nursing process as it applies to practice within the school system, it is helpful to begin with a comparison of the nursing situation in a hospital and a school. Following are excerpts from an article[7] written for the *Journal of School Health* in which I reminded the reader that an administrator's understanding of the nursing role is frequently the result of personal encounters with nurses:

> In the hospital, the patient knows he is ill and wants to get well. In the school, the patient and his family often do not recognize that he has problems, and not only do not seek help, but may resent and resist any effort to assist him.
> In the hospital, patients are assigned to a particular nurse for care. One of the basic responsibilities of the school nurse, however, is case-finding.
> In the hospital, the main goal of nursing care is cure. In school nursing, the goal is to build and maintain optimal physical, mental, and social health for each student.[7]

Nursing time is limited to school hours, so it is essential that students learn the skills and acquire the information which will enable them to make responsible decisions regarding their own health.

American Nurses Association standards

The American School Health Association, the National Association of School Nurses of the National Education Association (NEA), and the American Nurses Association (ANA) have all published standards that the school nurse can use for self-appraisal. The professional school nurse wants to guarantee quality, cost-effective service that is efficient. Adaptations of the ANA's *Standards: Community Health Nursing Practice*[8] in the school setting follow:

Assessing

The collection of data about the health status of the consumer is systematic and continous. The data are accessible, communicated and recorded (Standard I).

The cumulative health record is started when the student first enrolls in school. Information is gathered for the data base by a history from the parents and students, by physical assessment, and by developmental evaluations. With signed releases the nurse can also obtain data from other health care providers. The record-keeping system should allow for frequent update of information as well as easy retrieval of important data. The "Tickler" file of public health fame is a good method to use in the school system and is organized by date using a subsidiary color code system. The file should be set up with primary monthly guides and one or two sets of secondary guides. Planned follow-ups of health problems are listed day by day so the nurse can have ready reference to whatever problems require her attention.

Color coding, the subsidiary system, is used to identify a particular problem or concern. For example, if blue means polio, then a child who is due for his second oral polio vaccine would have a card in the file with a blue tag. If purple is assigned to vision problems, the child who is being observed because of a vision referral would have a purple tag.

To clarify the use of this system, we will suppose that Henry Silverman has a problem with hearing. During the hearing screening program, Henry did not respond to all the tones on the audiometer. The nurse will plan to recheck him in two weeks in case this failure resulted from a cold or allergy. A card is made out with Henry's name, grade, and teacher and is placed in the Tickler file at the appropriate date. It will be color coded orange, since that color has been assigned to hearing problems. As the nurse checks the Tickler each morning, she will retest Henry as originally planned. If he fails again, this will be noted on his cumulative record, and his parents will be notified. On the Tickler file card will be a simple notation: "Written notice to parents of possible hearing loss." The nurse will file the card for contact in a week. When the time arrives, she will check with the parent to determine what action has been taken. With this contact the nurse finds that the pediatrician has removed some earwax from Henry's ears. The nurse charts this on the cumulative health record, plans a recheck with the audiometer, and places Henry's card at the date decided on in the Tickler file. This process is repeated until the problem is resolved.

This system allows the school nurse to keep up with many concurrent cases. Information may be communicated as long as confidentiality remains secure. Written parental permission must be obtained before information is shared.

Nursing diagnoses

Nursing diagnoses are derived from health status data (Standard II).[8]

After exploring health problems and health needs through observation, interviews, and review of data that have been collected, the school nurse will analyze the information and arrive at a diagnosis. She will not rule out or make a differential diagnosis but will describe the student's state of health and her positive findings.

Nursing care plan

Plans for nursing service include goals derived from nursing diagnoses (Standard III).[8]

The school nurse arranges a conference with parents and student to discuss positive findings and to plan with them a course of action to alleviate or remedy the health problem. The nurse must estimate the abilities and readiness of the family members to recognize and cope with their own health problems. She must be aware of the family's resources or community resources that may be useful. Within the framework of available human and material resources, realistic goals are mutually set. A time period for achievement is agreed on by all. Sometimes the implementation of the agreed-on health goals can be accomplished by means of a contract.

Order set priorities

Plans for nursing service include priorities and nursing approaches or measures to achieve the goals derived from nursing diagnoses (Standard IV).

Nursing actions provide for consumer participation in health promotion, maintenance, and restoration (Standard V).[8]

The school nurse may give preventive or therapeutic treatment in the school setting with medical direction. By giving the family data necessary to make informed decisions, she may assist them to accept and assume responsibility for providing care and guide them toward self-help. She will help them to understand normal patterns of growth and development, and she and the family will share information about changes in health status. The nurse may have to assist in effecting change in the environment, particularly in relation to elimination or modification of health and/or safety hazards. In some instances she will help students and their families to adjust to their limitations.

Evaluate

Nursing actions assist consumers to maximize health potential (Standard VI).

The consumer's progress toward goal achievement is determined by the consumer and the nurse (Standard VII).[8]

The school nurse should evaluate whether opportunity was provided for the student and family to learn and to participate in the nursing process. Were nursing actions based on scientific principles? Using baseline data as well as current data on both nursing and consumer action, progress should be measured toward goal achievement.

Reorganize plan

Nursing actions involve ongoing reassessment, reordering of priorities, new goal setting, and revision of the nursing plan (Standard VIII).[8]

During a conference with the student and family, the nurse can discuss goal achievement or the lack of it. The decision to set new priorities and goals is jointly made by the family and the nurse. Determinations to try alternative actions or to terminate nursing service are mutually arrived at after reassessment and evaluation.

STUDY AND RESEARCH

The school nurse has a professional responsibility to keep abreast of change. To actively participate in professional organizations, read professional journals, attend continuing education programs, and to enroll periodically in formal classes are necessary to maintain a high level of competency. The nurse can identify and define problems for study in the school health field. She also should participate in conducting surveys, studies, and research related to her clinical and functional responsibilities.

QUALITY ASSURANCE

Just as adherence to nationally recognized standards ensures a professional approach to school health, the adoption of evaluation techniques leading to quality assurance also is of major concern. The tight budget situation in schools calls for accountability of expenditures. School boards have a right and a responsibility to demand cost-effective services, and nurses must prepare to prove that they are giving high-quality service for the lowest possible price. For the most part, cost effectiveness is not being measured in school systems. In many schools nurses are evaluated by the principal, who has little ability to judge quality nursing practice. The evaluation should include strengths and recommendations for improvement and should be done by someone who is in a position to evaluate *nursing* practice. The nurse must explain to school administrators the methods available, developed by nursing, to evaluate the practice objectively. The nurse must also look for ways to use nonprofessionals in the school health program when cost containment is a factor.

To determine what method of audit will be used, nursing service must decide what is to be evaluated: the nursing process, the outcome for the client, or a combination of the two.

After this decision is made, criteria for the evaluation must be established. Such criteria may be agreed on by the nursing staff or by a committee of administrators and nurses. Criteria should be objective and realistic for the particular school system and community. Each criterion should state the element to be measured, the standard (percentage), and any exceptions allowable. Once the criteria are established, actual practice is measured against them. This measurement must show the degree of compliance with the criteria. Following are several examples evaluating client outcome:

1. At the end of four weeks, 98% of the children enrolled in Edward School will have an established cumulative health record containing a medical, developmental, and immunization history.
2. Students who are prescribed glasses shall wear them as designated twenty out of any twenty-two observation days.
3. Adolescents who are pregnant, regardless of whether they are married, will have supportive prenatal care for the most healthful outcome for both mother and baby.

The audit may be done by the administrator or by peer review after a sample size has been determined. Actual practice findings should be analyzed in order that corrective action can be taken. After a reasonable time, corrective action must be followed up to assure that the deficiencies are really being rectified. For identified deficiencies, corrective action must not be punitive but should provide constructive suggestions to correct the deficiencies. These deficiencies may be remedied through in-service education, change in policies or proce-

dures, additional equipment, or in some instances one-to-one counseling.

The National Association of School Nurses of the NEA published an instrument for evaluation of the nursing process in the schools. It was designed to be used with the *Standard for School Nurse Services,* a companion publication. Following is an example of one criterion:

Health appraisal

1. Has conducted all required health assessment screening programs;
2. Uses information gathered from health assessment techniques to identify health problems;
3. Makes valid referrals to pupils, parents, and teachers.[9,p.6]

This method of evaluation has no time frame or quantitative measurement; the professional nurse can use her own judgment about time and measurement techniques.

If the nurse desires to evaluate both nursing process and student outcome according to functions, the following example might be helpful:

Function: Prevention of disease.
Expected outcome: Student will be fully immunized as early as possible and will participate in immunization booster clinic.
Time line: Within first semester or as arranged by local health department.
Nursing process: Provide parent and student with education regarding the value of immunization within the first ten weeks of school.
Criteria statement: Record audit shows that 90% of all students are immunized.
ANA standard: No. I.

SUMMARY

School nursing is an important service provided to our children. Society, however, has expressed a growing concern about the quality and effectiveness of many school health programs. Nurses must examine the role they play by asking themselves questions. Have I assessed the health needs of the children in my care? Am I providing a program that is basically preventive, and am I encouraging health promotion? Can I claim a reduction in the significant health problems of children such as accidents, emotional problems, obesity or undernutrition, pregnancy, venereal disease, and drug use? Obsolete practices must be eliminated. Perhaps a time-and-activity study would reveal the programs that need a revision.

In May, 1977, a national school health conference was held in Minneapolis. During the proceedings, a message was delivered by Joseph A. Califano, then Secretary of the Department of Health, Education, and Welfare, who said, "The President is interested in exploring these possibilities for using schools to provide a full range of services to children and families, including health and social services as well as education."[10] The theme of this message was that the federal government will be focusing existing and future resources for more equitable and proficient care to all school-age children. No other setting has the captive population, the educational resources, and the continuity of contact with vast numbers of youngsters that the school has.

The nurse who chooses this specialized field within community health practice can take credit for the future members of society who have increased health knowledge, follow good health maintenance habits, and practice responsible health behaviors.

NOTES

1. Cromwell, Gertrude E.: The nurse in the school health program, Philadelphia, 1963, W.B. Saunders Co.
2. Freeman, Ruth B.: Community health nursing practice, Philadelphia, 1970, W.B. Saunders Co.
3. Lowe, Charles U.: Health opportunities in schools, presented at the National School Health Conference, Minneapolis, May, 1977.
4. Fine, Louis, L., and Bellaire, Judith M.: The school nurse—an obsolete professional revisited, Pediatric Nursing 1(1):25-29, 1974.

5. McAtee, P.A.: Nurse practitioners in our public schools: an assessment of their expanded role as compared with school nurses, Clinical Pediatrics 13:360-362, 1974.
6. Hilmar, N.A., and McAtee, P.A.: The school nurse practitioner and her practice: a study of traditional and expanded health care responsibilities for nurses in elementary schools, Journal of School Health 43:431-441, 1973.
7. MacDonough, Georgia P.: Comparison of nursing roles, Journal of School Health 42:481-482, 1972.
8. Standards: community health nursing practice, Kansas City, Mo., 1973, American Nurses Association.
9. Evaluation instruments for school nursing services, Department of School Nurses, National Commission on Standards, Washington, D.C., 1972, National Education Association.
10. Califano, Joseph A., Jr.: School health, presented at the National School Health Conference, Minneapolis, May, 1977.

BIBLIOGRAPHY

Califano, Joseph A., Jr.: School health, presented at the National School Health Conference, Minneapolis, May, 1977.

Cromwell, Gertrude E.: The nurse in the school health program, Philadelphia, 1963, W.B. Saunders Co.

Evaluation instruments for school nursing services, Department of School Nurses, National Commission on Standards, Washington, D.C., 1972, National Education Association.

Fine, Louis L., and Bellaire, Judith M.: The school nurse—an obsolete professional revisited, Pediatric Nursing 1(1):25-29, 1974.

Freeman, Ruth B.: Community health nursing practice, Philadelphia, 1970, W.B. Saunders Co.

Hilmar, N.A., and McAtee, P.A.: The school nurse practitioner and her practice: a study of traditional and expanded health care responsibilities for nurses in elementary schools, Journal of School Health 43:431-441, 1973.

Lowe, Charles U.: Health opportunities in schools, presented at the National School Health Conference, Minneapolis, May, 1977.

Macdonough, Georgia P.: Comparison of nursing roles, Journal of School Health: 42:481-482, 1972.

McAtee, P.A.: Nurse practitioners in our public schools: an assessment of their expanded role as compared with school nurses, Clinical Pediatrics 13:360-362, 1974.

Standards: community health nursing practice, Kansas City, Mo., 1973, American Nurses Association.

Wold, Susan J.: School nursing: a framework for practice, St. Louis, 1981, The C.V. Mosby Co.

16

HEALTH NEEDS AND NURSING CARE OF THE LABOR FORCE

MARJORIE J. KELLER

The occupational setting is one area of nursing in which great latitude is available for health promotion and maintenance and disease prevention. Since World War II, tremendous strides have been made in implementing employee health programs in manufacturing, service, and commercial establishments. A majority of programs, however, tends to concentrate on providing emergency care. With the current pressure to study hazards to health from within the work setting and to expand the nursing contribution to health care, the role and functions of the nurse are enlarging and changing.

Occupational health nursing is the application of nursing and public health philosophy and skills to the relationship of people to their occupations for the purpose of prevention of disease and injury and the promotion of optimal health, productivity, and social adjustment. This definition is a modification and combination of statements made by Brown[1] and Page.[2] Page goes on to identify five branches of health care that are essential to the practice of a health professional in industry: (1) preventive, (2) educative, (3) constructive (promotive), (4) curative, and (5) habilitative.[2] A sixth area should be added: prospective, that of predicting the potential for development of disease and illness based on one's exposure to risk factors. These statements are the dimensions used in discussing the role of the occupational health nurse in this chapter.

A broad approach has been used here to describe the current state of occupational health nursing and its potential for nurses to make a full contribution to the health of employees. There is great diversity in the level of care provided by nurses in the work setting. The range is from strictly emergency care for occupational injuries and illnesses to full-scale programs for prevention and treatment of disease using innovative means of care. Nursing is changing, and nurses are recognized for their contributions in planning and implementation of health care for individuals. Several reasons are forcing these changes in philosophy:

1. Emphasis on developing the area of primary health care delivery
2. Need to decrease health care costs
3. Evolving philosophy of early detection of illness and disease and initiating alternative modalities of treatment
4. Increasing focus on promotion of health and prevention of disease

5. Increasing recognition of the detrimental influences in a work setting on worker-family-community health
6. Availability of nurses prepared to intervene in physical, emotional, social, economic, and spiritual needs of individuals
7. Rapid increase and acceptance of nurses prepared in expanded roles
8. Proven cost effectiveness of prevention programs and health education in the labor force

INFLUENCES ON THE PRACTICE OF THE NURSE

The scope of practice of an occupational health nurse is influenced by a number of characteristics within the work setting. Probably the overriding influence is the policy established by management and administrative personnel within the occupational health program. The philosophy and vision of these administrative persons can make or break the contribution of the nurse and the development of her full potential. A key question here is, how much input does the occupational health nurse have in establishing policies relating to the scope of the health program?

The nurse has the opportunity for having the best knowledge of and insight into the health of the employees, both as persons *and* as employees and usually is the first health professional contacted within the health program. The ability of the nurse to hear, see, and sense beyond the chief complaint of the individual worker is crucial to developing a depth of comprehension about health needs of the plant. It follows that one with this information must have input into determination of planning, implementing, and evaluating the occupational health program.

Several barriers may prohibit the nurse's participation. A major barrier may be the inability of the nurse to interpret and communicate health needs to business administration. This problem may be a factor particularly in business establishments with only one or two nurses. In plants in which a number of nurses are employed, their input may be limited, or, if welcomed, may be minimized in its importance. The ability to identify health needs, communicate these needs, and develop strategies for intervention is an essential skill for the occupational health nurse. Management, labor, and professional nurses can work together to establish

Table 16-1. Major characteristics of the work setting

People factors	Environmental factors
Essentially a well population	Purpose of setting other than health-oriented
Long-term contact	Deal with increasingly mobile population
Specific age grouping	Period of rapid change due to social and technological factors
Population in setting for major portion of waking hours	Major influences from the environment on the health of the population
Care influences families by dealing with one family member	Community-based
Influence on growth and development of an individual	Independent functioning of nurse from other health and nursing personnel
Major contribution of nurse through teaching and counseling	Large population groups for mass programs, i.e., screening and immunizations
Need for knowledge about behavioral, emotional, and clinical deviations of employees, especially those directly affecting the working process	Use of one or two nurse units or a large health team composed primarily of nonhealth professionals
	Associate with top management

Combined factors
Promotional, preventive, and curative function
"Captive" population in circumscribed geographical area

health policies. The health service is usually a part of personnel services and is considered a consultant resource for both management and labor. Also appropriate is that the occupational health nurse have an ongoing working relationship with the person who is responsible for plant safety.

Other characteristics that influence the role of the nurse fall into three categories: people-oriented factors, environment-oriented factors, and a combination of the two (Table 16-1).

GOAL OF AN OCCUPATIONAL HEALTH PROGRAM

Tinkham[3] has set forth one goal for occupational health programs as ''the promotion and maintenance of the highest degree of physical, social, and emotional well-being of workers in all occupations.'' She identifies three basic steps that enable a nursing program to move in this direction: (1) full acceptance of a workable broad definition of health, (2) the need to know and understand what nursing can contribute to the health of employees and their families by thinking in terms of groups of workers and their health needs, and (3) the need to serve as a health advocate for workers in all health matters.[3]

The format for this chapter includes the responsibilities of an occupational health nurse shown in terms of competencies needed by the nurse with suggested actions for breaking out of the traditional mold. Following this information, selected current concepts relevant to the occupational health nurse will be discussed, including the expanded role of the nurse (health assessment, screening, monitoring, health education, and counseling), family health care, the self-responsible consumer, growth and development of adults, and alternative modalities leading to high-level wellness.

PRESENT AND POTENTIAL CONSUMERS OF CARE

As dull as statistics can be, I believe that one must grasp the extent of the population to be served. According to Bureau of Census[4] data, in 1980 there were nearly 102 million persons in the civilian labor force in the United States. The projected number of employees for 1990 is 116 million. Of the 102 million persons, approximately 61% were men, and 39% were women. The breakdown according to race was 88% white and 12% black and other. The number (in millions) according to age distribution follows:

Ages	Males	Females
16-19	5.1	4.1
20-24	8.2	6.1
25-34	14.5	8.5
35-44	10.6	6.5
45-54	10.5	6.7
55-64	7.0	4.2
65+	1.9	1.0

Projected figures for 1990 indicate significant increase of both male and female employees in the age range of 25 to 44. These employees work in establishments ranging from one and two employ-

Table 16-2. Employees by type of industry*

TYPE OF INDUSTRY	PERCENT OF EMPLOYEES IN 1975
Professional, technical, and kindred workers	15.0
Managers, officials, and proprietors	10.5
Clerical and kindred workers	17.8
Salesworkers	6.4
Craftsmen and foremen	12.9
Operatives	15.2
Nonfarm laborers	4.9
Private household workers	1.4
Service workers, except private households†	12.4
Farmers and farm managers	1.9
Farm laborers and foremen	1.6

*From U.S. Department of Labor: Employment and training report of the president, 1976, Washington, D.C., 1976, U.S. Government Printing Office; U.S. Department of Commerce, Bureau of the Census: Social indicators, 1976, Washington, D.C., 1977, U.S. Government Printing Office.
† Includes repair, business, and personal services; entertainment and recreation; professional; and related, that is, health education, welfare, and religious.

ees to a population group of thousands. Frequently when one thinks of employees, the first thought is of large manufacturing plants, large insurance companies, and federal, state, and local governmental facilities. How is the labor force actually distributed according to numbers of employees by size of establishment? Social and Economic Statistics[5] from the Bureau of Census reveal that approximately 75% of all employees work in settings with fewer than 500 employees, approximately 9% in settings with between 500 and 1,000 employees, and 16% in settings with over 1,000 employees.

What are the categories of types of business endeavors in which people work and have health needs? Table 16-2 shows the broad range of sources of income for the working population of the United States in 1975. An estimate of numbers of employees for each category is noted.

Such a diverse population presents the potential for a great variety of health problems. For example, a look at the age breakdown reveals late adolescents with their many maturational crises; young adults facing the basic need to establish a family and to select and pursue a career; middle-aged adults with the need to support a family, develop community ties, and rise in the pursuit of a career, while coping with biological/psychological changes associated with menopause in women and midlife crisis in men; the older age group of employees with a chronic illness already present or the possibility of developing one; and retired employees.

One can already begin to identify some of the

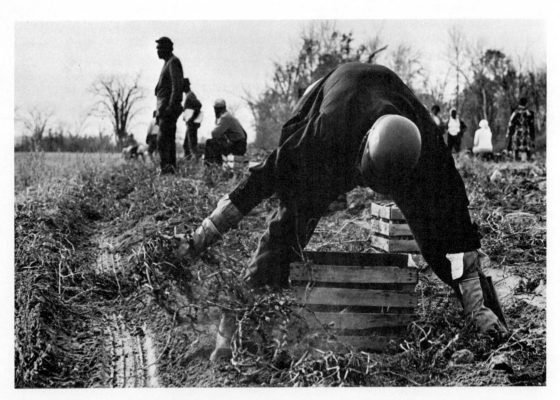

Fig. 16-1. Migrant farm workers have traditionally been denied access to health care and health insurance as employment benefits. (Photograph by Roger B. Smith; courtesy Editorial Photocolor Archives, Inc., New York.)

many health needs of these 102 million people that are based only on sex or race.

The Department of Health, Education, and Welfare estimated in the mid-1960s that only approximately 20% of the employed population had access to health services in the work setting. In spite of interest in the environment and much money being directed into health services, it is open to question whether this figure has been improved.

Moreover, business establishments of fewer than 500 employees generally do not have access to organized health services in the work setting (Fig. 16-1). When one hears ''occupational health'' and ''health of employees,'' the tendency is to focus one's thinking on large industrial plants that have developed health departments. But what of the plants with between 200 and 500 employees? In greater need of consideration are the small concerns with fewer than 200 employees. Another facet is the strong possibility that no nurse is available to the employee, as in establishments with fewer than 500 persons. Some health departments and visiting nurse services have developed part-time nursing services for small industry, but this is a model that has not caught on. I believe that this concept should be developed in every community health agency in order to begin meeting the needs of all employees. Nurses have much work to do to come close to meeting the health needs of employees.

INFLUENCES ON THE HEALTH OF EMPLOYEES IN THE WORK SETTING

The employment site has been and will continue to be influenced by increasing development of high technology, automation, and computerization. This will result in ever increasing physical, chemical, and biological hazards, especially in view in high rates of worker mobility and employment turnover. Kahn and Weiner[6] have projected a hundred significant technological innovations by the year 2000.

Two major sets of factors influence the health of workers at the work site: environmental factors and policy factors. Both sets have health-promoting and health-deterring elements (Table 16-3). The positive influences have tended to receive much publicity from management, and it is right that they

Table 16-3. Influences on the health of employees at the work site (not all-inclusive)

ENVIRONMENTAL		POLICY	
HEALTH-PROMOTING	**HEALTH-DETERRING**	**HEALTH-PROMOTING**	**HEALTH-DETERRING**
Meaningful, purposeful work	Injury/illness-causing conditions, i.e., unprotected machinery, toxic substances (gases, fumes, dusts, chemicals), heavy lifting, exposure to sun, exposure to cold, noise/vibration, radiation, welding, prolonged sitting/standing, poor ventilation	Adequate health-medical insurance	Mobility: frequent transfers necessitating family or inplant relocation
Satisfaction-producing work		Job security	Work shift rotation
Adequate financial reward with fringe benefits		Application of principles of ergonomics	Philosophy of crisis health care
Growth-producing work, both personal and professional		Opportunity for personal and professional growth	Bypassing/side-stepping regulations and standards established by governmental/industrial researchers
Safe environment	Emotional/intellectual stressors, i.e., routine repetitive tasks, unemployment, hazardous tasks, inplant/department conflict, excessive mobility/travel	Philosophy of health promotion and health maintenance	
Congenial co-workers		Compliance with standards established by governmental and industrial researchers	

Table 16-4. Means of contact and entry of toxic agents*

MODE OF CONTACT/ ENTRY	ACTIONS	EXAMPLES
Skin contact (very common)	Toxic agent may 1. React with skin surfaces and cause primary irritation 2. Penetrate skin, conjugate with tissue protein, and effect skin sensitization 3. Penetrate skin through folliculosebaceous route, enter bloodstream, and act as systemic poison 4. Enter through open wounds	Acids/alkalis Soaps Bacteria Waxes Inks/dyes Solvents Heat/cold
Inhalation (very common)		

Particles	Toxic agent contacts or enters through respiratory system
	Degree of toxicity affected by
	1. Size, density, and solubility of particles
	2. Rate and depth of breathing; anatomy and dimensions of respiratory system
	3. Amount of physical activity occurring during inhalation
	4. Temperature of environment and humidity
	5. Biochemical productivity of components
		Particulate matter
		  Dusts: silica, coal dust
		  Fumes: volatization
		    from molten metals
		  Mists: sprayed paint, oil
		    mists
		  Fog: supersaturation of
		    water vapor in air

Gas, fumes, and vapors	Toxic agent contacts or enters through respiratory system
	Degree of toxicity affected by
	1. Solubility of gas in aqueous environment of respiratory tract
	2. Absorption into bloodstream determined by concentrate of agent in inhaled air
	3. Rate of elimination by body
	4. Nature and degree of exposure
		Gas: carbon disulfide,
		  volatile hydrocarbons,
		  saturated ketones
		Vapor: gasoline, iodine

Ingestion (less common than skin contact and inhalation)	Toxic agent may be 1. Absorbed from gastrointestinal into blood 2. Passively ingested from inhaled substances that lodge in upper respiratory tract and are swallowed by ciliary action	Lead Arsenic Mercury

*Modified from Stokinger, Herbert E.: Routes of entry and modes of action. In Key, Marcus M., et al., editors: Occupational diseases— a guide to their recognition, Washington, D.C., 1977, U.S. Government Printing Office.

should; however, the health-deterring factors had been glossed over until the past decade. Attention to identifying and resolving the hazards to health in industry has mushroomed as a result of the consumer advocate movement and increased union interest. Almost daily the news media report on another hazard to health, such as vinyl chloride and its relationship to carcinoma of the liver, kepone and its influence on the nervous system, and stress as a causative factor in cardiovascular disease.

The DHHS[7] carried out much work on identi-

fication of toxic substances causing occupational disease in three major categories—chemical, physical, and biological—and in development of permissible exposure limit standards for safe use of these substances. Table 16-4 describes action of toxic agents. More recently much work has been done to establish toxicity levels and standards for use of toxic agents. Reports of these studies are readily available in most libraries, state health departments, and relevant industries.

Stellman and Daum[8] list exposures to hazards

by occupation. For example, the following exposures are listed for hospital workers, including physicians and nurses: anesthetics (ethyl bromide, ethyl chloride, ethyl ether, halothane, methoxyflurane, and nitrous oxide), antibiotics, antiseptics, beryllium, cobalt, detergents, disinfectants and germicides, drugs, fungicides, infections (bacteria and viruses, especially hepatitis), iodine, isopropyl alcohol, moisture, radiation, and tricresyl phosphate (in sterilizing surgical instruments). These are only the agent types of exposures; what about such hazards as excessive stress, lifting, overwork, interpersonal conflicts, lack of satisfaction, shift work, long hours, dealing with difficult patients and their families, and facing terminal illness?

The 1977 conference of the American Public Health Association was a forum for many presentations about hazards to the health of employees. The discussion included such topics as health hazards in the arts and crafts, occupational cancer, and estimating the magnitude of occupationally related mortality.

Shift work was studied for effect on family, social life, and physical and mental health. Results showed that

the time of the day or night and the time of the week designated for work bore a direct relationship to certain aspects of family life and social participation . . . and that the greater the difficulty he experienced in adjusting his time-oriented body functions [sleeping, eating, bowel habits] to his shift, the poorer his physical health.[9,pp.297-298]

The World Health Organization has proposed several activities for the period of 1978 to 1989 related to the work environment. These activities are (1) early detection of health impairment in occupational and work-related diseases, (2) evaluation and control of occupational health and safety hazards, (3) evaluation of toxic substances and development of maximum permissible limit standards, and (4) promotion of knowledge and use of work physiology, psychology, and ergonomics.[10]

The technology of ergonomics will play an in-creasing part in the relationship of the worker and his job. Ergonomics, an applied science combining knowledge of biomedicine and engineering, has several dimensions: (1) recognition of a person's structure, functions, and abilities and using them to design methods of work, tools, and the working environment with resulting decrease in effort and fatigue; (2) modification of work rather than adjustment of people to work; and (3) focus on protecting the worker rather than increasing production, although the change could result in greater production.[11] Nurses as workers could begin to think about how they could redesign some aspects of their work to make the job easier and more satisfying.

In 1970, the overall responsibility for assuring a safe and healthful work environment was relegated to a newly created agency within the United States Department of Labor: the Occupational Safety and Health Administration (OSHA). In addition, the National Institute of Occupational Health and Safety (NIOSH) within the structure of the DHHS (Department of Health and Human Services) was given the responsibility for research and education related to influences on health within the work setting. State governments, usually within the departments of health and/or labor, have the charge of carrying out enforcement at the local level. However, these agencies usually are under fire from consumer advocate groups for lack of an aggressive stance in enforcing standards for the protection of employee health. In addition, continual efforts are made to undermine and weaken the breadth and responsibilities of OSHA, particularly by the Reagan administration, which appears to believe that OSHA and other similar regulatory agencies are not performing an essential or even necessary function. The nurse should become aware of the movements underway among consumer advocate groups for modifying this situation. It is not necessary to spell out specific strategies because national meetings and the mass media perform that service adequately.

Data collection forms abound to survey an environment. Tinkham[12] has developed a tool relevant to nursing for studying the work setting. Another form for collecting data about a specific condition is described by Stellman and Daum.[8] This particular form was developed for use by unions but could be of use to the occupational health nurse.

The reader is encouraged to look around the environment and identify positive and negative influences on health. A description of such an exercise for learning has been discussed previously in the literature.[13]

Occupational health nurses must know about the influence on the health of employees in their work setting. Unless they know potential health-promoting and health-deterring factors, their approach to care could well center on curative or emergency care only.

RESPONSIBILITIES OF AN OCCUPATIONAL HEALTH NURSE

A variety of books and chapters have been written over the years about the role of the occupational health nurse and have served as the basis for present day practice.[1,14-16] Unfortunately, much of the role as described in these publications remains to be fully implemented.

The most recent publication spelling out the role of the nurse was done in the late 1960s as a component of a larger project.[17] Leavell and Clark's[18] levels of prevention and Maslow's[19] hierarchy of needs system were selected for defining the competencies of the professional nurse in occupational health. Table 16-5 and Fig. 16-2 are taken from the monograph and show the dimensions used in defining competencies.[17] The resultant framework that was developed from the meshing of these two theories is composed of twenty-five categories, each labeled with one level of prevention and one need. The categories range from "Health Promotion—Physiological" to "Rehabilitation—Self-actualization" (Table 16-6).[17] To further increase the scope of the identified competencies, the concept of a health cycle was used (Fig. 16-3). The

health cycle begins with the "well-productive citizen"; moving counterclockwise, there is a recognition of some need for health care. This need may range from a splinter or dental caries to chest pain or even a malignant growth. Care/treatment may be sought from health providers such as physicians, dentists, nurses/nurse practitioners, and osteopaths. There may or may not be hospitalization. After this, the consumer returns home to the care of his family or friends. The next stage is socializing outside the home: going to the market, to church, to meetings, and to social functions. This stage may prove to be the hardest step of the entire process. The return to work/school is the final step before the consumer again becomes a well-productive citizen. The occupational health nurse may be involved with the consumer at any stage in this cycle, including hospital or home visits.

Now look in Table 16-6 at the category labeled "Health Promotion—Physiological." Three identified competencies are noted with actions that a nurse can implement to meet the competencies. For example, she uses the well-recognized step in the problem-solving process (data collection), then moves forward to the planning and implementing/intervening stages of the process. The competencies and suggested nursing actions of the evaluation phase have been identified with the self-actualization component for each level of prevention. Table 16-6 should be reviewed carefully. The professional nurse should be held accountable by the employer, employees, and public for performance of these competencies.

In addition to the identification of competencies and suggested nursing actions, the same monograph[17] delineated the knowledge and skills needed by a nurse to practice the competencies.

For detailed discussion of the activities of the occupational health nurse, the reader is referred to the references cited at the end of this chapter; for information concerning Workman's Compensation, to the state or local workman's compensation office. *Text continued on p. 417.*

Table 16-5. Levels of prevention applied to occupational health*

HEALTH PROMOTION (DIRECTED CHIEFLY AT HOST, SECONDARILY AT AGENT)	SPECIFIC PROTECTION (DIRECTED AT CONTROL OF ENVIRONMENT)	EARLY DIAGNOSIS AND PROMPT TREATMENT (DIRECTED AT ADULT POPULATION)	DISABILITY LIMITATION	REHABILITATION
1. Fitting job to worker Preplacement examination including physical and emotional evaluation 2. Health counseling 3. Mental health aspects Satisfactions Morale Attitude 4. Physiological machine design Safety features Ease of using 5. Worker hygiene Cleanliness Food handling and service Rest service	1. Toxic hazards Route: skin, GI tract, respiratory system Agent: liquids, solids, mists, vapors, aerosols, fumes, dusts 2. Radiation 3. Accident prevention (physical hazards) 4. Communicable disease control (immunizations) 5. Environmental health promotion Ventilation Lighting Temperature Noise 6. Plant housekeeping and sanitary facilities	1. Occupational disability revealed in first aid records and medical reports 2. Nonoccupational disability based on absenteeism for minor illness	1. Preplacement and periodic examinations 2. Referrals 3. Proper handling of cases found with disease or disability 4. Estimation of productive capacity of worker (follow-up and such supervision as needed to limit disability and enable continuing to work until retirement)	1. Psychological trauma 2. Reevaluation of capabilities and placement accordingly

*From Keller, Marjorie J., in association with May, W.T.: Occupational health content in baccalaureate nursing education, Cincinnati, 1971, National Institute of Occupational Safety; modified from Leavell, Hugh Rodman, and Clark, E. Gurney: Preventive medicine for the doctor in his community—an epidemiologic approach, ed. 3, New York, 1965, McGraw-Hill Book Co.

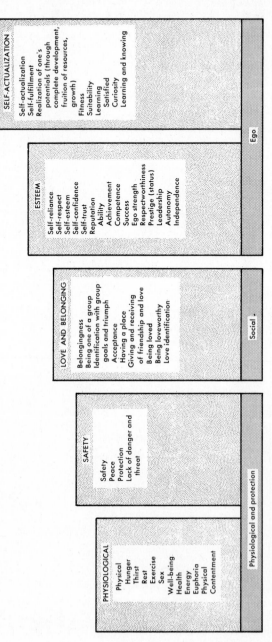

Fig. 16-2. Common human needs based on Maslow's hierarchical motivation theory. (Modified from Maslow, Abraham H.: Motivation and personality, New York, 1954, Harper & Row, Publishers; Keller, Marjorie J., in association with May, W.T.: Occupational health content in baccalaureate nursing education, Cincinnati, 1971, National Institute of Occupational Safety and Health.)

Table 16-6. Competencies and suggested nursing actions of the occupational health nurse*

MASLOW'S NEEDS	Competency	LEAVELL AND CLARK'S LEVELS OF PREVENTION
		HEALTH PROMOTION
		Suggested nursing action
Physiological	Assesses physical health needs of employees	Identifies physical health needs by observation, interview, analysis of records, reports, examinations; correlates identified needs and age grouping; identifies groups of employees with special physical health needs
	Collaborates in planning for health promotion and maintenance in work setting	Participates on health team in formulating philosophy and objectives for meeting needs of employees based on current standards and established policies; communicates health needs of employees to health team; interprets occupational health nursing as a member of the intraplant and extraplant health team
	Intervenes to promote health maintenance	Organizes nursing aspects of health screening and evaluation program; conducts health interview; conducts screening tests, e.g., vital signs, electrocardiogram, laboratory tests, vision and hearing tests; assists physician in physical examination procedures, e.g., draping, chaperoning; maintains records and reports for well employees; interprets examination findings to employee; guides employee to improved health habits through counseling, teaching, and demonstration, e.g., personal hygiene, diet, dental and general health care, rest, recreation; promotes positive attitudes toward health and health care among employees, family; interprets health-related information
Safety	Collaborates in assessing safety needs of employee and family	Identifies safety needs through observation, interview, and analysis of records and reports; identifies patterns of accident susceptibility; evaluates employee's environment for effectiveness of safety measures
	Intervenes to promote security of employee and family from economic stress due to occupational injury	Interprets health and medical insurance plans; identifies patterns of health needs from analysis of records and reports and utilization of health care services; assists in compiling medical insurance claims; estimates impact of illness on family from claim data
Social	Assesses social health needs of employee and family	Identifies health need relating to social adaptation of employee and family through observation, interview, analysis of records and reports; correlates identified needs and developmental level and age grouping of employee; analyzes employee-employee relationships; analyzes employer-employee relationships; analyzes employee-family relationships; identifies groups of employees with special needs
	Collaborates in planning and intervenes to promote social adaptation of employee and family	Collaborates in providing setting conducive to adaptation; interprets effect of total environment on health of employee and family; guides employee and family in social adaptation through counseling, interviewing, teaching, demonstration

Continued.

*From Keller, Marjorie J., in association with May, W.T.: Occupational health content in baccalaureate nursing education, Cincinnati, 1971, National Institute of Occupational Safety and Health; modified from Leavell, Hugh Rodman, and Clark, E. Gurney: Preventive medicine for the doctor in his community—an epidemiologic approach, ed. 3, New York, McGraw-Hill Book Co.: and Maslow, Abraham H: Motivation and personality, New York, 1954, Harper & Row, Publishers; Public Health Service Publication No. 2176.

Table 16-6. Competencies and suggested nursing actions of the occupational health nurse—cont'd

MASLOW'S NEEDS	LEAVELL AND CLARK'S LEVELS OF PREVENTION	
	HEALTH PROMOTION—cont'd	
	Competency	**Suggested nursing action**
Social—cont'd	Collaborates in planning health maintenance activities for total community health program	Interprets occupational health nursing to community; communicates health needs of employee and family; coordinates occupational health program with organized community health program
Psychological	Assesses emotional health needs of employees	Identifies needs of employees through observation, interview, analysis of records; correlates identified needs and developmental level and age grouping; identifies groups of employees with special health needs
	Collaborates in planning and intervening to promote emotional health	Communicates identified needs to health team; interprets effects of total environment on emotional health of well, productive citizen; guides employee and family through counseling, interviewing, teaching, demonstration; collaborates in providing setting conducive to good emotional health
Self-actualization	Assesses growth needs and health potential of employees	Identifies growth needs and health potential of employee through observation, interview, analysis of records; correlates identified needs and developmental level
	Collaborates in planning and intervenes to promote growth	Communicates identified needs to health team; guides employee to attainment of growth through interviewing, counseling, teaching, and demonstration; provides nursing leadership in planning recreational and self-development programs in plant and community; promotes self-responsibility for health and health care; recognizes health team as members of the labor force and as individuals
	Participates in and conducts systematic studies relating to health of employees	Identifies health problems of employee and family in need of study; initiates studies and projects using systematic research methodology
	Collaborates in evaluating the total health promotion and health evaluation program	Appraises program and services based on philosophy, objectives, current standards, and policies; predicts future health needs and problems of employee, family, community, work environment; revises program and services based on changing needs and utilization of services; analyzes relationship of nursing to other health team members—in-plant and community; evaluates nursing program based on philosophy, objectives, policies, legally recognized practice standards, and independent and dependent nursing functions; evaluates own performance and personal and professional development; estimates budget needs for nursing program; keeps abreast of current thinking and direction of changes in nursing and delivery of health care
	SPECIFIC PROTECTION	
Physiological	Collaborates in assessing the work setting for hazards to physical health	Identifies physical hazards to employee and family; observes and examines employee to prevent toxicity from environmental exposure; observes work environment for needed control measures; correlates relationship of employee health and physical environment; identifies aspects in work setting promoting health of employee

Safety	Collaborates in providing a safe environment	Serves as a member of the safety team; communicates safety needs and effect of environmental hazards on employee and family to safety and health team; recommends and promotes use of protective side measures and equipment; observes adherence to sanitation and food-handling regulations; guides employee and family in developing positive attitudes toward safety and protection; guides employee and family in safety education through counseling, teaching, and demonstration; analyzes patterns of symptomology from records and reports; communicates health needs for transcontinental and intercontinental travel to health team and individuals involved
	Collaborates in providing program to control communicable disease in work setting	Identifies need for immunizations based on travel regulations, agency recommendations, and inplant data; administers immunizing agents as prescribed; evaluates and refers employees with communicable disease conditions for medical care
	Collaborates in planning control programs for community health problems	Recognizes influence of work environment on community health; analyzes community-plant relationship; communicates need for control programs to inplant and extraplant health teams; assists in planning inplant and community programs for disasters
Social	Collaborates in assessing influence of social aspects of work environment on health	Identifies influences on health of employees from work setting; analyzes social influences from work setting and employee-family relationships on health of employee
Psychological	Collaborates in assessing influences on employee emotional health from work environment	Observes work environment for influences on emotional health of employee and family; identifies personal characteristics of employees in hazardous, stressful, and routine job operations; communicates special health needs of employees in hazardous, stressful, and routine jobs; analyzes emotional influences from work setting and employee-family relationships; predicts psychological effects of change in work environment on employees and families
Self-actualization	Participates in and conducts systematic studies relating to environment	Identifies health problems present in environment; initates studies and projects using systematic research methodology; applies findings in environmental control; communicates findings to health team and interested individuals and groups; participates in interdisciplinary studies and projects
	Collaborates in evaluating total program for environmental control	Appraises program based on philosophy, objectives, legal requirements, and policies; predicts future environmental problems; revises program based on health needs and utilization and results of program; evaluates nursing contribution to environmental control program based on philosophy, objectives, and independent and dependent functions

EARLY DIAGNOSIS AND PROMPT TREATMENT

Physiological	Provides emergency care for physical injury and illness	Recognizes legal limitations for nursing; recognizes signs and symptoms of pathological conditions; carries out nursing diagnostic procedures to establish need for care; administers emergency care, e.g., aseptic techniques for lacerations, removing foreign bodies, splinting, administering oxygen, administering medication; communicates by interpreting pathological processes and implications to health team or appropriate individuals; provides for continuing care, e.g., medical treatment, return visits, transportation; begins rehabilitation process; maintains appropriate records and reports; organizes nonprofessional first-aid services
	Intervenes to assist employee seeking medical care for identified disease process	Communicates with health facility; refers employee for continuing health and nursing care; guides employee in obtaining and carrying out medical care; follow-up on employee with illness

Continued.

Table 16-6. Competencies and suggested nursing actions of the occupational health nurse—cont'd

MASLOW'S NEEDS	LEAVELL AND CLARK'S LEVELS OF PREVENTION	
	EARLY DIAGNOSIS AND PROMPT TREATMENT—cont'd	
	Competency	**Suggested nursing action**
Safety	Collaborates in providing safe environment for employee with limited health problem	Identifies the demands on employee's health of job operation, e.g., stress, heavy lifting, walking, toxic materials; communicates health status of employee to health team or appropriate individuals; recommends placement of employee for employee's and co-workers' safety; observes employee for satisfactory placement
	Collaborates in promoting security of employee and family from economic stress due to occupational illness or injury	Complies with Workman's Compensation Act; maintains appropriate records and reports
Social	Collaborates in assessing and providing service to control influence from employee and group disorganization or social change on health of employee	Identifies health problems of employees related to disorganization or social change; recognizes effects of disorganization or social change on employee; work setting and community; analyzes influence of social change or disorganization on health and behavior patterns of employee and family; communicates to health team effects of social change causing disorganization; guides employee and family in coping with effects of social change or disorganization
	Collaborates in assessing and providing services for control of short-term absence	Identifies employee with high rate of absences from records and reports; identifies causes of behavior patterns from study of total environment; guides employee in seeking remedial care; determines causes of absence of employee and interprets to appropriate individuals
Psychological	Provides emergency care for emotional crisis of employee	Identifies immediate stressors and symptoms of and reactions to crisis; establishes and maintains therapeutic nurse-patient relationship; reduces anxiety level of employee, family, co-workers; provides emotional support; refers employee for continuing health and nursing care; communicates needs of employee to health team or appropriate individuals
	Assesses effect of stress on employee	Identifies signs and symptoms of stress and tension; communicates needs of employee to health team or appropriate individuals
Self-actualization	Creates climate conducive for employee to seek health care	Demonstrates attitude of acceptance of employee; provides assistance needed for employee to recognize and meet own health needs
		DISABILITY LIMITATION
Physiological	Provides care to relieve signs and symptoms of illness and injury	Identifies employees with long-term illness; develops nursing care plan based on identified needs; carries out medical directives, e.g., dressing changes, administration of medication, rest periods; performs technical nursing skills, e.g., checking vital signs, heat or cold applications; observes employee for progressing signs of disease process; communicates employee's condition to health team or appropriate individuals; collaborates in providing continuing health and nursing care; evaluates employee's and family's understanding of physical aspects of disease conditions, their understandings

Safety	Collaborates in providing safe environment for employee with disease process	of medical orders and ability to carry out; teaches skills and provides information relating to care of employee, e.g., temperatures, administration of medications, dressing changes
		Identifies the demands on employee's health of job operations; communicates health status of employee to health team or appropriate individuals; recommends placement of employee for employee's and co-worker's safety; observes employee for satisfactory job placement; recognizes effect of prescribed drugs on employee
Social	Assesses socioeconomic needs of employee and family with disease process	Observes employee and family for effects of illness; observes effect of employee's illness on work setting; identifies problems of employee and family coping with disease process, economic stress, social limitations; assists in compiling insurance claims
	Collaborates on planning and intervenes to enable adaptation of employee and family to illness	Observes employee and family in their total environment; guides employee and family in coping with effects of illness; communicates needs of employee and family to health team or appropriate individuals; guides employee and family in establishing new socialization patterns; collaborates in continuing health and nursing care through guidance, follow-up, support; assesses employee's and family's socioeconomic needs during absence from work
Psychological	Assesses emotional needs of employee and family where employee has disease	Observes psychological effect of illness on employee and family; observes psychological effect of employee's illness on co-workers; identifies employee and family problems in coping with disease process, emotional stress; evaluates employee's and family's understanding of emotional aspects of illness
	Plans and intervenes to enable employee and family to cope with emotional aspects of illness	Provides emotional support; guides employee, family, and co-workers in adjusting to illness; guides employee and family during terminal illness
	Provides care for employee with mental illness	Recognizes psychopathological process; communicates needs of employee and family to health team or appropriate individuals; guides employee and family in obtaining medical care; collaborates in providing continuing care, e.g., provision of meaningful activity, transportation, follow-up, emotional support; guides employee and family in meeting physiological and safety needs; guides co-workers associated with employee
Self-actualization	Collaborates in providing opportunity for meeting growth potential needs of employee	Identifies opportunity for continued growth of employee; communicates identified needs of employee
	Collaborates in evaluating total program for ill and injured employees	Appraises program based on philosophy, objectives, and policies; predicts future needs and changes in health care delivery; revises program based on changing needs and utilization of service; evaluates nursing contribution based on nursing philosophy and objectives, policies, legally recognized practice standards, independent and dependent nursing functions

REHABILITATION

Physiological	Collaborates in assessing physical needs	Identifies remaining abilities through observation, interview, records and reports, and testing; communicates abilities to appropriate individuals; interprets philosophy of rehabilitation
	Plans and intervenes to promote fullest functioning	Applies principles of activities of daily living to work setting; administers selected physical therapy, e.g., exercises, hydrotherapy, heat applications, supportive equipment; teaches self/help skills, e.g., transportation, housekeeping, personal care, transfer; com-

Continued.

Table 16-6. Competencies and suggested nursing actions of the occupational health nurse—cont'd

MASLOW'S NEEDS	Competency	LEAVELL AND CLARK'S LEVELS OF PREVENTION REHABILITATION—cont'd Suggested nursing action
Physiological—cont'd		municates identified needs to health team or appropriate individuals; collaborates in providing continuing health and nursing care
Safety	Collaborates in providing safety of environment	Observes employee's total environment for safety and adaptation for independent functioning; analyzes attitudes of employee toward safety; collaborates as described under disability limitation safety and protection in placement of employee; observes employee for suitable placement in work setting
Social	Assesses socioeconomic needs of employee and family	Identifies problems of employee in work setting and of employee and family in home and community; observes employee and family in coping with the social setting; identifies needs of co-workers in assisting with rehabilitation process
	Plans and intervenes to promote social adaptation of employee	Communicates needs of employee, family, and co-workers; counsels with employee, family, and co-workers; recommends environmental adjustments to meet employee needs; observes employee for adjustment to disability and social setting
	Collaborates with community health facilities	Interprets occupational health nursing contribution to restorative program; interprets community rehabilitation services to health team or appropriate individuals; communicates employee and family needs to health team or appropriate sources
Psychological	Assesses emotional needs of employee and family	Identifies needs of employee in work setting and of employee and family in home and community; observes employee and family in coping with effects of disability; identifies needs of co-workers in accepting employee
	Plans and intervenes to promote emotional adjustment of employee, family, co-workers	Counsels employee and family in adjustment to disability; counsels co-workers in expectations and acceptance of employee; communicates identified needs; provides emotional support for employee and family
	Plans and intervenes to promote fullest restoration potential	Communicates and interprets growth needs; guides employee and family to positive actions and attitudes by counseling, teaching, demonstration; recognizes productive work as a means of self-actualizing
Self-actualization	Collaborates in evaluating rehabilitation program	Appraises program based on philosophy, objectives, and policy; predicts future needs and changes in rehabilitation process; revises program based on nursing philosophy, objectives, and independent and dependent nursing functions

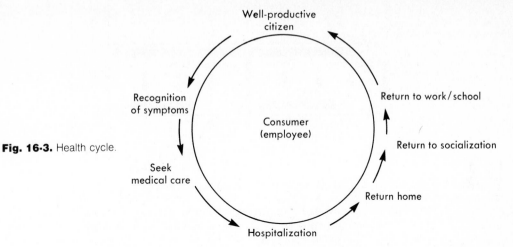

Fig. 16-3. Health cycle.

CONTEMPORARY CONCEPTS RELEVANT TO OCCUPATIONAL HEALTH NURSING

A majority of the concepts learned in nursing programs are relevant to all nursing, including occupational health. Occasionally, because of the site of practice, implementation of the concept must be modified. The modification and application of selected concepts will now be explored.

Holistic health

Today occupational health nurses, as well as other health professionals, have the opportunity and reinforcement for activating the concept of high-level wellness. Travis[20] presents a version of the concept that has much relevance for the work setting. His general philosophy is one of holistic health and is diagrammatically expressed in Fig. 16-4. Ardell[21] has also added to the definition of high-level wellness. He discusses five dimensions: self-responsibility, nutritional awareness, stress management, physical fitness, and environmental sensitivity. Holistic health as it emerges in the future will play an increasing part in the concepts of occupational health nursing.

Expanded role of the nurse

Occupational health nurses have always done history taking, partial physical examination, and the ordering of diagnostic tests as a part of their practice. Unfortunately, the preparation for this responsibility was frequently inadequate. During the 1940s through 1960s, they were severely criticized by nursing colleagues for not "practicing nursing"; however, occupational health nurses went about meeting health needs in the way they thought most appropriate.

Four common situations from before 1965 follow:

1. An employee arrives at a one-nurse unit with a complaint of abdominal pain. Questions elicit a history involving the quality of pain, mobility of the pain, appetite changes, bowel changes, and relationship of the symptoms to body functions and other activities. Some of the more secure nurses palpate the abdomen in a superficial manner prior to referral to the private physician.

2. An employee arrives complaining of "strain" of his wrist. A history relating to the characteristics of the symptoms and relationship of possible injury is recorded. An examination involving range of motion of the wrist, hand, and fingers follows, perhaps even an x-ray film of the area prior to referral if needed.

3. An employee arrives with a "rash" on his arms. The record reveals that he works in a department in which certain cleaning agents are used. A careful questioning includes whether exposure has occurred, when, how, length of time, duration of symptoms, quality and quantity of symptoms, and self-

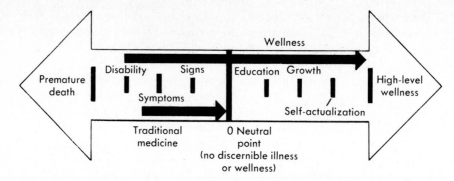

Fig. 16-4. Wellness-illness continuum. Moving from the center to the left shows a progressively worsening state of health. Moving to the right of center shows increasing levels of health and well-being. Traditional medicine is oriented toward curing evidence of disease, but usually stops at the midpoint. Wellness education begins at any point on the scale with the goal of helping a person to move as far to the right as possible. (From Travis, John W.: Wellness workbook, Mill Valley, Calif., 1977, Wellness Resource Center Press.)

treatment carried out. Using written orders, the nurse initiates appropriate treatment and requests follow-up visits.

4. An employee arrives with a headache. The nurse inquires about duration, location of pain, dizziness, medications taken, relationship to stress at home or work, exposure to chemicals, and his general physical state (i.e., fatigue, hunger, recent alcohol intake, etc.). Then she might perform simple neurological tests, maybe a gross vision test. Perhaps a more thorough examination by the company physician will be indicated for a decision regarding company versus personal responsibility for securing care.

The occupational health nurse was called on to make critical decisions about need for treatment and sources of referral. Community nurses and school nurses have always made decisions on these types of data, and occupational health nurses are doing the same.

Further elements of this expanded role of the occupational health nurse are health assessments, screening, monitoring, health education, and counseling.

HEALTH ASSESSMENTS

An occupational health nurse has the opportunity for carrying out the preemployment, periodic,

and terminal health histories and perhaps physical examinations of employees. During this contact with the employee, much relevant data about himself as a person, his family, his health behavior and patterns of health care, and his knowledge about health and illness can be obtained. To supplement skilled interviewing, numerous history-taking and assessment forms are available for use by the nurse.[20,22-24] It is essential that the history extend beyond the symptoms, illnesses, and diseases. The interview is conducted in a manner guaranteeing that the data will not be used in a detrimental way to the employee. Such assessments may also be a part of any contact with an employee for assisting the individual in moving in the direction of high-level wellness. Interpretation of the results of the assessment must be a planned activity within a series of employee-nurse visits.

The physical examination, frequently an anxiety-producing event, can be conducted in an atmosphere as relaxed as possible. Many physical examinations have been carried out in the past in a rapid look-see-feel manner. An occupational health nurse has the responsibility to spend time with the person, conducting the examination in a systematic and standard manner, while using the meeting to help the person learn about himself and some health measures, as in the following:

1. During inspection of the ears with the otoscope, after noting the presence of cerumen or evidence of "picking," use this teachable moment to tell the person about ways of removal of cerumen with means other than hairpins, crochet hooks, or fingernails.

2. During inspection of the mouth, recommend needed dental care or oral hygiene measures. Look also for signs for bruxism. After assessing overall evidence of stress of the individual, time can be taken to discuss this finding about stress and tension and its implications. Recommendation of relaxation exercises and other stress-reduction modalities may follow.

3. Routinely teach women the why and how of self-examination of their breasts and the importance of routine pelvic examinations with Pap smears.

4. Discuss height and weight norms with the individual, and advise regarding dietary habits as necessary. A review of sound basic nutritional priciples with the individual is usually well received and appreciated. I have found both men and women responsive to discussing nutritional needs and obtaining the highest value for each dollar spent on food. There are innumerable opportunities available for educating the individual, including bringing a health problem with the future implications (i.e., smoking and chronic obstructive lung disease, stress, and lack of exercise) to his attention. The nurse can work out with the employee alternatives for treatment with the consequences of each alternative, as well as how and where to secure help.

Factors to be considered in the administration of health assessment tools include (1) the employee's perception of the reason for administration, (2) the perception of management and union of the reason for and use of data collected, (3) the projected use of data, and (4) the capability of the occupational health personnel to use the tool and interpret the results to the employee.

Health needs can be looked at from individual employees' and employee groups' points of view. For an individual the data can be secured and results shared with the employee with minimal interruption in the daily work routine. Most employees are willing to share needed information about themselves if they understand that it will not adversely affect their job status and will ultimately benefit them. After the data are analyzed and interpreted to the employee at his level of comprehension, a care plan or contract can be arranged jointly by nurse and employee for modifications in health behavior and life-style. Administration of tools to groups of employees, by department, by job category, or by location, may be difficult to plan, with far more interpretation needed by management, union, and employees about the rationale and benefit of such study.

Other approaches to the study of health needs of groups within the work setting are through environmental survey of hazards to health; analysis of accidents, injuries, and illnesses of an occupational and nonoccupational nature; and compilation of results of individual health histories and physical examinations. This type of survey can be carried out by representatives of the industrial hygiene or safety department with input from the nurse.

SCREENING

On almost every visit of an employee to the health service, opportunity is available to the nurse for screening for selected health problems. Such screening techniques include blood pressure, pulse, evidence of excess stress, dermatoses on exposed areas of the body, posture, color, appearance, ability to communicate, color of conjunctivae, foot problems, and weight. Evidence of deviations from normal can be brought to the attention of the employee and can be noted in the record for further follow-up. Evidence of normal findings can be also conveyed.

Mass screening programs are useful with large population groups. In collaboration with established groups that have organized programs (i.e., American Heart Association, American Lung Association, American Diabetes Association, National Podiatry Association, local and state health departments, and the local Lion's Club), mass screening can be conducted with minimal demand on the nurse. Another source of screeening data on employees is blood banks. Each donor is screened for conditions including weight, height, blood pressure, hemoglobin and hematocrit, unexplained weight loss, shortness of breath, and chest pain.

MONITORING

Although employees have private medical care available to them outside the work setting, the occupational health nurse has the opportunity for assisting them in coping with and adapting to long-term illness conditions. The nurse is in an ideal setting to monitor the health of employees with the potential for a continuing relationship, sometimes twenty to thirty years. It is possible to establish a contract with employees to assist them with compliance with treatment regimens prescribed by their private physicians and to help them to cope with illness by adjusting and adapting work and lifestyles to meet the situation. The occupational health nurse is able to observe physical, emotional, and intellectual changes in an employee and intervene as needed. Frequently the employee needs support and assistance in handling problems if the spouse or a child has a long-term illness.

Occasionally occupational health physicians are reluctant to encourage nursing follow-up of employees because of the potential for objection by the medical community. This barrier may be present, but it is exaggerated in importance. Experience is showing that the private physician is cooperative when contacted by the occupational health nurse who uses the approach, "How can I help this employee comply with the regimen you have prescribed?" Most physicians are willing to share a bit of information about their clients (the employees) and frequently finish the conversation by saying to call anytime. An explanation of the occupational health nurses's contribution to the care of the physician's client is usually sufficient. Frequently the physician is "pulling his hair out" about how to get the employee to comply with his prescribed regimen.

Types of conditions conducive to such monitoring include the following:

Health promotion: Teaching and counseling about managing life-style problems; nutrition, physical fitness; stress reduction; increasing self-responsibility for one's own health; recreational and leisure time patterns

Long-term illness: Hypertension, chronic obstructive lung disease, renal disorders, diabetes, anemia

Emotional disorders: Mild depressions, situational anxiety, acute chronic stress

Growth and development: Adolescence, pregnancy, middle-aged crises, menopause, retirement

HEALTH EDUCATION

Nearly every contact with an employee presents the opportunity for some health teaching. The teaching does not have to be formal and planned; it can be informal, as during the taking of blood pressure of a black employee to inquire if he knows why blood pressure checks, particularly among black people, are important. The next sentence could be something like, "Does anyone at home have high blood pressure?"; then periodic checks at the employee health unit or at checking stations set up at shopping centers, fairs, and churches could be suggested. Another easily introduced topic is that of eating "junk foods." Most employees respond to this topic quickly. After such discussion several employees reported to the occupational health nurse that they were now more aware of their eating patterns and trying to change them. One man lost 10 pounds. Another example is that of medications in the medicine cabinet at home. This subject can be casually discussed when the occupational health nurse is dispensing the proverbial "two aspirins." The potential dangers of outdated drugs can be mentioned.

Not all situations are appropriate for teaching. The nurse's observational skills and common sense can identify such occasions with the severely injured, ill, or disturbed employee.

Group teaching is a method of reaching large numbers of employees. Whether it is as effective as is hoped is open to question. The primary function of an industry is production or provision of a service. For this reason a major deterrent to group teaching is securing time for such a program. A group approach that may be feasible is a health fair during shift changes. In addition to screening employees for signs and symptoms, booths can be set aside for private discussion with the nurse about a particular problem. Planning and conducting a health fair would be an excellent vehicle for collaboration between practicing occupational health nurses and school of nursing faculty and students.

Leaflets and written materials that are attractive, accurate, easily read and understood, and readily available are useful. These materials should be related to health promotion.

COUNSELING

The opportunity for a long-term relationship with an employee is a decided advantage for effective counseling. In addition, much counseling can be done on a one-visit contact with appropriate rapport and cues. All the principles and techniques for effective counseling in other nursing work sites apply in industry. Perhaps the most important principle to carry out is that of confidentiality. A misplaced word or leakage of information can be disastrous for nurse *and* employee.

A factor associated with counseling that must be worked out between the nurse and management is how confidential information will be handled. Management may expect to receive confidential information about employees, and it is up to the nurse to make management aware that all health information received pertaining to employees is confidential unless the employee himself gives written permission to release the information. Confidentiality is an essential ingredient of an effective employee health program.

Developing responsible, self-aware consumers of health care

The concept of consumerism in health care was discussed in Chapter 1. The occupational health nurse is able to put into operation this concept in health teaching. The focus of all teaching and counseling should be on developing a responsible,

self-aware consumer of health care. With access to well, productive individuals, the occupational health nurse can help employees learn simple skills such as taking temperatures and reading the thermometer, counting a pulse, and checking a blood pressure. A comprehensive list of do-it-yourself medical tests is available in a lay periodical.[25] Included are the following conditions and tests:

Blood pressure

Physical fitness

Obesity

Cancer (examination of breasts in women, testes in men, face, neck, mouth, skin, and stool)

Urine

Eyesight

Hearing

Teeth

Scoliosis

The occupational health nurse can arrange for first-aid classes for emergency care to be given immediately before or after a shift at the work site. A health activation course could be developed that is similar to the model used at the Georgetown University Department of Continuing Education.[26] The occupational health nurse can write short articles on health and health promotion or identification and care of common acute health problems for the company newsletter. Another technique might be to distribute forms for consolidating data about one's family health, for example, the *Family Medical Record* distributed by the local branch of March of Dimes.[27] An important component of creating the self-aware employee is to encourage questions from him about his body and its functioning and to interpret and discuss results of examinations and laboratory work with him. Everyday terminology should be used to convey what the normal and abnormal results mean to the individual.

Probably the most important aspect is for the employee to fully comprehend the hazards to which he is exposed in the work setting (Fig. 16-5). With a full understanding he can then decide whether he wishes to risk development of the disorder associated with the hazard. Employees respond in a positive manner to such an approach. It is with this kind of knowledge that employees can begin to

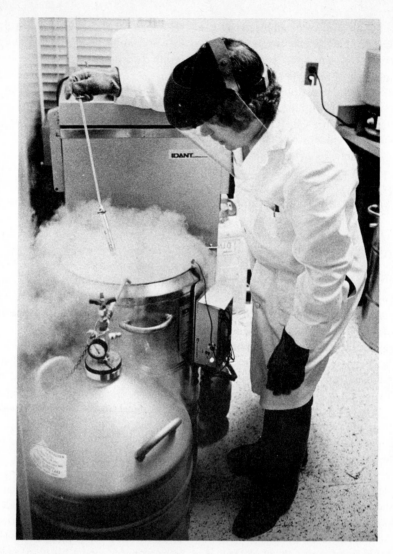

Fig. 16-5. The employee should fully understand the hazards to be faced on the job. This person should know what he is inhaling. (Photograph by Andrew Sacks; courtesy Editorial Photocolor Archives, Inc., New York.)

make conscious decisions about their health behavior and patterns of care.

Family health care

It is generally accepted that the health of a family can affect the health and job performance of an employee. The number of emotionally troubled employees is very large and only minimally recognized. The prevailing belief has been that the employer has no responsibility for home problems: the employee is there to work. This myth is dying, fortunately. Distraction, preoccupation, irritability, unreliability, and excessive stress symptoms are signs of the potentially "unsafe" employee.

The nurse may have difficulty in identifying family health problems because the employee may be reluctant to reveal them. Reasons for this reluctance may be (1) fear that the information could be used against him, (2) fear of lack of confidentiality, (3) inability to verbalize the problems, (4) lack of privacy during contact with the nurse, (5) established policy of employee health service to deal with employees on an episodic basis only, and (6) fear of the use of information that is recorded in his company health record.

The nurse herself may be a barrier to revelation of personal information for several reasons: (1) she may give the impression of disinterest or lack of concern; (2) her interviewing/counseling skills may need strengthening; (3) her job description may prohibit such conferences; or (4) she may be faced with a rushed pace of providing care to employees.

Reaching female employees may be more advantageous when the need is for change in life-styles within families. Topics such as nutrition, use of leisure time, development of hobbies and outside interests, assessing the health of family members, and exercise patterns may be more influenced by the female figure in the family than the male figure, but not necessarily. One-parent families may be particularly receptive to assistance from the occupational health nurse. These men and women have many of the problems of single persons plus the responsibility of bringing up children. Absence from work poses a serious threat.

Evidence of child abuse and wife beating may be identified among employees. Each occupational health program should have a protocol to give direction in dealing with this information.

How much detail of the information revealed by an employee should go into the employee's record is still to be determined. A rule of thumb that has been used with success is to record such observations as ''Employee vented feelings,'' ''Employee discussed past events in personal life,'' and ''Employee shared information regarding problems at home.'' The statement is then read to the employee, with no additional recording done unless it is read to the employee by the nurse.

Growth and development

The stages of growth and development of the adult years are now being studied to determine their characteristics. The nurse must be conversant with these stages to assist employees in coping with developmental changes. Application of the theories of Havighurst, Erikson, and Duval has been made by Burtt[28] in relation to the employed population.

The occupational health nurse cares for an individual from the ages of 18 to 65 or older with the opportunity to use her knowledge of the stages of growth and development during this time in order to understand behavior, verbalization, priority setting, values, and the need for anticipatory guidance of employees. For example, women need help in understanding what is happening physically, emotionally, and socially during the premenopausal and menopausal time of life. This period of development has been the target of twittering and jokes; it is not a stage of normal development to be taken lightly. It can be taken in stride more easily if a woman knows what is happening to her. Statistics show that in 1975 there were approximately 6.7 million women between the ages 45 and 54 in the labor force.

Another stage of development full of uncertainties and fears is that of retirement. Over the years efforts have been made to prepare the employee for the day after he stops working and the years that follow. Several approaches are in operation currently. One[29] is a series of audiovisual programs on retirement planning designed for use with persons 40 to 65 years old and includes the following topics: ''One-third of Your Life,'' ''Enough to Live On,'' ''A Place to Live,'' ''Time on Your Hands,'' ''Maintaining Health, '' ''Senior Citizenship,'' ''Consumerism, Fun, and Profit,'' and ''Friends and Relations.'' This concern has also led to a three-day seminar to help people plan for the remainder of their lives. Another approach is described in a study manual for retirement.[31] This group believes that planning should begin at least ten years before retirement and should include the spouse. The United Steelworkers of America has developed a brief series of sessions for retirement planning and is anticipating moving into a more extensive program.[31] Each of these examples appears to take a comprehensive approach to the planning, with health as a topic for one session.

What could the occupational health nurse contribute to a preretirement program? Activities might include securing a health history, physical examination, and appropriate diagnostic tests; encouraging repair of correctable conditions, especially the need for surgery; teaching about, providing anticipatory guidance for, and helping with coping mechanisms for physical and emotional changes; assisting the family, particularly the spouse, with life-style modifications; developing meaningful and cost-conscious leisure time endeavors; assisting with comprehension of Medicare benefits; and interpreting how the occupational health nurse can assist with health problems after retirement.

Alternative modalities for wellness

Hundreds of companies and agencies have initiated health and fitness programs for their employees. Most of these companies limit free use of these programs and services (many of them quite elaborate and extensive) to upper level executives, but they make them available to other employees at a nominal charge.

Such programs have been shown to influence employees in five ways: increased self-esteem, job performance, and satisfaction and decreased absenteeism and use of health services.[32] For example, Xerox Corp. reports a reduction in weight in 67% of their participants.[33]

Some occupational health nurses are helping employees to reduce stress. They are using in their practice such techniques as yoga, various relaxation techniques, mind control techniques, acupressure, touch therapy, and forms of biofeedback. At least one nurse has placed an easy chair in the health clinic in a quiet spot with dimmed lighting. After assessment of a distressed employee, the nurse encourages the employee to relax in the chair for a

period of time rather than dispensing a tranquilizer or other medication.

The employment site may prove to be one of the most appropriate locations for implementing a program leading toward high-level wellness.

INNOVATIVE APPROACHES TO HEALTH CARE IN THE WORK SETTING

With appropriate interpretation and use of personnel and facilities, experimental programs in occupational health nursing are possible. The nurse can be a major contributor to changing a traditional system using broad knowledge and skills of what needs to be done, what is possible, and how change can come about. Books and articles abound on the process of change, but prior to any change, there must be a kernel of an idea. Occupational health nurses have ideas. Some innovative programs have already been mentioned. Ardell has several thoughts still to be put into operation, such as company-subsidized quit-smoking clinics, conducting health screening with wellness inventories, or diet counseling programs. In addition, two other programs currently underway will be described in some detail.

Cardiovascular Health Services Center, Kimberly-Clark Corp., Neenah, Wisconsin

The purpose of this program[34] is to provide employees with detailed cardiac evaluation and individualized exercise therapy regimens. The scope of the program encompasses (1) a battery of screening tests for early identification of individuals relative to cardiovascular disease, (2) a battery of screening tests to support annual voluntary and preplacement physicals for salaried employees, (3) an exercise therapy program, and (4) an extensive education program for employee and spouse designed to analyze the participant's present knowledge regarding his cardiovascular condition. A family nurse practitioner with the program described the framework for her nursing practice[35]:

1. *Assessment* through health history, health screening procedures, and physical examination

2. *Planning* and employee health promotion by way of education, therapeutic management and maintenance, and further diagnostic evaluation and consultation
3. *Implementation* of innovative modalities and creative health promotion and management; identification of health risk factors; and awareness of physical, emotional, and cultural factors and problematic health behavior with noncompliance
4. *Evaluation* of outcome of intervention with flexibility in revising goals based on employee needs

Winston-Salem Health Care Plan, Inc., Winston-Salem, North Carolina

The Winston-Salem Health Care Plan[36] began in 1976 and is sponsored by R.J. Reynolds Industries for its employees and their families. It is a group health plan unrelated to the occupational health program for the company. The team is made up of physicians, nurse practitioners, and physicians' assistants. The chief responsibility of the nurse practitioners and physicians' assistants is the coordination and management of client care. They interpret illness for the clients, follow up to see if they have complied with directions, and counsel as needed. In addition, they assess clients' problems, perform necessary examinations, request diagnostic tests, and prescribe selected medications with the guidance of a physician. It appears that there is much potential for collaboration between the group health plan and the ongoing occupational health programs for improving the health care of the employees and their families.

SUMMARY

Occupational health nursing is a relatively new and ever-developing field of endeavor for the professional nurse. Her practice need not be limited by the walls of the business in which she works, and she can, in cooperation with labor and management, develop a program of health promotion and maintenance, as well as innovative ways to provide disease prevention and screening for employees. Her major function is to identify the health needs of employees, which may include the identification and resolution of health hazards on the work site. In order to plan and evaluate occupational health programs, the nurse works closely with all members of the community health team, most especially with the community health nurse.

CASES FOR DISCUSSION

The data in these cases for discussion are based on actual employee situations. All the data needed for the nurse to work with the employee are given; however, the actual plan implemented by the nurse is omitted. The goal is to bring the employee to the highest level of physical, social, and emotional well-being of which he is capable. If community agencies are needed, the reader should consider the appropriate local ones.

Study questions for all cases

1. What additional data are needed? What is the least threatening manner to use in securing these data?
2. What are the health problems for the occupational health nurse to identify?
3. What health teaching/counseling is needed? Who should be involved?
4. How can compliance be evaluated?
5. What other health professionals should be involved?
6. Which concepts relevant to nursing were used in responding to the preceding questions?

CASE 1

Name: Mr. Kenneth
Sex: Male
Age: 61
Marital status: Married; children married and out of state
Height: 6 feet 1 inch
Weight: 175 pounds
Habits: Smokes one package of cigarettes daily; social drinker (not excessive)
Job: Truck driver; good work record; infrequent absences
Diagnoses: Healthy male
Medications: None
History of visits
  First visit
    NURSE: May I help you?
    EMPLOYEE: I believe the retirement age in this company is 65.

NURSE: Yes, it is, Mr. Kenneth.

EMPLOYEE: What do I need to do to get ready for that day?

CASE 2

Name: Ms. Evans
Sex: Female
Age: 53
Marital status: Widowed two weeks ago; two children in another city 350 miles away
Height: 5 feet 4 inches
Weight: 134 pounds
Habits: Smokes two packages of cigarettes daily; occasional drinker
Job: Assembly line worker; good work record; infrequent absences
Diagnoses: Healthy female
Medications: None
History of visits
  First visit
    Arrives and just sits and looks at the wall. The occupational health nurse gently probes for the reason for the visit. After a minute or two of silence interspersed with sighs, the employee begins sobbing.

CASE 3

Name: Mr. Danilowitz
Sex: Male
Age: 56
Marital status: Divorced, wife remarried; children married
Height: 5 feet 5 inches
Weight: 155 pounds
Habits: Smokes one and a half packs of cigarettes daily, occasionally cigars; drinks three to four bourbons and water each evening; frequent martini before business luncheons; denies alcohol intake in the morning
Job: Executive—a workaholic; good work record
Diagnoses: Healthy male
Medications: None
History of visits
  First visit
    Has recently seen a movie on TV about alcoholism and wishes to discuss own habits with occupational health nurse.

CASE 4

Name: Ms. Lillian
Sex: Female

Age: 34
Marital status: Married; no children
Height: 5 feet 4 inches
Weight: 130 pounds
Habits: Nonsmoker; social drinker, not excessive
Job: Secretary; fair to poor job record (frequent absences)
Diagnoses in record
  Headache
  "Flu"
  Cold
  Sore throat
  Puncture wound from staple
Medications: Occasional aspirin or acetaminophen (Tylenol)
History of visits
  First visit
    Complains of headache, feeling weak and tired, aches all over; T, 98.4; P, 80; BP, 120/84. Has felt this way for 24 hours. Looks at floor. A review of her health record reveals visits to the employee health service three to four times a month for similar vague symptoms for the past year. Is usually given aspirin and returned to work or sent home. No statements from her own physician regarding visits to him.

CASE 5

Name: Mr. Neuman
Sex: Male
Age: 21
Marital status: Married; two young children
Height: 5 feet 9 inches
Weight: 210 pounds
Habits: Nonsmoker; drinks two packs of beer weekly
Job: Laboratory technician (3 to 11 shift); fair work record; absent ten to twelve days each year
Diagnoses: Healthy male
Medication: Occasional aspirin
History of visits
  First visit
    Referred to nurse by company physician for counseling. BP, 140/92; triglycerides (blood), 250 points above maximum normal range. Mr. Neuman says he has no particular health problems. Asks perceptive and pointed questions about laboratory report.
  Second visit

Weight, 208; BP, 134/88. Continues to ask questions about meaning of laboratory report.

Third visit

Weight, 209, BP, 132/88. Mentioned infant daughter has been hospitalized for severe lung infection. Is worried about costs of hospital care.

Fourth visit

Weight, 208; BP, 140/94. Seems preoccupied. Daughter is home and recovering well. Asked again about laboratory report; blood triglycerides to be repeated before next visit. Reveals tension between himself and his wife.

Fifth visit

Weight, 207; BP, 138/90. Second laboratory report (also elevated) reviewed with him, ruling out disorder associated with increased triglycerides. Reveals three bouts of substernal, squeezing chest pain in past five months.

CASE 6

Name: Ms. Edward
Sex: Female
Age: 49
Marital status: Married; one daughter
Height: 5 feet 5 inches
Weight: 165 pounds
Habits: Nonsmoker; social drinker (?) slightly to excess
Job: Machine operator (3 to 11 shift), standing most of time; good work record
Diagnoses of private physician
  Diabetes mellitus
  Hypertension
Medications
  Chlorpropamide (Diabinese) tablets, 250 mg daily
  Diazepam (Valium), 5 mg bid
  Hydrochlorothiazide, 50 mg bid
  Conjugated estrogens tablets (Premarin), 1.25 mg daily (added by private physician two days before first visit)
  All medications taken in the morning for the first dose.
History of visits
  First visit
    Requests BP check weekly. BP, 170/ 110. Conversation reveals tension at home with divorced daughter who works during the day.

Ms. Edward cares for daughter's 1-year-old child when she is away from home.

Second visit

BP, 160/108; weight, 165½ pounds. Feels weak and "not quite with it" for the past couple of days late in the morning.

Third visit

BP, 148/108; weight, 164. Appears tense, speaks rapidly, and moves in jerky movements. Conditions at home difficult.

CASE 7

Name: Ms. Gordon
Sex: Female
Age: 35
Marital status: Single; lives alone
Height: 5 feet 8 inches
Weight: 165 pounds
Habits: Nonsmoker; social drinker, not excessive
Job: Staff nurse in local hospital; good job record
Diagnoses: Low-back injury
Medications: Aspirin for back pain and frequent headaches
History of visits
  First visit
    Arrives with beads of perspiration on forehead, dragging her right leg, unable to sit without falling into chair, and, once sitting, unable to rise without great discomfort.
  Second visit
    Has been examined by employee health service physician. No physical defect is found on x-ray film. Was told to use bed rest, heat, and aspirin for pain. Condition is much better, but still has back pain on walking, standing, and rising from and sitting on chair. Told by physician to "go home and learn to live with the condition." The nurse notes that Ms. Gordon's posture is fair with her abdomen somewhat protruding.

CASE 8

Name: Ms. Silverman
Sex: Female
Age: 38
Marital status: Separated; responsible for her four children
Height: 5 feet 11 inches
Weight: 175 pounds

Habits: Nonsmoker; nondrinker

Job: Supervisor

Diagnoses

 Total hysterectomy for removal of fibroids two months ago

 Hypertension

Medications: Diuretic daily

History of visits

 First visit

  Cleared for return to work following hysterectomy; no problems. BP, 138/86

 Second visit

  (Two weeks after first visit) Generalized trembling, quivering voice, barely able to walk without assistance. Two past entries in record other than reinstatment note: (1) a cold over a year ago and (2) a small laceration of finger ten months ago. Reveals extreme agitation and fear of what is happening to her. No psychiatric history in past or evidence of psychotic episode on this visit. No particular stress at home. BP, 134/86. Is unable to concentrate, has insomnia, feels "on edge." Is considering committing herself to a psychiatric institution.

CASE 9

Name: Mr. Sosnovsky

Sex: Male

Age: 39

Marital status: Married; three teenage sons

Height: 5 feet 11 inches

Weight: 232 pounds

Habits: Smokes two packs of cigarettes daily; beer drinker, several packs weekly

Job: Laborer (7 to 3 shift); poor work record, absent four or five days each month

Diagnoses by private physician

 Asthma

 Emphysema

 Hypertension

 Peptic ulcer

 Frequent respiratory infections

Medications

 Hydrochlorothiazide, 50 mg bid

 Chlordiazepoxide (Librium), 5 mg qid

 Theophyllin expectorant, 4 cc qid

 Methyldopa (Aldomet), 2 gm tid

 Prednisone, 30 mg daily

 Gelusil tablets, prn

History of visits

 First visit

  Review of above history. BP, 148/106; P, 84. Pulmonary function test and chest x ray requested (company has laboratory facilities).

 Second visit

  Weight, 232 pounds; BP, 104/106. Pulmonary function test shows 40% lung function; chest x ray shows beginning evidence of chronic obstructive pulmonary disease (COPD).

 Third visit

  Weight, 233; BP, 150/96; P, 80. Reveals he has few outside interests except gardening in the summer.

 Fourth visit

  Weight, 231; BP, 140/90; P, 80. Asks about Life and Breath Clinic through local Lung Association. Classes are held three days a week for ten sessions from 2 to 4 P.M. Charge is about $100.

 Fifth visit

  Weight, 230; BP, 142/90; P, 78. To start at Life and Breath Clinic classes.

 Sixth visit

  Weight, 230; BP, 140/90; P, 80. Has attended Life and Breath Clinic classes. A telephone call to Lung Association reveals lack of cooperation, smoking during sessions, and argumentative regarding smoking and weight.

CASE 10

Name: Ms. Wolomraj

Sex: Female

Age: 27

Marital status: Married; lives with husband and four children, ages 6, 4, and 2-year-old twins

Height: 5 feet 9 inches

Weight: 195 pounds

Habits: Nonsmoker; drinks alcohol "socially"

Job: Machine operator (3 to 11 shift); good job record

Diagnoses by private physician

 Gastroreflex esophagitis

 Hiatal hernia

 Obesity

 "Nerves"

Medications

 "Diuretic" 50 mg qd

 Valium, 5 mg tid

Amitriptyline (Elavil), 1 capsule qn
"Antibiotic," 250 mg qid for sore throat (second renewal)
Theragran, 1 capsule tid
"Amphetamine," 1 qd
Gelusil, 1 tablet tid
Tylenol No. 4, prn for cramps
Dimetapp Extentabs, 1 tablet prn for allergy
History of visits
First visit
Brings statement from private physician that she can return to work after a ten-week absence for above diagnoses. Says she feels dizzy, has intermittent nausea. BP, 144/96; throat slightly reddened; no exudate; T, 98.4

CASE 11

Name: Ms. Brahms
Sex: Female
Age: 32
Marital status: Married; two children, ages 6 and 9
Height: 5 feet 6 inches
Weight: 140 pounds
Habits: Smokes one pack of cigarettes daily; "social" drinker
Job: Quality control inspector; absent sixty days in past year for virus, colds, nerves, laceration on hand
Diagnoses: None
Medications: None
History of visits
First visit
Asks to talk with particular nurse. Reveals vague home problems and feelings of fatigue. Stares at floor. CBC and urinalysis requested.
Second visit
Laboratory reports reviewed. CBC was within normal limits; urinalysis indicated 20 to 30 RBCs. Requests repeat urinalysis. BP, 128/76; P, 82.
Third visit
Repeat urinalysis unchanged. Appears depressed by still-present vague home and job stresses. Has lost 4 pounds since first visit one month before. Referred to urologist.
Fourth visit
Stares at floor. Responds only to direct questions. Scheduled for intravenous pyelogram by urologist.

Fifth visit
Has been absent ten days in past month. Admits to gross hematuria. Canceled scheduled cystoscopy because of "nerves," and her eye had been injured. Reveals her husband had beaten her; he is now taking heroin and has "strange" people coming to her house. States she found a bullet hole in driver's side of her car. Has lost 4 more pounds.

Health problems identifiable in cases

Case 1: Information about retirement program, health assessment, anticipatory guidance for employee and wife regarding physical, psychological, and social changes associated with aging and retirement
Case 2: Grieving, need for emotional support, adaptation to life-style change
Case 3: Alcoholism, loneliness, smoking, need for social activities
Case 4: Depression, frequent absences, tension at home or work
Case 5: Increased blood triglycerides, overweight, dietary habits, absenteeism rate, tension at home, evaluation of chest pain, knowledge regarding health insurance benefits, need for relaxation exercises
Case 6: Hypertension, overweight, dietary habits, anxiety, tension in home, drug interaction of diuretic and estrogen, diabetes mellitus, menopause, drinking habits
Case 7: Low-back disorder, weak back and abdominal muscles, poor posture, anxiety, slightly overweight, need for relaxation exercises
Case 8: Menopause, mild hypertension
Case 9: COPD, smoking, obesity, dietary habits, compliance, use of leisure time
Case 10: Anxiety, drug overdosage and interactions, obesity, dietary habits, hypertension
Case 11: Depression, anxiety, hematuria, being beaten by drug-addicted husband, anxious about children, fear of own and childrens' safety, absenteeism problem

NOTES

1. Brown, Mary Louise: Occupational health nursing, New York, 1956, Springer Publishing Co.
2. Page, Robert Collier: Occupational health and mantalent development, Berwyn, Ill., 1963, Physicians Record Co.
3. Tinkham, Catherine W.: The Catherine R. Dempsey Memorial Lecture. Occupational health nursing in the 1980's, Occupational Health Nursing **25:**7-13, June, 1977.

4. U.S. Department of Commerce, Bureau of the Census: Statistical abstract of the United States, 1976, ed. 97, Washington, D.C., 1976, U.S. Government Printing Office.

5. U.S. Department of Commerce, Bureau of the Census: Social indicators, 1976, Washington, D.C., 1977, U.S. Government Printing Office.

6. Kahn, Herman, and Weiner, Anthony J.: The next thirty-three years: a framework for speculation, Daedalus **96:**711-716, Summer, 1967.

7. Stokinger, Herbert E.: Means of contact and entry of toxic agents. In Gafefer, W.M., editor: Occupational diseases—a guide to their recognition, Washington, D.C., 1964, U.S. Government Printing Office.

8. Stellman, Jeanne M., and Daum, Susan M.: Work is dangerous to your health—a handbook of health hazards in the workplace and what you can do about them, New York, 1973, Pantheon Books, Inc.

9. Mott, Paul E.: Shift work—the social, psychological, and physical consequences, Ann Arbor, Mich., 1965, The University of Michigan Press.

10. Occupational health problems and their control, WHO Chronicle **30:**323-334, August, 1976.

11. Karvonen, Martti J.: Fitting the job to the worker, World Health, p. 30, July-August, 1974.

12. Tinkham, Catherine W.: The plant as the patient of the occupational health nurse, Nursing Clinics of North America **7:**99-107, March, 1972. (See Nursng Clinics of North America **7,** June, 1972, for correction to text previously cited for pp. 99-100.)

13. Keller, Marjorie J.: The student program—participation, not observation, Occupational Health Nursing **18:**17-19, November, 1970.

14. McGrath, Bethel J.: Nursing in commerce and industry, New York, 1946, The Commonwealth Fund.

15. Freeman, Ruth B.: Community health nursing practice, Philadelphia, 1970, W.B. Saunders Co.

16. Leahy, Kathleen M., et al.: Community health nursing, ed. 3, New York, 1977, McGraw-Hill Book Co.

17. Keller, Marjorie J., in association with May, W.T.: Occupational health content in baccalaureate nursing education, Cincinnati, 1971, National Institute of Occupational Safety and Health.

18. Leavell, Hugh Rodman, and Clark, E. Gurney: Preventive medicine for the doctor in his community—an epidemiologic approach, ed. 3, New York, 1965, McGraw-Hill Book Co.

19. Maslow, Abraham H.: Motivation and personality, New York, 1954, Harper & Row, Publishers.

20. Travis, John W.: Wellness workbook, Mill Valley, Calif., 1977, Wellness Resource Center Press.

21. Ardell, Donald B.: High level wellness—an alternative to doctors, drugs, and disease, Emmaus, Pa., 1977, Rodale Press, Inc.

22. Francis, Gloria M., and Munjas, Barbara: Manual of social psychologic assessment, New York, 1976, Appleton-Century-Crofts.

23. Malasanos, Lois, Barkauskas, Violet, Moss, Muriel, and Stoltenberg-Allen, Kathryn: Health assessment, ed. 2, St. Louis, 1981, The C.V. Mosby Co.

24. Sorochan, Walter D.: Personal health appraisal, New York, 1976, John Wiley & Sons, Inc.

25. Scott, Michael P.: Do-it-yourself medical tests, Better Homes and Gardens **55:**70-77, December, 1977.

26. Sehnert, Keith, W.: How to be your own doctor—sometimes, New York, 1975, Grosset & Dunlap, Inc.

27. Family medical record, New York, 1972, The National Foundation–March of Dimes.

28. Burtt, Elizabeth A.: Employee assessment of the young and the older worker, Nursing Clinics of North America **7:**109-119, March, 1972.

29. Preparation for retirement, Minneapolis, American Manpower and Aging Advisory Services.

30. Arnold, Suzanne, et al.: Ready or not—a study manual for retirement, New York, 1974, Manpower Education Institute.

31. When you quit work—a pre-retirement course for steelworkers, Washington, D.C., United Steelworkers of America Education Department (AFL-CIO-CLC).

32. Jaffe, Russell M.: Science and wellness: the new medicine, presented at the One hundred fifth Meeting of the American Public Health Association, Washington, D.C., November 3, 1977.

33. Arnold, W. Brent: Empirical findings of an employee health maintenance program at Xerox Corporation, presented at the One hundred fifth Meeting of the American Public Health Association, Washington, D.C., November 3, 1977.

34. Dedmon, Robert E.: Description of health services center, Neenah, Wis., February 3, 1976, Kimberly-Clark Corp. (mimeographed).

35. Bauer, Rosalia R., et al.: The role of a family nurse practitioner in a cardiovascular health program, presented at the One hundred fifth Meeting of the American Public Health Association, Washington, D.C., October 31, 1977.

36. Winston-Salem Health Care Plan, Inc., Newsletter **1,** April, 1977.

BIBLIOGRAPHY

Ardell, Donald B.: High level wellness—an alternative to doctors, drugs, and disease, Emmaus, Pa., 1977, Rodale Press, Inc.

Arnold, W. Brent: Empirical findings of an employee health maintenance program at Xerox Corporation, presented at the One hundred fifth Meeting of the American Public Health Association, Washington, D.C., November 3, 1977.

Arnold, Suzanne, et al.: Ready or not—a study manual for retirement, New York, 1974, Manpower Education Institute.

Bauer, Rosalia R., et al.: The role of a family nurse practitioner in a cardiovascular health program, presented at the One hundred fifth Meeting of the American Public Health Association, Washington, D.C., October 31, 1977.

Brown, Mary Louise: Occupational health nursing, New York, 1956, Springer Publishing Co.

Burtt, Elizabeth A.: Employee assessment of the young and the older worker, Nursing Clinics of North America 7:109-119, March, 1972.

Dedmon, Robert E.: Description of Health Services Center, Neenah, Wis., February 3, 1976, Kimberly-Clark Corp. (mimeographed).

Family medical record, New York, 1972, The National Foundation–March of Dimes.

Francis, Gloria M., and Munjas, Barbara: Manual of social psychologic assessment, New York, 1976, Appleton-Century-Crofts.

Freeman, Ruth B.: Community health nursing practice, Philadelphia, 1970, W.B. Saunders Co.

Garvin, William: Occupational hazard, Saturday Evening Post 243:102, Winter, 1971.

Jaffe, Russell M.: Science and wellness: the new medicine, presented at the One hundred fifth Meeting of the American Public Health Association, Washington, D.C., November 3, 1977.

Kahn, Herman, and Weiner, Anthony J.: The next thirty-three years: a framework for speculation, Daedalus 96:711-716, Summer, 1967.

Karvonen, Martti J.: Fitting the job to the worker, World Health, p. 30, July-August, 1974.

Keller, Marjorie J.: The student program—participation, not observation, Occupational Health Nursing 18:17-19, November, 1970.

Keller, Marjorie J., in association with May, W.T.: Occupational health content in baccalaureate nursing education, Cincinnati, 1971, National Institute of Occupational Safety and Health.

Leahy, Kathleen M., et al.: Community health nursing, ed. 3, New York, 1977, McGraw-Hill Book Co.

Leavell, Hugh Rodman, and Clark, E. Gurney: Preventive medicine for the doctor in his community—an epidemiologic approach, ed. 3, New York, 1965, McGraw-Hill Book Co.

Malasanos, Lois, Barkausakas, Violet, Moss, Muriel, and Stoltenberg-Allen, Kathryn: Health assessment, ed. 2, St. Louis, 1981, The C.V. Mosby Co.

Maslow, Abraham H.: Motivation and personality, New York, 1954, Harper & Row, Publishers.

McGrath, Bethel J.: Nursing in commerce and industry, New York, 1946, The Commonwealth Fund.

Mott, Paul E.: Shift work—the social, psychological, and physical consequences, Ann Arbor, Mich., 1965, The University of Michigan Press.

Occupational health problems and their control, WHO Chronicle 30:323-334, August, 1976.

Page, Robert Collier: Occupational health and mantalent development, Berwyn, Ill., 1963, Physicians Record Co.

Preparation for retirement, Minneapolis, American Manpower and Aging Advisory Services.

Scott, Micahel P.: Do-it-yourself medical tests, Better Homes and Gardens 55:70-77, December, 1977.

Sehnert, Keith W.: How to be your own doctor—sometimes, New York, 1975, Grosset & Dunlap, Inc.

Sorochan, Walter D.: Personal health appraisal, New York, 1976, John Wiley & Sons, Inc.

Stellman, Jeanne M., and Daum, Susan M.: Work is dangerous to your health—a handbook of health hazards in the workplace and what you can do about them, New york, 1973, Pantheon Books, Inc.

Stokinger, Herbert E.: Means of contact and entry of toxic agents. In Gafefer, W.M., editor: Occupational diseases—a guide to their recognition, Washington, D.C., 1964, U.S. Government Printing Office.

Stokinger, Herbert E.: Routes of entry and modes of action. In Key, Marcus M., et al., editors: Occupational diseases—a guide to their recognition, Washington, D.C., 1977, U.S. Government Printing Office.

Tinkham, Catherine W.: The plant as the patient of the occupational health nurse, Nursing Clinics of North America 7:99-107, March, 1972.

Tinkham, Catherine W.: The Catherine R. Dempsey Memorial Lecture. Occupational health nursing in the 1980's, Occupational Health Nursing 25:7-13, June, 1977.

Travis, John W.: Wellness workbook, Mill Valley, Calif., 1977, Wellness Resource Center Press.

U.S. Department of Commerce, Bureau of the Census: Social indicators, 1976, Washington, D.C., 1977, U.S. Government Printing Office.

U.S. Department of Commerce, Bureau of the Census: Statistical abstract of the United States, 1976, ed. 97, Washington, D.C., 1976, U.S. Government Printing Office.

When you quit work —a pre-retirement course for steelworkers, Washington, D.C., United Steelworkers of America Education Department (AFL-CIO-CLC).

Winston-Salem Health Care Plan, Inc., Newsletter, 1, April, 1977.

17

AGING

Seneca, the Roman philosopher and playwright, said, "Old age is an incurable disease." In the United States about 23 million people have this "disease" (10% of the population), and in many it is compounded by poverty, starvation, physical illness, and depression.

Most people are affected by mandatory retirement, and although in 1977 Congress raised the mandatory retirement age from 65 to 70, the benefits of these extra five working years are rapidly being eroded by an inflation rate that is rising faster than most had anticipated. Many people have participated in pension programs and there is still Social Security, but the payments derived from these sources are fixed while the inflation rate is not. Some people are wealthy and will continue to be in old age and some have had the foresight to build large retirement annuity accounts for themselves (usually those who were self-employed and had a large income while they were working), but most old people live on the edge of poverty and some are so grindingly poor that a well-fed lion in a progressive zoo lives in conditions that the elderly poor could envy.

It is true that there are many elderly who lead happy, satisfying, and healthy lives. This should be a goal of old age. And although it is frightening and depressing to contemplate, we must acknowledge that for many older Americans, life is not the cheery fantasy of a Norman Rockwell painting. Those who live in the inner cities are constant prey to the young hoodlums who roam the streets looking for the defenseless to assault and rob. The elderly fill this bill so well that many are terrified to venture out, even in the daytime, to the supermarket a few blocks away. The chance of their returning home with their bodies, their wallets, and their bag of groceries intact is less with each passing day of increasing personal violence. The police, for a variety of reasons, seem powerless to stop this flood of muggings and assaults, and many of the elderly cannot afford to pay the higher rents of safe neighborhoods. Nursing homes, although providing a measure of personal security, are frequently depressing, understaffed, and uncaring.

Those that make an effort to provide a homelike and cheerful atmosphere with professional thought given to the needs of the elderly are often so expensive that only the very wealthy can afford them.

Elderly people tend to think poorly of themselves, which is reinforced by society's demonstration that it has no further use for them. There are logical reasons for the elderly to feel bleak about themselves and their future: they are likely to be widowed and going through periods of grief and mourning. Even when the pain of death is no longer fresh, the loneliness of the half-empty marital bed remains forever. Couples who remain together into old age can face readjustment problems, such as being alone together for long periods of time. The feeling of not being needed, of not being a participatory member of the work force, is more than some people can bear. The nearness of death is a source of depression for many elderly people. They fear death itself, but even more they fear the process of dying and the possibility of pain and debilitating illness. As the years pass, the opportunities to fulfill one's dreams and ambitions diminish, and with this realization comes the thought of all that could have been done but was not; regret can be acute. Guilt feelings may play a significant role in the summing-up process of preparation for death. Past sins—real, exaggerated, or imagined—weigh heavily. But by far the greatest cause of misery and alienation is loneliness, caused by physical and social isolation, widowhood, disease and disability, and a sense of futility about the future.

The reality of old age in America is unpleasant; there is often not enough money to live on, certainly not for the little luxuries that make us smile, such as a bar of sweet-smelling soap, a warm new sweater, or dinner in a candlelit restaurant. Henry David Thoreau said that men lead lives of quiet desperation; this is especially true of the elderly. "Death is not the greatest loss of life. The greatest loss is what dies inside us while we live. The unbearable tragedy is to live without dignity or sensitivity."[1]

Age 65 is the arbitrary point (originally established by Chancellor Otto von Bismarck in determining nineteenth century social policy in Germany) at which a person is considered old or elderly in that it is the age for receiving Social Security and other social benefits. But the age at which a person becomes old depends almost entirely on the person himself—on his physical, social, and emotional functioning. Everyone knows people who are hopelessly old at 55 and those still sprightly and youthful at 80. This chapter will discuss some of the factors involved in aging, what can be done to alleviate the problems, and what the role of nursing should be in the care of the elderly.

The demographics of aging point out indications of social trends and possible solutions. About 45% of the people over 65 are over 73 years old, and 5% are 85 years or older; the elderly are the fastest growing age-group in the United States, and there is reason to believe that their numbers will increase proportionately.[2] Females live longer than males; for every 100 males over age 65 there are 142 females, and whites live longer than blacks (the death rate for blacks ages 65 to 74 is 56.6% and for whites in the same age-group it is 37).[2,pp.5-7] As could be assumed from demographic data, most elderly men are married, and most elderly women are widowed, which makes widowhood a particularly female state of affairs. If a man is widowed, he has a wide range of future wives from which to choose, but women are likely to remain widows until they die.

The myth that most elderly persons live in some kind of institution (nursing home, old age home, etc.) is false; only about 5% live permanently in institutions;[2,p.8] the rest live in the community—alone, with spouses, with their children's families, or with nonrelatives. The way an elderly person lives is one of the most crucial aspects of his life and can spell the difference between loneliness and helplessness and a satisfying life-style. Living with one's children has been the traditional solution for a widowed person who needs help and companionship but who resists the idea of a nursing home. This is not necessarily the best solution because in many instances children ask their elderly parents to live with them more out of a sense of duty, obligation, and an effort to avoid guilt than out of a sincere desire to share their lives with their parents. This situation is extremely likely to engender resentment and animosity. Worse still, if parents move in with children without being expressly invited, the situation is potentially explosive. As a result one sees an increase in the number of nonrelated elderly who are living together in small groups to provide each other with physical, emotional, and financial support. This kind of arrangement can provide a sense of human contact in a life that may be otherwise isolated. Housemates can care for each other and provide physical and emotional security. Moreover, the "pooling" of Social Security checks can be a major advantage. The movie "Going in Style" depicted just such an arrangement, although it is more likely that three healthy elderly men would have married, and three women would have shared an apartment and each other's lives.

The elderly are concentrated in inner cities and in rural areas; few live in suburbia,[2,p.9] but there is reason to believe that this trend is changing, especially with the enormous spurt in growth of retirement communities in the suburbs (a group of apartments or homes designed specifically for the elderly, not to be confused with a nursing home). These retirement communities offer the quiet and relative safety of suburbia and provide services such as on-call health personnel, community activities, and transportation to shopping and entertainment. They are, however, usually expensive and are therefore not available to the elderly poor who must continue to cringe behind locked doors in crime-ridden cities. One must also be mobile to live comfortably in the suburbs. If one cannot drive, suburban living can lead to an even greater sense of isolation. Public transportation in most suburbs is poor, if it exists at all.

Butler and Lewis,[2,pp.28-30] in describing aging and mental health, define some characteristics that are common to most elderly people:

1. The desire to leave a legacy. Human beings want to leave behind something of themselves, perhaps to mark their existence or to prove their lives had meaning. Legacies consist of people (children and grandchildren); creative accomplishments in art, business, or the professions; and money.

2. The "elder" function. The elderly have a natural propensity to share knowledge and wisdom with the young. This function forms a connection between generations and increases the self-esteem of the old when younger people are interested in what they have learned. Communication between the generations is sometimes hampered by envy and distrust of the young and impatience and boredom with the old.

3. Attachment to familiar objects. Things that have sentimental value—pictures, clothes, furniture—take on increasing value as discontinuity with other aspects of life takes place. Loss of possessions can be equated with loss of everything that is familiar and thus increases the fear of the un-

known future. One's own possessions can also signify a sense of security: the feeling that one's entire life is not disintegrating in front of one's eyes.

4. A change in the sense of time. Time is running out for the elderly, and they tend to develop a strong sense of the "here and now" and do not postpone plans for the future. Old people, if they are emotionally and spiritually sensitive, develop an even keener sense of what is important in their lives and is to be continued and what is not important and can be discarded as irrelevant.

5. A sense of the life cycle. The elderly have personal experience with the entire life cycle and frequently tend to develop interests in philosophy and religion. A sense of history and human perspective is more a characteristic of the old than of the young.

6. Creativity, curiosity, and surprise. Creativity does not necessarily decline in old age, and many people become creative for the first time when they grow older. Well known artists, diplomats, and business people remain creative and productive into old age.

7. A sense of consummation or fulfillment in life. A sense of satisfactorily completing a cycle can be characteristic of the older person, especially if he has a loving relationship with his children and has found some gratification in life (Fig. 17-1). Material success is not necessarily a component of this sense of fulfillment and may even detract from it if some aspects of life were neglected in favor of others.

One might, in the course of reading this chapter, conclude that old age is totally depressing and negative. It is not, nor does it have to be. The chapter is, however, written as realistically as possible, not with the intent of frightening the student or causing her not to want to have anything to do with the elderly, but to point out areas of need and ways in which the community health nurse can brighten the lives of the elderly. Problems do exist, and it will soon become obvious to the careful reader that most of the problems stem from the social and economic system in which we live. The nurse works within this system and does what she can to alleviate the problems of individual elderly persons or small

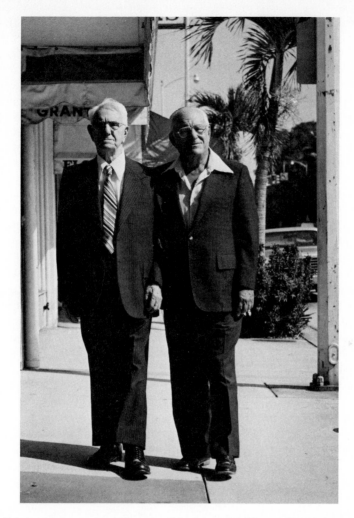

Fig. 17-1. Elderly people can lead lives of satisfaction and fulfillment. Here father and son enjoy each other's company and love.

groups; she cannot, however, change the fundamental social structure of the United States, which is the cause of many of the problems we will be discussing.

DEVELOPMENTAL ASPECTS OF AGING
Physical

The purpose of this section is to provide a brief overview of the physical aspects of aging. The reader is referred to medical-surgical nursing and pathophysiology texts for more definitive descrip-

tions of particular diseases. We are mainly concerned here with how the aging body affects the human being as he lives, thinks, and feels. It is safe to say that the elderly are not as frail and debilitated as popularly believed, nor do they cease functioning when one body system falters. Old age need not be a time of frail health or a rocking chair existence. I used to have some neighbors, an elderly couple who appeared to be in their 80s, who every evening after dinner would take a brisk walk, hand-in-hand around the neighborhood, even in cold winter weather. They appeared in excellent health and seemed to enjoy the exercise and each other's company. Perhaps they had physiological problems; surely their bodies were beginning to deteriorate, but they made full use of the physical functions not affected by age. They also had a positive effect on their younger neighbors; we enjoyed their health and vitality.

Each body system is characterized by particular signs of aging. The cardiovascular system is marked by a thickening and loss of elasticity of blood vessels. Heart valves undergo similar changes, but the heart itself remains the same size or shrinks slightly. Common cardiovascular conditions associated with old age are arteriosclerosis, hypertension, and myocardial degeneration. Since cardiovascular diseases are the leading cause of death for all adult Americans, many older people bring cardiovascular problems with them into old age and have adapted with varying degrees of success to cardiovascular insufficiency. Cardiovascular problems affect the lives of the elderly in that they tire more easily, their hearts take a longer time to recover from periods of stress, and they sometimes suffer from periods of mental confusion due to decreased oxygenation of brain cells from reduced cardiac efficiency. Hypertension is generally asymptomatic except in severe cases when it causes visual disturbances, headache, and perhaps even loss of full cerebral function.

Changes in the central nervous system cause the most unhappiness and embarrassment to the elderly. The brain shrinks in size and weight, and individual cells atrophy and die. Cerebral vessels also show arteriosclerotic changes, which lead to further loss of cells. Deterioration of the central nervous system has a profound effect on lives. Memory is affected, but not in a uniform way; recent memory is sometimes fuzzy, but recollection of distant events is sharp. This produces a classical picture of an old person who cannot remember what he ate for dinner last night but can describe in full detail a party he attended in adolescence. This quirk of memory tends to disconnect the elderly from the present and strengthen ties with the past. The abil-

ity to conceptualize and solve complex problems is not significantly impaired unless there is pathology of the central nervous system. Sleep patterns change; the elderly do not sleep as much as the young. One wonders if there are not strong psychological components to the decreased amount of sleep: perhaps a reluctance to spend precious remaining time asleep or the fear that sleep may turn to death. Changes in the central nervous system also produce changes in gait, muscle function, facial expression, and reflexes. All this leads to decreased mobility and speed of movement, which can cause a safety hazard. An older person cannot run from a mugger on the street or move quickly out of the way of an oncoming automobile. In the event of fire, old people are likely to be trapped in buildings because they cannot exit quickly enough, and they are easily knocked down by crowds.

Musculoskeletal changes tend to produce similar reactions and result from a general wasting of muscle tissue and loss of strength. Degenerative diseases of the musculoskeletal system are characterized by weakness and loss of coordination and control. The entire body skeleton changes so that it appears shrunken and diminutive, the "little old lady" syndrome. Joints are not as loose and mobile, muscles and tendons shrink, and the vertebral column itself changes shape and loses flexibility. Many of the age-associated musculoskeletal changes cause loss of mobility to some extent and drastically affect life-style.

The respiratory system is *relatively* free from the ravages of age, except that preexisting conditions such as emphysema, lung cancer, bronchitis, and tuberculosis will increase in severity. The elderly tend to be more affected by environmental conditions such as air pollution. When Mt. St. Helens erupted in 1980 the elderly of the region were more seriously affected by atmospheric ash than were younger persons.

Age affects the gastrointestinal system to widely varying degrees. Many people lose their teeth (due more frequently to gum disease than to dental caries), and certain digestive processes slow, such as esophageal dilatation and emptying and peristalsis.

Constipation is a common complaint among the elderly and is due to slowing of digestive processes, diminished physical activity, ingestion of less roughage because of poor chewing ability, and the relatively high price of foods that tend to prevent constipation (fresh produce, whole grains, meat). The elderly may experience poor appetite for the same reasons as do younger persons: anxiety, depression, loneliness, and the necessity to eat alone much of the time.

Among the most disturbing changes that take place in old age are those of sensory functions; sooner or later most of the senses diminish in acuity. Vision dims because of cataracts, glaucoma, and the aging process of retinal cells. Poor vision in the elderly becomes more than a nuisance; it can be a handicapping defect that leads to loneliness and isolation. Deafness is an even greater cause of isolation because the ability to hear is a major part of almost all forms of communication. Decreased vision and hearing also constitute a safety hazard, as do diminution of the senses of touch and spatial relationship. The skin of old persons loses turgor and elasticity and grows wrinkled in appearance; it sags and loses subcutaneous fat. This loss of fat makes the elderly person more sensitive to temperature changes; they find it difficult to tolerate extremes of heat and cold. This is one of the reasons why the elderly tend to move to the Southern and Southwestern states. Those persons who have worked outdoors most of their lives tend to have more aged skin than those who held indoor jobs. Wrinkled skin is one of the first signs of aging, and the size and strength of the American cosmetic market indicates just how frightened we are of appearing old and to what lengths we will go to prevent that appearance. Greying, brittleness, and thinning of the hair also occur.

The most obvious effects of an aging endocrine system appear in the hormones. Menopause occurs well before old age, but noticeable decreases in testosterone levels occur much later in men. Sexual function may be tempered by decreased Bartholins secretions and diminished erectile power, but sexual ardor does not decrease with age, and it is a mistake to assume that the elderly cannot have and do not want active and fulfilling sex lives.

Emotional

If one had to characterize the emotional component of old age in a single phrase, the one that fits best is loss and grief. The combination of losses faced in old age is tremendous: spouse, job, a sense of productivity and belonging, home, the active role of parent, close friends, physical health, and all or part of one's previous income. All the components of a satisfying life are drastically changed, and some are gone forever. The task of coping with that much loss is difficult, and it is no wonder that depression is a serious problem of the elderly. Although the number of research studies pertaining to the emotional coping mechanisms of the elderly is increasing, there is no direct evidence to show that certain coping techniques work better than others. Health professionals can contribute most to easing the trauma of loss and grief by recognizing specific problematic areas and providing care that is both anticipatory and therapeutic.

The elderly react to the emotional problems of aging in as wide a variety of ways as the young react to their unique problems, but major categories or reactions can be identified. Grief or mourning occurs as a result of loss and may happen several times during old age. Grief is both a personal process and one that is defined by culture and religion. It is characterized by shock, which may be accompanied by physical symptoms such as a feeling of emptiness in the stomach or shortness of breath; feelings of disbelief, unreality, sadness, and anger; disorganization of usual thought processes and lifestyle; and anxiety and loneliness that last anywhere from a few months to a year. The many studies that have been done on grief reactions show a fairly predictable chain of events, although individual differences occur. When distortion of the typical grief process occurs, immediate family may not notice it or, if they do, they may assume it to be mere idiosyncrasy and not suggest that the ''morbidly'' grieving person seek help.

Guilt is a common emotional reaction of aging.

It stems from feelings about dead spouses, parents, and other relatives and toward children who unfortunately sometimes encourage guilt in parents and are unable to accept past resentments and hostilities. Guilt may provoke a renewed interest in religion, which can have the unexpected benefit of increased social activities as the old person becomes a regular churchgoer. Loneliness is an emotion that attacks all people of all ages; no one is protected from it, but it seems to affect old people in ways different from younger ones, most likely because they see themselves as having fewer opportunities for release from loneliness. This feeling may be grounded in reality, especially if the old person is physically isolated, shy, or has experienced many losses of friends and family. It is difficult to admit to loneliness; the need for companionship can be interpreted as self-pity (it may not be, but the elderly can feel this to be so). Asking for help may not have been part of the person's character in youth, and habits tend to grow more strongly entrenched as age increases.

A sense of anxiety in some form is always present in old age. Adapting to drastic changes in lifestyle and circumstances can be frightening; in reality there is much to be frightened or anxious about. The person's future is uncertain, both in terms of its existence and the way it will be lived. It is a common phenomenon to look ahead from retirement and feel a sense of helplessness or impotence. This is particularly true of men who have traditionally held much of society's power and who in retirement become almost powerless. Problems specific to retirement will be discussed in more detail later in this chapter.

Many old people experience a tremendous amount of anger, even rage, much of which is well-founded. Society treats old people as generally worthless, a nuisance, not particularly physically attractive, and a blot on the landscape of American youth and vigor. It seems perfectly natural and healthy to react with anger to being treated so shabbily, but much of this anger is directed inward and turns to depression. More and more, however, anger is being directed toward the system that per-petuates the poor treatment of the elderly, and old people have become a political force with an increasingly loud voice. One sees street demonstrations by the elderly in response to a variety of discriminatory acts, and organizations like the Grey Panthers are becoming increasingly active in securing civil rights for the elderly.

Whatever emotional aspects of aging exist, adaptive techniques match them. The reader is referred to the many excellent books on psychiatric nursing for a full description of how people use psychological adaptive techniques. A brief overview of those common to the elderly is appropriate here. It is sometimes easy to spot denial in the excessively youthful way an old person dresses or in the fact that an effort is made to continue the level of physical activity of youth or middle age. It is not uncommon for people of advancing years to view themselves as much younger than they are, despite the way in which they are viewed by others. Regression to earlier, less stressful phases of the developmental continuum is often an adaptation of aging. The phrase ''second childhood'' is used to describe such a reaction, but senility is not necessarily always implied.

Old people develop selective memories and tend to discard those parts of their lives that were unpleasant or somehow painful. Many develop what is called a counterphobia, that is, ''staring down'' the frightening or dangerous aspects of aging. For example, a woman who is subject to shortness of breath will venture out on a walk to a place where she knows there will not be a convenient spot to sit down and rest. Or a man who suffers dizzy spells will climb a stepladder to hang curtains. Counterphobias are another form of denial and a way of refusing to adapt to the inevitable deterioration of the flesh.

There are many healthy and productive reactions to aging: participation in social and political activities that directly benefit the elderly; seeking work (both paid and voluntary) that will in some way compensate if retirement is perceived as emptiness; and development of a rich inner life, augmented by reading, further education, and a healthy life view. ''The elderly individual who has a steady comprehension of the life process from birth to death is thereby assisted in his efforts to decide what to oppose and what to accept, when to struggle and when to acquiesce, and, ultimately, to understand the limits of what is possible.''[2.p.48]

Sexuality

One developmental aspect of aging that encompasses both the physical and emotional realms is sexuality. Masters and Johnson,[3] during the course of their extensive research on sexuality, found that what is generally believed to be true about sex and the elderly is not necessarily true. Their work shed much light on sexual functioning of all humans, including those who are no longer young. One of the most commonly believed sexual myths is that old people are ''beyond all that,'' that they have no sexual desire, and even if they did, they do not have the adequate physiological response to act on the desire. Sexual need and function come to a halt only with death, but changes do occur with aging. In both men and women physiological changes result in changes in sexual function. Women experience decreased sexual stimulation and muscular response, and genital tissues are less likely to engorge with blood and become lubricated. Orgasm still occurs, but the muscle contractions may be less intense, and the preexcitement phase is reached more rapidly after orgasm. Men achieve erection more slowly but are often able to maintain it for longer periods of time without ejaculation than can a younger man. The force of penile contractions during orgasm is less intense in the elderly man, as is the strength of ejaculation. The resolution phase (the time it takes for the penis to become completely detumescent) takes place more quickly, and an elderly man requires a considerable rest period before he is again capable of erection.

Both men and women report decreasing incidence of both intercourse and masturbation;[8] sexual activity decreases proportionately to increasing age. Several factors are responsible for lessening sexual activity: death of the spouse, illness, lack of interest due to grief, depression, loneliness, and lack of partners. The latter factor is responsible for a great deal of unrequited sexual longing; one hesitates to seek out and ask for an activity that is so frowned on by the rest of society. Today's elderly tend to have more conservative sexual attitudes than today's youth and thus may shy away from sexual fulfillment outside the marital bond. On the other hand, the process of aging and the ability to place values in perspective, if that ability exists, may help the old person place less stress on what other people think he *should* feel or need. This decreased concern for the opinion of others may help the elderly make sexual advances in their old age that they never would have dared in their youth.

In Western culture sexuality, youth, and beauty have been so closely allied with each other that it seems amazing to the young that an old person has sexual desires. By the same token, if one regards the primary purpose of sex as procreative, then sex has no real purpose after menopause has taken place; however, this is not a popular view. It is interesting to note here that a woman is not capable of reproduction after menopause, but she is perfectly capable of sexual response. A man's capability for both reproduction and sexual response (the two phenomena are interdependent) have no upper age limit. Therefore, if the main purpose of sex is reproductive, then a man would not be morally or socially castigated for continuing sexual activity as far into old age as he desires, while sex for a woman would be considered useless and therefore impermissible. Thus, sexual repression of women follows them even into old age. If, however, the purpose of sex is seen as pleasure, communication, or a way to strengthen the bonds of love and affection, then the sexual taboos of old age are less strong and more easily disregarded.

One way older people compensate for a lack of sex partners is to choose younger people. This, however, is easier discussed than accomplished and is frequently accompanied by societal ''punishment.'' An older woman who takes a young man as a lover is often looked at with disgust and ridicule (if he is very young and handsome, he is assumed to be a gigolo), whereas an old man with a young woman is better tolerated, but the assumption is made that he has money or another form of influence to offer as an inducement to sex. Lovers of widely disparate age groups are almost never viewed with societal equanimity. There is suspicion, envy, embarrassment, and outright hostility.

Financial

The elderly are one of the most economically disadvantaged groups in the United States. Because they are poorer than younger people, major (or even minor) health care expenditures are proportionately more financially devastating. Health care expenditures for the elderly are about four times what they are for persons under age 65.[5] This is due to the fact that the elderly are ill more frequently, have a wider variety of illnesses, and take longer to recover from each bout of illness than do younger persons. Hospital stays are longer, and the elderly take more prescription and nonprescription drugs. The elderly cannot afford this significantly greater extent of illness.

Poverty in general, not just as it relates to health care expenses, is a condition of many elderly. People who were always poor will grow poorer with age, and they will be joined by those middle income persons who depended on a regular paycheck to keep the wolf from the door. The elderly represent about 10% of the population but about 25% of American poor. Although in terms of numbers there are more poor whites than blacks, the poverty of the latter is more profound, and a greater percentage of blacks than whites are elderly poor. More elderly persons starve to death in America (or die of diseases where malnutrition is a strong contributory factor) than any other single age group.[2,pp.10-11] Another common myth about the elderly is that they can live on less money than younger people. Facts prove this to be false; food, clothing, transportation, housing, and health care are not benefited by ''senior citizens''' discounts. If elderly people live on less money, it is because they are forced to subsist on only the bare necessities of life. The American dream of a comfortable and relaxed retirement filled with books, travel,

and entertainment has been turned into a nightmare by inflation. The difference in the standard of living provided by the fixed income of a pension and the standard provided by the flexibility of a constantly escalating salary is enormous. There are some middle income and even rich elderly people, but they are in the minority: those persons whose income is derived from invested assets and who do not need to worry about inflation. Unless they are very wealthy and have incomes that are self-perpetuating, the nonpoor elderly are in constant danger of becoming poor when continuing inflation eats into their spendable income.

The elderly earn 20% of their aggregate income from continuing employment, while 46% comes from retirement, 4% from public assistance programs, and the remainder from investments (15%), veterans benefits (3%), and contributions from relatives (3%). It is commonly believed that the aged are adequately provided for by Social Security and Medicare. But these programs have not met the needs of the elderly.[2,p.12]

Social Security was never intended to be the primary source of income for retired elderly persons. When the Social Security Act was first passed in 1935, the tenor of the United States was far different than it is today. Working people were expected to save for their old age, and Social Security funds were to be used only in an emergency to prevent the kind of mass poverty that accompanied the Depression. The concept of Social Security was that it was (1) an insurance policy, that is, one is obligated to provide for one's old age; therefore government simply took a portion of one's paycheck to pay for that insurance, and (2) the young and middle aged contributed to the support of the elderly.

Of course, inflation, as well as fraud and government mismanagement, has made a mockery of that original intent. Every year or so the amount of Social Security benefits increases slightly but nowhere near as rapidly as the rate of inflation.

Poverty in old age causes and aggravates other problems of the elderly: malnutrition, inadequate health care, increased street crime, and violation of living spaces. It causes loneliness, depression, and isolation, and worst of all, it produces a hopelessness of spirit that nothing but money can relieve. Social Security contributions for salaried employees are mandatory (and probably will continue to be), but many people could have made wiser and more productive investments with the money deducted from their paychecks. This is a source of frustration and anger for those who know something about economic conditions and a reason for unknowing helplessness for those who do not understand what might have been. It is an example of government paternalism that began with good intentions but went awry.

COMMUNITY PROBLEMS SPECIFIC TO THE ELDERLY
Stress

The reader is referred to a discussion of the General Adaptation Syndrome in Chapter 8 for general organistic responses to stress. In an article written more than two decades after his initial work on stress and publication of the GAS concept, Hans Selye discusses the behavioral implications of stress.

It is a biologic law that man—like the lower animals— must fight and work for some goal that he considers worthwhile. We must use our innate capacities to enjoy the eustress of fulfillment. Only through effort, often aggressive egoistic effort, can we maintain our fitness and assure our homeostatic equilibrium with the surrounding society and the inanimate world. To achieve this state, our activities must earn lasting results; the fruits of work must be cumulative and must provide a capital gain to meet future needs.[6]

Selye goes on to describe a rather egoistic means to adapt to the behavioral manifestations of stress, and some of his ideas will be adaptable to the stress of aging. His philosophy is comprised of three major guidelines, which I shall state and then interpret as they can relate to the elderly.

1. Find your own natural predilections and stress level. Selye suggests that everyone has tolerable limits of stress and will tolerate more stress in activities considered valuable and worthwhile. He also suggests that desired changes can result in a break with tradition and thus decrease stress. The elderly frequently have no choice in the amount and kind of stress they must endure, and surely they cannot avoid certain stresses altogether. But the suggestion to increase self-knowledge about endurable stress levels is excellent. The elderly can examine their lives, isolate and identify particular stressors, and thus, and this is the crucial part, identify which stressors can be eliminated, which can be decreased, and which are immutable. The knowledge of what, if anything, can be done to alleviate stress, and action on that knowledge, can in itself be an effective stress reducer.

2. Learn altruistic egoism. Selye suggests that one build up and hoard the good will, love, and affection of others in order to enjoy a more creative, energetic, and beautiful life. This philosophy can be translated to the lives of the elderly by a seemingly simple maneuver: emphasize the positive. It is true that there are many aspects of old age that are humiliating, demeaning, and depressing. But there are also parts that can be pleasurable, even joyful. They exist in *everyone's* life, even those lives that are seemingly filled with nothing but misery. If an elderly person cannot find the pleasure in his life, it is up to the nurse to help him do so. One of the best "cures," albeit perhaps temporary, for depression is to list, with pencil and paper if necessary, all the positive aspects of one's life, no matter how seemingly insignificant. The community health nurse who sits down at the kitchen table with an elderly depressed person and encourages him to draw up such a list will be providing nursing care of the most professional and caring kind.

3. Earn your neighbor's love. "Who would blame him who wants to assure his own homeostasis and happiness by accumulating the treasure of other people's benevolence toward him?"[6] Selye could almost be promoting a kind of Golden Rule for the elderly. An old person who provides service, comfort, love, and affection for others will surely receive it in return, in increased measure and in increased self-esteem and happiness.

It is a common belief that certain factors such as stress in one's physical and social environment lead to an increased incidence of certain diseases.

Despite increased efforts, however, attempts to document the role of social factors in the genesis of disease have led to conflicting, contradictory, and often confusing results. There is today no unanimity of opinion that social factors are important in disease etiology, or if they are, which social processes are deleterious, how many such processes there are, and what the intervening links between such processes and disturbed physiologic states may be.[7]

Stress is one of the environmental factors about which there has been much research, little of it conclusive but a great deal indicative, that stress does cause some diseases and increase the severity of others. All stress results from a stimulus or a combination of stimuli, referred to as stressors. Individuals' ability to tolerate stressors vary so widely that it is difficult to pinpoint precisely what role, if any, stressors play in physical diseases. Determining whether the intrinsic or extrinsic effects of stress are the causative agents is also difficult. For example, if a person lives on a street that is frequently used by motorcyclists racing up and down, one cannot know if the noise itself is the stressor, if it is the person's reaction to the harshness of the noise, or if it is a combination of the two. Cassel[7,p.45] believes that a reasonable approximation between the psychosocial process and physical disease is that environmental stressors alter the body's endocrine balance, thus increasing susceptibility to disease organisms. The psychosocial processes can be seen as enhancing susceptibility, even if they cannot be proved to be a specific causative factor.

The stress to which the elderly are subject can sometimes be considered a causative factor in physical disease. Having to live in poverty and fear, with not enough food to eat surely is a stressor of the most humiliating and life-threatening kind. Drastic changes in life-style also produce stress. Scotch[8] found that blood pressure levels among Zulus who had recently moved to a city were higher than among the Zulus who had remained in the rural tribal surroundings *or* among those who had been living in the city for more than ten years. The stress factor was change, not the fact of city living. Those elderly who receive most of their protein intake from dog food risk not only severe protein malnutrition and disease from the dangerously high (for humans) bacteria content in dog food, they also face the stress of drastically changing their diet *and* from the unbelievable sadness and humiliation of having been reduced to such circumstances.

Cassel[7,p.51] further reports that family and social disorganization is a stressor that leads to increased rates of tuberculosis, mental illness, stroke, hypertension, and coronary disease. Since these are diseases that have a particularly high incidence among the elderly, it seems clear that an interrelationship, if not a definite causal relationship, exists between the social disorganization that always accompanies aging and these diseases. Holmes and Rahe[9] developed a rating scale of major and minor life changes (points are "scored" according to the severity or seriousness of the life changes); the higher the score, the more likely it is that physical illness will follow, within six months to a year. It seems logical to assume that because the elderly experience severe life changes, they will be more prone to physical illness. It also appears logical that coping with stress is a major developmental task of the elderly. Any health professional who neglects to take stressors into consideration when assessing and evaluating the health status of an elderly person is missing a major area of potential and actual health problems that *could be prevented*.

Loneliness

The physical and psychological isolation of the elderly is one of the most important problems that the community faces, even though most members of the community are not aware of the problem, and, when on rare occasions they must face it, it is so distressing that the most common reaction is to shudder in horror and then put it out of mind. The problem of lonely elderly people in the community is monumental.

Most elderly people have family, and 80% of them have living children; 67% live with some family member.[2,pp.8,119] However, the fact that a person lives in a family does not necessarily mean that loneliness is not a problem, although the potential for its alleviation exists. Many old people who live in families are ignored *as persons;* they are sometimes seen as crotchety, slow, and a general nuisance. The loneliness that results from this kind of attitude may be even harder to bear than living alone because expectations of warmth and companionship are dashed. It is analogous to the loneliness of an empty marriage as opposed to that of being single; hopes and expectations differ.

It is a common belief that Americans abandon their elderly, that is, put them into nursing homes when they become ''too much trouble,'' or simply leave them to fend for themselves. The general picture of the breakdown of American family life and increased societal emphasis on youth and vigor contribute to this belief. However, research has shown that it is not true. Most old persons who live alone are in contact with their families, and the majority actually live within the family fold. There is economic help, as well as varying degrees of support and affection, for most American elderly. Shanas[10] believes that the myth of the abandoned elderly is perpetuated by professional health and social workers who tend to come in contact with those old people who do not have adequate family supports, and by childless old people who believe that most elderly are neglected by their children. We might add a third factor that perpetuates the myth: the media. Newspaper and television ''magazine'' programs are fond of presenting investigative reports on the condition of the elderly in the United States. The reports are sad, dramatic, and true for those situations reported. However, frequently the reports are not placed in their realistic perspective in terms of comparison with the total. Thus the person reading the article in the Sunday paper, complete with heart-rending pictures, will assume that this is typically what happens to the elderly. Certainly, instances of horrifying abuse and neglect exist. Nursing home owners do bilk clients out of their financial assets; old people are starved and tortured by their families. More subtle forms of cruelty are more common. But they occur in a minority of instances.

Another myth is the wholesale ''dumping'' of old persons into nursing homes and other institu-

tions. Only 5% of the elderly in the United States live in institutions; why then, when the facts so clearly prove otherwise, is this myth so popular? One reason is probably because many of the nursing homes that do exist are appalling and the treatment of the elderly demeaning and inhumane. There are a few nursing homes that treat residents with dignity and respect, but they do not represent the average institution for the elderly. The ironic, but not unexpected, fact is that only the very wealthy can afford these few nursing homes. The others generally show a disrespect for personhood in the way the personnel treat clients. Many homes are physically pleasant and have more than adequate facilities, but the clients are viewed as mouths to be fed or beds to be changed, and more clients are patronized and condescended to (calling persons ''Pop'' or ''Hon'') than are not.

Another reason the myth persists is because health personnel and the media tend to emphasize the poor conditions in most nursing homes. Again, the facts are mostly accurate, and life is indeed bleak to the point of hopelessness for most nursing home residents, but 95% of persons over age 65 do not live in nursing homes. It is with this majority that community health nurses are concerned. Not all those 95% are lonely, and as we have seen, only a minority live in physical isolation, but loneliness in the elderly is a common enough phenomenon to make it a major problem. Loneliness compounds all other problems: physical illness sometimes becomes unmanageable; mental illness tends to increase; appetite decreases and nutrition suffers. Often continuing as a functional member of the community becomes impossible; it is to the prevention of this state of affairs that the community nurse should direct her efforts.

Retirement

Retirement is a psychological, financial, and social jolt from which many never recover. No matter how eagerly anticipated retirement was and no matter how many new activities there are to occupy time, the world of work is so unique that no other experience is the same. Even those business executives and academic and other professionals who are assured of work as consultants, advisors, and members of boards of directors find that life changes drastically upon retirement. Retirement is in many ways unfair because it is based on the arbitrary milestone of age and has nothing to do with competence, productivity, health, or even the desire to work. Those who argue for mandatory retirement point out that the business and professional world must provide employment for younger people who would not find jobs if mandatory retirement did not exist. However, no statistics exist to show the number of people who would not have retired if they were not forced to by company policy. One possible solution to the problem of unemployment of the young and mandatory retirement of the old is to restructure the work situation during the entire course of a person's working life, that is, work fewer hours per week for a greater number of years. The logistics of such an arrangement would be difficult but not impossible. American industry has not, however, shown much of an interest in this kind of flexibility in employment practices.

In a just and humane society workers should retire only if they choose to (or if they are incompetent because of age, but then that would not be considered retirement in the usual sense of the word). In American society where work is a major component of societal usefulness, mandatory retirement is particularly cruel if the person preferred to continue working. It can be accompanied by a sense of loss of self-worth and identity, increased idleness, and even a social stigma. In all instances it is a source of stress. The American Medical Association's Committee on Aging found that mandatory retirement inflicts a disease-producing condition that compares in severity with cancer, tuberculosis, and heart disease. The enforced idleness, according to the AMA, robs people of the will to live and deprives them of opportunities for compelling physical and mental activity. It encourages atrophy and decay and "narrows physical and mental horizons."[11] It is interesting to note that the vast majority of physicians are not subject to mandatory retirement.

As mandatory retirement is a fact of life (raising the age from 65 to 70 helped somewhat), the most effective way to cope with it and adapt to it is by anticipatory planning and counseling. The person in late middle age can engage in certain activities that will make retirement less stressful:

1. One should assess psychosocial needs with a realistic appraisal of how retirement will affect mental health. For example, a person who rarely spends an evening or weekend not working should know that retirement will be a particular source of stress. That person should begin to look for work opportunities outside the usual and traditional employment channels. Self-employment opportunities are almost limitless. If work is so integral a part of one's life that psychological health and survival are doubtful without it, then plans should be made to continue working, although perhaps in a different mode.

2. Financial planning is a necessity. All pension plans provide workers with information about what the pension benefits will be, and most people have a fairly accurate idea of their living expenses. True, the rate of inflation may continue to increase, and one cannot plan for every eventuality, but there should be an attempt to determine what future financial needs will be.

3. Persons facing retirement need to become familiar with the wide variety of government and private agencies available to help the elderly (these agencies and services will be discussed in more detail later in the chapter).

4. Planning for creative use of those extra 40 hours a week is essential. If an individual does not want to work at all or wants to work only part-time, the bulk of one's time must be filled to forestall the sense of hopelessness and uselessness mentioned previously. Persons living with a spouse must become used to many more hours of being together than had been their habit when one or both were working. Some marriages benefit from the increased companionship, but some founder from the strain of too much "togetherness."

5. The state of the person's physical health

should be assessed prior to retirement. Whatever physical problems exist, or seem likely in the future, should be known to the person so he can take whatever action seems most appropriate.

Unfortunately the role of the community health nurse in this anticipatory planning is usually minimal because most people in late middle age who should be engaging in the planning are relatively healthy and generally do not require the services of community health professionals. It is more likely that the nurse will come in contact with people who are already retired and who suffer from some health problem. She is then in a position to assess whatever damage retirement has done and to offer suggestions for reestablishing equilibrium and for increasing activities that provide meaning to life.

In developing a program of work, activity, and living for the retired person, the nurse should take into account his total personality, life-style, physical condition, and most important, what he wants to do with the rest of his life. Many old people want to spend their retirement years doing "nothing": sitting in the sun, visiting with friends, reading, and contenting themselves with their own thoughts. It is easy for the nurse to make the mistake of sweeping into people's lives and galvanizing them into action when they would prefer to plant a few tulip bulbs and then sit back and watch television. There is nothing essentially wrong or unhealthy about these activities as long as they are a result of conscious *choice* and not depression or hopelessness. A person who has worked for 50 years and has not derived much emotional or intellectual pleasure from it has every reason in the world never to want to work again. Retirement can be a time when responsibility for earning a living is gladly put aside and new and different activities explored. Although the independence that a regular paycheck provides might diminish to some degree, the absence of job and family responsibility can result in increased social and emotional independence. The goal of retirement should be to make it an occasion of choice, increased possibilities, and excitement.

Chronic illness

Any illness can exist in a chronic form; the elderly, especially the poor, are more susceptible to chronic illness than any other group of people. These two observations contribute to making chronic illness a major community health problem for the elderly. Added to this is the fact that the chronic illnesses seen most frequently in old people, such as arthritis, rheumatism, congestive heart failure, osteoporosis, and various degenerative neuromuscular diseases, are not "dramatic" enough to draw attention to themselves and therefore do not generate as much research interest and money as do more acute diseases from which people either suffer and die or recover dramatically. The slow wearing out of the body and the chronic debilitating diseases that accompany it do not interest the media, nor do they interest most scientists who want to make a "major" discovery. Not only are the elderly discriminated against, their diseases even take a back seat to those of younger people. Gerontology and gerontologic nursing are not popular specialities of health professionals.

The National Health Survey in 1974 indicated that about 14% of the general population suffer from chronic disease (11% were limited in their activity), but the number jumps to 39% in persons over 65. Of these chronic diseases, the most prevalent involve lesions of the central nervous system, closely followed by heart disease, hypertension, arthritis and other orthopedic conditions, and sensory impairment. The distribution of conditions resulting in visits to physicians' offices follows a similar pattern.[12]

More people suffer from chronic disease now than in the past, but it is not clear whether the increase is absolute or relative. Morbidity and death rates are not necessarily an accurate reflection of actual incidence and prevalence of chronic disease among the elderly. When death rates are calculated on an age-specific basis (a different rate for each year of life instead of a rate for an age range), it can be seen that the increase in death from chronic disease is not increasing as rapidly as had been thought.

On the other hand, some have pointed out that the population is not now aging as rapidly as before World War II and that the increase in chronic disease cannot be linked as closely to increased age of the population as previously assumed. Granted that older populations have more chronic diseases than do others, careful analysis indicates that there are not really enough of them proportionately to alone account for the difference. The sheer number of older persons who are better educated and more apt to be examined, and with improved diagnostic methods, must be considered.[12,p.497]

Because cure of most chronic diseases is unlikely in the near future, the basic way to manage the problem in the elderly must be prevention. Here the community nurse plays a vital role, both as a member of the community health team in attacking certain environmental and community problems that tend to cause or aggravate chronic diseases and as a nurse working with individual clients and families. The wider community approach is more difficult because it involves encouraging people to do things about which they are traditionally resistant: thinking about growing old and changing some practices that almost inevitably lead to chronic illness. Those changes might include suggestions to stop smoking, change basic nutritional habits, walk a few city blocks instead of taking the bus, and the like. Detection, early diagnosis, and adequate treatment of some acute diseases in youth, middle, and old age can sometimes prevent chronicity. Examples are rheumatic fever, kidney diseases of various types, musculoskeletal deformities, and some forms of respiratory disease. Some chronic diseases, although they may be unavoidable in and of themselves, such as diabetes or some cardiovascular diseases, can have their effects minimized by taking action to either delay their onset or lessen the severity. Mass screening procedures can frequently detect propensity for or early stages of chronic disease: diabetes, cardiovascular and respiratory diseases, cancer of some systems (colon, breast, lung, cervix), glaucoma, and others. There is some screening done today, and public education about chronic illness in relation to aging does exist, but both screening and education is done on a sporadic basis. A national commitment to prevention of chronic disease would require a major allocation of funds and somewhat of a change in national priority from emphasis on curing acute illness to preventing chronic disease. This would necessitate a major policy shift and would likely involve much sociopolitical debate.

Generally, one could say that in many instances the prevention of certain types of disease rests with the individual, and surely the responsibility for seeking health care is the individual's. But in the elderly this generalization is not easy to make. The choice of food that an old person eats may be limited by finances, and exercise could be difficult or impossible. If an elderly person detects an ache or pain that worsens or will not disappear, his inclination may be to visit a physician, but if transportation is inadequate or too complicated or if the weather is bad, the trip to the physician may be postponed or neglected. Finances are also a reason why symptoms are ignored or tolerated in silence; illness if expensive, and no matter how much government assistance is available, an outlay of cash is almost always necessary.

Old people generally react to the beginning of illness in two distinct ways: by exaggerating the symptoms and using them as a source of attention and seeking health care immediately, or by ignoring them and assuming that whatever is wrong is simply a manifestation of aging. Both reactions have problems. Those old people who seek attention for every ache or pain will soon be ignored or taken less seriously by health professionals who may fail to understand that old people imbue physical symptoms with more than physical qualities (a trip to the physician's office can be seen as a social occasion and something to relieve monotony). Of course, those symptoms that are ignored for whatever reason may not disappear spontaneously and may herald the beginning of a serious illness. Either way, the elderly person's health risk increases.

Substandard living conditions

Elderly persons live in as great a variety of places as do younger people, but because there is a higher percentage of poor people among the elderly than among the rest of the population, the elderly are more likely to live in substandard conditions, either alone or with others. This places them in double jeopardy, that is, not only are the homes or apartments themselves rundown, dirty, and unsafe, they are likely to be in city neighborhoods where the crime rate is exceptionally high, and the elderly are trapped indoors, unable even to escape the misery of their living environment. In Philadelphia, and probably in other major cities, organizations of adolescent boys provide an escort service for the elderly in some neighborhoods, walking with them to the bus stop, supermarket, or physician's office—to protect them from gangs of other adolescent boys who prey on the elderly. The necessity of living this way reminds one of the Old West where outriders "rode shotgun" to protect stagecoaches from bandits. This vigilante mentality is more appropriate to criminals who require bodyguards because they lead violent lives than to elderly persons who have done nothing to deserve the fear in which they are forced to live.

Those elderly persons who live in the suburbs with family or who have sufficient money to maintain a decent living standard do not constitute a community problem, at least in regard to their living conditions. Aside from acknowledging that the problem exists and suggesting ways in which life could be made a bit safer, there is little the community nurse can do about substandard living conditions because only one thing will alleviate the problem: money. Most times the source of the money must be private, but increasingly the federal government is becoming involved in aid to housing for the elderly. All the preventive health care in the world, all the nutritional advice the nurse can offer, and even all the sympathetic caring she provides will not change the facts of a dilapidated building, broken stairs, burnt out light bulbs, and muggers lurking on the streets and in the hallways.

Only legislative action and changes in people's attitudes about aging will improve the living conditions of the elderly poor.

ALLEVIATION OF PROBLEMS
Attitude changes

Old age has a negative connotation in the United States as it does in most of Western culture. We panic at the first grey hair and spend hard earned dollars on wrinkle potions. We fear growing old and try to postpone it for as long as possible. Old age itself is seen as an undesirable existence; only death follows. Death *always* follows old age. We fear death; therefore, we fear old age.

A middle aged man of my acquaintance plays tennis well and frequently. In fact, he would rather play tennis than do almost anything else. But what provides his greatest joy and satisfaction, and produces the most glowing smile, is winning games from young men. Winning against his contemporaries is not the triumph that winning against the 22-year-old tennis pro is. Aging is thus postponed for at least another little while.

American culture perpetuates the idea that old people are relatively useless. They are not permitted to work; health care research ignores them to a great extent; they are treated with impatience and a patronizing attitude by some younger people; and many elderly find themselves outside the mainstream of productive life.

The general almost phobic dislike of aging remains the norm, with healthy older people being ignored and the chronically ill receiving half-hearted custodial care. Only those elderly who happen to have exotic or "interesting" diseases or emotional problems or substantial financial resources ordinarily receive the research and treatment attentions of the medical and psychotherapeutic professions.[2,p.19]

What, then, can be done to change this negative view of old age? Correction of myths is a good beginning. Butler[2,pp.25-26] cites several common ones, which are listed below with some added suggestions about correcting misconceptions:

1. All aging occurs chronologically. Compare the picture of the man on the left in the photograph on p. 435 with other 98-year-old men you have seen, and it becomes obvious that not everyone ages at the same rate. The man's 75-year-old son looks healthier and sturdier than do many men at age 60.

2. All old people are senile. This is as untrue as the statement that all adolescents are sexually promiscuous or all homosexuals seduce children or the generalization that all members of any group engage in a particular activity or behavior. The term *senility* is not a precise descriptor and is frequently used in a perjorative way to describe those characteristics of the elderly that appear negative or irritating to others. It is not an accurate label of a disease or syndrome.

3. The tranquility myth portrays the elderly as calmly sitting and rocking on the front porch, enjoying life, and calmly accepting the inevitability of death. This myth is akin to the popular one of several decades ago that slaves were content to pick cotton and to be cared for by white masters. Many old people are angry to the point of rage about society's treatment of them, and many are forming politically active groups to improve the life of the aged.

4. All old people are unproductive. A list of names should be sufficient to dispel this myth: Pablo Picasso, Averill Harriman, Albert Einstein, Leopold Stokowski, Louise Nevelson, Grandma Moses, Arthur Rubinstein, Pablo Cassals, Helen Keller, David Ben Gurion, Henrietta Szold, Florence Nightingale, Golda Meir.

Another way of counteracting the negative image of aging is by viewing old age not only as a condition, but as another developmental phase of the life cycle. The final decade or two of life can be as full of learning about the world as the first decade. There is joy to be gained in fulfilling life goals and setting new and different ones. Grandparenthood has rewards and pleasures that are denied to parents. An understanding of what it means to be a person and to have endured, survived, and gained from a variety of life experiences is a benefit that accrues *only* to the elderly. Growing old is a transition to a new phase of existence, a rite of passage to what can be an exciting and fulfilling experience.

Nursing, if it is to fulfill its responsibility to the elderly, must contribute to changing negative attitudes. One way to do this is for the nurse herself to examine her own attitudes about aging and to assess the ways in which she provides nursing care to elderly clients. The nurse needs to ask herself what her own feelings, fears, and anticipations are in regard to her own old age. How does she relate to her grandparents (or to her parents if she is in middle age), and how does she perceive their lives? Another profitable experience for the community nurse is to compare the amount of time she spends with elderly clients with the amount spent with younger ones. Although this is not the only measure of attitudes, nor is it always precise, it can provide some indication that attitudes differ depending on the age of the client. If the nurse notices that she is spending significantly less time with elderly clients, she can be reasonably certain her nursing care is less professional and less caring than it should be. She can be absolutely certain that her motivations, attitudes, and practices need to be closely examined.

Services and benefits

Services and benefits for the elderly generally fall into five categories: (1) health maintenance, which includes private physicians, health maintenance organizations (HMO), and government and private screening programs; (2) prevention of disease or injury, which has components of health maintenance, but is not the same; (3) early detection and treatment of illness, which involves all agencies providing tertiary health care as well as health education programs; (4) limitation of disability and preservation of maximum function, which includes all rehabilitation services; and (5) restoration of as much independent activity as possible. Services for the elderly should include formal and informal education related to both health and general topics; research on needed services;

distribution of resources according to research indicators; health assessment and maintenance; ambulatory or follow-up care; high quality custodial care when necessary; nutrition counseling and actual provision of food; and financial resources.

The federal government is increasing its activities and allocating more resources as the proportion of elderly persons in the population increases and as the elderly become more vociferous in their demands to have their needs met. In terms of political power, the elderly constitute quite a sizable number of votes, and if they should ever vote as a bloc, their political power would increase. In 1958 the President's Council on Aging issued a report that led to formation of the Administration on Aging (AOA), which is part of the Department of Health and Human Services (DHHS). The AOA provides grant money to establish and maintain community services for the elderly, to conduct research, and to establish pilot or demonstration projects that are believed to hold potential value. The AOA also sponsors a wide variety of other projects, such as the Foster Grandparents Program, which matches (and pays for) the elderly poor with the children of the younger poor while their parents work or attend manpower development training programs. The Retired Senior Volunteers Program (RSVP) provides for travel and meal expenses for elderly people who wish to volunteer their services for a variety of community projects.

The Older Americans Act, passed in 1965 and amended in 1973 as a result of a second White House Conference in Aging in 1971, provides funding and consultation for a wide variety of state and local agencies that are charged with the task of improving services to the elderly. In 1974 the Research on Aging Act (PL 93-296) authorized establishment of the National Institute on Aging (NIA) of the National Institutes of Health. This guaranteed provision of funds for research on the biomedical, social, and behavioral aspects of aging and provides funds for the further training of gerontologic nurses and physicians. The philosophy of the NIA is that aging is not a disease but a life process. As a result, NIA research projects extend into many avenues of inquiry that are not specifically disease related, such as cellular biology and chemistry, the effects of stress on aging, all types of nutritional research, and the sociology of aging.

Increasing public awareness of the problem of aging has led to much legislation in the past two decades. This legislation provides benefits in several major categories: financial aid from the Old Age Assistance amendment to the Social Security Act; medical assistance provided by the legislatures in all 50 states, although in varying degrees and amounts; and a hospital insurance program under the Social Security Act that provides for several hospitalization plans.

Health services for the elderly are not as adequate as those provided for the young just as health services for the poor are not as adequate as those for the nonpoor. This may seem a broad and perhaps unwarranted generalization, but just as we have demonstrated how and in what ways the poor receive short shrift from the health care system, so do the elderly for a variety of reasons: they are unable to get to the places where health care is delivered; they may not understand the complexities of Medicare and fear that illness will be too costly; they may not understand the meaning of various signs and symptoms; and health care professionals tend to take people's physical complaints less seriously than those of younger people. In 1970 Congress passed the Emergency Health Personnel Act (PL 91-623), administered by the National Health Service Corps of the United States Public Health Service (USPHS). The act authorizes assignment of health personnel of the USPHS to areas where they are in short supply: usually inner cities and rural areas. In addition, various community health agencies provide both nursing services and homemaker care to the elderly, and hospital discharge planning services, if they function as they are designed to, should communicate potential problems and areas of need to the appropriate community agency.

Private funds and foundations also provide economic assistance both to the elderly themselves and to health and social welfare professionals to carry out research and service activities. For example, in 1980 the Robert Wood Johnson Foundation provided $4.6 million in grants to benefit the elderly in the areas of case-finding, rehabilitation, delivery of meals at home, university based research, and education of health professionals.

MEDICARE

Medicare has had a greater influence on the health care of the elderly than any other single public or private act. Medicare is officially known as Title XVIII of the Social Security Act, ''Health Insurance for the Aged and Disabled'' (PL 89-97) and became effective on July 1, 1966. It has two major components: Part A, which provides hospital insurance benefits, and Part B, which provides supplementary medical insurance benefits, that is, medical expenses incurred outside the hospital. Part A is automatically provided to all persons at age 65 who are receiving Social Security benefits; Part B is optional and must be purchased by the individual. Medicare is essentially an insurance policy whose premiums are paid by the federal government (all of Part A) or are shared by the government and the beneficiary (Part B). It is administered by the Health Care Financing Administration of the DHHS.

Generally, the home health services covered by Medicare are short-term, skilled services utilized by persons recovering from an acute illness or injury. Part A, in fact, requires that the client has had a prior hospital stay of at least 3 days. Home health aide services are provided only in addition to skilled nursing care, speech therapy, or physical therapy. As it is now, Medicare has essentially no coverage for long-term, maintenance, or preventive home health care services.[13]

Not only is Medicare not the panacea for the health needs of the elderly that was hoped for, it has caused a multitude of problems in health care delivery. Because of health provider fraud, political decisions, and bureaucratic snafus, the Social Security Administration has repeatedly denied payment to providers of service, with a resultant cutback in the services they are willing to offer. Home

health agencies were among the most drastically affected. Opportunities for graft in the Medicare system are almost limitless, and those physicians and other health care providers who have been indicted and convicted of Medicare fraud represent only a tiny fraction of actual fraudulent practices. The shaky financial position of the Social Security Administration itself perpetually jeopardizes provision of Medicare benefits as well as other Social Security benefits. The paperwork involved in processing claims is so voluminous that all hospitals and even some private physicians employ personnel to do nothing but work with Medicare claims. For this reason many nonhospital providers of care are loathe to accept ''Medicare patients.'' Processing the forms consumes so much of the office overhead that providers frequently react in one of two ways: they reject the clients, or they cheat Medicare.

Whatever the shortcomings of the administration of Medicare, the fact remains that it provides health service to hundreds of thousands of elderly persons who ordinarily would have received no care or fewer health benefits than Medicare now provides. Eligible persons are grouped in two categories: those who are over age 65 and who are eligible for Social Security benefits and disabled persons under age 65 who meet Social Security disability regulations and who have been disabled for more than 24 months. The vast majority of Medicare beneficiaries fall into the first category. The rules, regulations, definition of terms, eligibility requirements, and statements of benefits are a bureaucratic nightmare; those readers who require details are referred to the appropriate government documents, but the following is a general picture of nonhospital benefits: skilled nursing care in the home after acute illness that required at least three days hospitalization; home health aide service to prevent or postpone institutionalization; speech, physical, and occupational therapy; social service; and various consultative services such as a nutritionist. Medicare will provide 100 days of skilled nursing care in an extended care facility (ECF) *only* if it is justified by the ECF and agreed to by Medicare auditors. Most people believe the 100 days are an automatic right and do not realize that Medicare can refuse payment if the need for skilled care is not documented. Many people find the Medicare reviewers to be arbitrary and capricious, often refusing to justify denial of claims. Medicare does not provide extended services to the elderly and chronically ill, that is, to those people who most require home care, unless there has been a prior hospitalization. Home health benefits generally provide for early discharge from a hospital or prevent or delay the need for institutionalization. Stewart[13,p.110] recommends several needed Medicare reforms: the range of services should be expanded, especially for homemaking and transportation; eligibility for service should not be tied to the need for another service (for example, only those who have been hospitalized are eligible for skilled nursing service at home); the number of allowed home visits should be increased; the physician requirement for determination of eligibility for service should be removed and any qualified health professional should be permitted to recommend need for services; regulations could be interpreted less strictly, although this last recommendation might lead to an even greater amount of fraud. Medicare appears to be a fine piece of liberal legislation that has gone slightly awry and at times seems to cause as many problems as it solves.

Improved nutrition

Diets of the elderly are by and large deficient in both quantity and quality. Both problems are due mainly to shortage of money, although they are complicated by decreased appetite, poor cooking facilities, and chronic illness and fatigue that make cooking too much of a chore. Older persons generally require fewer calories per pound of body weight because they tend to exercise less (calorie requirements would, of course, increase if exercise increased) and because tissue grows and develops at a much slower rate. Many older people are overweight for several reasons: poor eating habits that do not change as calorie requirements decrease; boredom, frustration, and loneliness sometimes lead to eating as "something to do"; high carbo-

hydrate foods such as potatoes, rice, pasta, and junk food tend to be less expensive and more filling than foods with high concentrations of protein, vitamins, and minerals.

Nutritional services are provided by Medicare, and one of the functions of a home health aide is helping the client with meal preparation and grocery shopping. The Older Americans Act provided for one hot meal a day to be served to the aged, either in community centers or at home through such agencies as Meals on Wheels. One important way for the elderly to improve the quality of their nutritional intake and to maintain the social activities that surround food and eating is the communal sharing of meals, which can be accomplished in several ways. One is for elderly people to live together in communal houses or apartments. In addition to the obvious social, emotional, and financial benefits of such an arrangement, the responsibility and pleasure of cooking for others almost guarantees well-balanced and enjoyable meals. Those who would tend to live on cold sandwiches and junk food because they did not have the energy and inclination to cook for themselves would be encouraged by their housemates to eat. A way to encourage communal cooking and eating without communal living is for a number of elderly persons in a neighborhood to form a "cooking cooperative" in which they come together for one or two meals a day. A schedule is arranged for periodic responsibility for shopping, cooking, and dishwashing. Yet another arrangement is to take meals at a local community center. The point in sharing meals is that everyone, no matter what one's culture, associates eating with socializing, and although a solitary meal while reading a good novel or watching television is frequently pleasurable, the necessity of having to eat alone all the time is depressing and lonely. Communal eating can be an appetite stimulant.

Another important way in which nutrition can be improved is for the nurse to accurately assess the elderly client's nutritional habits and patterns. The diet history should include not only the kinds and amounts of foods eaten (a written nutrition ''diary'' is helpful for this, as is a 24- or 48-hour nutrition recall if the client's memory permits this), but what the person's shopping habits are, what supplemental vitamins he takes, and how and with whom the person usually eats. The nurse should also note existing cooking facilities; a hot plate and tea kettle are most assuredly not the same as a full kitchen and can be a clue to poor nutrition. A diet history must be obtained with the utmost kindness and discretion. A person whose protein requirement comes from dog food and who has not had a piece of fresh fruit or a salad in years is likely to be ashamed and humiliated by that fact. Whatever lies a client might tell the nurse about his eating patterns will be out of unwillingness to admit the truth and a desire not to be a ''bother'' to the nurse. Nutritional lies told by the elderly are frequently seen as necessary to protect their dignity and whatever self-esteem remains. The nurse must never ''catch'' the person in a lie; it would be an act of cruelty. Consider the picture of a student nurse, whose rosy cheeks and bursting good health proclaim her good nutrition, sitting at a kitchen table talking to an elderly person who eats mostly watered canned soup and pasta. If the student can put herself in the client's position for a moment, she would see the unfairness and tragedy of the situation and will increase her sensitivity to the plight of the elderly.

One way the student might be able to gain an idea of how the elderly are forced to eat is to eat what her clients do for a week. She can base her week's menu on either one client's nutritional pattern or on a composite of several clients. She should also, as far as possible, try to prepare and eat her meals in circumstances similar to the client. In all likelihood the student will be eating alone, foregoing late-night pizza snacks, and may be thoroughly bored and depressed by the end of the week.

Research

Research on aging has as its primary goal increased knowledge about the aging process itself. Secondary goals include extending the human life span and making the process of aging more physically, psychologically, and socially comfortable. Research on extending the life span investigates areas such as nutrition, cellular biology, living arrangements, past life habits and practices, and more elusive qualities such as the will to live and perceptions of the future. Shock[14] found four major factors that affect the length of the life span: environmental conditions; disease, particularly cardiovascular, respiratory, and cancer; obesity; and reserve capacity for organ function and regeneration.

The reader is referred to various research and gerontologic journals for details of research findings; a general overview will suffice for our purpose here. Scientists at the Rand Corporation have predicted that in only half a century the aging process will be chemically controlled, and biochemicals will be used to stimulate growth of new cells to make regeneration of some organs and systems almost limitless. Research findings on diseases that are the major causes of death in all adult age groups can be related to the aging process. Surgical techniques have been developed to replace organs and parts of organs, and it is assumed that organ transplant research will continue so that ''spare part surgery'' will become commonplace, as will replacement of some body parts with synthetic ones. Social research continues in the area of the effects of retirement and alternative plans if developing technology leads to more people choosing early retirement. Leisure or ''empty'' time and its effect on the elderly is being studied, as is the possibility of beginning a new career in mid-life and basing retirement on the number of years worked in a particular field, not on chronological age. Research also needs to be done on the role of the older person in society, the places they occupy, the contributions they make, and the ways in which they are perceived by the nonelderly.

One particularly interesting and significant study is ''The Effects of Aging on Attitudes and Activities.''[15] It had been assumed that aging changes persons' attitudes and activities, but Palmore and his associates found that this was not always necessarily the case. At three-year intervals over a period of more than ten years, 127 participants were examined and interviewed, using a variety of physical and psychological measures. The men showed almost no overall reduction in activity in the ten years; the women showed more reduction, but it was still relatively small. At the end of the study the age range was 70 to 93 with a mean age of 78. Two plausible explanations are offered for the results: first, although the elderly may decrease activity in some spheres of life (work and social organizations), they tend to compensate by increasing activity in other spheres, such as family contacts and religious activities. Second, the participants were relatively healthy and managed to survive for the ten years of the study; the fact of being healthy would tend to assure continued activity and more positive attitudes toward life than would the fact of being unhealthy. Thus the study did not represent an accurate cross-section of the elderly in the community. Another finding was that activity was positively correlated with attitudes; that is, the more positive one's attitude, the greater and more varied the activity level.

Research on the length of human life should be closely associated with research on the quality of that life. It seems absurd to increase an existence marked mainly by poverty, isolation, and misery. Although all human life has value, and some believe that life should be preserved and continued no matter what the circumstances of that life, it seems counterproductive of dignity and pleasure to ignore life's quality in favor of only quantity.

NURSING CARE

The major goal of the community nurse when caring for the elderly should be in improvement of all aspects of the person's life. If a person, no matter what his age, is encouraged to achieve his maximum potential for living, the quality of his life must improve. Nursing assessment of the elderly person or couple should include physical assets and liabilities and what is currently being done to alleviate or control physical health problems; the interactions that the elderly person has with the people with whom he lives, with family and friends, and with the community as a whole, or at least those segments of the community that relate to his life; economic status and possible sources of financial assistance; nutritional status and shopping, cooking, and eating habits; exercise and the capacity for physical mobility, including how mobility restrictions affect the person's daily life; the individual's general outlook on life, how he feels about himself and the future; and the activities in which the person participates and what his life interests and goals are.

The reader is referred to the detailed description of the nursing process to determine how the process can be specifically applied to the elderly, but some general suggestions for interventions are in order here:

1. Arrange for attention to whatever physical problems exist by suggesting health care services in the client's neighborhood if a family physician is not available. This may include arranging for transportation or for escort service.

2. Help with the bureaucratic paperwork that is involved in association with any public or private agency. Forms to be filled out may loom as a monumental task, especially if the print is too small to be easily read. The complexities of social organizations can sometimes defeat even the most persistent person (a phone call to obtain routine information may involve being transferred to two or three different departments); the elderly may give up rather than persevere and suffer frustration.

3. Establish goals in maximizing physical and psychosocial potential based on the desires and needs of the client. If the person wants to find part-time work, help him write a resume and suggest ways to obtain job interviews. If the person wants to get out and take walks in the neighborhood, organize groups of older persons, perhaps with an adolescent escort, for regular exercise. Help the client achieve his own goals, not those that his family and health professionals may have for him. If the nurse does not think she is qualified to do this, she can refer the client to agencies that specialize in this kind of action, such as the National Association of Retired Persons.

4. Spend time with the person if he is lonely. This may be difficult to accomplish if the nurse works for an agency that has a quota of home visits she is expected to make each day. But there will be creative ways to cope with even this obstacle. For example, assuming that the permission of all those involved is obtained and the client is physically able, the nurse might take the client along with her on another home visit. There is nothing to prevent the nurse from introducing clients to each other. If at the end of the work day, the nurse finds she has extra time because many of her clients were not at home, she could stop in to play a game of cards with a lonely elderly client. The creative, caring nurse will devise many more ways to increase time spent with clients. If the nurse finds she absolutely can spend no more time with clients than she is presently giving, it would be worthwhile to put the client in contact with various community groups of elderly people.

5. Work toward increasing social and legislative benefits for the elderly. This may involve political action or volunteering one's time or financial resources toward that end. It could mean participation in community education activities or serving as a consultant to a variety of public and private community agencies.

6. If possible, the nurse should strive to increase the client's interaction with his family, even if it is only an occasional telephone call. Sometimes old persons misperceive families' attitudes and feelings. The statement, ''What do these young kids want with an old lady like me?'' may be more of a reflection of the elderly's decreased self-esteem and an expression of hope than an accurate depiction of the family's real attitude. A visit to the client's children or other relatives might be in order for the nurse. One woman had a sister in a nursing home with whom she had been very close throughout her whole life, but she never visited her sister. When the nurse asked why, the woman replied, ''When the people in the home see what a tottery old woman I am, they'll want to keep me there too.'' No amount of persuasion could make the woman believe this was not true, so one morn-

ing the nurse called from the office and ''ordered'' the client to have her hat and coat on in an hour. She put the client in her car and drove her to visit her sister. The reunion was so joyous that the two sisters were able to reestablish their former closeness.

The point to all nursing care of the elderly, as the point to all care of all human beings, is to help them improve the quality of their lives, to maximize happiness, and to create the feeling that it is good to still be alive.

SUMMARY

Old age in America is frequently unpleasant, lonely, and filled with unhappiness, but the saddest part is that this state of affairs is, by and large, unnecessary. The social and economic facts of life for the elderly are unduly harsh, frequently because of negative attitudes toward old people. Developmental aspects of aging are not all negative, but problems do exist. The physical person deteriorates to some degree at vastly different individual rates, and certain physical problems such as degenerative musculoskeletal diseases tend to be characteristic of the elderly. Sleep and eating patterns change, and exercise usually decreases, as does sensory acuity. The emotional component of aging varies as much as the emotional reactions of younger persons. One's outlook on life generally reflects one's living conditions: the more of everything that one has in old age (money, health, comfort, family, friends, and activities), the more likely one is to be content and filled with a sense of a positive future. The major emotional problems faced by old people are loneliness and isolation, which are frequently compounded by poverty and poor health.

The elderly are often poor and are more likely to be poor than younger people. Poverty for the elderly is more serious than for others because there is no possible way out. The elderly poor live on fixed incomes which, for the most part, cannot keep pace with the constantly spiraling inflation; therefore the elderly grow even poorer each year. The two major results of poverty are substandard living conditions and inadequate nutrition.

Community problems exist that affect everyone but are especially problematic for the elderly. Stress is one that the elderly find more difficult to adapt to because they tend to have less flexibility of action and are less future oriented than the nonelderly. Loneliness is a problem that is surmountable, but it takes persistence, creativity, and imagination on the part of those who wish to help. Loneliness is also compounded by poverty; they have an interdependent causal relationship.

Retirement, especially when it is mandatory, can be a blessing or a curse. It can provide the freedom to do all the things one planned for, or it can create a sense of emptiness and uselessness. The best way to achieve positive retirement is to plan for it during middle age. Chronic illness affects the elderly more than any other group and is frequently aggravated by isolation, poor nutrition, and poverty. The single most important way to manage chronic illness is by prevention, both of the disease itself and of chronicity. A national commitment to the prevention of chronic illness, which implies allocation of large sums of money, would significantly decrease its incidence.

Alleviation of the problems of the elderly include attitude changes on the part of health professionals and the lay public; provision of public and private services and benefits, including a major overhaul of Medicare benefits and regulations; improved nutrition; more and wider-ranging research on the physical and psychosocial components of aging; and competent, professional, and creative nursing care.

NOTES

1. Cousins, Norman: The right to die, Saturday Review, p. 4, June 14, 1975.
2. Butler, Robert N., and Lewis, Myrna I.: Aging and mental health, ed. 2, St. Louis, 1977, The C.V. Mosby Co., p. 5.
3. Masters, William H., and Johnson, Virginia E.: Human sexual response, Boston, 1970, Little, Brown & Co.
4. Woods, Nancy F.: Human sexuality and the healthy elderly. In Brown, Mollie, editor: Readings in gerontology, ed. 2, St. Louis, 1978, The C.V. Mosby Co., p. 80.
5. Weaver, Jerry L.: National health policy and the underserved, St. Louis, 1976, The C.V. Mosby Co., p. 23.
6. Selye, Hans: Stress without distress. In Garfield, Charles A., editor: Stress and survival, St. Louis, 1979, The C.V. Mosby Co., p. 15.
7. Cassel, John: Psychosocial processes and 'stress': theoretical formulation. In Garfield, Charles A., editor: Stress and survival, St. Louis, 1979, The C.V. Mosby Co., p. 45.
8. Scotch, N.A.: A preliminary report on the relation of sociocultural factors to hypertension among the Zulu, Annals of the New York Academy of Science **84**(17):1000-1009, 1960.
9. Holmes, T., and Rahe, R.: The social readjustment rating scale, Journal of Psychosomatic Research **11**:213-218, 1967.
10. Shanas, E.: The unmarried old person in the United States: living arrangements and care in illness, myth, and fact, paper prepared for the International Social Science Research Seminar in Gerontology. Marbaryd, Sweden, August, 1963.
11. Retirement: a medical philosophy and approach, Chicago, 1972, American Medical Association.
12. Hanlon, John J., and Pickett, George E.: Public health administration and practice. ed. 7, St. Louis, 1979, The C.V. Mosby Co., pp. 495-496.
13. Stewart, Jane E.: Home health care, St. Louis, 1979, The C.V. Mosby Co., p. 97.
14. Shock, Nathan W.: Age with a future. In Brown, Mollie, editor: Readings in Gerontology, ed. 2, St. Louis, 1978, The C.V. Mosby Co.
15. Palmore, Erdman B.: The effects of aging on activities and attitudes. In Brown, Mollie, editor: Readings in Gerontology, ed. 2, St. Louis, 1978, The C.V. Mosby Co.

BIBLIOGRAPHY

Bahr, Sr. Rose Therese: The family facing retirement. In Hymovich, Debra P., and Barnard, Martha U., editors: Family health care, ed. 2, New York, 1979, McGraw-Hill Book Co.

Brown, Mollie, editor: Readings in gerontology, St. Louis, 1978, The C.V. Mosby Co.

Busse, Geraldine, and Simpson, Roger: Dentistry and nursing work together to improve care of the aged, Journal of Gerontological Nursing **6**(5):280-283, May, 1980.

Butler, Robert N., and Lewis, Myrna I.: Aging and mental health, St. Louis, 1977, The C.V. Mosby Co.

Cassel, John: Psychosocial processes and 'stress': theoretical formation. In Garfield, Charles A., editor: Stress and survival, St. Louis, 1979, The C.V. Mosby Co.

Chow, Rita K.: Quality of care: a present and future challenge for all nurses, Journal of Gerontological Nursing **6**(5):255-259, May, 1980.

Dickman, Sherman R.: Nutritional needs and effects of poor nutrition in elderly persons. In Reinhardt, Adina M., and Quinn, Mildred D.: Current practice in gerontological nursing, St. Louis, 1979, The C.V. Mosby Co.

Garfield, Charles A., editor: Stress and survival, St. Louis, 1979, The C.V. Mosby Co., 1979.

Gelein, Janet L.: Improving distributive health care for the elderly through continuing education for nurses. In Hall, Joanne E., and Weaver, Barbara R.: Distributive nursing practice: A systems approach to commuity health, Philadelphia, 1977, J.B. Lippincott Co.

Grants to coordinate community services for elderly, Journal of Gerontological Nursing **6**(5):284-285, May, 1980.

Gress, Lucille D.: The family with an elderly member. In Hymovich, Debra P., and Barnard, Martha U., editors: Family health care, ed. 2, New York, 1979, McGraw-Hill Book Co.

Hall, Joanne E., and Weaver, Barbara R.: Distributive nursing practice: a systems approach to community health. Philadelphia, 1977, J.B. Lippincott Co.

Hanlon, John J., and Pickett, George E.: Public health administration and practice, ed. 7, St. Louis, 1979, The C.V. Mosby Co.

Hymovich, Debra P., and Barnard, Martha U., editors: Family health care, ed. 2, New York, 1979, McGraw-Hill Book Co.

Marley, Margaret S.: The making of a group, Journal of Gerontological Nursing **6**(5):275-279, May, 1980.

Masters, William H., and Johnson, Virginia E.: Human sexual response. Boston, 1970, Little, Brown & Co.

Murray, Ruth, and Zentner, Judith: Nursing assessment and health promotion through the life span, Englewood Cliffs, N.S., 1975, Prentice-Hall, Inc.

Palmore, Erdman B.: The effects of aging on activities and attitudes. In Brown, Mollie, editor: Readings in gerontology, St. Louis, 1978, The C.V. Mosby Co.

Reiff, Theodore R.: The essentials of a geriatric evaluation, Geriatrics May, 1980, pp. 59-68.

Reinhardt, Adina M., and Quinn, Mildred D.: Current practice in gerontological nursing, St. Louis, 1979, The C.V. Mosby Co.

Retirement: a medical philosophy and approach, Chicago, 1972, American Medical Association.

Riffle, Kathryn L.: Physiological changes of aging and nursing assessment. In Reinhardt, Adina M., and Quinn, Mildred D.: Current practice in gerontological nursing, St. Louis, 1979, The C.V. Mosby Co.

Robischon, Paulette, and Akan, Alice M.: The family and its role with the elderly parent. In Reinhardt, Adina M., and Quinn, Mildred D.: Current practice in gerontological nursing, St. Louis, 1979, The C.V. Mosby Co.

Selye, Hans: "Stress without distress. In Garfield, Charles A., editor: Stress and survival, St. Louis, 1979, The C.V. Mosby Co.

Shock, Nathan W.: Age with a future. In Brown, Mollie, editor: Readings in gerontology, St. Louis, 1978, The C.V. Mosby Co.

Spradley, Barbara W.: Contemporary community nursing, Boston, 1975, Little, Brown & Co.

Stanford, E. Percil: The politics of providing health and mental health care for the aged. In Reinhardt, Adina M., and Quinn, Mildred D.: Current practice in gerontological nursing, St. Louis, 1979, The C.V. Mosby Co.

Stewart, Jane E.: Home health care, St. Louis, 1979, The C.V. Mosby Co.

Sullivan, Therese: The subculture of the aging and its implications for health and nursing care to the elderly. In Reinhardt, Adina M., and Quinn, Mildred D., Current practice in gerontological nursing, St. Louis, 1979, The C.V. Mosby Co.

Troll, Lillian E.: Eating and aging. In Brown, Mollie, editor: Readings in gerontology, St. Louis, 1978, The C.V. Mosby Co.

Wahl, Patricia R.: Therapeutic relationships with the elderly, Journal of Gerontological Nursing **6**(5) May, 1980. pp. 260-66.

Weaver, Jerry L.: National health policy and the underserved, St. Louis, 1976, The C.V. Mosby Co.

Wells, Thelma J.: Nursing committed to the elderly. In Reinhardt, Adina M., and Quinn, Mildred D., Current practice in gerontological nursing, St. Louis, 1979, The C.V. Mosby Co.

Woods, Nancy F.: Human sexuality and the healthy elderly. In Brown, Mollie, editor: Readings in Gerontology, St. Louis, 1978, The C.V. Mosby Co.

18

CULTURAL DIVERSITY IN THE COMMUNITY

The United States has often been described as a melting pot, an expression used to describe its enormous cultural diversity. Once when I was a child on a trip around New York harbor, my mother pointed out Ellis Island where so many hundreds of thousands of immigrants had been processed through the bureaucracy to begin a new life in the United States. I asked if we could stop to see the big pot where they melted the people. When my mother asked what I meant, I explained that since America is a melting pot, I had assumed that all the people who came here were transformed, melted, from whatever they had been into Americans and that the pot must be on Ellis Island. An avid tourist, even as a child, I wanted to see the process. My mother explained what the phrase meant, and later she took me to visit some of New York's ethnic neighborhoods so I could see for myself that cultural differences were indeed not ''melted'' out of people. This chapter will be a celebration of the fact that the giant pot of my childhood fantasy does not exist.

The community nurse must first recognize the great cultural diversity that exists in any community; she then must learn how the fact of belonging to a particular culture can affect health and attitudes that surround health. We shall begin with definitions. One's culture is usually defined in terms of one's ethnic background. Ethnicity pertains to a social group within a cultural or social system that

stands apart from the larger system on the basis of one or more several distinguishing variables: religion, language, ancestry, or physical characteristics. Within an ethnic group are many degrees of ethnicity. For example, Jews are generally considered to be an ethnic group in the United States. Yet there is much diversity among American Jews: Chassidic Jewish men are easy to recognize because of their characteristic dress and appearance; they are strictly Orthodox in their religious observances and stand out sharply against the backdrop of American life. Other Jews are not the least bit Semitic in appearance and have become so assimilated into American life that it is impossible to distinguish them from other Americans. Yet all Jews share a common ethnic and religious heritage that sets them apart from all other people, and it is the fundamental part of their existence, second only to the fact of their personhood. Other common examples of ethnic groups in the United States are people who share a common national origin such as Polish Americans, those who speak a common language such as Ukranian, and those with distinguishing physical characteristics such as black Americans.

The phrase *ethnic group* or *ethnicity* has, from time to time in American history, raised both strong positive and strong negative feelings. Members of ethnic groups have been used and abused, both by each other and by those Americans who claim to belong to no particular ethnic group. Politicians court ethnic groups for votes by acknowledging that they are groups with special interests and needs and then tend to ignore campaign promises. The serious abuse and repression of ethnic groups has always been, and continues to be, a problem in the United States, although at the present time it is exhibited at a different and more subtle level. A few examples illustrate this abuse: when the Irish came to this country in huge immigration waves as a result of famine in Ireland in the early part of the nineteenth century, it was common to see the phrase "INNA" on help-wanted advertisements in newspapers and on placards in windows advertising for employees. The acronym meant "Irish need not apply" and was testimony to the severe employment discrimination of the new Irish immigrants.

When the United States was first being criss-crossed with railroad tracks, Orientals laid the tracks a good part of the way. They were totally subject to the employment practices of the railroad companies, and benevolence was not one of the railroads' characteristic ways of treating lower level employees. The Oriental laborers were fed insufficiently and were worked until many of them dropped dead from malnutrition and overwork. Because most of them spoke no English and were living in a culture so foreign to their own, they were almost totally at the mercy of others.

Blacks were brought to this country in chains and lived for a century and a half as slaves. Although slavery has been illegal for 120 years, blacks in the United States are among the most disadvantaged and discriminated against groups.

Within a culture or ethnic group there are norms that constitute standards of acceptable behavior for the members of that group or rules of conduct for what may and may not be done. The rules frequently apply to courting and mating behavior, particularly as they relate to marriage outside the culture or ethnic group.

The *beliefs* of the society are its collective sense of what is real. Beliefs are descriptive statements. To the

extent that they are shared . . . they constitute a distinctive world view for the group or society under consideration.

The importance of both norms and beliefs lies in the enforcement. Adherence to the belief system of the group and its standards of behavior will be rewarded, and deviations will be punished. These *sanctions* can vary in intensity from mild (e.g. a nod of approval or shake of the head) to severe (e.g. a formal award of a title or honor on the one hand to the death penalty on the other). The intensity of sanctions is governed by seriousness with which the deviation is regarded, norms regarding the appropriateness of response by others, and beliefs in the effectiveness of the response in altering behavior.[1]

Values are often a component of culture; they are defined as criteria to be used in the event that a conflict arises over behavioral norms. Values are generally seen as both good in and of themselves (intrinsic value) and good for what they can achieve or accomplish (instrumental value). The "Protestant work ethic" is an example of a value; that is, work is seen as both good in and of itself and good because it can help to obtain other desirable values, such as career advancement, greater social status, increased income, and the like. Education is highly valued among Jews for the same reasons. Female virginity until marriage is prized among some Latin cultures because it is seen as a badge of honor and purity, a marital gift for one's husband.

Before we continue to describe cultural or ethnic differences, a word should be said about the dangers of stereotyping and making generalizations about groups of people. Stereotypes exist because many people in a particular culture or ethnic group *do* exhibit certain physical, social, or psychological characteristics. The stereotype would not exist if this were not true. However, the issue in stereotyping is not that it exists, but how it is used. More people use racial, cultural, or ethnic stereotypes for negative purposes than for positive ones. None are harmless, but some are more harmful than others. For example, the common belief that Jews are good at business really does not do any major harm, although some Jews are hurt, especially if they have been using a great deal of red ink at work. But the stereotype that blacks commit more crimes than whites is tremendously harmful because it creates a negative impression in people's minds, particularly the police who might be tempted to arrest a black person when there are no reasonable grounds for doing so.

Although there are characteristics that are common to members of certain ethnic groups, those groups are composed of individual human beings who should be treated as such. For example, a common belief about Puerto Rican families is that they are very patriarchal; that is, the father is dominant and expects to be accorded subservience and respect from his wife and children. This may be an important piece of information for the community nurse to have if she works in a Puerto Rican neighborhood, but it does not mean that every Puerto Rican family she sees will be characterized by a dominant father. Not all Cubans like to dance the *salsa* to Caribbean music; some find the waltz more to their liking; surely many Mexicans would prefer a meal of meat, vegetables, and a salad to refried beans. There are American Indians who have never been near a reservation and would hardly know what to do with a feathered headdress if one were put into their hands.

Cultural stereotyping can be a dangerous practice, especially when judgments are made on the basis of seeing behaviors through eyes not accustomed to the beliefs, norms, and values of the group under consideration. First impressions, and conclusions drawn from those impressions, can be both wrong and biased to the point of serious prejudice. Consider the following description of a particular cultural practice: a certain tribe of people live near the shore of a large body of water that often has dangerous waves and is subject to strong tidal pulls. The tribe knows about the forces of the water and even listens to a chief describe the ferocity of nature's forces each day. The voice of the chief is projected through a listening box around which members of the tribe gather to hear the chief speak about the forces of nature. After each announcement they talk quietly among themselves as though

intending to internalize the chief's words and to relate them to their own lives. The members of the tribe then remove most of their clothes, covering only those parts of the body that have to do with reproduction, and annoint themselves with holy oils. At times they rub the oils into each others' bodies and at other times they perform this sacred ritual for themselves. A great deal of preening and grooming behavior accompanies this ritual annointing of oils. When this ceremony is complete, the members of the tribe congregate on the shore, and there many of them hurl themselves into the ferocity of the waves and permit themselves to be subjected to the forces of the tide and current. They do this even though the voice of the chief on the listening box warned them of the nature of the water and wind.

The description of this cultural practice is the description of something that many Americans of all cultural and ethnic groups do evey summer: they listen to the weather forecast and go to the beach, an innocuous, pleasurable activity that does not carry the somewhat sinister and masochistic overtones described by the fantasy "anthropologist." One must be wary of overly academic and detached descriptions of real people.

Another danger in stereotyping is that generalizations may be made about an entire culture from observing the behavior patterns of only a few individuals or families in that culture. For example, getting to know a group of Navajo Indians in Arizona means that one can learn a great deal about those particular Navajos, not about Indians in general or perhaps not even about Navajos who live in South Dakota or elsewhere. Climatic conditions alone may make the life-style of Navajos in South Dakota very different from Navajos living in Arizona. Even members of a culture who live in the same geographic area may hold different sets of beliefs and values.

Health workers themselves should be wary of assuming that people in their own local area all believe and do pretty much the same thing and should be skeptical of any anthropological treatises that seem to tell them that this is the case. If you get out and investigate things for yourself, making a point of talking with a variety of people and looking at a number of differing situations, you will be much less likely to be trapped by these pitfalls of stereotyping and generalization.[2]

The set of preconceptions and misinformation that a community nurse can bring with her when she works with ethnic groups or cultures that differ from her own contribute to stereotyping, generalizations, bias, and prejudice. *Everyone* has biases, even strong prejudices, that contribute to negative attitudes and feelings about strangers and other groups of people. The recognition that the nurse is subject to these thought processes is the first step in eliminating them and replacing them with the ability to see clients as individual persons with beliefs, practices, and values that are both different from and similar to her own. Following are some mental exercises that the nurse might engage in to facilitate this process:

1. Examine the attitudes about health and illness that sprang from your cultural background. How does illness affect your life, and what steps do you take to stay healthy? Do you hold certain beliefs about what contributes to healthy or unhealthy states, and do you have empirical evidence that these beliefs are in fact true? Which of your beliefs are your own and which were unthinkingly adopted from your parents and grandparents?

2. How do you feel about strangers in general and members of different ethnic or cultural groups in particular? Do you like to meet new people or do you prefer to stay with your "own kind"? When you go to a party or other gathering and you see someone very different in appearance from most of the others (because of either certain physical characteristics or mode of dress), do you shy away from that person, or are you eager to meet him?

3. When you find yourself in conflict with someone about culture or ethnicity in general, how do you react? For example, if when you and a friend are driving through a part of town that is predominantly Hispanic and your friend says, "Those people always play the radio so loud the whole neigh-

borhood can hear it," how would you respond? If you know this to be an erroneous generalization, would you keep silent simply to avoid an argument, or would you correct your friend's misconception?

4. How do you feel about belonging to your own particular ethnic group (everyone belongs to an ethnic group, no matter how large or small or in what proportion to the rest of the population), and how strong is your sense of participation in its cultural practices and beliefs? How do you feel when you are the butt of an ethnic joke or racial slur?

5. Do you tell ethnic jokes and do you find them funny when you hear them?

6. Examine your prejudices by identifying the groups of people you dislike and think about why you dislike them. Try to isolate disliked characteristics that are based on fact and those that are based on a stereotype or generalization. Identify the differences.

When writing about cultural diversity in the community, it is impossible to treat separately every cultural minority that exists in the United States; if an attempt were made, a group would always be inadvertently forgotten. There are many excellent anthropological and sociological texts that fill that need; there are also increasing numbers of nurse-anthropologists who are writing scholarly works on cross-cultural nursing. This chapter will concern itself with the way in which the variety of cultures in the community affects the practice of community health nursing and how nurses can enhance their professional practice when clients belong to a culture different from their own.

The four major cultural groups generally included in discussions of this sort are Asian Americans, black Americans, native Americans, and Hispanic Americans. According to the 1970 United States Census,[3] these four minority ethnic groups comprise a total of 16.8% of the population, although many demographers believe this number is unrealistically low because the vast majority of persons uncounted in each census come from these four minority groups. A problem with writing about culture is that within each of the four traditionally named groups, there are tremendous varieties of subcultures that may be as different from each other as the four major groups are from each other and from the white majority. For example, the Asian American population includes (according to the United States census) Koreans, Filipinos, Chinese, Japanese, and Hawaiians. The large influx of Vietnamese in the mid to late 1970s will add another major subculture to the group of Asian Americans. In certain circumstances it can be a grave error to speak of Asian American culture when the subcultures can be so different from each other (for example, the Chinese and Japanese). Another example: the Hispanic American population is comprised of Cubans, Puerto Ricans, Mexicans, Spaniards, and those from Central and South America. These subcultures may be as different from each other as Asians are from each other. The community nurse who automatically assumes that a client who speaks with a Spanish accent will hold a particular set of cultural values or beliefs runs the risk of being mistaken and alienating that client and family.

The community nurse must also understand the concept of racism if she is to work effectively with cultural minorities. Racism is the ideology that holds that one race is either inferior or superior to another or to all others simply because of the characteristics of the race. It always results in oppression of the race considered inferior. In the history of the world racism has always worked against those races with dark skin who have been oppressed by races with light skin. In the United States racism works mainly against blacks, but sometimes Asians, Hispanics, and Indians are swept up into the racist ideology. An important characteristic of racism is that it is based *solely* on the fact of being of a particular race and not on the moral or behavioral attributes of members of that race. In fact, negative attributes are ascribed to members of a particular race *because* they are members of the race, not because the individual person has the attributes so described. Racism frequently, but by no means always, is exhibited on the part of the majority race toward the minority. Apartheid in South Africa is a clear example of a racial minority

subjugating the majority, as was the situation during the earliest part of American history when American Indians were in the majority.

Racism exists on a continuum of evil (evil is not too strong a word to use; no benefit can possibly accrue to either the oppressor or the oppressed when racism is practiced), and behaviors range from a slight dislike (e.g., curling of the lip) to enraged hatred (resulting in genocide). Some persons are open about their racism and seem almost proud of it (for example, members of the Ku Klux Klan), and others try to conceal it because outward manifestations of racism may not be acceptable in their social or business circles or because they experience guilt feelings about it.

The term *institutional racism* is increasingly used to refer to operation of the health care system as well as other business or government institutions. Institutional racism implies that a particular organization such as a hospital, community health agency, township, or even a state government condones and encourages acts of individual racism by failing to punish it or perhaps by not even officially acknowledging it. Examples of institutional racism include sterilization of black women without their fully informed consent; the Tuskegee Syphilis Study (see Chapter 5); the generally lower quality of health care provided by the Bureau of Indian Affairs; and the police department of a city assigning more officers to investigate the murder of a white person than of a Hispanic person. Institutional racism exists at all levels of society, and the community nurse will see it throughout her entire professional career. Because the phenomenon exists, the way she conducts her personal and professional life is an extremely crucial factor and is even more important than if institutional racism were not the case. Because if each individual nurse conducts her professional practice in a nonracist manner, others might be encouraged to do the same, and institutional racism could lose some of its power to hurt and destroy. This is not to say that institutional racism will be eliminated by an individual's personal and professional nonracist behavior, but the fewer people in any given institution who do not reinforce the institution's racism, the less power the institutional policy (overt or tacit) has. Policy makers are affected by the beliefs and practices of subordinates, although admittedly to a lesser extent than subordinates are affected by policy makers.

ASPECTS OF CARE THAT DIFFER WITH CULTURE
Communication

Nurses have learned, practically from their first day as a student, that interviewing technique is an essential skill, a tool without which an accurate nursing assessment and diagnosis cannot be made. This is even more true when the clients come from different cultures; interview techniques must be adapted and modified to conform to other people's modes of communication. For example, in some cultures asking a direct question is considered an insult and an invasion of privacy. For example, asking "What do you put into that stew?" may be seen as a rude way of obtaining nutritional information, whereas saying, "That stew smells wonderful" may produce a recipe and an open discussion of nutrition. (If the stew does not smell wonderful and the nurse still wants to know what is in it, she can make some other appropriate nonjudgmental remark, such as, "That stew smells interesting and very different.") Matters of health are often considered highly personal and private, and asking a question about bowel habits may be as shocking an affront to an Asian as asking questions about one's sex life may be to a white person or some other cultural minority.

Within each culture certain situations are appropriate and others are not. And even within situations where inquiry is acceptable, the time at which the questioning should begin may vary greatly. For example, in certain situations in the Anglo culture, an interviewer may be expected to 'come to the point' and get his questioning over with. In similar circumstances in Papago culture the interviewer . . . may be expected to engage in an appropriate amount of small talk before coming to the business at hand.[2,p.17]

The way clients feel about direct questioning and other forms of interviewing can sometimes be learned from other more experienced health workers and sometimes by simply getting to know the family.

One nurse was having a particularly frustrating time with an elderly Cuban woman who had moved to her district from a refugee camp in Florida where she had lived for four months after having escaped from Cuba. She spoke only the few words of English she had picked up at the camp, but the nurse spoke Spanish well; thus a language barrier was not the source of frustration. When the nurse first met Ms. Olivera, who lived on the fourth floor, it was the middle of summer, and by the time the nurse got to her apartment, she was drenched in sweat. Ms. Olivera was always delighted to see the nurse and hugged her. The nurse hugged back because it was impossible not to be drawn to Ms. Olivera's warmth and affection. Ms. Olivera always offered the nurse a cup of hot *cafe con leche* (a mixture of half coffee and half milk sweetened with sugar). The nurse, still sweating and mopping her brow, always refused and instead drank a glass of ice water or somtimes cold juice. Then the frustration began because Ms. Olivera refused to discuss any of her health problems (her medical record indicated that she had several). She was always very friendly and polite but refused to discuss her problems, and the nurse left without having accomplished anything. One day by chance she and Ms. Olivera were at the clinic at the same time, but Ms. Olivera did not know the nurse was there. Ms. Olivera and the physician (also a Cuban) were talking about *her!* Ms. Olivera commented on the nice nurse who always came to visit—so young and eager, but she didn't know *anything* about proper health. The physician seemed surprised because he knew the nurse to be quite competent. Ms. Olivera stated that anyone who didn't know that hot *cafe con leche* stopped sweating in hot weather didn't know much. The next time the nurse visited Ms. Olivera, she accepted the hot drink, and Ms. Olivera mentioned how badly her toe swelled when she held it in a certain position. That was the beginning, and from then on the nurse was able to help Ms. Olivera with many of her problems.

This example provides an illustration, not just of reasons why people might be hesitant to discuss health, but also of a professional dilemma. What if the nurse had not happened into the clinic that day, what if she never drank coffee or was allergic to it, or what if she just did not *want* to drink the *cafe con leche* offered? The frustration would have continued, and Ms. Olivera would not have received the help she eventually did, all because of a belief in the "healing" power of *cafe con leche*. The point is one of responsibility; that is, the nurse and other health professionals have a responsibility to understand a client's culture and to communicate with them within the social and ethnic bounds of that culture. But the client also has a responsibility for his own health, and part of that responsibility may be to widen the horizons of one's culture in order to facilitate communication with mainstream health workers. Ms. Olivera's refusal to discuss health problems with the nurse unless she drank the *cafe con leche* might have led to more serious problems, and there would have been nothing the nurse could have done about it.

Other difficulties in communicating with people from other cultures involve trust and misinterpretation. Nurses, because they wear their uniforms as a "badge of officialdom," often assume that their clients will trust them because they *should* trust them. This is not always the case, and it may be particularly true if the nurse is from another culture. Xenophobia can be strong. Some people will not trust others of another culture until the latter prove their trustworthiness. This places the burden of proof on the nurse, whose only way of proving trust is to practice in a professional manner. Persons from another culture may also tell the nurse and other health professionals what they think the professionals want to know. This is done in an effort to please, to avoid insulting those who are trying to help, and in an effort to gloss over facts that may be painful or unpleasant. This is frustrating for the health professional who frequently knows when a client is making an effort to please rather than being honest about the problem. It is counterproductive, sometimes dangerous, for the client. Saying that everything is all right when in reality it hurts like hell can create a worse problem than the one that already exists. If the nurse confronts the client with what she knows to be happening, the client may retreat further into subterfuge, and the problem will worsen. In this situation the nurse can only open all the doors to communication that she can and leave the decision up to the client.

Brownlee[2,pp.20-22] lists some further barriers to cross-cultural communication:

1. The interviewer may be asking the wrong people for the desired information. Sometimes the information is not known, and sometimes the person asked will deliberately confuse the questioner for reasons of his own.

2. The interviewer may be asking the wrong questions and thus receive incorrect or incomplete information. The questions may not be phrased in a way the respondent can understand, or technical terms might not be understood.

3. The questions may be asked at the wrong time or place. A crowded clinic might not provide the privacy the client requires, or the nurse may have to wait while the client finishes a particular activity, such as a religious ritual.

4. People may have difficulty in reflecting on what is second nature to them; that is, many aspects of health care are seen as so integral a part of life that it is difficult to think about them objectively. Some questions might be perceived as not worth asking. For example, if a nurse asks a young Chinese woman who lives in a very traditional home, how she feels about an impending arranged marriage, the young woman might not see the subject as integral to her mental health. Arranged marriages are the norm of the culture and are neither healthy nor unhealthy.

5. Translation may alter the meaning of a question or response.

6. The questioner's own characteristics and demeanor may influence the response. This is true also of intracultural communication, but the hurdle

is higher in cross-cultural communication. A Hispanic man might not respond well to questions that involve sexuality if they are asked by a woman, and a male nurse may receive a blank stare if he asks a Hopi Indian woman questions about breastfeeding.

7. Respondents may mistake the ideal for the real. In all cultures there exists a gap between what the members of the culture believe should happen and what actually does happen. For example, a particular Indian tribe may believe that God will provide food resources in the form of plentiful fish and game when in reality many members of the tribe may be starving.

> Your informants, in many cases, may not be consciously trying to lead you astray, but may be simply describing to you the ways they have always been taught that things are. They may never have realized that what they tend to do most often is actually quite different. Keep in mind that you may also tend to mistake the ideal for the real, and search beneath the layer of the ideal for the somewhat different reality.[2,p.22]

The communication problem caused by the inability of the client and nurse to speak the same language is solved only by a translator. In areas that have a high proportion of clients speaking a foreign language, agencies usually try to employ nurses who speak that language. The most common example is Spanish. In many cities that have a high concentration of Hispanic Americans, publications of many government and private agencies are available in both English and Spanish, and signs in clinics and even on the street are bilingual. Some health agencies will not hire nurses unless they are bilingual. This is a commendable attitude on the part of the government and the health care system, but the nurse, even while she is speaking Spanish to the client, should encourage him to learn English if he is planning to live in the United States for any length of time. English is the language of the United States, and all business transactions, professional life, higher education, and socializing outside the immediate cultural group are conducted in

English. If the client plans to move in any of these circles, to climb a career ladder, or to seek employment in the society of the majority, he must learn fluent English. The nurse who does not encourage the client to learn English if he expresses a desire for any of these goals is as remiss as the nurse who neglects to encourage childhood immunization simply because the client does not understand the complexities of germ theory.

An interesting and politically sensitive aspect of the language problem is the federally mandated program of bilingualism in the public schools.* There are about 3.5 million schoolchildren in the United States for whom English is a second language, and in 1968 Congress passed the Bilingual Education Act, which gives non–English-speaking children the choice of attending classes in any one of 70 native tongues. The number of children affected has risen steadily from 25,000 in 1969 to more than a half million in 1980. The cost to the American taxpayer is about $700 million a year. Both the cost and the number of children participating are expected to increase. There are advantages and disadvantages to the program. Children are encouraged to maintain connections with and positive feelings about their cultural heritage, and the school dropout rate for non–English-speaking students has decreased. But the program is expensive and an ineffective way to absorb children into the American culture. It also hinders the necessity of learning English; there are second and third generation Puerto Ricans in bilingual classes in New York City. There is almost no empirical evidence to show whether or not the program is effective in the long run, but supporters and opponents are equally vociferous about their positions. It is an emotional issue.

Family structure and function

The family is the basic structure of society in almost every culture of the world, certainly in all the cultures that the American community

---

*From Time, pp. 64-65, September 8, 1980.

nurse is likely to meet. It is important, then, for the nurse to learn that a wide variety of family structures and functions exist within any culture and, of course, between cultures. Some of the ways in which the nurse can familiarize herself with the characteristics of family life are by answering the following questions and others that are pertinent.

1. What is the composition of the family; that is, how many generations are considered to be a single family, and which relatives comprise the family unit?

2. What is the source of family power and cohesion? Families are usually defined as either matriarchal or patriarchal, but this does not mean that *all* family power lies with *either* the man or the woman. For example, a man may have the economic power to determine the family's standard of living, but the woman may control the actual running of the family and the way in which intrafamilial relationships are conducted.

3. What marriage customs prevail, and what is the attitude toward separation and divorce? Is the sanctity of the marital bond to be preserved at all costs, no matter how unhappy the family, or is divorce permitted if all else fails?

4. What is the role of children in the family? How much respect are they accorded, and are they viewed as full persons even within the limitations of their developmental stage? When the children need to be disciplined or punished, how is it done? If physical means are used, in what way? Do the parents demonstrate physical affection for each other in front of the children, and do the children receive physical affection from their parents?

5. Is there time spent as a family unit, and if so how? What modes of communication are used and what leisure activities are engaged in? How much time is spent watching television; what are the favorite programs?

6. What major events are important to the family, how are they celebrated, and which family members play a role in the celebration?

Traditional family practices and beliefs can change when the family moves to a new cultural environment. For example:

A Japanese family who recently moved to San Francisco maintained a traditional mode of existence for several months. They all wore Western clothes, but they had done that in Japan. The two adolescent girls came immediately home from school every day, and the mother never left the house except to shop, and then she was always accompanied by her husband. The family, except for the father, was quite isolated from the mainstream of American life. One evening the elder daughter, 15-year-old Moshika, came to the dinner table with her hair in curlers. Her father was horrified almost beyond speech, but he managed to ask why his daughter was engaged in such behavior. Her reply was, "Johnny's picking me up right after dinner." The father, a sophisticated businessman, was familiar with American dating behavior, although in a detached kind of way. He now faced a dilemma: should he insist on maintaining the traditional style of family life and thus create unhappiness for his wife and daughters, plus the family conflict that he knew would ensue, or should he allow his family to assimilate into American life and thus lose part of the culture that was dear to him? He decided on a compromise, in part, by permitting his daughters to date (but not to wear hair curlers to the dinner table), but he insisted on meeting the boys first and to impose strict rules on dating behavior.

These kinds of changes occur in all individuals and families when they move to a new culture, but adaptation in varying degrees takes place. A certain amount of compromise in modes of behavior is necessary for survival, but the fact that it *is* necessary creates conflict. American society is different from all others, and it can be seductive in its emphasis on materialism and violence. It is difficult enough for a family who has lived here for several generations to succeed in not being swallowed up by the homogenization of beliefs and practices that seems desirable to so many; it is even more difficult for a family that is accustomed to different cultural behaviors. A common reaction is to settle in an area of the city or country that has a high proportion of persons of one's own culture and then be tempted not to move out of that small cultural enclave. There is a sense of security in this, in hearing one's own language spoken on the street, and in knowing one's neighbors will have familiar food in the refrigerator. The sense of continuity and stability, however, is always threatened because eventually children will want to explore the larger community beyond, and they will bring home both positive and negative behaviors that have been learned outside the culture. Thus, living in a cultural enclave has advantages and disadvantages.

The strain and tension of living in a new culture can sometimes prove disastrous for a family. There may not be enough money. If both parents are out of the house working or looking for work, and if day-care is not available or is too expensive, children are left alone to fend for themselves—and to get into trouble. Schoolchildren are caught between the traditions at home and the temptations of "the American way" at school. They may experiment with drugs and sex or allow themselves to be drawn into the kind of activities that would be severely disapproved of at home. All children play "I dare you" in which some kind of risky activity is involved. Consider the child from a different culture: he wants to fit in with his new friends and thus is vulnerable to their taunts and dares. Many cars are stolen in this way, drugs are taken for the first time, or an item is shoplifted from a store.

Many families when they come to the United States (with the exception of Puerto Ricans who are not subject to immigration laws because they are American citizens) are separated from close relatives, even spouses, because of the vagaries of immigration laws and are suffering from the grief of separation and loss. The difficulties of being a single parent are then compounded by the difficulties of living in a strange culture. One of the primary functions of the community nurse in such situations is to put the newcomer in contact with people in the cultural community who are well established and who "know the ropes" about functioning in the larger society outside the culture.

The problems of living in a strange culture, either alone or with only a part of one's nuclear family, are extremely complex. The community nurse can help, but only to a limited extent unless health problems are a major part of the family's difficulty. She can learn family structure and functioning and can be aware of other, more established people in the community. But this instance is an excellent example of where the nurse may experience frustration at not being able to help with all problems. This is also a case where knowledge of other community resources is essential. For example, a phone call to the United States Immigration and Naturalization Service would probably be highly fruitful, as would a call to a local service organization. In fact, sometimes an hour in the office on the telephone ends up being more beneficial for the client than does a two-hour home visit. Professional judgment is again the most vital ingredient when deciding which intervention technique is most appropriate.

Attitudes about health

Attitudes about health vary widely from culture to culture, and stories of stereotypes, not all of them told in a tolerant manner, abound among health professionals. Recent statistical surveys indicate that physical illness is the norm among all Americans, even those who are not aware that they have currently significant symptoms.[4] Previously it had been believed that relative health was the norm among the vast majority of the population. How is it, then, that so many people are walking around clinically ill and are not aware of it or can ignore it sufficiently to carry on with their usual lives?

A great deal has to do with cultural perceptions of illness and attitudes about health. Zola[4,pp.86-88] speculates that there are two major ways in which signs that would ordinarily indicate illness in one population may be ignored in others. The first is actual prevalence of the sign, and the second is congruence with dominant value orientations. If a sign or symptom is so prevalent among a particular population that it affects a majority of the people, then it is viewed as part of everyday life and is thus ignored. Among Mexican Americans in the Southwest, for example, diarrhea, sweating, and coughing are so common that they are not considered aberrations. "In the second process, it is the 'fit' of certain signs with a society's major values that accounts for the degree of attention they receive. For example, in some nonliterate societies there is anxiety-free acceptance of and willingness to describe hallucinatory experiences."[4,p.87] In Western society, which emphasizes rationality and control, hallucinations would be seen as indicative of severe mental illness. Fatigue is a sign that precedes many major, even fatal illnesses, but it is seen as a normal aspect of life among many populations: for example, women who work as domestics and take care of their own homes as well, students, business executives who work long hours in an effort to get ahead in careers, and persons who farm under the sun every day. Fatigue is assimilated into the lifestyle of these and other groups of people. Dysmenorrhea is an example of a symptom that is congruent with societal expectations. American women tend to complain of dysmenorrhea because it is accepted and even encouraged in American society (note the advertisements for a wide range of medications supposedly designed specifically for dysmenorrhea). It is difficult to find references to dysmenorrhea in physical anthropology reports either because it is not expected by the vast majority of cultures or because it is expected as an ordinary part of a woman's life and is thus considered normal or usual.

It is worthwhile to select two examples of cross-cultural views of health and illness, although the illustrations are by no means exhaustive and there are surely exceptions to the descriptions that follow.

According to Spector, the Chinese view health as a state of spiritual and physical harmony with nature. The major task of the traditional Chinese physician is to keep the person healthy, and indeed he is paid by the client as long as he stays healthy; when illness occurs, payment stops. In fact, the physician is required to pay for whatever medications are necessary to restore health. The Chinese

view of the universe is that it is a vast indivisible entity with each individual being (both human and nonhuman) in the universe having a separate function that is interdependent on all other individual beings and their functions. The universe is in total harmony, and individuals must adapt themselves to this harmony. Illness violates the harmony, as does war and other catastrophes.

The Chinese view their bodies as a gift from their ancestors; therefore care must be taken to return the bodies whole and in good condition when the person has no further use of it. The organs maintain the harmony of the body, which in turn maintains the harmony of the universe. The major powers that regulate the universe, and thus the body, are *yin* and *yang*. *Yang* is the male, or positive, energy that produces light, warmth, and fullness. *Yin* is the female, or negative, and is the force of darkness, cold, and emptiness. Various parts of the body correspond to the dualistic nature of *yin* and *yang;* for example, the inside of the body is *yin,* and the surface is *yang;* the front is *yin,* and the back is *yang.* Some organs are *yin* and some are *yang.* Illness is a disruption in the balance of *yin* and *yang,* and diagnosis is usually accomplished by examination of the tongue, listening to body sounds, asking questions of the person, and feeling the pulses. Healing is accomplished in a variety of ways, most commonly by acupuncture, which is puncturing the body with special metal needles at predetermined points known as meridians where the forces of *yin* and *yang* merge. The goal of the treatment is to restore the balance of *yin* and *yang,* and acupuncture is a highly specialized and ancient art. Western medical practitioners have only recently begun to investigate its value. This traditional form of healing is practiced in both China and in the United States.

Chinese Americans have a higher death rate for both men and women than does the white population; this is due mainly to the high incidence of tuberculosis and the great degree of poverty among the Chinese. Many work in laundries and restaurants where they are not protected by unions and frequently work in extremely unhealthy conditions for low wages. Primary health care is far too expensive for most Chinese Americans, who when they do fall ill, often seek the help of Chinatown herbalists, sometimes but not always in conjunction with Western medicine. Western diagnostic procedures are seen as painful and unnecessary (although immunizations and x rays are acceptable), particularly the practice of drawing blood. Blood is seen as a source of life for the entire body, and it is believed not to regenerate. Because no medical diagnosis is made without blood tests, the Chinese tend to be wary of Western health care.

They do not react well to the often-painful procedures used in diagnostic workups. Some people—because of their distaste for this kind of procedure—leave the Western system rather than tolerate the pain. . . . The Chinese have deep respect for their bodies and believe it is best to die with their bodies intact. For this reason, many people refuse surgery or consent to it only under the most dire circumstances.[5]

It is difficult to describe black Americans' attitudes toward health because blacks, although they do form a cultural and ethnic group, are so much a part of the fabric of American society in all classes and at all levels of socioeconomic life that their attitudes are no different in many respects from white Americans. However, there are some clear differences, and more black Americans are now closely emotionally attuned to their African heritage than they have been in recent years. The upsurge in black studies in high schools and universities has encouraged this ancestral link, and it is important for the community nurse to understand some African attitudes about health, although the great variety of African cultures and tribes makes generalization difficult. To the African, life is a process rather than a state of being, and a person is viewed in terms of energy rather than matter. All beings (both living and dead) influence each other through both behavior and knowledge. Mind, body, and spirit are not separated, and when one possesses health, one is in harmony with nature. Disharmony, or illness, is attributed to a variety of sources, primarily demons and evil spirits. The

spirits enter the body on their own accord, and the goal of treatment of ill health is to remove the spirits, most commonly by voodoo.

This is a belief system that is poorly understood but is still practiced in many parts of Africa and Central and South America. The name *voodoo* comes from the god *Vodu* who presided over a cult of snake worshippers from the West African coast. They came to the new world as slaves, having been sold through the West Indies. Voodoo came to the United States with the slaves, and eventually its practice was outlawed because it was so feared by whites. Voodoo consists of a number of ceremonial rituals, held at night in open country and attended by large numbers of people. The ceremony involves sacrifice and the drinking of blood (one of the reasons voodoo was outlawed was because it was commonly believed that children were sacrificed, but there is no evidence to support this belief). The ceremonies are frequently conducted by women, and voodoo can be used for evil means as well as to heal illness. A ''fix'' can be placed on a person whereby evil spirits enter the body and cause illness. *Gris-gris* are oils and powders that that can prevent illness or give it to others; there are both good and evil *gris-gris*.

There are also a number of Catholic saints or relics to whom or which the practitioners of voodoo attribute special powers. Hence there may be a prominent display of portraits of St. Michael, who makes possible the conquest of enemies; St. Anthony de Padua, who brings luck; St. Mary Magdalene, who is popular with women who are in love; the Virgin Mary whose presence in the home prevents illness; and the Sacred Heart of Jesus, which cures organic illness. These *gris-gris* are available today and can be purchased in stores in many American cities.[5,p.234]

Those who might be tempted to dismiss voodoo as irrational or merely useless are urged to consider the above quotation *and* the fact that every known system of spiritual belief is based to some extent on irrationality and occult happenings. There is ritual in every religion that appears bizarre to the outsider.

Many black Americans also believe in the power of certain individuals to heal illness; this is a reflection of deep religious faith. The Pentecostal movement has always been popular with blacks, and they have traditionally participated in faith healers' tent meetings. Geophagy, or the eating of clay or dirt, is another common practice, particularly among pregnant women. It is believed that clay is rich in iron, and when it was not available dirt was substituted. Today's city dwellers rely on grocery store starch. Anemia gave rise to the practice of geophagy, which is today the cause of much anemia.

Black Americans avail themselves of traditional health care to a great extent, but many forms of folk medicine, both to prevent and to heal illness, are practiced today, particularly in rural areas. Asafetida, or rotten flesh that looks like a dried sponge, is worn around the neck to prevent contagious diseases, and in the spring a sulfur and molasses preparation is taken because it is believed that at the beginning of a new season people are more susceptible to illness. Copper or silver bracelets are a general protection against harm and are an indication of an impending illness when the skin around the bracelet turns black. The most common method of treating illness is prayer and the laying on of hands, but there are many potions and remedies that are also believed to be beneficial: for example, sugar and turpentine mixed together and drunk to get rid of worms; a potato poultice applied to the affected area to draw out disease; an herb tea made from goldenrod root drunk to treat pain and reduce fever; two pieces of silverware in the shape of a cross to cure a "crick in the neck"; sour milk placed on stale bread and wrapped in a cloth to treat cuts and wounds; colds treated with hot lemon water and honey; a sprained ankle healed with clay wrapped in a dark leaf and applied to the sprain; and raw onions placed on the feet and then wrapped in a blanket to break a fever.

It is again extremely easy and tempting for practitioners of Western health care to laugh at or simply dismiss as foolish these folk remedies. Some are indeed useless but harmless, and some are downright harmful, both in and of themselves and because they prevent people from seeking care that might prove beneficial or even life-saving. Others, however, have medicinal value that has been empirically demonstrated. For example, the potato poultice depends on the rotting process of the potatoes that produces a penicillin-like mold, which can destroy certain infectious organisms. Sour milk produces enzymes that can be very effective in wound healing, and the clay wrapped in a dark leaf produces a cooling and drawing effect that can reduce the swelling and pain of a sprained ankle.

Blacks who enter the traditional health care system have had unique experiences because they are black. Blacks are subject to more patronization and condescension than are whites because they are seen as less intelligent. They are insulted, either overtly or subtly, more frequently and generally wait longer for treatment than whites. A generalization can be made that blacks receive health care inferior to whites in kind, amount, and the way it is provided, just as the poor receive health care that is inferior to that of the nonpoor. Blacks tend to feel alienated from the health care system, which is controlled by whites, and there have been numerous cases of blacks suffering death or increased illness because of discrimination by whites. Many blacks view the efforts of white health care professionals to provide them with information about contraception as genocide and will resist all such efforts. For these and other reasons the tensions between blacks and whites in the health care system can run high. Community nurses can become more familiar with black Americans' attitudes toward health by understanding why some attitudes exist and why they persist.

These two illustrations provide only a small sample of the great variety in people's beliefs and attitudes about health. It is important that the nurse understand that the meaning of health and its importance in people's lives can vary greatly with culture. For example, the white American upper middle class is generally very conscious of health, considers good health essential, and will spend vast sums of money to ensure continuing good health (for example, the American craze for tennis is expensive; tennis racquets, balls, clothing, other paraphernalia, and club membership can cost upwards of $1,000 a year. Moreover, the tennis player needs to spend money on high quality protein foods to maintain fitness). The upper middle class American also does not work at a job that is known to be particularly hazardous to his health, such as coal mining or steel manufacturing. These people tend to consider wellness to be optimum health functioning, whereas other groups may consider wellness to be merely absence of disease. A coal miner who does not have black lung disease may consider himself well (and lucky!) even though he may be suffering from a number of other less life-threatening ailments. The meaning of health to him may revolve around the fact that he is well enough to work and feed his family.

Health is a cultural value, just as education, religious training, and career advancement are cultural values. For example, in the Navajo culture congenital dislocation of the hip is a fairly common phenomenon, but the Navajos do not seem particularly concerned about it. The child so affected has a limp, but it is not considered a major disability, especially when compared to other disasters that could occur. As the child grows older, arthritis of the hip joint is likely to result; this is painful and can be corrected only by surgical fusion of the joint. However, for the Navajo this is an impractical procedure because he would not be able to take meals with his family, which are eaten on the ground on a sheepskin, nor would he be able to ride horseback. These consequences of corrective surgery are so serious that the child continues to limp. The meaning of the health problem is thus directly related to the group's life-style, as is the decision for treatment.

The community nurse can begin to understand the meaning of health for a particular cultural or ethnic group by observing how the members of the group react to illness, how far they will let the symptoms continue before they seek some type of health care, what steps they take to remain healthy, what they see as an actual health problem and not

simply a fact of life, what quality of health care they see as desirable, and what their usual forms of health care are.

Concepts of hygiene are sometimes an indication of attitudes about health. Cleanliness is an attitude that varies greatly with culture. The typical middle class American attitude is that it is absolutely essential, and dirty hair, clothes, and fingernails are considered disgusting and a social stigma. We sanitize and deodorize ourselves in an effort to banish all body odors and secretions. People from other cultures believe this effort to be slightly crazy and certainly unnecessary; body secretions and odors are a part of nature and thus should be left alone. White American women who shave their legs and underarms are among the very few women in the world who do so. It is frequently difficult to draw a clear line between hygiene practices that contribute to disease and those that do not, but there is empirical evidence for some linkages between hygiene and disease, such as water contaminated with feces containing the danger of typhoid or cholera. Community nurses who insist on a certain standard of cleanliness *for* clients run the risk of alienating them, but because certain degrees and kinds of poor hygiene lead to certain diseases, she should promote cleanliness to some extent. The difficulty lies in determining when hygiene is a matter of personal preference and when it is a matter of disease prevention.

Religion

We have already looked at two examples of cultures in which health is closely related to, or a part of, the harmony of the universe, and in which to be in good health means to continue that harmony. This is an essentially religious belief because the vast majority of people on earth believe in God, gods, or some other spiritual force that controls the universe. Religion and health are closely allied. Faith healing is an example of this alliance, and the upsurge in the popularity of the Pentecostal movement will provide some indication of attitudes about religion and health. Christianity, and to a lesser extent Judaism, have traditionally used prayer as a powerful adjunct to the healing process, although prayer, of course, presupposes a belief in God or gods. Although attendance at formal religious services is decreasing in the United States, many members of cultural minorities find comfort and solace in the familiarity of religious rites and ceremonies; frequently the clergyman is the first member of the health care team to be sought for advice and help.

The community nurse should know something about the religion of the cultural groups with whom she comes in contact most frequently. Christianity is, of course, the most common religion in the United States, and the nurse is most likely herself a Christian; but many forms of Christianity exist, and there is a great difference between Roman Catholicism and the various types of Protestantism. A religion that has had enormous impact on the history of civilization but about which most Christians know almost nothing is Judaism. There are about six million Jews in the United States today, and they tend to live in major metropolitan areas. Most nursing texts, when they discuss meeting the religious needs of clients, mention two or three major Jewish holidays and make a vague reference to dietary laws, and that about covers the topic of Judaism.

The community nurse, however, needs to know more when she cares for Jewish clients, particularly in their homes. She needs to know what the laws of *kashruth* are (the word has been anglicized to *kosher* and literally means clean) and why observant Jews do and do not eat certain foods at all and others only at certain times. For example, a Jew who maintains a strictly kosher home cannot buy meat at the local supermarket; he must go to the kosher butcher shop, which may not be nearby and which will always be more expensive (kosher meat is usually about double the price of nonkosher meat because of the higher cost of preparation and because a small butcher shop usually has a higher proportional overhead than does a large supermarket). Therefore, when the nurse blithely suggests to the poor Jewish family that they increase their daily intake of meat, she might be suggesting some-

thing that is almost impossible for them to accomplish. If she has a poor or incomplete understanding of the laws of *kashruth*, she will not be able to deal effectively with the family's nutritional problems.

Another example is that of a Jewish family who is being forced to move out of their apartment in a large city because the building has been sold to a condominium developer and they do not want to buy the apartment. In fact, the family is expecting its third child, and they need a larger place to live. However, they want to stay in the city and because they are Orthodox Jews, they need to be within walking distance of their synagogue and must find either a private house or an apartment on a low floor (Orthodox Jews do not ride in cars or elevators on the Sabbath). House-hunting with these requirements and a middle income salary can be almost an insurmountable problem, and if the community nurse is to be of help, she must know why these restrictions exist. It should be noted, however, that the number of Jews who maintain these Orthodox traditions is small in comparison to the total number in the United States; most observe religious traditions in a more relaxed and haphazard manner.

The nurse can familiarize herself with the religious practices and beliefs of her clients in several ways: reading about the religion, attending religious services, learning which holidays and feast days are important and what the ceremonies attached to them are, and asking what role religion plays in the life of the individual client and family. Religious beliefs can affect health care in that individuals may refuse to avail themselves of secular health care (that not provided by a clergyman, healer, or some other religious authority) because religious faith is so strong and unshakable. This poses a dilemma for the nurse: she has a desire to provide the person with the most effective care possible, but she must respect his religious beliefs. She cannot force or coerce him to seek traditional care, and he has the legal right to choose his own mode of care or even to refuse treatment altogether even if that refusal is likely to result in his death. How far can the nurse go in trying to persuade a client to seek "proper" health care, and when does that persuasion turn to coercion? When the client refuses her entreaties, what should she do? She cannot simply abandon him because he prefers a faith healer to a board certified cardiologist, but it is difficult for her to provide the kind of care she sees as necessary when he rejects that care. This is a difficult position for the nurse and one that will require all her professional judgment. The best course of action seems to be to establish sufficiently open and honest communication with the client so that "opposing" positions can be identified and discussed. It then becomes the client's choice whether he wishes to continue receiving the services the nurse offers. She cannot and should not lower her standards of practice (adapting standards of practice to meet the differing cultural needs of clients is not the same as lowering those standards), and it must be the client who decides whether he wishes to continue the professional relationship with the nurse.

Nutrition

Eating habits vary with culture almost more than any other human activity. Human beings have evolved and continue to do so because they have been able to adapt their nutritional requirements and habits to the environmental conditions in which they find themselves.

Many models of cultural evolution have been developed that focus primarily on the stages of evolution, rather than on the process of change. The stages are generally either based on the technology available or on the social structure, with some common categories being big-game hunting, hunting-gathering, horticulture, agriculture, and industrialization. These stages are seen as having distinct forms of social organization as well as different technologies. An obvious point generally overlooked is that all of these frames of reference in some way refer to food procurement. Several of the critical changes in human cultural evolution have been in food procurement and processing. Sharing and distribution are central characteristics of the feeding behaviors of humans; thus it makes sense that the ways in which food is procured, processed, and utilized are central to many other aspects of human social organization.[6]

This is a crucial concept for the community nurse to understand; many of the differences that the nurse observes in food procurement and processing will depend on where she is practicing and who her clients are. The nurse who works on a Sioux reservation in South Dakota may see her clients eat what they have personally hunted and killed, and she may share their meals. The closest that Cubans in Miami will come to hunting is looking for the grocery store with the lowest prices. The nurse who practices in Iowa may have clients who eat nothing except what they grow on their own farms; a black American living in Chicago will probably confine his farming to caring for a few philodendron on the windowsill.

Food habits are among the most culturally ingrained and the hardest to change, but there is usually no reason to do so unless the dietary patterns are definitely harmful. Cultural practices and attitudes in regard to food are shaped by many factors such as the following:

1. Certain kinds of food are seen as more desirable than others; those that are the most desirable will go to those who rank the highest in the social system of the culture. Distribution can also be done on the basis of gender, that is, males, who are seen as contributing more to the continuation of the culture than females, receive the more desirable foods. Generally, animal foods are more desirable than plant foods.

2. Pregnancy and lactation are conditions that require special consideration in food consumption in almost all cultures. Most cultures will give a pregnant or lactating woman added benefits in food, although some cultures prohibit certain foods to pregnant women in an effort to protect the fetus from the inherent risks they contain.

3. The weaning of children involves highly specific cultural beliefs, thus ingraining certain food practices in children at an early age. Most cultures believe that certain foods are appropriate or not as weaning foods (a weaning food is that which is first given to the child when he stops breast-feeding). For example, in many parts of Africa bananas are considered the best weaning food; consequently

many black American babies eat bananas as their first "real" food.

4. Certain illnesses have a high correlation with the dietary practices of a particular culture. For example, in Western countries diets are particularly high in animal fat and butterfat foods; as a result the incidence of cardiovascular disease in the West tends to be higher than elsewhere. In India polished rice is considered preferable to unpolished rice even though the former has a much lower concentration of thiamine than the latter. Therefore, those persons who eat polished rice have a greater likelihood of contracting beriberi.

5. Sociocultural and technological change contribute to changes in dietary practice. For example, the amount of carbonated soft drinks consumed by American children far outstrips the amount of milk and fruit juices consumed,[6,p.118] resulting in a higher consumption of "empty" calories and the acquisition of poor nutritional habits at an early age. Processed and prepared foods are also consumed in the West (particularly in the United States, although Western Europe is quickly developing the processed food habit), resulting in a higher percentage of the food budget being spent for items that are not edible (processing and packaging).

6. People tend to eat the way their parents ate. Food habits are usually the last process to be changed in the acculturation to a new society. A black American who has "made it" in the business world and goes to work in a three-piece suit may have his most pleasurable eating experiences when he rolls up his sleeves to enjoy a meal of ribs, black-eyed peas, and greens. The process of acculturation in regard to food sometimes involves learning whole new eating patterns and sometimes adapting existing patterns to the new culture. In any event, change will take place which will cause some degree of distress.

The nurse should assess the nutritional patterns and habits of her clients. She can do this best by sharing meals with families, but this is not usually practical over a long period of time. In lieu of being present at mealtime, she may be present during meal preparation, or she may accompany clients when they shop for food. She needs to know what percentage of the family budget is spent on food and what proportion of the purchases are "ethnic" foods and which are "American." Although it might be said that this information is none of the nurse's business (and if clients feel this is true, many are likely to say so), the amount of money spent on food can give the nurse an indication of how well the family is able to budget its disposable income and whether or not they are shopping as economically as possible in view of their circumstances. The proportion of ethnic to American food is simply one (and surely not the only) indication of the degree to which the family has become assimilated into the general American culture.

She should also know the amount of time devoted to shopping and who is responsible for food purchases. What does the family like to eat, and does everyone in the family have similar tastes in food? Does the family generally eat breakfast and/ or dinner together, and who is mainly responsible for food preparation. Do children share responsibility for food preparation and clean-up? How much food is wasted, and are the family members encouraged to eat everything on their plates? Which family members have health problems that make it difficult or impossible to share the eating patterns of the rest of the family? How are these problems accommodated, and do they increase the family's food expenditures? Are ethnic foods readily available in the neighborhood, or does their purchase require a major expedition to another part of town? What about the family's alcohol intake: is wine used in cooking and is it drunk during the meal? Do children drink diluted wine at meals with their parents? Are there any foods that are expressly forbidden by the culture or are a cultural requirement in observance of a rite or ceremony?

Social class

Hispanic Americans, black Americans, Asian Americans, and native Americans belong to all social classes, although the greatest majority of them are poor, which places them in the lower class. Those so described are considered lower class, *not* because of the fact of their ethnic or cultural minority but because they are poor. However, because minorities tend to be discriminated against on the job and by potential employers, they are more likely to be unemployed and poor. Therefore, culture and social class tend to be related, although there is not necessarily a direct causal relationship.

Social class in the United States almost always has money as its prime consideration, although family background, education, social accomplishments, mode of dress, and speech patterns are strong contributing factors and indicators. Someone with a meager income can be considered upper class if he comes from an upper class family, demonstrates appropriate values and behaviors, and engages in expected activities. By the same token, a person of lower class will always remain lower class, no matter how much money he may suddenly earn, if he continues to exhibit lower class values and behaviors and especially if he is a member of a cultural minority.

One of the most brilliant writers about class was Karl Marx, and the term ''class struggle'' came out of Marxist theory. Marx's system of class, however, was based on economic production: all society was composed of the proletariat and the bourgeoisie, or the workers and the owners.

Thus, economic position leads to the development of class consciousness, or the complex of attitudes, opinions, even distinctive life styles, which are the action components of social change. It is the position that the individual occupies in the social organization of production that indicates to which social class that individual belongs. Indicators of the distribution of material good and prestige symbols, such as education, income, or occupation, while they may reflect in some way the organization of production, are not identical with it.[7]

Although the United States is not a Marxist society and few people hold a Marxist philosophy, one has only to compare the structure of society with the organizational structure of big business to realize that Marx's observations were quite accurate. Marx's vision was to bring about social change by the formulation of class consciousness and the free-

dom of the masses from dependence on economic authority. Marxism is a purist approach to democracy, which does not work well in practice when large numbers of people are involved.

The sociologist Max Weber saw the distribution of power within a community as a function of three distinct orders: the economic, social, and political. In Weber's view social class is not the only route to power in a community, and we see evidence of this in the United States. Politicians frequently spring from the lowest social classes, as do members of the military who wield enormous power. However, power always revolves around economic status, and according to Weber one is either a debtor or creditor, buyer or seller, worker, or employer. Those who are debtors, buyers, and workers will never have the power of their opposite numbers. Most members of minority groups belong to the former category, and although opportunities exist to change economic status (these opportunities exist in greater measure in the United States than elsewhere), they are rare. The number of rungs of the occupational, economic, and social ladders are fewer and further apart the higher one climbs on the ladder. There is less room at the top and always plenty of room at the bottom. There are, however, ways for ethnic and cultural groups who are at the bottom of the power heap to move up: entry into local politics and achievement of subsequent political success; a vocational or academic education that will provide entry into an occupation or profession; or a talent or particular skill that is so outstanding that it provides for economic success. The most important of these, because it is the most widely available, is education. In fact, the lack of an education almost guarantees stagnation in the lower class and in a poor and dependent economic position.

In Chapter 11 we saw how poverty contributes to both poor health and health behaviors that contribute to an unhealthy life-style. Poverty also changes and affects the way people are treated by the health care system and how they relate to it and feel about the system. Many of those observations can also be applied to persons from cultural and ethnic minorities who also happen to be poor.

In addition to being divided into classes with the rest of the American population, each culture has its own definition of class or caste, which is in turn viewed differently by various members of the cultural group. Following is one person's description of Mexican Americans:

One informant, a Mexican-American wife of a construction foreman, divided members of the colony into four groups: *"la alta sociedad"*, or high society, *"los medianos"*, or middle class, *"los de abajo"*, or the lowly ones, and the *"braceros"*, low-class workers from Mexico. She placed herself and her family within the second group. An American-born Mexican-American businessman who was classified by those below him as a member of high society could only see two classes: "those of us who are trying to get ahead and make a decent life", and "most of the people", who "just don't even seem to care".[2,p.35]

Economics

The economic conditions of a particular cultural community usually apply only to a particular segment of the culture, based on geography, occupation, and the like. For example, the economic conditions of black Americans living in Washington, D.C., are extremely varied because of the nature of the city. About 75% of Washington is black (blacks are about 11% to 12% of the total American population), which is in itself an unusual phenomenon. Because of the enormous number of white collar government jobs in the city, there is a large black middle class, which is also unusual. And because Washington is the center of political power, there are many more upper class blacks there than in any other city. Washington also has lower class blacks, but their proportion is lower than in most other American cities.

Persons of particular cultures tend to congregate in certain areas of the country, such as Cubans in Southern Florida, Hispanics in the Southwestern states, and Orientals on the West coast. This geographic concentration tends to affect the economy of the cultural group. For example, in Texas and Arizona Mexican Americans usually hold the most menial jobs and are, for the most part, among the lowest income group. This is true for a number of reasons: racism is as pervasive against Mexican Americans in this part of the country as it is against blacks in other parts of the country; a number of Mexican Americans are illegal aliens, or "wetbacks" (the name derives from the practice of swimming across the Rio Grande in an effort to evade border patrols), who are almost totally at the mercy of white employers and who receive no employee benefits other than a low wage, usually paid in cash; Mexican Americans in the Southwest have almost no education and their rate of illiteracy is high. All these factors combine to make the Mexican American in that area one of the most economically deprived groups in the United States.

There are several ways that the community nurse can assess the economic situation of the cultural community in which she works: by noting if there is some group of occupations or businesses that seem to be most prevalent (such as restaurants in Chinatown); assessing the motivational level of her clients, that is how badly they want to improve their economic status; noting the amount of crime in the area and the prevalence of various kinds of crime—drugs, prostitution, numbers running, and the like; determining who the economic "heroes" are, that is, to what level and kind of economic status do the members of the community aspire; and determining the gender orientation of occupations, that is, do women work as frequently and in the same kind of occupations as men? Are the people satisfied with their economic lot in life? If one comes across the attitude of shrugging one's shoulders and accepting life as a "second class citizen" because one belongs to a minority group, the nurse has little basis on which to encourage and strengthen motivation. If there is some degree of dissatisfaction and anger (too much anger tends to be counterproductive, as was clearly demonstrated in the race riots of the 1960s and early 1970s), the nurse can encourage change and improvement by a variety of techniques: teaching people how to recognize and capitalize on their natural talents; stressing the importance of education;

showing clients how to look for a job and how to present themselves in the best possible light; using the political process to the client's advantage; and teaching them how to increase and improve their self-image.

Members of many poor minority groups live in ghettos. This adds to their economic and health problems. Ghetto living affects one's entire life and outlook on the future. It is more than just a matter of an address or an apartment in a certain part of the city. It is living one's entire life within a few blocks, never venturing out into the larger community, and becoming so entrenched in the way of life in the ghetto that any other life-style constitutes severe culture shock. Behaviors that may be acceptable in the ghetto may not be in the outside world, and sometimes ghetto dwellers are unable to function anywhere except in the ghetto. Existence of a ghetto does not *necessarily* mean that all those living in it are poor (European ghettos of the recent past encompassed all socioeconomic groups but only one cultural group), but in the United States this is usually the case, and ghetto living has become associated with poverty. Ghettos are not necessarily bad or negative in and of themselves because they frequently provide a sense of nurturance and a way to continue cultural patterns and practices without the homogenization of outside assimilating forces. In times of adversity ghetto residents can depend on and support one another against a common enemy (the story of the Warsaw ghetto during World War II is a story of both tragedy and incredible courage). The ghetto can, however, be a stultifying influence, providing so much support and catering to all aspects of the fulfillment of a ghetto life-style that one's sense of motivation and determination can flag, and ennui can become overpowering.

IMPLICATIONS FOR NURSING: A SUMMARY

This chapter has discussed the wide diversity of cultures the community nurse will meet, in which ways they are similar to each other and to American society as a whole, and in which ways they differ. It must be emphasized that the nurse should learn as much as possible about the culture she is working with, but even more important, she must learn as much as she can about the individual persons within that culture because it is with the individual client and family that the community nurse is primarily concerned.

There are probably as many irresponsible and incorrect labels and stereotypes about cultural minorities as there is correct information. Labeling a group of persons as exhibiting a particular character trait is as counterproductive as it is wrong. Even "positive" lables ("all Jews are rich,"; "the Chinese don't commit crimes") are harmful because they frequently are not accurate and are demeaning to members of the group *as persons*. Covering one's racism with a thin layer of "tolerance" and patronization ("some of my best friends are Jews"; "you're not like those other blacks") is *always* demeaning and insulting to the person addressed and to the cultural or ethnic group as a whole. Leininger sums it up well when she speaks of the nurse working with Spanish Americans:

Spanish-Americans like to view health workers as friends rather than formal, indifferent, and cold strangers. If the nurse gets to know the Spanish-American family and shows signs of genuine respect and empathy for them, they will be apt to cooperate with her. One can say that the most important professional skill that Spanish-Americans look for in a nurse is her interpersonal skills and her genuine interest in them as a cultural group. This significant professional attribute is possible only when health personnel understand the dynamic cultural context of human behavior and specific cultural groups.[8]

The community nurse should take into consideration the cultural group's traditional attitudes and beliefs about health care when she makes a nursing assessment and diagnosis and when she presents suggestions to the client for interventions. The client may or may not act on her suggestions, and the nurse will have a variety of feelings and reactions if the client chooses to ignore traditional health care or to refuse treatment altogether. The client has every legal and moral right to make his own decisions about care and treatment, and it is likely that if the nurse "pushes" too hard, the client will run faster in the opposite direction to what the nurse would prefer. It is often possible to involve indigenous caregivers into the traditional or mainstream mode of treatment, such as seeking a faith healer to speed recovery from surgery or consumption of various herbs and roots along with the antibiotics. As long as the cultural practice is not known to be harmful, there is no reason why the nurse should not encourage it. Ways of healing that are peculiar to that culture can provide a familiar comfort during illness.

One further word must be said about the conflict between minority cultures and the majority white American society. Hatred, fear, and suspicion travel in two directions. Most often the one against whom these feelings are directed is the member of the minority group, but minorities sometimes see racism and persecution when little or none exists, blame all their life failures on the white society, and generally assume that they are disliked and distrusted by whites when they do not know this to be true. The poem "I am Joaquin" by Rondolfo Gonzalez[9] echoes these sentiments. Following is the opening passage from the poem:

I am Joaquin
Lost in a world of confusion,
Caught up in a world of a
    Gringo society.
Confused by the rules,
Scorned by attitudes,
Suppressed by manipulation,
And destroyed by modern society.
My fathers
    Have lost the economic battle
And won
    The struggle of cultural survival.
And now!
    I must choose
        Between
    The paradox of

Victory of the spirit
Despite physical hunger
    Or
    To exist in the group
Of American social neurosis,
Sterilization of the soul
    And a full stomach.

It is true that Hispanic Americans are frequently victims of the white society, and they *are* confused and scorned. Choices do indeed have to be made, but there is no reason why Hispanic Americans and all other minorities cannot have the best of both worlds—if they are motivated to take the opportunities presented in this country. The anger, bitterness, defeatism, and self-pity expressed in this poem are counterproductive, and if the community nurse can work toward preventing these kinds of feelings in the culturally diverse groups she serves, she will have behaved in an exceptionally professional manner. She cannot, however, instill a sense of pride, strength, and responsibility where none exist. These characteristics must spring from the soul of the individual; the nurse can only fan the flame of hope and desire.

NOTES

1. Twaddle, Andrew C., and Hessler, Richard M.: A sociology of health, St. Louis, 1977, The C.V. Mosby Co., p. 41.
2. Brownlee, Ann T.: Community, culture, and care, St. Louis, 1978, The C.V. Mosby Co., p. 24.
3. United States Census. United States Department of Commerce, Bureau of the Census, Washington, D.C., 1970, U.S. Government Printing Office.
4. Zola, Irving, K.: Culture and symptoms—an analysis of patients presenting complaints. In Spector, Rachel E.: Cultural diversity in health and illness, New York, 1979, Appleton-Century-Crofts, p. 85.
5. Spector, Rachel E.: Cultural diversity in health and illness, New York, 1979, Appleton-Century-Crofts, p. 222.
6. Ritenbaugh, Cheryl: Human foodways: a window on evolution. In Bauwens, Eleanor, editor: The anthropology of health, St. Louis, 1978, The C.V. Mosby Co., p. 112.
7. Weaver, Jerry L.: National health policy and the underserved, St. Louis, 1976, The C.V. Mosby Co., p. 3.
8. Leininger, Madeleine: Nursing and anthropology: two worlds to blend, New York, 1970, John Wiley & Sons, Inc., p. 121.

9. Gonzalez, Rodolfo: I am Joaquin. In Martinez, Ricardo, A., editor: Hispanic culture and health care, St. Louis, 1978, The C.V. Mosby Co., p. 17.

BIBLIOGRAPHY

Archer, Sarah E., and Fleshman, Ruth P.: Community health nursing: patterns and practice, ed. 2, N. Scituate, Mass., 1979, Duxbury Press.

Bauwens, Eleanor, editor: The anthropology of health, St. Louis, 1978, The C.V. Mosby Co.

Brownlee, Ann T.: Community, culture, and care, St. Louis, 1978, The C.V. Mosby Co.

Cassell, Eric J.: The healer's art, New York, 1979, Penguin Books.

Corey, Lawrence, Epstein, Michael F., and Saltman, Steven E.: Medicine in a changing society, ed. 2, St. Louis, 1977, The C.V. Mosby Co.

Davitz, Lois J., et al.: Suffering as viewed in six different cultures, American Journal of Nursing 76(8):1296-1297, August, 1976.

Hodgson, Corinne: Transcultural nursing: the Canadian experience, The Canadian Nurse pp. 23-25, June, 1980.

Kolasa, Kathryn: I won't cook turnip greens if you won't cook kielbasa: food behavior of Polonia and its health implications. In Bauwens, Eleanor, editor: The anthropology of health, St. Louis, 1978, The C.V. Mosby Co.

Kramer, Marlene, and Schmalenberg, C.: Path to biculturalism, Wakefield, Mass., 1977, Contemporary Publishing.

Leininger, Madeleine: Nursing and anthropology: two worlds to blend, New York, 1970, John Wiley & Sons, Inc.

Leininger, Madeleine: Cultural diversities of health and nursing care, Nursing Clinics of North America 12(1):5-18, March, 1977.

Leininger, Madeleine: Transcultural nursing: concepts, theories, and practices, New York, 1978, John Wiley & Sons, Inc.

Martinez, Ricardo A., editor: Hispanic culture and health care, St. Louis, 1978, The C.V. Mosby Co.

Rackovsky, Isaiah: Nurses, nursing, and culture, Supervisor Nurse, pp. 20-22, July, 1980.

Reinhardt, Adina M., and Quinn, Mildred D.: Current practice in family-centered community nursing, St. Louis, 1977, The C.V. Mosby Co.

Ritenbaugh, Cheryl: Human foodways: a window on evolution. In Bauwens, Eleanor, editor: The anthropology of health, St. Louis, 1978, The C.V. Mosby Co.

Shubin, Seymour: Nursing patients from different cultures, Nursing '80, pp. 79-81, June, 1978.

Spector, Manuel: Poverty: the barrier to health care. In Spector, Rachel E.: Cultural diversity in health and illness, New York, 1979, Appleton-Century-Crofts.

Spector, Rachel E.: Cultural diversity in health and illness, New York, 1979, Appleton-Century-Crofts.

Spradley, Barbara W., editor: Contemporary community nursing, Boston, 1975, Little, Brown & Co.

Twaddle, Andrew C., and Hessler, Richard M.: A sociology of health, St. Louis, 1977, The C.V. Mosby Co.

Weaver, Jerry L.: National health policy and the underserved, St. Louis, 1976, The C.V. Mosby Co.

Weeks, H. Ashley: Income and disease—the pathology of poverty. In Corey, Lawrence, Epstein, Michael F., and Saltman, Steven E.: Medicine in a changing society, ed. 2, St. Louis, 1977, The C.V. Mosby Co.

Wilson, Christine S.: Developing methods for studying diet ethnographically. In Bauwens, Eleanor, editor: The anthropology of health, St. Louis, 1978, The C.V. Mosby Co.

Zola, Irving, K.: Culture and symptoms—an analysis of patients presenting complaints. In Spector, Rachel E.: Cultural diversity in health and illness, New York, 1979, Appleton-Century-Crofts.

INDEX